Lippincott's
Review Series

Critical Care Nursing

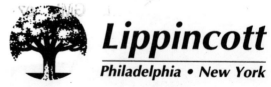

Lippincott
Philadelphia • New York

Lippincott's Review Series

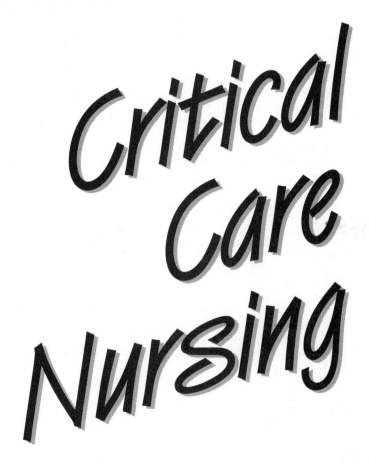

Critical Care Nursing

Linda M. Valenti, RN, CCRN
Staff Nurse
Episcopal Hospital
Philadelphia, Pennsylvania

Michele B. Rozinski, RN, MSN, CCRN
Instructor
School of Nursing
Episcopal Hospital
Philadelphia, Pennsylvania

Rosemary Tamblyn, MSN, CNS
Associate Professor
Bucks County Community College
Newtown, Pennsylvania

Acquisitions Editor: **Susan M. Glover, RN, MSN**
Developmental Editor: **Genell Hilton, MS, CRNP, CCRN, CNRN**
Assistant Editor: **Bridget Blatteau**
Project Editor: **Gretchen Metzger**
Production Manager: **Helen Ewan**
Production Coordinator: **Adina LoBiondo**
Design Coordinator: **Doug Smock**
Indexer: **Michael Ferreira**

9 8 7 6 5 4

Library of Congress Cataloging in Publications Data

Valenti, Linda M.
    Critical care / Linda M. Valenti, Michele B. Rozinski, Rosemary Tamblyn.
        p.   cm. — (Lippincott's review series)
    Includes index.
    ISBN 0–397–55455–9 (alk. paper)
    1. Critical care nursing—Outlines, syllabi, etc.   2. Intensive care nursing—Examinations, questions, etc.   I. Rozinski, Michele B.   II. Tamblyn, Rosemary.   III. Title.   IV. Series.
    [DNLM: 1. Critical Care—examination questions.   WY 18.2 V155c 1998]
    RT120.I5V35   1998
    610.73′61—dc21
    DNLM/DLC
    for Library of Congress   97–17480
                                                                                    CIP

Care has been taken to confirm the accuracy of the information presented and to describe generally accepted practices. However, the authors, editors, and publisher are not responsible for errors or omissions or for any consequences from application of the information in this book and make no warranty, express or implied, with respect to the contents of the publication.

The authors, editors, and publisher have exerted every effort to ensure that drug selection and dosage set forth in this text are in accordance with current recommendations and practice at the time of publication. However, in view of ongoing research, changes in government regulations, and the constant flow of information relating to drug therapy and drug reactions, the reader is urged to check the package insert for each drug for any change in indications and dosage and for added warnings and precautions. This is particularly important when the recommended agent is a new or infrequently employed drug.

Some drugs and medical devices presented in this publication have Food and Drug Administration (FDA) clearance for limited use in restricted research settings. It is the responsibility of the health care provider to ascertain the FDA status of each drug or device planned for use in their clinical practice.

To my husband Michael for sharing the excitement, frustration, anticipation, and joy of writing this book with me. A special thanks to my daughter Melinda for dragging me out of the computer room and into the sunshine for small trips to Ashley's house or "the field" (thereby saving my sanity), and to my son Michael for "hanging out" in the computer room just to keep me company when escape from the computer was impossible (thereby allowing for the completion of the book!).

To my brothers John and Joe and my sisters Kathy and Mary, thank you for your encouragement, guidance, and philosophical conversations. Each of you act as an inspiration by example.

To Mom-Mom and Pop-Pop (Mike and Claire Valenti), thank you both for your encouragement and for keeping me on my toes.

To my good friend Diane Winkler, thank you for being a great sounding board whenever procrastination kicked in!

Linda M. Valenti, RN, CCRN

To Tom, who has steadfastly remained by my side throughout the writing of this book; you have given me new direction in my career and in my life. Thanks for being strong when I needed to lean.

To my students, who have taught me much more about life and living than I could ever teach them about nursing.

To my kitties, who "helped" with the editing when I wasn't looking!

Michele B. Rozinski, RN, MSN, CCRN

Dedicated to my husband Jack, whose patience, love, support, and encouragement have made this giant step in my career a reality.

Also thank you to Linda Valenti for this opportunity and for her confidence in me.

Rosemary Tamblyn, MSN, CNS

CONTRIBUTING AUTHORS

Suzanne Adams, BS, RN, CCRN
Nurse Manager
Nurse Works, Inc.
Bala Cynwyd, Pennsylvania

Kathleen Aumendo, BSN, RN
Staff Development
Organizational Training and Development
Episcopal Hospital
Philadelphia, Pennsylvania

John J. Brennan, RN
Staff Nurse
Acute Hemodialysis
BMA–Abington
Willow Grove, Pennsylvania

Karen Csenteri, MSN, RN
Nursing Instructor
Helene Fuld School of Nursing in Camden County
Blackwood, New Jersey

Kelliann Donaghy, ADN
Staff Nurse
Intensive Care Unit
Episcopal Hospital
Philadelphia, Pennsylvania

Michael Kirkpatrick, RN
Staff Nurse
Intensive Care Unit
Episcopal Hospital
Philadelphia, Pennsylvania

Irene Mishinkash, RN, BSN
Registered Nurse—Staff
Episcopal Hospital
Philadelphia, Pennsylvania

Carol Okupniak, RN
Labor and Delivery/Postpartum
Episcopal Hospital
Philadelphia, Pennsylvania

Mary Jean Ricci, BA, BSN, MSN, RNc
Assistant Professor of Nursing
Holy Family College
Philadelphia, Pennsylvania

Janet Marie Riggs, MSN, RN, CCRN
Level III Staff Nurse
Cardiothoracic Telemetry Unit
Hospital of the University of Pennsylvania
Philadelphia, Pennsylvania

Frances E. Shuda, MSN, RN, CCRN, ET
Director
Staff Development Department
Episcopal Hospital/Episcopal Long Term Care
Philadelphia, Pennsylvania

Renee Stephens, RN
Assistant Clinical Manager
Intensive Care Unit
Episcopal Hospital
Philadelphia, Pennsylvania

Scott Strubinger, RD
Food Service Director
Multicare (Pennypack Nursing & Rehabilitation)
Philadelphia, Pennsylvania

REVIEWERS

Jo-Ann D. Barrett, RN, BSN, CDE
Center Director
Control Diabetes Services
Braintree, Massachusetts

Janice Boundy, RN, PhD
Associate Professor, Coordinator
Saint Francis College of Nursing
Peoria, Illinois

Patricia M. Dunphy, MSN, RNC
Perinatal Clinical Nurse Specialist, Lecturer
University of Pennsylvania School of Nursing
Philadelphia, Pennsylvania

Sandra G. Elkin, EdD, FNP
Assistant Professor of Nursing
Northern Arizona University
Flagstaff, Arizona

Mary K. Evans, MSN, CCRN, CS
Staff Nurse (Clinical Nurse II)
Surgical ICU
Georgetown University Medical Center
Washington, DC

Terri L. Jones, RN, CCRN
Clinical Supervisor
Intensive and Coronary Care Unit
Mary Greeley Medical Center
Ames, Iowa

ACKNOWLEDGMENTS

The authors would like to thank Lippincott-Raven editorial staff Sue Glover, Bridget Blatteau, and Deedie McMahon for guiding us with patience and understanding. Each of you went out of your way to make the writing of this book an enjoyable process. We would also like to thank our contributing authors Renee, M.J., Fran, Suzanne, Kathy, Janet, Kelli-Anne, Mike, John, Irene, Carol, Karen, and Scott for teaching us what it has taken them years of clinical experience to learn.

A very special thanks to our bosses and our co-workers for allowing us some slack during the deadline days and the staff nurses in the ICU/CCU at Episcopal Hospital for giving us ideas, telling us what absolutely "must be included" and what was "not so important" with a lot of creative ideas on how to get the theories across. We would also like to acknowledge those physicians, Dr. Craig Carter and Dr. Barry Weinberger among others, who have the natural ability and love for teaching and who routinely take time out of their busy schedules to teach the complexities of various disease processes and technological advances to the nursing staff.

Finally, we would like to thank our patients for reminding us why we ever became nurses, for continually teaching us new lessons, and for pushing us to strive for excellence in nursing. Ernie, when this book hits the bookshelves, I hope that you are out walking Sandy.

Linda M. Valenti

INTRODUCTION

Lippincott's Review Series is designed to help you in your study of the key subject areas in nursing. The series consists of nine books, one in each core nursing subject area:

Community and Home Health Nursing   *Mental Health and Psychiatric Nursing*
Critical Care Nursing   *Pathophysiology*
Fluids and Electrolytes   *Pediatric Nursing*
Maternal-Newborn Nursing   *Pharmacology*
Medical-Surgical Nursing

Each book contains a comprehensive outlined content review, plus chapter study questions and answer keys with rationales for correct and incorrect responses, and a comprehensive examination and answer key with rationales for correct and incorrect responses.

Lippincott's Review Series was planned and developed in response to your requests for outline review books that address each major subject area and also contain a self-test mechanism. These books meet the need for comprehensive subject review books that will also assist you in identifying your strong and weak areas of knowledge. Each book is a complete source for review and self-assessment of a single core subject—all nine together provide an excellent comprehensive review of entry-level nursing.

Each book is all-inclusive of the content addressed in major textbooks. The content outline review uses a consistent nursing process format throughout and addresses nursing care for well and ill clients. Also included are necessary additional concepts such as growth and development, nutrition, pharmacology, and body structures, functions, and pathophysiology. Special features of each book are Key Concepts and Nursing Alerts, which are identified by distinctive icons. Key Concepts ✹ are basic facts the nurse needs to know to perform his or her job with ease and efficiency. Nursing alerts ⚕ are fundamental guidelines the nurse can follow to ensure safe and effective care.

You can use the books in this series in several different ways. Overall, you can use them as subject reviews to augment general study throughout your basic nursing program and as a review to prepare for the National Council Licensure Examination (NCLEX-RN). How you use each book depends on your individual needs and preferences, and on whether you review each chapter systematically or concentrate only on those chapters whose subject areas are particularly problematic or challenging. You may instead choose to use the comprehensive examination as a self-assessment opportunity to evaluate your knowledge base before you review the content outline. Likewise, you can use the study questions for pre- or post-testing after study, followed by the comprehensive examination, as a means of evaluating your knowledge and competencies of an entire subject area.

Regardless of how you use the books, one of the strengths of the series is the self-assessment opportunity it offers, in addition to guidance in studying and reviewing content. The chapter study questions and comprehensive examination questions have been carefully developed to cover all topics in the outline review. Most importantly, each question is categorized according to the components of the National Council of State Boards of Nursing Licensing Examination (NCLEX).

► Cognitive Level: Knowledge, Comprehension, Application, or Analysis
► Client Need: Safe, Effective Care Environment (Safe care); Physiological Integrity (Physiologic); Psychosocial Integrity (Psychosocial); and Health Promotion and Maintenance (Health Promotion)
► Phase of the Nursing Process: Assessment, Analysis (Dx), Planning, Implementation, Evaluation

For those questions not related to a client need or to a phase of the nursing process, NA (not applicable) will be used, as in questions that test knowledge of a basic science.

Unlike the NCLEX examination, which tests the cumulative knowledge needed for safe practice by an entry-level nurse, these practice tests systematically evaluate the knowledge base that serves as the building block for the entire nursing educational process. In this way, you can prepare for the NCLEX examination throughout your course of study. Good study habits throughout your educational program are not only the best way to ensure ongoing success, but also will prove the most beneficial way to prepare for the licensing examination.

Keep in mind that these books are not intended to replace formal learning. They cannot substitute for textbook reading, discussion with instructors, or class attendance. Every effort has been made to provide accurate and current information, but class attendance and interaction with an instructor will provide invaluable information not found in books. Used correctly, these books will help you increase understanding, improve comprehension, evaluate strengths and weaknesses in areas of knowledge, increase productive study time, and, as a result, help you improve your grades.

MONEY BACK GUARANTEE—Lippincott's Review Series will help you study more effectively during coursework throughout your educational program, and help you prepare for quizzes and tests including the NCLEX exam. If you buy and use any of the nine volumes in Lippincott's Review Series and fail the NCLEX exam, simply send us verification of your exam results and your copy of the review book to the address below. We will promptly send you a check for our suggested list price.

Lippincott's Review Series
Marketing Department
Lippincott-Raven Publishers
227 East Washington Square
Philadelphia, PA 19106-3780

CONTENTS

Introduction to the Critical Care Setting

1

I. **Critical care environment: The intensive care unit (ICU) environment is stressful to health care professionals and patients alike. Listed below are some of the things that make the ICU so stressful:**
  A. 24-hour activity: overly bright lights and loud noises result in sleep deprivation
  B. Communication barriers

C. Crowded surroundings (patients, families, nurses, doctors, technicians, and ancillary personnel)

D. Equipment: large and overbearing (monitors, pumps, ventilators, EKG machines, cardiac output machines, etc.)

E. Close working conditions: often cause the staff to either conflict or work exceptionally well together

II. ICU psychosis

A. Definition: Term pertaining to a temporary alteration in the patient's perception of reality directly related to the ICU environment

B. Etiology and incidence
   1. Higher incidence in the geriatric population
   2. Seen in instances of serious illness, trauma, anesthesia, and use of narcotics
   3. Increased incidence when patients spend more than 24–48 hours in the ICU

C. Pathophysiology and management
   1. While in the ICU, patients experience a lack of sleep in addition to whatever stressors caused the ICU admission.
   2. Constant light and noise prevent the patient from remaining oriented to day/night.
   3. Patients develop an altered state of perception and may become paranoid or delusional.
   4. ICU psychosis is self-limiting and resolves usually within 48 hours of being transferred out of the ICU.
   5. Management while in the ICU is aimed at reorienting the patient to reality and promoting a safe environment.

D. Assessment findings: Patients generally exhibit the following symptoms:
   1. Emotional lability, decreased attention span, confused conversation, and memory problems.
   2. Paranoia, delusions, and hallucinations.

E. Nursing diagnoses
   1. Sensory Perceptual Alterations: Visual, Auditory, Tactile
   2. Fear
   3. Anxiety
   4. Risk for Injury

F. Planning and implementation
   1. Plan nursing care to allow at least 90- to 120-minute sleep cycles at night. Dim lights at night.
   2. Limit the number of people (hospital personnel included) at the bedside at one time.
   3. Do not talk over the patient: either talk to the patient or go out of earshot. *Never discuss one patient at another patient's bedside.*
   4. Always answer the patient's questions with honesty.
   5. Try to follow a daily routine; this will decrease fear of the unknown.
   6. Reorient patient as necessary.
   7. Administer prescribed medications (for pain, anxiety, sedation) before the pain, anxiety, or sleep deprivation escalates.
   8. The patient is usually aware of a change in perception. Offer reassurance and explain that it is only temporary.
   9. Keep all bed rails up and the call light within reach. Do not allow patient out of bed alone.

    G. Evaluation
1. The patient will resume previous level of orientation.
2. The patient will not incur any injuries during hospitalization.
3. The patient will not suffer undue anxiety or fear during hospitalization.

III. Stress on the nurse (burnout)

    A. Description: Physical and emotional exhaustion resulting in an onslaught of physical symptoms as well as feelings of hopelessness and depression at work.

    B. Etiology and incidence: Causes of nurse burnout include:
1. Noisy, crowded working environment
2. Long work days, with few breaks
3. Understaffing
4. Complexity and management of highly technical equipment
5. Close working conditions
6. Conflicts regarding patient care
7. Malfunctioning equipment and inadequate supplies
8. Perceived mismanagement of patients
9. Managing combative and agitated patients
10. Ethical dilemmas
11. Dealing with family members
12. Perceived lack of control in the work place
13. Incidence is dependent on the overall health and coping mechanisms of the individual nurse in addition to any additional personal stressors.

    C. Pathophysiology and management
1. The stress response is a physiologic response to a real or perceived threat to the self.
2. Hormones are released and the heart rate and blood pressure rise temporarily.
3. In a long-term situation, as with a stressful life-style, anxiety and nervousness occur and contribute to a dysfunctional immune system and chronic illness.
4. Too little stress is considered a stressor in itself and is as detrimental to the health as too much stress.
5. Management is aimed at learning to live a healthy life-style and improving coping mechanisms.

    D. Assessment findings
1. Nurse may experience fatigue, malaise, and show an increase in use of sick/late days.
2. Depression and feelings of hopelessness may be expressed.
3. Nurses may be bored with work and exhibit apathy and an inability to concentrate.
4. Negative attitudes with frequent complaints about work and co-workers may be expressed.
5. Irritability; loss of appetite; or overindulgence in food, alcohol, caffeine, and tobacco may occur.

    E. Nursing diagnoses
1. Anxiety
2. Powerlessness
3. Self-Esteem Disturbance
4. Ineffective Individual Coping

F. **Planning and implementation**

1. Limit empty calories, sugar, caffeine, tobacco, alcohol, and drugs. These may all increase stress and decrease self-esteem and energy. They may also decrease ability to concentrate and cope with stressful situations.

2. Exercise! Regular exercise increases energy and endurance, promoting the ability to cope with stressful situations.

3. Get enough sleep, but not too much.

4. Arrive to work on time. Lateness increases the stress level before even getting to work.

5. Take breaks! Inefficiency at the bedside increases as stress increases.

6. Keep up with the most current nursing practices. Knowledge and preparedness will increase the self-confidence necessary to care for critically ill patients. It will also enable you to feel in control of any situation, lessening some of the stress when the worst possible scenario occurs.

7. Join committees. Committee membership offers control, and control offers a higher comfort and a lower stress level.

8. Learn the resource people in other departments. Communication between departments will lower everybody's stress level.

9. Evaluate your own coping techniques and alter them if they are ineffective.

10. Practice relaxation techniques.

G. **Evaluation**

1. The nurse will demonstrate effective coping mechanisms.

2. The nurse will notice a decrease in anxiety, nervousness, irritability, and an increase in self-esteem.

3. Optimal patient care will be provided.

IV. Legal and psychosocial considerations

A. **Advance directives: Legal documents written to allow competent individuals to indicate their consent or refusal for health care treatment when they are no longer able to make or convey decisions.**

1. The admission process and acuity of the critical care patient does not always allow sufficient time to discuss information and address concerns about advance directives.

2. Ideally the discussions and decisions regarding advance directives should be made by the patient with the family and the attending physician before admission.

3. The Patient Self Determination Act requires that patients be asked if they have advance directives or would like information on advance directives on admission to any health care facility.

4. A Living Will instructs health care providers not to use life-sustaining measures if the person becomes terminally ill, or in some states in an irreversible coma. It must be signed by the person executing it in the presence of two witnesses and two doctors must agree in writing that the patient is terminally ill or in an irreversible coma for the living will to go into effect.

5. A Durable Power of Attorney for health care decisions authorizes someone who is chosen by the person executing the document to make health care decisions when the person is no longer capable to do so. It allows the person to state the kind and type of care the person

wants or does not want. It also states the scope of decisions the person's designee is able to handle. This document must be signed by the person executing it and it must be notarized.

6. The Living Will and the Durable Power of Attorney can be revoked at any time, either verbally or in writing if the person who has executed the document is competent.

7. A lawyer is not required for executing either document.

8. Do not resuscitate (DNR) is an order stating that the patient should not be resuscitated in the event of a cardiopulmonary arrest. This order must be written in the chart by a doctor and signed by the attending physician within 24 hours.

   a. Nurses acting against the wishes of the patient are guilty of negligence and battery.

   b. The decision to discontinue any therapy initiated before to the DNR order can be determined by asking the following questions:

      ▶ Is the therapy more burdensome to the patient than beneficial?

      ▶ Does the therapy provide any benefit aside from prolonging death?

   c. Nourishment can be held/withdrawn if desired because it may cause aspiration pneumonia, pulmonary edema, sinusitis, and nausea. There is no difference between withholding and withdrawing therapy.

9. According to the Nurse Practice Act, under no circumstances do nurses play a role in active euthanasia.

10. Relieving pain in a terminally ill patient, even if the medication may cause death, is allowed because the goal is to relieve the pain, not kill the patient.

B. Religious considerations

1. Religious beliefs must always be taken into account when providing care to a patient and their family.

2. Believing in a religion may give the patient the hope and positive attitude necessary to improve physically.

3. At the very least the familiarity of a religious ceremony will relieve some of the patient's anxiety.

4. Allow the clergy to visit with patient as requested.

5. Allow prayer, readings, or other religious ceremonies as tolerated by the patient's condition whenever possible.

6. Show respect for the patient's religious articles, beliefs, and prayers.

C. Communication barriers

1. These may be secondary to language barriers, oral endotracheal tubes, mistrust between patient and nurse, talking above the patient's level of understanding, or treatment with paralytic drugs.

2. Inability to communicate greatly increases anxiety, leading to the release of catecholamines and an increase in heart rate in an already compromised patient.

3. Use hospital interpreters, family, or friends to assist with communication and decrease the patient's feelings of isolation.

4. Always answer the patient's questions honestly and assess for any misunderstandings.

5. Attempt to foresee and meet the needs of a patient being treated with paralytic drugs. Explain all procedures as you would to anyone else to minimize his or her fear. Explain that the medication will be weaned off when appropriate and he or she will be able to move again.
6. Keep a call light, picture board, notepad, and pencil within reach of the ventilated patient at all times. Answer the call light right away even if only to say that you'll be right over. Let the patient know that you know he or she is frustrated.

V. Nutritional issues in critical care
A. General information
1. Nutrition support has become an accepted part of medical care and special techniques have been developed for the delivery of nutrients.
2. Nutritional care of patients can be accomplished by integrating principles of nutrition support into daily care of patients.

B. Criteria
1. Newly accepted criteria for dietary efficacy include length of intensive care unit stay, infectious morbidity, and survival.
2. Lab values that predict nutrient efficacy remain elusive. However, preventing loss of lean body mass during critical illness is an important therapeutic end point in any case.
3. No specific disease process appears to benefit from starvation.
4. The goal of nutrition support is either repletion of nutritional deficit or maintenance of the patient's present nutritional status.

C. Nutrition intervention decision tree (Fig. 1-1)

D. Evaluation
1. The patient will meet energy and protein needs.
2. The patient will maintain/gain weight.
3. The patient will maintain normal fluid and electrolyte balance.
4. Optimal organ function will be maintained.

VI. Blood components
A. Whole blood: provides all components, including platelets and coagulation factors
1. Whole blood is only used for acute massive blood loss.
2. Preservation is via citrate-phosphate-dextrose (CPD) which is an anticoagulant preservative that binds calcium to prevent clotting.
3. Massive transfusions may cause hypocalcemia.
4. Shelf life is 21 days. Increased storage time causes increased acidity and hyperkalemia related to release of potassium into plasma.
5. Hypothermia can occur with massive transfusions, so blood should be warmed before administration.
6. Once warmed, blood may not be refrigerated again.
7. Flush line only with normal saline solution to prevent lysis.
8. Administration time is not to exceed 4 hours.

B. Packed red blood cells (PRBCs)
1. This is the component of choice for severe anemia, chronic anemia, congestive heart failure, and in the elderly.
2. The advantages to PRBCs over whole blood include:
   a. decreased chance of fluid overload;
   b. decreased antigenicity to plasma antigens;
   c. increased hematocrit up to twice as much as does whole blood.
3. Same nursing considerations as for whole blood administration.

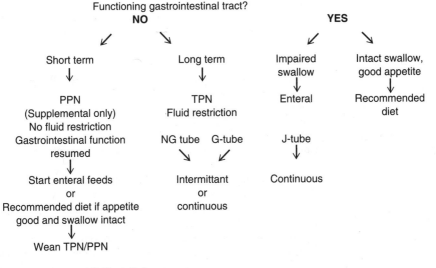

Assessment:
  Weight loss?
  Gastrointestinal function? (motility, absorption)
  Impaired swallow?
  Appetite?
   Fluid restriction?
Cost/benefit justification
Laboratory tests: albumin, major/minor profiles, 24-hour creatinine, 24-hour urine nitrogen

FIGURE 1-1.
Nutrition intervention decision tree. NG—nasogastric, PPN—partial parenteral nutrition, TPN—total parenteral nutrition.

4. With all RBC products, check vital signs before starting, 15 minutes later, and hourly until completed or a reaction occurs.
C. Washed RBCs: contain lower levels of platelet and leukocyte antigens.
D. Fresh frozen plasma (FFP): contains all coagulation factors.
  1. FFP provides volume expansion or replaces deficient coagulation factors in critical care patients.
  2. FFP is also given in conjunction with massive packed RBC transfusions to provide clotting factors missing from RBC products.
  3. Store up to 12 months frozen and 4–6 hours if thawed.

       4.   If not frozen, FFP may contain adequate amounts of factors VII, IX, X, and XI, but not V and VIII.

E. **Cryoprecipitate: contains factors VII, XIII, and fibrinogen**

       1.   Indicated for hemophilia and von Willebrand's disease.

       2.   Taken from a single donor rather than from a donor pool.

       3.   Can receive up to 75 units of factor VIII per donor.

       4.   Dose is 1 unit per 6 kg initially, then one-half that amount every 6–12 hours.

       5.   Administration rate is 1 unit over 5 minutes.

F. **Platelets**

       1.   Indicated for thrombocytopenia.

       2.   One unit is derived from 500 mL whole blood via centrifuge method.

       3.   Shelf life is 8–10 days in recipient's circulation. This is dependent on patient's clinical condition.

       4.   One unit usually increases count by 12,000–15,000.

       5.   Administered quickly, sometimes IV push, to rapidly increase circulating platelets.

       6.   Requires special tubing and filters.

       7.   Do not refrigerate (if possible).

G. **Nursing measures**

       1.   Ensure compatibility when administering any blood products (see Table 9-1).

            a.   Check patient ID number, making sure that blood bracelet number correlates with information on the unit of blood.

            b.   Have two RNs check blood before administration.

            c.   Administer RBC products slowly for the first 15 minutes to minimize the severity a reaction, if one develops.

            d.   Ensure type and screen of blood occurs before administration. This tests for potential compatibility in order to avoid transfusion reactions.

       2.   Ensure that blood is properly stored in blood bank until needed. This will decrease incidence of contamination.

H. **Volume expanders**

       1.   Albumin has an oncotic pressure of plasma and is the main determinant of plasma volume.

       2.   Plasmanate/Hespan are hyperosmolar solutions of albumin and amino acids.

I. **Transfusion reactions**

       1.   Hemolytic reaction:

            a.   Due to ABO or Rh incompatibility

            b.   May lead to disseminated intravascular coagulation or death

            c.   Renal complications common and are dose-dependent

            d.   Initial signs and symptoms include fever, chills, and urticaria

            e.   Later symptoms include back pain, dyspnea, vomiting, diarrhea, hematuria, chest pain, circulatory collapse, hypotension, and renal failure.

       2.   Bacterial reaction:

            a.   Develops after transfusion of contaminated blood products.

            b.   Usually resulting from gram-negative pathogens, which release endotoxin if not properly refrigerated.

    3.   Allergic reaction:
        a.   Symptoms include urticaria and itching.
        b.   Circulatory overload can occur.
    4.   Treatment of all transfusion reactions include:
        a.   Discontinue unit immediately.
        b.   Stay with patient. Have someone else notify physician.
        c.   Send blood and tubing to lab.
        d.   Collect blood and urine samples to check for renal complications.

Bibliography

Huth, J. (1995). Advance directives and the Patient Self-Determination Act: What is a nurse to do? *J Post Anesth Nurs* 10(6), 336–339.

North American Nursing Diagnosis Association (NANDA). (1996). *Nursing diagnoses: Definitions & classification 1997–1998*. Philadelphia: Author.

Reigle, J. (1995). Should the patient decide when to die? *RN* 58(5), 57–61.

Ross, P., & West, D. (1995). Advance directives: The price of life. *Nurs Econ* 13(6), 354–360.

Schwartz, D.B. (1996). Enhanced enteral and parenteral nutrition practice and outcomes in an intensive care unit with a hospital-wide performance improvement process. *J Am Diet Assoc* 96, 484–489.

Simpson, T., Lee, E. R., & Cameron, C. (1996). Patients' perceptions of environmental factors that influence sleep after cardiac surgery. *Am J Crit Care* 5(3), 173–181.

Talton, C. (1995). Touch—of all kinds—is therapeutic. *RN* 58(2), 61–64.

Zaloga, G.P. (1984). *Nutrition in critical care*. St. Louis: Mosby.

STUDY QUESTIONS

1. Which of the following statements about ICU psychosis is false?
   a. Risk factors include serious illness, elderly status, and narcotics use.
   b. It may cause the patient to require treatment with anti-psychotic medications for up to 1 year following an ICU admission.
   c. Environmental factors include 24-hour lighting/noise and unfamiliar environment.
   d. Allowing 90- to 120-minute sleep cycles may assist in prevention.

2. Which of the following does not apply to an ICU nurse?
   a. experiences a lot of on-the-job stress
   b. does not require additional training
   c. must be able to prioritize
   d. should take breaks and lunches in the unit due to the high acuity of their patients

3. Signs and symptoms of job burnout include:
   a. increased frequency in sick and late days
   b. depression, apathy, over- or under-eating
   c. frequently complaining about job, boss, co-workers, patients, families
   d. all of the above

4. Which of the following statements is false?
   a. It is difficult to find time to stay fit because a nurse's schedule is so irregular.
   b. An effective coping tactic is to go home, eat a candy bar, and relax on the couch until bedtime everyday after work.
   c. Relaxation techniques require practice initially, but become effective stress reducers with regular use.
   d. Tobacco and caffeine increase the heart rate, contributing to stress and anxiety.

5. Which of the following statements is true?
   a. The Nurse Practice Act allows nurses to assist the physician with assisted suicide in some states.
   b. An end-stage cancer patient in extreme pain with a respiratory rate of 12 breaths/minute and a DNR order may not be treated with large doses of morphine.
   c. Nurses going against the wishes of a patient regarding a DNR request are guilty of negligence and battery.
   d. If a patient has made a DNR request after being placed on vasopressor drips, it would be unlawful to discontinue the drips.

ANSWER KEY

1. *Correct response: b*

   ICU psychosis is temporary and usually resolves within 24–48 hours after discharge from the ICU.

   a and c. These environmental and risk factors are associated with ICU psychosis.

   d. Uninterrupted periods of full sleep cycles decrease the risk of psychotic episodes.

   Knowledge/Health promotion/ Evaluation

2. *Correct response: d*

   ICU nurses should physically leave the unit especially when stress levels are high.

   a. Being an ICU nurse can be extremely stressful

   b. Additional training is needed to be an ICU nurse.

   c. An ICU nurse must be able to make rapid accurate assessments and prioritize the appropriate interventions.

   Application/Safe care/Implementation

3. *Correct response: d*

   All are manifestations of stress and job burnout.

   Knowledge/Health promotion/ Evaluation

4. *Correct response: b*

   Once in a while relaxing with a candy bar and laying on the couch all night can be very effective, but on a daily basis it would contribute to an unhealthy life-style, increasing calories and stress levels and decreasing self-esteem and ability to cope.

   a. Nurses' schedules are variable, making it difficult to find a regular time to work out.

   c. Relaxation techniques require learning a new skill, but become invaluable with regular use.

   d. Believe it, it is TRUE!

   Health promotion/Application/ Intervention

5. *Correct response: c*

   It is legally as well as ethically wrong to go against the wishes of a patient regarding a DNR order.

   a. It is against the Nurse Practice Act to play any role in euthanasia.

   b. If the intent is to relieve pain, not to kill the patient, morphine can legally be given.

   d. Any intervention that offers no benefit to the patient other than prolonging life can be discontinued after the patient has made a DNR request.

   Application/Safe care/Implementation

Central Nervous System: The Brain

I. **Anatomy and physiology**
  A. Structures and functions
  B. Cerebral hemispheres
  C. Cerebral arterial circulation
  D. Cerebral venous circulation

II. **Overview of neurologic disorders**
  A. Assessment
  B. The Monroe–Kellie theorem
  C. Intracranial pressure monitoring
  D. Nutrition
  E. Psychosocial implications
  F. Commonly used medications
  G. Medications affecting the brain

III. **Increased intracranial pressure**
  A. Description
  B. Etiology and incidence
  C. Assessment
  D. Nursing diagnoses
  E. Planning and implementation
  F. Evaluation

IV. **Closed head injury**
  A. Description
  B. Etiology and incidence
  C. Pathophysiology
  D. Assessment
  E. Nursing diagnoses
  F. Planning and implementation
  G. Evaluation

V. **Skull fractures**
  A. Description
  B. Etiology and incidence
  C. Pathophysiology
  D. Assessment
  E. Nursing diagnoses

F. Planning and implementation
G. Evaluation

VI. **Hematomas**
  A. Description
  B. Etiology and incidence
  C. Pathophysiology
  D. Assessment
  E. Nursing diagnoses
  F. Planning and implementation
  G. Evaluation

VII. **Transient ischemic attacks**
  A. Description
  B. Etiology and incidence
  C. Pathophysiology
  D. Assessment
  E. Nursing diagnoses
  F. Planning and implementation
  G. Evaluation
  H. Home health considerations

VIII. **Cerebrovascular accident**
  A. Description
  B. Etiology and incidence
  C. Pathophysiology
  D. Assessment
  E. Nursing diagnoses
  F. Planning and implementation
  G. Evaluation
  H. Home health considerations

IX. **Arterial-venous malformations**
  A. Description
  B. Etiology
  C. Assessment
  D. Nursing diagnoses
  E. Planning and implementation

I. Anatomy and physiology

  A. Structures and functions

    1. Scalp: first layer of protection

    2. Skull: rigid cavity that houses the brain

      a. Bones: frontal, parietal, temporal, and occipital

      b. Fossae: three broad, shallow depressions in the base of the skull; anterior, middle, and posterior

      c. Tentorium cerebelli: forms a roof over the posterior fossa

    3. Meninges: three separate layers of connective tissue covering the brain

      a. Dura mater: outermost covering of tough fibrous tissue

      b. Arachnoid mater: middle layer; fine, fibrous layer: "spider web"

      c. Pia mater: innermost layer

    4. Falx cerebri: infolding of the inner dural layer between the two cerebral hemispheres

     5.   Spaces: these are considered potential spaces because there is nothing in them under normal circumstances:
   a.   Epidural
   b.   Subdural
     6.   Subarachnoid space: real space between the arachnoid and pia mater
   a.   Contains the larger blood vessels
   b.   CSF flows in this space
   c.   Arachnoid villi: projections of arachnoid matter that serve as channels for CSF absorption

B. **Cerebral hemispheres: Consist of two cortexes of gray matter, separated by a longitudinal fissure and joined by the corpus callosum**
     1.   Lobes of the cerebral hemispheres:
   a.   Frontal lobe: responsible for voluntary motor function, higher mental functions such as judgment and personality, and contains Broca's area, which controls the motor aspect of speech
   b.   Parietal lobe: responsible for all sensory functions and body awareness
   c.   Temporal lobe: responsible for hearing, speech in the dominant hemisphere, vestibular sense or balance, emotion and behavior
   d.   Occipital lobe: responsible for vision and visual interpretation
     2.   Basal ganglia is made up of white matter. Functions include:
   a.   Integration of voluntary movement and posture
   b.   Inhibition of skeletal muscle tone
   c.   Serves as the center of the extrapyramidal motor system
     3.   Limbic system
   a.   Biologic rhythms
   b.   Sexual behaviors
   c.   Emotions
   d.   Some aspects of memory
     4.   Diencephalon
   a.   Thalamus: relay station for sensations and conscious awareness of sensations
   b.   Hypothalamus: general function of homeostasis; temperature regulation, water regulation, appetite, sleep, and regulation of hormone secretion from the pituitary gland
   c.   Pituitary gland:

      ▶ anterior lobe: secretion of hormones
      ▶ posterior lobe: storage of antidiuretic hormone (ADH), and origin of cranial nerves I and II

     5.   Cerebellum
   a.   Coordination of fine motor movement
   b.   Balance and equilibrium
   c.   Unconscious proprioception
     6.   Brain stem
   a.   Midbrain is located between the pons and diencephalon. It contains the reticular activating system (RAS), which is responsible for sleep and wake cycles and is the origin of cranial nerves III and IV (Table 2-1).

TABLE 2-1.
Cranial Nerves

CRANIAL NERVE	TYPE	FUNCTION
I (Olfactory)	Sensory (afferent)	Smell
II (Optic)	Sensory	Sight
III (Oculomotor)	Motor (efferent)	Eye and upper eyelid movement
	Autonomic	Pupillary constriction/ accommodation
IV (Trochlear)	Motor	Eye movement
V (Trigeminal)	Sensory	Sensation of face, opthalmic, maxillary, and mandibular branches
VI (Abducens)	Motor	Eye movement
VII (Facial)	Sensory	Taste (sweet and salty)
	Motor	Facial expression
	Autonomic	Tear and saliva secretion
VIII (Acoustic)	Sensory	Hearing and equilibrium
IX (Glossopharyngeal)	Sensory	Taste (sour and bitter)
	Motor	Swallow, phonation, and gag
	Autonomic	Saliva secretion
X (Vagus)	Sensory	Sensation around ears and visceral structures
	Motor	Swallow, cough and gag
	Autonomic	Regulation of smooth and cardiac muscle, glands, and carotid reflex
XI (Accessory)	Motor	Swallow, head and shoulder movement
XII (Hypoglossal)	Motor	Tongue movement in swallow and phonation

      b.   The pons connects the midbrain and the medulla. It is a relay center, pneumotaxic center, and contains the origins of cranial nerves V, VI, VII, and VIII.

      c.   The medulla is located at the base of the brainstem and is continuous with the spinal cord. It contains the cardiovascular and respiratory centers, crossover center for motor fiber tracks, and is the origin of cranial nerves IX, X, XI, and XII.

   7.   Openings

      a.   Tentorial notch: opening within the tentorium to accommodate the brain stem

      b.   Foramen magnum: site of brain stem connection with the spinal cord

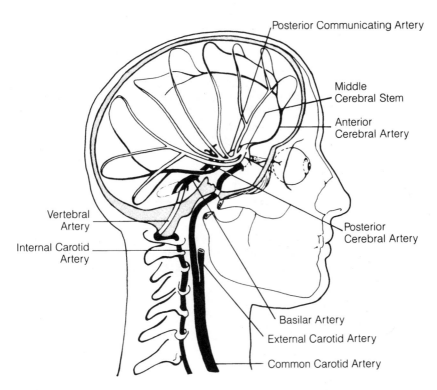

FIGURE 2-1.
The major vessels of the brain. The internal carotid, anterior, and middle cerebral arteries constitute the anterior circulation. The vertebral, basilar, and posterior cerebral arteries and branches comprise the posterior circulation.

        c.   Foramina (various): allow for entrance and exit of blood vessels and cranial nerves

C.   **Cerebral arterial circulation (Fig. 2-1)**

      1.   Anterior circulation (carotid arteries)

          a.   Left common carotid: rises from the aortic arch and bifurcates to form the internal and external carotids

          b.   Right common carotid: rises from the innominate artery

          c.   Cerebral arteries: anterior cerebral and middle cerebral

          d.   Communicating arteries: anterior and posterior

          e.   Middle meningeal artery: site of epidural bleeds

      2.   Posterior circulation (vertebral arteries)

          a.   Ascends from the subclavian artery

          b.   Two vertebral arteries join to form the basilar artery

          c.   Includes the posterior inferior cerebellar artery (PICA) and the posterior cerebral artery

      3.   Circle of Willis

          a.   Vessels form a ring at the base of skull

          b.   Located in the subarachnoid space

          c.   50% of the general population has an incomplete circle of Willis

D.   **Cerebral venous circulation**

      1.   Venous sinuses:

          a.   Drain through the internal jugular system

    b.   Largest is located in the dura mater

    c.   **Superior sagittal sinus also drains CSF from the arachnoid villi**

2.   Ventricular system: series of connected cavities filled with CSF:
    a.   Right and left lateral ventricles are located in the cerebral hemisphere
    b.   Third ventricle joins the laterals at the foramen of Monro
    c.   Fourth ventricle joins the third ventricle via the aqueduct of Sylvius
    d.   Central canal of the spinal cord rises from the fourth ventricle

3.   Blood–brain barrier
    a.   Protects neural cells via selective permeability
    b.   Regulates and maintains the internal environment

    c.   **Highly permeable to water, carbon dioxide, oxygen, and most lipid-soluble substances**
    d.   Restricts large molecules, heavy metals, some antibiotics, and toxins

4.   Cerebral blood flow (CBF)
    a.   Components are blood and CSF

    b.   **Flows at a rate of 50–60 mL/100 g brain tissue per minute, for a total of 750 mL/min**
    c.   Is regulated by baroreceptors (pressure) and chemoreceptors (ions)

    d.   **Autoregulation is the ability of cerebral vessels to change their diameter in order to maintain constant blood flow despite changes in perfusion pressure**

    e.   **Cerebral perfusion pressure (CPP) is the CSF pressure that reflects cerebral blood flow. 80–100 mm H2O is needed for optimal flow in the average adult. Mean arterial pressure (MAP) minus intracranial pressure (ICP) equals CPP (MAP – ICP = CPP)**

5.   Cerebral metabolism: Normal metabolic processes are dependent on:

    a.   **Carbon dioxide, oxygen, and hydrogen ions, which have a potent effect on CSF**

       ► Arterial dilation, resulting in increased flow, occurs secondary to decreased oxygen.
       ► Vasodilation, resulting in increased flow, occurs secondary to increased carbon dioxide.

    b.   **Glucose: cerebral metabolic need requires serum glucose level 70–110 mg/100 mL. The brain is unable to store glucose, though, so need is constant.**
    c.   Serum osmolarity is maintained at 285–295 mOsm/kg. Alterations are associated with abnormal metabolic states, such as HHNK and hepatic encephalopathy.
    d.   Body temperature: Increased cerebral metabolic activity sec-

ondary to fever leads to increased CBF and consumption of oxygen and glucose.

II. Overview of neurologic disorders

A. Assessment

1. Past health history

   a. In assessing the client with a neurologic deficit, one must not suggest symptoms to the client. The health care provider must obtain an accurate description of the illness. Always remember to assess the client's mental status before obtaining a health history.

   b. Neurologic dysfunction symptoms should dictate the assessments to be performed. For instance, if the client is complaining of weakness, then a complete assessment of motor and sensory functions should be performed.

   c. Question the patient about smoking, safe recreational activities, nutrition, sleep–rest patterns, and stress.

    d. **The nurse should pursue an in-depth history of all dysfunctions.**

   e. Medication history: Assess for current medication use. Many drugs have a direct effect on neurologic functioning. Pay particular attention to mood-elevating drugs, sedatives, tranquilizers, anticoagulants, aspirin, anticonvulsants, alcohol, and illicit drug use.

   f. Past surgical history: The nurse should interview the client for a history of surgery to the nervous system.

2. Clinical manifestations

   a. If there is a dysfunction in the cerebrum, the nurse should assess for a history of personality changes, changes in level of consciousness (LOC), and changes in speech patterns. The Glasgow Coma Scale is the standard for assessing LOC.

   b. If there is a pupillary change, loss of gag reflex, or asymmetry, perform a cranial nerve assessment.

   c. If there is a dysfunction in the cerebellum, the nurse will assess for a history of uncoordinated movements in the client.

   d. If there are complaints of muscle weakness, abnormal movements, numbness, tingling or other abnormal sensations, then the nurse should assess for a history of sensory-motor system problems as well as checking all reflexes.

3. Physical Examination

   a. Assessment of cerebral functioning

      ► Appearance and behavior: Assess the dress, grooming, hygiene, motor activity, and language ability of the client.

      ► Level of consciousness: Assess the orientation to time, place and person. Memory, insight, judgment, attention span, and general knowledge should be evaluated.

      ► Emotional responses: Observe the mood and affect of the individual:

         (1) Thought patterns: Note the presence of illusions, hallucinations, and delusions.

(2) Intelligence: Observe for dementia and ask questions about presence of developmental delays.

b. Assessment of the cranial nerves (see Table 2-1)

c. Motor function assessment

▶ Ask the client to raise arms and feet and look for weakness. Move limbs through range of motion (ROM). Observe tone and tremors.

▶ Assess balance and coordination by having client touch their nose and examiner's finger alternately as nurse repositions finger so client must adjust for distance. Balance can be assessed by performing knee bends on alternate legs. All movements should be smooth.

▶ The heel shin test is another test for the assessment of coordination. The client places one heel on the opposite shin and moves heel toward the ankle. All movements should be smooth.

d. Sensory function assessment

▶ Assess for discriminatory sense, eg, sharp versus dull, on all extremities.

▶ Light touch is then employed by the nurse again asking client to identify the location.

▶ Assess for temperature sensation.

▶ Vibratory sense: Use a 128-Hz tuning fork, placed on bony prominences, and have client identify the location with eyes closed.

▶ The Romberg test may be performed by having client stand with feet together and eyes closed.

▶ Two point discrimination is assessed by placing two points of compass on the client's fingers and extremities. Two point discrimination can be recognized at 4 mm on the fingers and at larger distances on the extremities.

▶ Stereognosis: tested by placing familiar objects in the client's hand and having the client identify the object.

▶ Graphesthesia: tested by tracing letters or numbers on the client's hand and having them identify the letter or number with eyes closed.

e. Reflexes

▶ Reflexes are assessed by striking the end of various muscles with a reflex hammer. The reflexes must commonly tested are those of the biceps, triceps, brachioradiales patellar, and Achilles tendons.

▶ The normal response is contraction of the muscle.

4. Laboratory studies

a. Lumbar puncture: Cerebrospinal fluid (CSF) is aspirated through a needle inserted between L4 and L5.

 b. **Assist the client in maintaining a lateral fetal position without any movement so the client is not at risk for paralysis while the CSF is withdrawn.**

c.   **Post-procedure, position the client in a recumbent position, to prevent a spinal headache. Spinal headache results from CSF leakage at the puncture site.**

    d.   It highly recommended that fluids be forced to replace the fluids withdrawn.

    e.   If there is persistent CSF leakage, as evidenced by complaint of headache, then a blood patch may be performed.

5.   Diagnostic studies

    a.   Cerebral angiography: performed to assess for lesions of blood vessels, abscesses, or tumors.

> ► The procedure consists of catheter insertion, either brachially or femorally, with maneuvering to either the carotid or vertebral artery.
> ► A radiopaque dye is injected and radiologic films are evaluated.
> ► Post-procedure: observe for reactions to the dye as well as bleeding and infection at the puncture site.

    b.   Computer tomography (CT scan): performed to visualize blood vessels and the brain via computer-assisted radiologic films and assists in diagnosing tumors, brain infarctions, hemorrhages, abscesses, and atrophy.

    c.   Magnetic resonance imaging (MRI): Magnetics are employed with computer-assisted radiologic techniques to visualize edema, blood vessels, neoplasms, and bony structures.

    d.   Skull series: X-rays that aid in the diagnosis of skull fractures, degenerative processes, and calcification of the head.

    e.   Spinal Series: X-rays that aid in the diagnosis of fractures, dislocations, or degenerative processes in the spinal vertebrae.

    f.   Myelography

> ► This procedure is similar to a lumbar puncture in that the client is placed in a lateral fetal recumbent position.
> ► A catheter is inserted between L4 and L5 into the subarachnoid space, and a radiopaque dye is injected.
> ► This aids in the diagnosis of spinal tumors, herniation of disks, and arteriovenous lesions.
> ► Post-procedure: elevate the head of the bed to a semi-Fowler's position to prevent the dye from accumulating in the brain.
> ► Headache, nausea, and vomiting are frequent side effects.

    g.   Carotid Doppler and ultrasound study

> ► A Doppler and ultrasound scan is a noninvasive study which evaluates carotid occlusive disease.
> ► A probe is transversed along the carotid artery and produces an ultrasound signal that records reflected blood movement while the sound signal is evaluated.

h.   Transcranial Doppler sonography (TCD): The TCD study is useful in diagnosing any defects in blood flow or embolic phenomena. A probe is placed on the skull and sonar waves are recorded in a noninvasive manner.

i.   Electroencephalography (EEG): Electrodes are attached to the scalp to record brain voltage. This is useful in diagnosing brain tumors, epilepsy, and coma.

j.   Electromyography (EMG): Electrodes record impulses from muscle. EMGs aid in the diagnosis of myopathy and enervation.

B.   The Monroe–Kellie theorem

1.   **The skull is a nonexpandable cavity that contains CSF, blood, and brain tissue.**

2.   **The Monroe–Kellie theorem states that if there is an increase in either CSF, blood, or brain tissue then there will be an increase in ICP.**

3.   The body can compensate for increasing ICP by the following mechanisms:

   a.   Increasing CSF absorption.

   b.   Shifting blood into the subarachnoid space.

   c.   Inhibiting CSF production.

4.   When the body can no longer compensate, the following sequelae occur: (Fig. 2-2)

   a.   Cerebral blood flow is decreased.

   b.   Hypoxia develops as PCO_2 increases and PO_2 decreases.

   c.   Cerebral edema increases.

   d.   ICP increases.

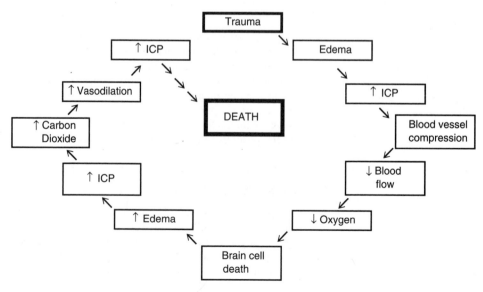

FIGURE 2-2.
Pathophysiologic changes occurring with increased intracerebral pressure.

5. As ICP rises, the brain may herniate, leading to eventual death. The signs and symptoms of increased ICP are:

   a. **Change in the LOC: the Glasgow Coma Scale measures eye opening response, verbal response, and motor response. A score of 7 or below is indicative of coma.**
   b. Pupillary changes: fixed, dilated, and/or unequal.
   c. Bradycardia, bradypnea.
   d. Systolic blood pressure rises as diastolic blood pressure decreases.
   e. Visual changes, weakness, decreased response to pain.
   f. Headache.
   g. Vomiting.
   h. Decerebrate and decorticate posturing:

   ▶ Decerebrate posturing is more serious. In decerebrate posturing the arms are extended, adducted, and pronated, whereas the legs are extended and the feet are in plantar flexion.

   ▶ Decorticate posturing is internal rotation and adduction of the arms with extension of the legs.

C. ICP monitoring (Fig. 2-3)
   1. Components of ICP monitoring system include a sensor, transducer, and a recording device.
      a. ICPs impinge on the sensor which transmits this information to the transducer.
      b. Finally, an electrical signal is displayed via oscilloscope.
      c. ICP monitoring techniques include: intraventricular catheter, subarachnoid screw/bolt, epidural/subdural catheter or sensor, and fiberoptic transducer-tipped catheter (FTC).
   2. Types of ICP catheters/monitoring devices:
      a. Intraventricular catheter

      ▶ A cannula is inserted into the ventricle of the nondominant hemisphere via a hole in the skull.
      ▶ The cannula is connected via pressurized tubing to a transducer.
      ▶ This catheter measures ICP directly and permits CSF to be withdrawn as needed.
      ▶ This catheter places the client at risk for CSF loss and infection.

      b. Epidural catheter

      ▶ A transducer is placed between the skull and the dura or may be placed subdurally.

      ▶ **A major drawback with this type of catheter is that CSF samples cannot be obtained.**

      c. Subarachnoid screw

      ▶ A burr hole is made in the skull and screw is placed in the subarachnoid space. This is attached to a transducer, which directly measures pressure.

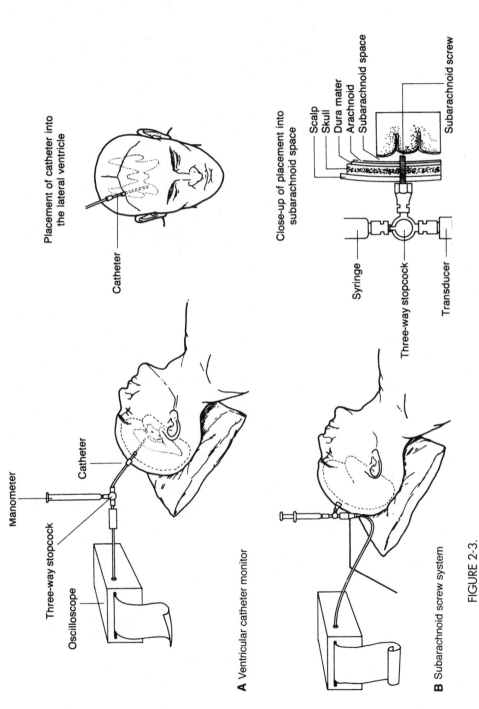

Placement of catheter into the lateral ventricle

Catheter

Close-up of placement into subarachnoid space

Scalp
Skull
Dura mater
Arachnoid
Subarachnoid space
Subarachnoid space
Subarachnoid screw

Syringe

Three-way stopcock

Transducer

Manometer

Catheter

Three-way stopcock

Oscilloscope

A Ventricular catheter monitor

B Subarachnoid screw system

FIGURE 2-3.
Intracranial pressure monitoring devices: *A,* ventricular catheter and *B,* subarachnoid or hollow screw. These devices are connected to a pressure transducer and display system.

▶ CSF sampling cannot take place.

3. ICP monitoring values:

   a. **Normal ICP less than 10 mm Hg.**
   b. **Mild ICP elevation 10–15 mm Hg.**
   c. **Moderate ICP elevation 15–20 mm Hg.**
   d. **Severe ICP elevation greater than 20 mm Hg.**

4. ICP monitor wave formations:

   a. An A wave is associated with pressures between 50 and 100 mm Hg which lasts several minutes.
   b. A B wave is associated with respiratory and circulatory pressure changes.
   c. A C wave is associated with respiratory and circulatory pressure changes.

5. Nursing care of the client with ICP monitor:

   a. Ensure continuous neurologic assessment of the client.
   b. If ICP monitoring equipment is in place, maintain equipment:

     ▶ Maintain closed system sterility.
     ▶ Maintain transducer at the same level as the foramen of Monro or at level of the ear.
     ▶ Zero balance and calibrate whenever client's bed position is changed.
     ▶ Do not permit air bubbles to enter transducer or tubing to prevent wave dampening and inaccurate readings.

   c. Monitor pressures and wave formations as ordered.
   d. Assist with withdrawing CSF in clients with intraventricular cannulas.
   e. Report and document pressure changes.

 f. **Remember that coughing, sneezing, or Valsalva maneuvers may cause a temporary change in pressure.**

   g. Elevate head of bed 15–30 degrees.
   h. Maintain a neutral position of head.
   i. Hyperoxygenation of clients requiring suction is essential.

 j. **Provide oxygen or ventilatory support to maintain $PaCO_2$ between 25–30 mm Hg and a PaO_2 of at least 100 mm Hg.**

   k. Limit suctioning to 15 seconds to decrease the risk of hypoxia.
   l. Teach client the importance of avoiding Valsalva maneuvers.
   m. Administer the prescribed medication regimen

     ▶ Osmotic diuretics: mannitol (Osmitrol), glycerol, ethacrynic acid (Edecrin), furosemide (Lasix), which reduce brain water tissue.
     ▶ Glucocorticoids: dexamethasone (Decadron) to control cerebral edema.
     ▶ Barbiturate coma: sodium methohexital (Brevital) to decrease pressure. These patients must be on ventilatory support.

> ▸ Neuromuscular blockage, such as pancuronium (Pavulon) to decrease the body's metabolic requirements.
> ▸ Provide the client with adequate sedation.

   n.   Maintain homeostasis of the client's temperature.

D.   Nutrition

1.   After brain injury, catabolic hormones and cytokine levels increase, and norepinephrine levels may rise as high as seven times normal.

2.   These are examples of the metabolic response to head injury and are speculated to be induced in part by the systemic and central surge of metabolites.

3.   This response is characterized by hypermetabolism, hypercatabolism, hyperglycemia, depressed immunocompetence, altered vascular permeability, and altered gastrointestinal (GI) function.

4.   The acute phase during head injury is noted by depressed albumin levels, poor drug transport, and intolerance of enteral feedings. The response is also noted for fever without evidence of infection or fluctuation in serum or urine zinc levels.

5.   Considerations for medical nutrition therapy:

   a.   The overall goal is to increase the nutrient intake to achieve caloric balance and meet intake needs.

   b.   Hypercatabolism: decrease nitrogen loss by increasing nitrogen intake.

   c.   Hypermetabolism: propranolol (Inderal) administration can produce a decrease in the metabolic rate and heart rate accounting for 25% of the hypermetabolism 3 to 12 days following removal from mechanical ventilation. This in turn could help to reduce ICP.

   d.   Acute phase response which is denoted by fever, low albumin, and loss of zinc and iron. Management involves an increase in nutrient administration and administration of exogenous albumin. Replace protein loss and other substrate deficiencies (eg, zinc, iron, fibrinogen).

   e.   Hyperglycemia: Provide insulin administration when the blood glucose level is above 200 mg/dL.

   f.   Immunology: Provide optimal nutrients. At this point there is no evidence that nutrient therapy improves immune status.

   g.   Altered gastric function: Bypass the stomach and feed into the small intestine using a naso-duodenal tube, for example. If enteral nutrition cannot be provided within 24 hours postinjury, the parenteral route should be used.

   h.   Nutrient modification: Ensure high nutrient and high protein intake. Parenterally fed patients have been found to have a better neurologic outcome.

E.   Psychosocial implications

1.   Nurses must aid in caring for the psychosocial well-being of the client and family.

2.   Nurses can decrease anxiety in the following ways:

   a.   Maintain a competent professional demeanor.

   b.   Provide reassurance as needed.

   c.   Offer concise responses and explanations to clients and families.

    d.   Allow for family participation and input into care if the client is unable to perform self-care.

    e.   Assist the client and family to accept the limitations of the disorder.

    f.   Assist the client to develop a positive self-concept.

    g.   Assist the client in adapting to lifestyle changes as a result of physical limitations and mental changes.

F.   Commonly used medications (medications used to treat neurologic problems are disease specific):

    1.   Corticosteroids, such as dexamethasone, reduce inflammation and decrease ICP.

        a.   Administer IV in life-threatening situations.

        b.   Always taper drug dosage to prevent adrenal insufficiency.

    2.   Anticonvulsants, such as phenytoin, control seizures.

        a.   Teach patient that anticonvulsants may cause drowsiness and stopping medication may cause seizures.

        b.   Instruct patient about the side effects of rash, cold or flulike symptoms, as well as oral problems and to report them to their health care provider immediately.

    3.   Anticholinergics, such as Cogentin, inhibit the action of acetylcholine.

        a.   Instruct patient to take with food to decrease the GI side effects and hard candy or ice chips to relieve dry mouth.

        b.   Teach patient that anticholinergics may cause drowsiness.

    4.   Cholinergics, such as neostigmine, inhibit the breakdown of acetylcholine.

        a.   Teach the patient to take medications at the same time each day and take with food to decrease the GI side effects.

        b.   Atropine is the antidote for overdose.

    5.   Antihistamines, such as diphenhydramine, inhibit acetylcholine.

        a.   Teach the patient to take with food to decrease the GI side effects.

        b.   Instruct the patient that it may cause drowsiness and dry mouth which can be relieved with ice chips or hard candy.

    6.   Antiparkinson drugs, such as carbidopa, make more dopamine available to peripheral tissues.

        a.   Monitor hourly intake and output.

        b.   Assess for signs and symptoms of dehydration.

        c.   Maintain systolic blood pressure of at least 90 mm Hg.

G.   Medications affecting the brain

    1.   General anesthesia: Anesthesia allows for a loss of sensation for a temporary period of time. During a painful experience the body experiences hormonal changes resulting in electrolyte disturbances, increased susceptibility to infection, and poor wound healing. Increased heart rate secondary to pain or fear predisposes the patient to cardiac disturbances. Anesthesia changes the patient's perception of pain by interrupting the pain impulse before it reaches the central nervous system. Other benefits of anesthesia include rendering the patient unconscious, decreasing anxiety, and producing an amnesiac effect.

        a.   All anesthetic agents have actions and side affects that may cause problems or be unpredictable.

        b.   Considerations must be made in choosing anesthetic drugs and their effect on cerebral metabolism, cerebral blood flow, and vasomotor tone.

    c.   Regard should be given to anesthetic agents that will contribute to brain relaxation and that are nonirritating so that coughing and retching are not precipitated.

    d.   Anesthetic agents with minimal side affects and adverse reactions on various body systems that are readily recognized should be preferred when selecting the actual agent.

    e.   During the immediate postoperative period the patient should be monitored closely for hypoxia, hypoventilation, hypotension, hypertension, cardiac dysrhythmias, hypo- or hyperthemia, malignant hyperthemia, nausea/vomiting, and pain. Any of the above may be side effects of the anesthetic agents used during surgery or the surgery itself. Prepare for immediate intervention.

  2. Narcotics

    a.   Narcotics are known to cause central nervous system changes.

    b.   The action of narcotics act by depressing pain impulse transmission at the spinal cord level by interacting with opioid receptors.

    c.   The use of narcotics are to control moderate to severe pain and are used before and after surgery.

III. **Increased intracranial pressure**

  A. **Description: an ICP exceeding 15 mm Hg due to an increase in one of the three intracranial components, blood (intracranial bleed), CSF (hydrocephalus), or brain tissue (brain tumor).**

  B. **Etiology and incidence**

    1. Common causes of increased ICP include tumors, abscesses, hemorrhage, edema, hydrocephalus, and hemorrhage.

    2. Because increased ICP is related to varied pathologic processes, the incidence is specific to the underlying cause.

  C. **Assessment**

    1. **The earliest signs of increased ICP are often transient and subtle. Early signs include restlessness, confusion, drowsiness, headache, seizures, and sensory deficits.**

    2. Later signs include widened pulse pressure, bradycardia, abnormal respiratory patterns, increased temperature, sluggish and dilating pupils, decreased LOC, vomiting, and impaired brain stem reflexes, such as a gag reflex.

    3. Motor findings may include contralateral hemiparesis and decorticate or decerebrate posturing.

    4. Papilledema may be present.

    5. ICP readings in excesses of 15 mm Hg will be present.

  D. **Nursing diagnoses**

    1. Ineffective Airway Clearance

    2. Altered Tissue Perfusion: Cerebral

    3. Altered Thought Processes

    4. Risk for Infection

    5. Risk for Impaired Skin Integrity

    6. Risk For Injury

    7. Decreased Adaptive Capacity: Intracranial

E. **Planning and implementation**
1. Assess neurologic status, including LOC, pupillary reactivity, ocular movement, and general sensory/motor function.
2. Monitor vital signs and note alterations from baseline.
3. Ensure that body temperature is maintained to prevent acceleration of O_2 consumption and prevent precipitous rise in ICP.
4. Maintain patent airway and adequate ventilation.
5. Assess respiratory rate and pattern.
6. Assess for cyanosis.
7. Auscultate lung fields to evaluate aeration.
8. Suction as needed. Hyperventilate with 100% oxygen before and after suctioning to prevent hypoxia.
9. Assess ventilator settings for accuracy.
10. Assist with mechanical hyperventilation to decrease CO_2 and promote cerebral vasoconstriction and decrease ICP.
11. Monitor blood gas levels to assure adequate oxygenation is present and to prevent hypercarbia which causes cerebral vasodilatation and subsequent increase in ICP.
12. Maintain optimal patient positioning.
    a. Elevate head of bed 30 to 40 degrees in neutral position to promote venous return.
    b. Turn patient q2hr.
    c. When the client is alert, have them exhale during turning and repositioning to block activation of Valsalva maneuver.
    d. Perform passive range-of-motion (ROM) exercises.
    e. Avoid having the client assist with repositioning or exercises. These activities initiate Valsalva maneuver and increase ICP.
13. Monitor fluid balance
    a. If ordered, ensure that fluid restriction is maintained.
    b. Measure urine outputs.
14. Prevent precipitous increases in ICP:
    a. Provide quiet environment.
    b. Prevent coughing.
    c. Avoid vomiting by administration of antiemetics as ordered.
    d. Prevent straining at stool by providing ordered laxatives.

     e. **Avoid grouping nursing activities together that may cause ICP spikes.**
15. Monitor ICP and assess ICP monitoring system:
    a. Pressure waves form analysis is documented.
    b. Ensure that baseline trending is performed.

     c. **A waves are initiated from an already increased ICP tracing; are usually of 5 to 20 minutes in duration; occur with an increase in BP of 50 to 100 mm Hg; and are more frequent when ICP >20 mm Hg. They are clinically significant because of underlying irreversible ischemia.**
    d. B waves usually occur q 1/2 to 2 minutes; are related to the respiratory cycle; are not sustained; and are not usually significant.
    e. C waves occur as a result of normal changes in arterial BP and are not clinically significant.

f. **Normal ICP reading is 0–10 mm Hg. A sustained reading of >15 mm Hg is considered abnormal.**

g. Obtain readings during "quiet" periods.

h. Ensure that the client's position and the position of the transducer is unchanged from previous readings.

 i. **For clients with a ventriculostomy catheter, ensure that drainage device is secured at the level ordered by the physician.**

j. For clients with a subarachnoid bolt/screw or an epidural or subdural sensor or a fiberoptic transducer-tipped catheter (FTC), ensure that the monitoring system has been assembled per hospital policy.

k. **Adhere to strict aseptic technique when manipulating system.**

l. Check insertion site for signs and symptoms of infection and ensure that site is appropriately dressed.

m. Assess system for signs of loose connections, air in line, CSF leakage or blockage.

16. Administer medications as ordered:

a. Osmotic diuretics (eg, mannitol) to decrease ICP.

b. Corticosteroids (eg, Decadron) to provide anti-inflammatory action and to decrease ICP.

c. Diuretics (eg, Lasix) to decrease cerebral edema.

d. Stool softeners (eg, Colace) to prevent initiation of Valsalva maneuver.

e. Anticonvulsants (eg, Dilantin) to prevent seizure activity.

f. Antacids (eg, Maalox) to prevent gastric irritation.

g. Histamine blocking agents (eg, Tagamet) to reduce stimulation of GI secretions.

h. Antipyretics (eg, Tylenol) to reduce temperature elevations which cause an increase in O_2 consumption.

i. Analgesics (eg, codeine) in small doses for headache relief. Analgesics are used with great caution, as they may cause respiratory and neurologic depression.

17. Be aware that barbiturate therapy:

a. may be administered IV to induce coma for clients unresponsive to other therapies;

b. decreases metabolic demands and therefore decrease ICP;

c. requires constant assessment of ICP, arterial BP, PA pressures, ABGs, serum barbiturate levels and ECG;

d. requires that the client receive all nursing measures necessary for the mechanically ventilated client.

F. Evaluation

1. The client's ICP remains within acceptable range.

2. The client's body temperature is within normal limits.

3. The client is free from infection.

4. The client exhibits a patent airway and adequate ventilation.

5. The client has no skin breakdown.

6. The client is free from injury and maintained in a safe environment.

7. The client is pain free.
8. The client's mentation is sustained and/or improved.
9. The client and his family demonstrate decreased anxiety.

IV. Closed head injury

A. Description: **A closed head injury is one in which some degree of damage occurs to the contents of the cranium without causing a break in the skull itself.**

B. Etiology and incidence

1. Closed head injuries are most commonly the result of motor vehicle accidents, falls, and assaults. Alcohol has frequently been found to be a causative factor.
2. Head trauma causes approximately 100,000 deaths annually in the United States.

C. Pathophysiology

1. Concussion: a severe blow to the head which causes temporary neural dysfunction.
2. Contusion: a more severe blow to the head which causes bruising of the brain's surface with resultant neural dysfunction.
3. Laceration: a traumatic tear of the cortical surface of the brain.
4. Diffuse axonal injury (DAI): extensive damage to the axons in the white matter, usually related to high velocity acceleration–deceleration accidents.
5. Hypoxic brain injury: the result of certain metabolic or cardiac events that contributes to cerebral oxygen deficits and subsequent injury.

6. **Management is aimed at perfusing the brain and preventing complications.**

D. Assessment

1. Concussions usually present with headache and transient loss of consciousness followed by post-traumatic amnesia, nausea, dizziness, and irritability.

2. **Contusions present clinically with neurologic deficits based on the site and severity of injury. Symptoms include decreasing LOC, aphasia, hemiplegia, and sensory deficits.**
3. Non-specific complaints may include headache, vomiting, and restlessness.
4. Evaluation of the precipitating event should include mechanism of injury.

E. Nursing diagnoses

1. Altered Thought Process
2. Altered Tissue Perfusion: Cerebral
3. Risk for Injury
4. Decreased Adaptive Capacity: Intracranial

F. Planning and implementation

1. Assess vital signs.
2. Monitor neurologic status and mentation, and compare to baseline.
3. Optimize cerebral perfusion pressure (CPP):
   a. Elevate HOB at least 30 degrees.
   b. Avoid initiation of the Valsalva maneuver.
   c. Provide psychological support to client and family.

        d.   Observe for deterioration in neurologic status: hemiplegia, aphasia and/or sensory changes.

    4.   Maintain patent airway and ventilation.

    5.   Maintain safe environment.

    6.   Evaluate thought processes and re-orient client as necessary.

    7.   Promote skin integrity by:

        a.   Turning and repositioning q2h using a written turning schedule.

        b.   Ensuring that skin is dry by the use of moisture barriers.

        c.   Preventing friction and shear during positioning by use of a pull sheet under the client.

    8.   When necessary, pharmacologic agents are administered to control brain swelling and maintain ICP within normal limits.

        a.   Diuretics, particularly osmotic diuretics, may be administered to minimize cerebral edema.

        b.   Steroids may be used to decrease inflammation.

        c.   Antacids or histamine-blocking agents may be administered to reduce the risk of gastric irritation from other pharmacologic agents.

G.   **Evaluation**

    1.   The client exhibits CPP and ICP within acceptable limits.

    2.   The client maintains a patent airway with adequate ventilation.

    3.   The client remains free from injury.

    4.   The client's neurologic status remains stable.

    5.   The client's skin remains intact.

V.   **Skull fractures**

    A.   **Description: a skull fracture is a disruption in the integrity of the cranial vault.**

    B.   **Etiology and incidence**

        1.   Common causes include blunt or penetrating trauma.

        2.   Between 80,000 and 100,000 deaths occur annually as a result of head trauma.

    C.   **Pathophysiology**

        1.   Basilar fracture:

            a.   involves the base of the skull.

            b.   usually stems from an extended area of linear fracture.

            c.   often involves paranasal air sinuses or the middle ear.

            d.   can involve the orbit of the eye.

        2.   Depressed skull fracture:

            a.   involves inward displacement of the outer skull table to at least the inner table of surrounding skull.

            b.   can occur with open or closed head injuries.

        3.   Linear skull fracture:

            a.   most common type of fracture.

            b.   no actual displacement of bone occurs.

        4.   **Management is aimed at relieving pressure/ischemia and preventing complications.**

    D.   **Assessment**

        1.   Clinical manifestation are based on location and type of injury.

2. The presence of rhinorrhea (CSF drainage from the nose), sub-conjunctival hemorrhage, and periorbital ecchymosis (raccoon's eyes) may indicate a fracture of the paranasal sinuses.

3. Otorrhea (CSF drainage from the ear), vertigo, and nystagmus may be present.

4. Ecchymosis over the mastoid bone is referred to as Battle's sign and may occur 24–48 hours post-injury.

5. Headache and pain over the fracture site is common.

6. Altered LOC and possible sensory deficits may occur.

E. Nursing diagnosis
1. Risk for Injury
2. Decreased Adaptive Capacity: Intracranial
3. Risk for Infection
4. Altered Tissue Perfusion: Cerebral

F. Planning and implementation
1. Assess client for specific deficits based on site and type of fracture.
2. Note presence of rhinorrhea and/or otorrhea.
3. Evaluate fluctuations in vital signs and LOC.
4. Assess motor function.
5. Monitor and report any complaints of headache.
6. Prevent injury by providing a safe environment.
7. Inspect fracture site and perform dressing changes as ordered using sterile technique.
8. Observe for signs of increased ICP related to bone displacement and subsequent edema.
9. Provide psychological support to client and family.
10. Maintain client on bedrest.
11. Be aware of potential complications.
   a. Internal carotid artery injury and CSF Leakage are associated with basilar fractures
   b. Infections are associated with depressed skull fractures
   c. Hemorrhages
   d. Sequela from increased ICP, including herniation.

G. Evaluation
1. Client will be free from injury.
2. Client will exhibit no signs of infection.
3. Client will demonstrate coping skills to decrease anxiety level.

VI. Hematomas

A. Description: Hematomas are intracranial hemorrhages that produce bleeding into the epidural, subdural, subarachnoid space or ventricles.

B. Etiology and incidence
1. The usual causes of hematomas include motor vehicle accidents, assaults involving blunt or penetrating trauma and falls.
2. Up to 15% of all head injuries are subdural hematomas.
3. They may also occur spontaneously in patients with coagulopathies.

C. Pathophysiology (Fig. 2-4)
1. Subdural hematoma: an accumulation of blood between the dura and the arachnoid that involves venous bleeding and forms slowly.

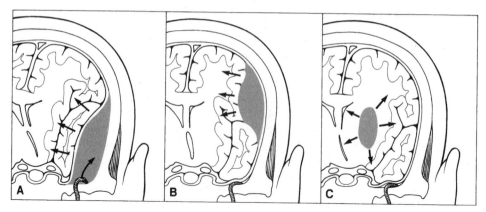

FIGURE 2-4.
Cerebral hemorrhage or bleeding. *A,* Epidural or extradural hematoma—bleeding between the inner skull and the dura, compressing the brain underneath. *B,* Subdural hematoma—bleeding between the dura mater and arachnoid membrane. *C,* Intracerebral hemorrhage—bleeding in the brain or the cerebral tissue with displacement of surrounding structures.

    a. **Acute form becomes symptomatic within 48 hours of injury and is usually associated with underlying cerebral contusion.**

    b. **Subacute form becomes symptomatic from 2 days to 2 weeks from the time of injury. The contusion to the underlying tissue is less severe than in the acute form.**

       c. Chronic form becomes symptomatic within 2 weeks to several months from time of injury.

   2. Epidural hematoma: a collection of blood between the dura mater and the skull which usually results from laceration of the middle meningeal artery with a rapid accumulation of blood.

   3. Subarachnoid hemorrhage: bleeding into the subarachnoid space which is a common finding in severe head injuries.

   4. Intracerebral hematoma: an accumulation of blood into the brain parenchyma.

D. **Assessment**

   1. Specific clinical symptoms are based on the type and site of the injury.

       a. Epidural hematomas generally produce a brief loss of consciousness, followed by lucidity and progression to vomiting, severe headache, rapid decrease in LOC, seizures, and ipsilateral pupillary dilation.

       b. Subdural hematoma manifests with altered LOC, headache, focal neurologic deficits, and personality changes.

       c. Intracerebral hemorrhage produces headache, decreased LOC, and contralateral hemiplegia.

       d. Subarachnoid and intraventricular hemorrhage produces nuchal rigidity, decreased LOC, headache, hemiparesis, and ipsilateral dilated pupil.

E. **Nursing diagnoses**
1. Ineffective Airway Clearance
2. Altered Tissue Perfusion: Cerebral
3. Altered Thought Processes
4. Decreased Adaptive Capacity: Intracranial

F. **Planning and implementation**
1. Maintain patent airway.
2. Monitor vital and neurologic signs.
    a. Observe for signs of increased ICP and seizures.
    b. Observe for hemiplegia, aphasia, and sensory problems and plan for care accordingly.
3. Provide a safe environment.
4. Provide psychological support to client and family.
5. Re-orient client to surroundings as needed.
6. Provide measures to prevent complications of immobility.
7. Ensure optimal skin integrity by use of appropriate positioning and product usage.

m 8. **Be aware of potential complications:**
    a. **Seizures**
    b. **Intracranial hypertension that, unresolved, may lead to herniation**
    c. **Death**

G. **Evaluation**
1. The client maintains a patent airway with adequate ventilation.
2. The client exhibits stable vital signs and neurologic signs that are within acceptable limits.
3. The client remains free from injury.
4. The client exhibits full ROM.
5. The client maintains intact skin.

VII. **Transient ischemic attacks**
A. **Description: A transient ischemic attack (TIA) is a brief neurologic deficit lasting minutes to 24 hours with no permanent deficits.**
B. **Etiology and incidence**
1. One-third of all people who have a stroke had a previous TIA.
2. Another third of all people who suffer a TIA will have another TIA.
3. The last third of people who have a TIA never have any other neurologic deficits

C. **Pathophysiology**
1. A TIA is a temporary disruption in blood flow due to spasm or microemboli.
2. Management is aimed at preventing complications and future TIAs from occurring.

D. **Assessment**
1. Signs and symptoms are dependent on the area of the brain affected.
2. Complete neurologic assessment is recommended to evaluate the full extent of the temporary cerebral injury.
3. If the TIA occurs in the right cerebral hemisphere then assess for the following temporary deficits:
    a. Left hemianopia: blindness on the left side of the client's visual field.
    b. Left hemiparesis or hemiplegia: numbness or paralysis.

     c.   Sensory deficits related to the inability to deal with familiar objects or situations.

4. If the TIA occurs in the left cerebral hemisphere, then assess for the following temporary deficits:
   a. Right hemianopia: blindness on the right side of the client's visual field.
   b. Right hemiplegia: numbness or paralysis.
   c. Aphasia: the inability to communicate

   ▸ Expressive: the inability to speak or use written language.
   ▸ Receptive: the inability to understand spoken or written language.
   ▸ Global: the inability to communicate or understand language in oral or written form.

   d. Temporary loss of consciousness, dizziness or garbled speech.
5. Diagnostic procedures
   a. CT scan: may reveal areas of ischemia or vasospasm.
   b. Angiography: may reveal vascular deficits.
   c. EEG: may reveal focal neurologic deficits.
   d. Doppler ultrasonography: performed to evaluate blood flow and cerebral perfusion
   e. Positron emission tomography (PET): utilizes the chemical makeup of the brain to evaluate brain tissue damage.
   f. MRI: utilizes magnetics to reveal brain tissue damage.

E. Nursing diagnoses
1. Self Care Deficit
2. Impaired Physical Mobility
3. Sensory/Perceptual Alterations
4. Ineffective Airway Clearance
5. Impaired Swallowing
6. Altered Nutrition: Less than Body Requirements

F. Planning and implementation
1. Assess for communication ability.
2. Assess for and prevent skin breakdown.
3. Assess for neurologic status.
4. Assess respiratory status.
5. Maintain fluid and electrolyte balance.
6. Provide for rest.
7. Apply antiembolic stockings.
8. Provide ROM exercises.
9. Instruct client on the use of assistive devices.
10. Manage pain with analgesics.
11. Teach proper use of medications such as warfarin (Coumadin) for anticoagulation.
12. Administer medications as indicated and appropriate, TIAs may be managed with ticlopidine (Ticlid), dipyridamole (Persantine), or acetylsalicylic acid (ASA). See discussion of CVA.
13. Offer nutritional support:

    a.   **Before any dietary consideration is made, ascertain for the presence of a gag reflex. If there is no gag reflex, consult speech therapist for swallowing exercises until the neurologic deficit passes.**

   b. Elevate the head of the bed.

   c. Provide balanced diet that is low in salt, calories, and choles-terol. Reposition food so client can see it.

   d. Pureed foods are the most easily swallowed although they are often bland.

   e. Offer foods that enhance elimination.

G. **Evaluation**

  1. The client will be able to optimally carry out activities of daily living.

  2. The client will maintain social interaction.

  3. The client will remain injury free.

  4. The client will be able to make all needs known.

H. **Home health consideration**

  1. Plan for rest.

  2. Decrease stress via relaxation techniques.

  3. Encourage weight reduction and a low-salt diet to assist in control-ling blood pressure.

  4. Teach client to seek appropriate care for headache, numbness, and visual changes.

VIII. **Cerebrovascular accident**

 A. **Description: A neurologic deficit that is the result of damage or disease in the cerebral blood vessels.**

 B. **Etiology and incidence**

  1. Affects more people over age 65. One-third of all people with a CVA die.

  2. Causes of CVA include:

   a. Thrombosis (the most common cause)

   b. Embolism

   c. Intracranial hemorrhage related to a ruptured cerebral blood vessel. The middle cerebral artery is the most common artery affected.

  3. Risk factors include:

   a. Advancing age

   b. Race: African Americans are at greater risk than Caucasians

   c. Genetics: strokes sometimes follow hereditary patterns

   d. Cardiovascular disease

   e. Hypertension

   f. Hypercholestronemia

   g. Stress

   h. Smoking

   i. Diabetes mellitus

   j. Oral contraceptive use

 C. **Pathophysiology**

  1. An area of the brain becomes hypoxic, secondary to edema or an obstructed blood vessel.

  2. Deficits will be varied depending on the area of the brain affected

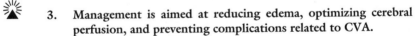

  3. **Management is aimed at reducing edema, optimizing cerebral perfusion, and preventing complications related to CVA.**

 D. **Assessment**

  1. Signs and symptoms are dependent on the areas of the brain affected.

2.   A complete neurologic assessment is recommended to evaluate the extent of injury.

3.   If a CVA occurs in the right cerebral hemisphere then assess for the following deficits:

   a.   Left hemianopia: blindness in the left half of the visual field.

   b.   Left hemiparesis or hemiplegia

   c.   Astereognosis: the inability to recognize familiar objects when placed in the hand.

   d.   Proprioception: the inability to determine body positions.

   e.   Apraxia: the inability to complete a task.

4.   If a CVA occurs in the left cerebral hemisphere, then assess for the following deficits:

   a.   Right hemianopia: blindness in the right half of the visual field.

   b.   Right hemiparesis or hemiplegia: numbness or paralysis.

   c.   Astereognosis

   d.   Proprioception

   e.   Apraxia

   f.   Expressive, receptive, or global aphasia

5.   Assess for familial or personal history of vascular disorders, hypertension, cardiovascular disease, or diabetes.

6.   Diagnostic procedures

   a.   Lumbar puncture: may reveal red blood cells and protein if CVA was due to intracranial hemorrhage.

   b.   CT scan may reveal ischemia, infarction, or hemorrhage.

   c.   Angiography: may reveal defects or spasms in cerebral blood vessels.

   d.   EEG may reveal focal neurologic deficits.

   e.   Doppler ultrasound: used to evaluate cerebral blood flow.

   f.   Positron emission tomography (PET): uses the chemical makeup of the brain to evaluate tissue damage.

   g.   MRI: uses magnetics to differentiate between CVA of hemorrhagic embolic or thrombotic origin.

E.   Nursing diagnoses

1.   Impaired Verbal Communication

2.   Impaired Physical Mobility

3.   Self Care Deficit

4.   Risk for Impaired Skin Integrity

5.   Social Isolation

F.   Planning and implementation

1.   Assess for communication ability and offer alternative methods of communication.

2.   Assess for and prevent skin breakdown.

3.   Assess neurologic status.

4.   Assess respiratory status.

5.   Provide for rest.

6.   Provide balanced diet as ordered.

7.   Maintain fluid and electrolyte balance.

8.   Apply antiembolic stockings.

9.   Provide ROM exercises.

10.   Instruct client on the use of assistive devices.

11. Teach proper use of medication.
12. Manage pain with analgesics.
13. Prepare the client and family for possible carotid endarterectomy.
14. Teach safety precautions.
15. Administer medications as indicated and ordered
    a. Administer osmotic diuretics if ICP is increased.
    b. Administer anticoagulants if patient had a thrombotic stroke.

    ▸ Heparin is given at a rate of 1000 units per hour or until the partial thromboplastin time is 1.5 to 2 times normal.

     ▸ **The antidote to heparin is protamine sulfate.**
    ▸ After heparin, the patient is usually placed on warfarin (Coumadin). Coumadin is usually given in a dose of 5–10 mg per day.
    ▸ The antidote to coumadin is vitamin K.
    ▸ The side effect of heparin and coumadin is bleeding.

    c. Administer platelet aggregation inhibitors to interfere with the platelet's ability to stick together or to the vessels walls.

    ▸ Acetylsalicylic acid (ASA): doses range from 80–1000 mg per day. The side effects are bleeding, GI upset, and bruising.
    ▸ Dipyridamole (Persantine): doses range from 50–75 mg four times a day. The side effect is GI upset.
    ▸ Ticlopidine hydrochloride (Ticlid): dose of 250 mg twice a day. The side effects of ticlid are neutropenia and diarrhea.
    ▸ Thrombolytic therapy-tissue plasminogen activator (TPA): used to lyse a clot. It must be given within 6 hours. The major side effect is bleeding.

16. Ensure adequate nutrition

     a. **Assess for gag reflex. If there is no gag reflex, consult a speech therapist and prepare for either a nasogastric feeding or total parenteral nutrition.**
    b. Elevate the head of the bed.

    c. **Liquids are the most difficult to swallow. Pureed foods are most easily swallowed although they are often bland.**
    d. Offer foods that enhance elimination.

G. Evaluation
1. The client and family will have a means to communicate.
2. The client will be able to carry out activities of daily living.
3. The client will show no evidence of skin breakdown.
4. The client will maintain social interaction.
5. The client will demonstrate knowledge of proper use of assistive devices.

H. Home health considerations
1. Teach family how to adapt home environment to accommodate to the needs of the client.
2. Teach family ROM exercise.
3. Teach family transfer techniques.
4. Teach family about the disease process.

5.   Teach family about medication routine.

6.   Teach family relaxation techniques.

7.   Refer family to appropriate support group.

IX.   Arterial-venous malformations (AVM)

A.   Description: A defect in the intima or wall of an artery or brain such as a rupture, aneurysm.

B.   Etiology: Caused by congenital defects in the walls of arteries and veins.

C.   Assessment: Symptoms associated with rupture of an AV malformation include headache, nausea and vomiting, and focal neurologic deficits.

D.   Nursing diagnosis (see CVA)

E.   Planning and implementation (see CVA)

1.   Craniotomies are sometimes performed to correct the defect via microsurgery.

2.   If the client undergoes surgery, nursing care must be directed to prevent infection and long-term complications.

X.   Cerebral aneurysms

A.   Description: An aneurysm is a weakness in an arterial wall. High arterial pressure leads to an out-pouching of the arterial wall, which can hemorrhage.

B.   Etiology and incidence

1.   Aneurysms arise from weaknesses in blood vessels as a result of a congenital defect, hypertension, or coronary artery disease.

2.   When an aneurysm ruptures, blood may leak into the subarachnoid space or brain tissue.

3.   As a result of a ruptured aneurysm, the brain tissue is damaged and increased ICP can ensue.

C.   Pathophysiology (as listed under CVA)

D.   Assessment

1.   The client with an aneurysm is usually asymptomatic or has mild complaints of headache or visual changes until the aneurysm ruptures.

2.   A ruptured cerebral aneurysm may produce signs and symptoms of increased ICP, headache, neck pain, photophobia, blurred vision, and restlessness.

3.   Signs and symptoms manifested as neurologic deficits are dependent on the area of the brain affected. A complete neurologic examination is advised to evaluate all deficits.

4.   Deficits produced by a ruptured aneurysm are similar to those of a CVA.

E.   Nursing diagnoses

1.   Impaired Verbal Communication

2.   Impaired Physical Mobility

3.   Self Care Deficit

4.   Decreased Adaptive Capacity: Intracranial

5.   Risk for Impaired Skin Integrity

F.   Planning and implementation

1.   Hourly neurologic examinations should be performed.

2.   **Provide a quiet environment. Darkness will provide comfort for photophobia.**

     3.   Place the patient in semi-Fowler's position.

     4.   Administer anticonvulsants to prevent seizures.

     5.   Employ measures to decrease ICP.

     6.   Prepare patient for surgical clipping of the aneurysm.

     7.   Maintain patient safety.

     8.   Nursing interventions for the patient with an aneurysm are similar to the care of the patient with a CVA.

     9.   Administer medications as ordered:
        a.   Osmotic diuretics to reduce ICP.
        b.   Corticosteroids to decrease cerebral edema.
        c.   Sedatives are used to help the patient rest.
        d.   Aminocaproic acid (Amicar) may prevent lysis of the clot.

     10.   **Be aware of potential complications:**
        a.   **Rebleeding can occur after the initial bleed of the aneurysm. Rebleeding usually occurs approximately one to two weeks after the initial rupture of the aneurysm.**
        b.   **Cerebral ischemia may result from vasospasm.**
        c.   **Neurologic deficits occur in response to injury of brain tissue.**

     11.   Cleanse craniotomy site with antiseptic solution and apply dry sterile dressing.

G.   **Evaluation**
     1.   The client will be able to make needs known.
     2.   The client will be able to carry out activities of daily living.
     3.   The client will have a mechanism to communicate.
     4.   The client will have a decrease in pain.
     5.   The client will maintain social interaction.

H.   **Home health considerations**
     1.   Teach the client and family communication techniques.
     2.   Teach the client's family how to provide care for the client.
     3.   Teach the client and family methods which will ensure safety.

XI.   **Brain tumors**

A.   **Description: An intracranial neoplasm either of primary or secondary origin.**
     1.   Primary lesions: tumors originating within the brain such as a gliomas, meningiomas, neurinomas or adenomas.
     2.   Secondary lesions: tumors resulting from a metastasizing neoplasm originating elsewhere in the body.

B.   **Etiology and incidence**
     1.   Etiology of primary tumors is unknown.
     2.   Etiology of secondary tumors may be due to exposure to carcinogens.

C.   **Pathophysiology**
     1.   Tumors apply pressure to brain tissue causing ischemia and necrosis to effected areas.

     2.   **Management is aimed at relieving pressure, when possible, and preventing complications associated with brain tumors.**

D.   Assessment
  1.   A complete neurologic examination should be completed.
       a.   Assess LOC.
       b.   Assess for seizures, nausea, and vomiting.
       c.   Assess characteristics of headache.
       d.   Assess for signs and symptoms of increased ICP.
  2.   Prepare patient for CT scan or MRI to locate tumor.

  3.   **If the tumor is located in cerebral area, assess for hemiplegia, gait disturbances, impaired judgment, visual disturbances, and personality changes.**
  4.   If the tumor is in the thalamus or is a sellar tumor, assess for diabetes insipidus.
  5.   If the tumor is located in the brain stem, assess for headache on rising.

E.   Nursing diagnoses
  1.   Altered Tissue Perfusion: Intracranial
  2.   Anxiety
  3.   Impaired Verbal Communication
  4.   Decreased Adaptive Capacity: Intracranial
  5.   Altered Thought Processes
  6.   Impaired Physical Mobility

F.   Planning and implementation
  1.   Prepare the client for a craniotomy by providing education.
  2.   Provide reassurance to client and family.
  3.   Prepare family for behavior changes.
  4.   Provide client safety measures.
  5.   Provide quiet environment.
  6.   Assist with activities of daily living.
  7.   Provide adequate nutrition.
  8.   Provide client and family with a means to communicate.
  9.   Assess for signs of increased ICP.
  10. Decrease ICP.
  11. Prepare client and family for potential change in body image.
  12. Permit client to verbalize feelings.
  13. Teach client stress reduction techniques.
  14. Provide adequate pain management.
  15. Administer medications, as ordered, to include osmotic diuretics, corticosteroids, narcotics, sedatives, and chemotherapeutic medications.
  16. Ensure cleanliness of craniotomy incision site.
  17. Be aware of potential complications:
       a.   Infection
       b.   Seizure
       c.   Change in mental status

G.   Evaluation
  1.   The client will not have an increase in ICP.
  2.   The client will remain free of injury.
  3.   The client will remain free of infection.
  4.   The client will be able to perform activities of daily living.

H.   Home health considerations

1. Foster communication between client and family.
2. Encourage client to maintain activity level.
3. Instruct family on importance of notifying health care provider of mental status changes.
4. Instruct family on safety precautions.

XII. **Status epilepticus**

- **A.** Description: abnormal electrical activity in the brain that interferes with normal functioning. This electrical activity produces life threatening seizures of a tonic–clonic nature. Tonic–clonic seizures are continuous.
- **B.** Etiology and incidence: The causes of status epilepticus can result from tumor, electrolyte imbalance, alcohol withdrawal, abrupt discontinuance of anticonvulsants, brain abscess or infection, hypoglycemia, head trauma, cerebral edema or disease.
- **C.** Pathophysiology

     1. During seizure activity, the brain and other organs are deprived of oxygen due to vasoconstriction. Brain tissue is lost with each episode, and replaced with scar tissue.

     2. Management is aimed at stopping the current seizure, providing safety during seizure activity, and preventing further seizure activity.

- **D.** Assessment
    1. Take an accurate history to assess for contributing factors.
    2. Assess characteristics of seizure activities.
    3. Assess electrolyte status.
    4. Assess for hypoglycemia as increased seizure activity increases glucose utilization.

- **E.** Nursing diagnoses
    1. Risk for Injury
    2. Reflex Incontinence
    3. Ineffective Individual Coping
    4. Bowel Incontinence
    5. Anxiety
    6. Ineffective Airway Clearance

- **F.** Planning and implementation
    1. Assess respiratory status.
    2. Employ methods to stop or control seizure activity.
    3. Maintain oxygenation.
    4. Provide for client safety especially avoiding head injury.
        a. Place client on floor if not in bed.

         b. **Do not insert objects into client's mouth.**
    5. It is essential to maintain adequate calories during seizure activity via IV route due to increased glucose needs.
    6. Administer medications as ordered:

         a. **Diazepam (Valium): administer diazepam to achieve a plasma level of 0.5 μg/mL. Valium increases neurotransmitter availability in an attempt to decrease seizures. The major side effect is respiratory depression.**

m b.   **Phenytoin (Dilantin): administer dilantin to achieve a plasma level of 10–20 µg/dL. Intravenous lines must be flushed with normal saline only to prevent crystallization Dilantin precipitates when in contact with glucose. Dilantin blocks neurotransmitters.**

m c.   **The major side effect of dilantin is cardiac dysrhythmia.**

    d.   Phenobarbital: administer to achieve plasma level of 20–40 µg/dL. Phenobarbital increases the seizure threshold. Side effects include cardiovascular and respiratory depression.

    e.   Carbamazepine (Tegretol), primidone (Mysoline), divalproex (Depakote), and clonazepam (Klonopin) are other commonly used anti-convulsants.

    f.   All medications given to control seizures cause drowsiness.

m 7.   **Clients are sometimes given barbiturates to induce coma to stop seizure activity or more importantly decrease metabolic needs.**

    8.   Be aware of potential complications:
        a.   Respiratory depression
        b.   Injury

G.   Home health considerations
    1.   Ensure prevention of seizures through medication compliance.
    2.   Seek appropriate treatment for any changes in seizure activity.
    3.   Refer to appropriate resources.
    4.   Teach family safety measures.
    5.   Instruct client on importance of wearing a medical alert bracelet.
    6.   Refer family to the Epilepsy Foundation of America.
    7.   Assist the family to identify coping measures.

XIII.   Encephalitis

A.   Description: Encephalitis is an inflammation of the brain which is caused by a virus, bacteria, fungus, or parasite.

B.   Etiology and incidence
    1.   Encephalitis may occur as a complication of other diseases, such as measles, mumps, and chicken pox.
    2.   Ingestion of toxic substances, including carbon monoxide, have been found to cause encephalitis.

C.   Pathophysiology
    1.   Pathophysiology varies with causative factors.

    2.   **Management is aimed at supporting body functions during acute phase and preventing complications.**

D.   Assessment
    1.   Symptoms are based on the specific site of invasion and the causative agent.
    2.   General findings include headache, fever, chills, vomiting, and alterations in LOC.
    3.   Later findings include convulsions, stupor, and signs of meningeal irritation, including nuchal rigidity.

E.   Planning and implementation
    1.   Monitor vital signs and neuro checks frequently.
    2.   Provide nursing measures for increased ICP, seizures, hyperthermia if they occur.

3. Assess fluid balance to assure optimal hydration status.
4. Maintain patent airway.
5. Protect the client from injury.
6. Assess and control pain.

 7. **Provide a quiet environment and stimulate client only as needed to decrease CNS irritation.**
8. Maintain skin integrity by providing appropriate skin care and adhering to a written turning schedule.
9. Prevent complications of immobility.

F. **Evaluation**
1. The client's vital signs and neurologic checks remain stable.
2. The client's optimal fluid balance is achieved.
3. The client's airway is patent and oxygenation is adequate.
4. The client is maintained in a quiet environment.
5. The client's skin remains intact.
6. The client retains full ROM.

XIV. Brain herniation

A. **Description: Protrusion of the brain from one compartment to another due to increased ICP.**
1. Uncal herniation, also called lateral transtentorial herniation, involves shifts in structures located above the tentorium.
2. Posterior fossa herniations involves an infratentorial shift and involves the area below the tentorium which includes the cerebellum and brain stem.

B. **Etiology**
1. **When the cerebral edema or a mass occurs in the brain, the pressure exerted by the lesion is not evenly distributed resulting in shifting or herniation of the brain from one compartment of high pressure to one of lesser pressure.**
2. As a result of these shifting structures there is pressure or traction on some structures, which is evidenced by malfunction of that area of cerebral tissue.

C. **Pathophysiology**
1. Herniation occurs when ICP rises to the extent that movement of brain tissue from one area to another occurs in an attempt to decrease ICP.
2. Brain compression results in distortion of other brain structures and vascular compromise.
3. Obstruction of CSF movement can also occur.
4. This results in brain damage and eventual death.

D. **Assessment**
1. Supratentorial or uncal herniation:
   a. Results from a laterally expanding mass lesion producing a shift which causes a compromise of the ipsilateral third cranial nerve and the ipsilateral posterior cerebral artery.
   b. This produces characteristic signs and symptoms:
      ► Decreased LOC
      ► Ptosis with fixed dilated pupil
      ► Outwardly downward-directed eyeball that becomes bilateral

       ► Contralateral hemiparasis

       ► Ipsilateral third nerve palsy

       ► Possible Cushing's response and cardiovascular decompensation causing ischemia to the medulla oblongata's vasomotor center

       ► Flexor posturing

       ► Extensor posturing

       ► Flaccidity

        ► **Frequent assessments help the health care team intervene early and appropriately.**

  2. Infratentorial herniation

    a. Lesions of the infratentorial compartment contributing to herniation are much less frequent that those involving the supratentorial region.

     b. **An expanding lesion creates increased pressure on selected structures which interferes with normal function of the involved tissue and causes edema, ischemia, infarction, and neurosis.**

    c. If the process is not reversed expansion causes eventual increasing pressure on the brain stem structures, particularly the medulla which contain centers for vital functions.

    d. The result is death from respiratory and cardiac arrest.

    e. Be aware of the following signs and symptoms:

        ► **Abnormal respiratory patterns, depending on the area involved**

       ► Pupillary changes: midposition and fixed in the midbrain area, small and fixed in the pontine area

       ► Loss of upward gaze

       ► Hemiparesis and hemiplegia

       ► Decortication or decerebration, which may progress to flaccidity in medullary injury

       ► Cranial nerve disfunction, such as trigeminal or facial paresis with pontine injury

       ► Coma

E. **Nursing diagnoses**

  1. Fluid Volume Excess

  2. Tissue Perfusion: Cerebral

  3. Pain

  4. Risk for Injury

  5. Impaired Physical Mobility

  6. Social Isolation

  7. Decreased Adaptive Capacity: Intracranial

  8. Altered Role Performance

F. **Planning and implementation**

   1. **Be aware that the goal is to spare the brain from injury that will result in permanent disability, reduced quality of life, and the possibility of death.**

2. **Perform neurologic checks at least every hour, more frequently when indicated by changes.**
3. Continually monitor vital signs.
4. Apply cooling blanket as ordered for hyperthermia, warming blanket for hypothermia.
5. Monitor respiratory rate and pattern.
6. Provide respiratory support as necessary.
7. Administer medications as ordered and appropriate:
    a. Osmotic diuretics are given to draw water from the extracellular space of the edematous cerebral tissue into the plasma.
    b. Antihypertensives may be ordered for hypertension.
8. Monitor ICP when applicable.
9. Maintain aseptic technique when doing invasive line/site care.
10. Perform body changes as tolerated by ICP.
11. Provide pain relief if applicable.

G. **Evaluation**
1. The patient will maintain optimal body functioning.
2. The patient will remain free of nosocomial infection.

XV. Brain death

A. **Description: A state of irreversible loss of both cortical and brain stem activity. The criteria for brain death is highly controversial. Diagnosis of brain death is based on the following criteria:**
1. **Absence of brain stem reflexes**
2. **Absence of cortical activity**
3. **Demonstration that this state is irreversible**

B. **Brain death protocol**
1. Absence of brain stem reflexes
    a. The patient is pre-oxygenated for 5 minutes with 100% oxygen and then disconnected from the ventilator.
    b. The patient receives 100% oxygen via the ETT at 8–12 L/min.
    c. The PCO_2 is allowed to rise to 55–60 mm Hg which should trigger the respiratory drive.
    d. The chest is observed and palpated for spontaneous respirations for 10 minutes.
    e. The patient is reconnected to the ventilator.
    f. If the patient takes even one spontaneous breath in that 10 minutes, he or she is not considered brain dead.
2. Absence of cortical activity as evidenced by a flat EEG in a comatose patient who is unresponsive to painful stimuli
3. State of irreversibility
    a. A neurologic diagnosis adequate to produce brain death must be present.
    b. A neurologic examination demonstrating the absence of brain stem function must be done. This exam must be reproducible.

    c. **Unusual factors which may account for loss of neurologic function must be absent, including: drug overdose, drug toxicity, hypothermia, shock, and a local disease involving the eyes or ears.**
    d. A period of 24 hours without clinical neurologic change must elapse.

XVI. Organ donation

A. **Legal aspects: varies as to physician's responsibility to request organ donation**

B. **Institutional policies:**
   1. Guidelines for request of tissue/organ donation by staff
   2. Identification of a regional agency to facilitate organ/tissue donation:
   3. Retrieval and matching process which validates donor eligibility
   4. Direction on how to obtain signed consents
   5. Determination of organs to be donated
   6. Pre-retrieval organ viability interventions

C. **Conflict of interest**
   1. The physician declaring death is protected from potential conflict of interest by:
      a. not being part of the transplant team
      b. not being a family member
      c. not having malpractice charges pending
      d. not having any special interest in the declaration of death

D. **Donor selection**
   1. The candidate must experience brain death from brain damage in a previously healthy person.
   2. Age is dependent on organ to be donated. There is no age limit for some organs.
   3. The donor must be free from communicable and metastatic diseases.
   4. The donor must have a satisfactory physical exam.

E. **Criteria for non-acceptance**
   1. **These are general guidelines only. Organ retrieval centers should be notified of all impending deaths.**
   2. Prolonged ischemia due to profound hypotension or asystole
   3. Trauma or disease of the potentially transplantable organs
   4. Selected malignant diseases
   5. History of IV drug use

F. **Organ retrieval process**
   1. ICU nurse, nurse manager, or physician identifies potential donor.
   2. Regional agency is notified (1-800-KIDNEY-1).
   3. Evaluation of donor suitability occurs.
   4. Discussion with family and physicians occurs and consents are obtained.
   5. Clearance from medical examiner and/or district attorney is sometimes needed.
   6. Continued observation/maintenance of donor by ICU nurse must occur.
   7. Physician pronounces patient dead.
   8. Transplant nurse ensures logistical arrangements for retrieval:
      a. Surgical team
      b. Site and time scheduling
   9. Notification of specialty areas must take place:
      a. Eye bank
      b. Skin bank

10. Transplant team participates in:
    a. retrieval surgery
    b. perfusion and preservation of donor organs
    c. transportation, tissue typing of donor organs
    d. identification of recipients
    e. transplantation of organs.

 11. **It is the responsibility of the ICU nurse to care for the patient and family as he or she would any other dying patient. The nurse from the organ donation agency may offer suggestions to the attending physician, who may be unfamiliar with organ donation, on interventions to maintain adequate perfusion to all organs while awaiting transplantation. After offering support to the family of the patient, organ perfusion is a priority.**

Bibliography

Bayley, E.W., & Turcke, S.A. (1992). *A comprehensive curriculum for trauma nursing.* Boston: Jones and Bartlett.

Bruder, N., Duman, J.C., & Francois, G. (1991). Evolution of energy expenditure and nitrogen excretion in severe head injured patients. *Crit Care Med* 19, 43–48.

Chin, D.E., & Kearns, P. (1991). Nutrition in the spinal injured patient. *Nutr Clin Pract* 6, 213–222.

Feldman Z., Narayan R.D., & Robertson, C.S. (1992). Secondary insults associated with closed head injury. *Contemp Neurosurg* 14, 1–8.

Kinney, M., Packa, D., & Dunbar, S. (1993). *AACN's clinical reference for critical-care nursing.* St. Louis: Mosby.

Marie, C., & Bralet, J. (1991). Blood glucose level and morphological brain damage following cerebral ischemia. *Cerebrovasc Brain Met Rev* 3, 29–38.

Marino, P.L. (1991). *The ICU book.* Malvern, PA: Lea & Febiger.

North American Nursing Diagnosis Association (NANDA). (1996). *Nursing diagnoses; definitions & classification 1997–1998.* Philadelphia: Author.

Ott, L., Young, B., & Phillips, R. (1991). Altered gastric emptying in the head injured patient: Relationship to feeding intolerance. *J Neurosurg* 74, 738–742.

Urden, L., Davie, J., & Thelan, L. (1992). *Essentials of critical care nursing.* St. Louis: Mosby.

Young, B., Ott, L., & Phillips, R. (1991). Metabolic management of the patient with head injury. *Neurosurg Clin North Am* 2, 301–320.

Zaloga, G.P. (1994). *Nutrition in critical care.* St. Louis: Mosby.

STUDY QUESTIONS

1. A client is admitted to the intensive care unit with a diagnosis of Status Epilepticus. The nurse knows that this is a life-threatening emergency that places the client at risk for which one of the following complications?
   a. head injury
   b. pneumonia
   c. spinal shock
   d. diabetes mellitus

2. In caring for a client with increasing ICP, which one of the following nursing interventions will decrease the ICP?
   a. immobilizing the client's head
   b. monitoring vital signs every 5 minutes
   c. raising the head of the bed
   d. limiting the client's caloric intake

3. The nurse should include which of the following when teaching the client about a computed tomography (CT) scan of the brain?
   a. "You will receive general anesthesia before the test."
   b. "During the test you will be asked to reposition yourself every 5 minutes."
   c. "The test will take about 5 minutes."
   d. "During the test you may have a metallic taste in your mouth when the dye is administered."

4. The nurse observes a slight facial tic in a client. The nurse should perform an assessment of which of the following cranial nerves?
   a. CN I
   b. CN VI
   c. CN VII
   d. CN XII

5. During a report, the nurse is told that a client has suffered a CVA in the left hemisphere of the brain. The nurse should expect that the client will have:
   a. left hemiplegia
   b. left hemianopia
   c. deviation of the eyes to the right
   d. aphasia

6. The nurse knows that all of the following define nursing implications for the client on anticonvulsants except:
   a. instructing the client that anticonvulsants may cause drowsiness
   b. teaching the client that to stop anticonvulsants abruptly may cause seizure activity
   c. instructing the client that atropine is the antidote in the event of overdosage
   d. informing the client that gum irritations are a side effect of the medication

7. The nurse should plan for which of the following, post-craniotomy?
   a. providing for diversional activity
   b. increasing ICP
   c. waking the client every 5 to 10 minutes
   d. preventing infection

8. A chronic subdural hematoma occurs:
   a. from bleeding between the dura mater and the arachnoid
   b. from bleeding in the vertebral artery
   c. rapidly with no change in the LOC
   d. from a space-occupying lesion

9. The family's caring for a client suffering from an intracranial tumor should be instructed by the nurse about:
   a. preventing infection
   b. reducing bleeding by direct pressure
   c. possible behavioral and personality changes
   d. increasing the LOC

10. Nursing care of the client with encephalitis includes all of the following except:
    a. decreasing fever through the use of an automatic cooling blanket
    b. replacing fluid and electrolyte imbalances
    c. waking the client hourly
    d. administering anticonvulsants as needed

11. The initial nursing goal for a client with an acute head injury is:
   a. to restore motor functioning
   b. to relieve head pain
   c. to maintain cerebral perfusion
   d. to assist the client to overcome self-esteem disturbances

12. The nurse instructs the clients on the signs and symptoms of post-concussion syndrome. The symptoms include all of the following except:
   a. headache
   b. infection
   c. lethargy
   d. personality changes

13. The nurse understands that the patient must be assessed for the presence of metal for which of the following neurologic diagnostic tests?
   a. lumbar puncture
   b. myelogram
   c. electromyogram
   d. magnetic resonance imaging

14. The nurse is caring for a client in the ICU with an ICP monitoring system. While providing hygiene measures for the client, the nurse observes that the ICP reading is 18 mm Hg. The *first* action that the nurse should take is to:
   a. raise the head of the bed to a 45-degree angle
   b. cease stimulating the client
   c. lower the head of the bed to a 10-degree angle
   d. continue with the hygiene measures, as the pressure reading is within normal limits

15. The nurse is assessing a client with a subarachnoid hemorrhage. Which of the following findings would the nurse most likely observe?
   a. constricted pupil on the ipsilateral side
   b. quadriplegia
   c. aphasia
   d. nuchal rigidity

16. When assessing a client with astereognosis, the nurse would expect to find that the client:
   a. cannot differentiate familiar objects by touch

   b. can only see objects with one eye
   c. cannot perceive sensation on the upper part of the body
   d. has decreased hair growth on the lower extremities

17. Subdural hematoma is:
   a. a collection of blood between the skull and the outer layer of the dura
   b. a bruising of the brain (without tearing)
   c. a collection of blood within the cerebral tissue
   d. usually caused by a tear in the bridging veins between the brain and the dura

18. Which of the following results in an increase in ICP?
   a. increased metabolic activity
   b. neutral head position at 30 degrees
   c. PaO2 of 80 mm Hg
   d. CO_2 retention

19. Which of the following is not a major risk factor for CVA?
   a. hypertension
   b. cardiac impairment
   c. diabetes mellitus
   d. obesity

20. Normal ICP can be defined as an ICP reading of:
   a. up to 10 mm Hg
   b. up to 20 mm Hg
   c. up to 25 mm Hg
   d. up to 30 mm Hg

21. What is the most important indicator of neurologic functioning?
   a. neuromuscular reflexes
   b. pupillary function
   c. LOC
   d. vital signs

22. When using the Glasgow Coma Scale to assess the client's neurologic status, which of the following statements is true?
   a. A Glasgow score of 10 is the highest possible score.
   b. Each institution establishes a normal score for their clients.
   c. A Glasgow score of 7 or less usually indicates coma.
   d. Glasgow score is the baseline tool to be used for a complete neurologic assessment.

ANSWER KEY

1. **Correct Response: a**
   Status epilepticus is a life-threatening situation consisting of violent seizures which could injure the clients head during the muscle contractions.
   b. Pneumonia is not an immediate complication. Pneumonia would be possible only if aspiration occurred.
   c. Spinal shock is a complication of a spinal cord injury.
   d. Diabetes mellitus is a result of pancreatic dysfunction.
   Comprehension/Physiologic/Assessment

2. **Correct response: c**
   Raising the head of the bed will decrease ICP by decreasing venous resistance.
   a. While decreasing extreme neck flexion is important for decreasing ICP, head immobilization is not necessary.
   b. Hourly vital signs and neurologic assessment are important for the care of the client but will not decrease ICP.
   d. Limiting caloric intake will not decrease ICP and may interfere metabolic processes.
   Analysis/Implementation/Physiologic

3. **Correct response: d**
   A computer tomography (CT) scan may be performed with contrast media. The client should be instructed that a metallic taste is a side effect of the dye.
   a. General anesthesia is not necessary for a CT scan. Mild sedation is sometimes given to reduce severe anxiety or in the case of the claustrophobic client.
   b. During a CT scan it is vital that the client remain absolutely still.
   c. The average length of time for the completion of an uncomplicated CT scan is 30–60 minutes.
   Application/Implementation/Safe care

4. **Correct response: c**
   The seventh cranial nerve innervates the facial nerves.

   a. CN I is the olfactory nerve.
   b. CN VI is the abducens. It controls eye movement and pupil size.
   d. CN XII is the hypoglossal. It controls tongue movement.
   Knowledge/Physiologic/Assessment

5. **Correct response: d**
   Aphasia is a common side effect of left CVA because this hemisphere is responsible for speech.
   a. Left hemianopia implies a right hemisphere injury.
   b. Left hemianopia means that a client is unable to see the left visual field.
   c. In a left CVA, the eyes would deviate to the right.
   Knowledge/Physiologic/Assessment

6. **Correct response: c**
   Atropine is not given to the client on discharge on anticonvulsant therapy. The client is instructed to comply with the therapy regiment.
   a. Anticonvulsants may cause drowsiness and should be instructed not to drive or operate machinery.
   b. It is imperative that clients adhere to medication regimen. Abrupt changes in medication could cause seizure.
   d. Anticonvulsants may cause gingival hyperplasia.
   Application/Physiologic/Implementation

7. **Correct response: d**
   A craniotomy involves a surgical opening in the cranial cavity and requires strict asepsis.
   a. A client post-craniotomy is usually too sick for excessive activity. Activity may increase ICP.
   b. Every effort is made to decrease ICP post-craniotomy.
   c. Hourly neurologic assessments are performed once the client stabilizes.
   Comprehension/Physiologic/Planning

8. **Correct response: a**
   A subdural hematoma is the result of bleeding between the dura mater and the arachnoid.

b. Bleeding from a vertebral artery would produce ischemia to vital centers of the brain.

c. A chronic subdural hematoma occurs slowly with event deterioration in the LOC.

d. A space-occupying lesion describes an intracranial tumor.

Knowledge/Physiologic/Assessment

9. *Correct response: c*
Intracranial tumors in the frontal lobe cause behavior and personality changes.

a. Unless surgery has been performed to evacuate the tumor then the client is not at risk for infection.

b. Intracranial tumors produce no external bleeding.

d. There are no interventions to increase the LOC.

Comprehension/Physiologic/Implementation

10. *Correct response: c*
Waking the client hourly would not be consistent with providing a restful environment for the client.

a. Cooling blankets are effective in decreasing body temperature.

b. Encephalitis produces fever which can cause dehydration, therefore adequate fluid replacement is necessary.

d. Clients with meningitis are at high risk for seizures, therefore anticonvulsants may be necessary.

Comprehension/Physiologic/Intervention

11. *Correct response: c*
Cerebral perfusion is crucial to all of life functions.

a. Restoring motor functioning is a tertiary intervention.

b. It is not president to administer narcotics to head injured clients as this may decrease the neurologic functioning.

d. Overcoming self-esteem disturbances is not an initial nursing goal in an acute head injury.

Application/Safe care/Planning

12. *Correct response: b*
Infection is not a sign of post-concussion syndrome.

a. Post-concussion syndrome is characterized by headache, lethargy, and personality changes.

c. Post-concussion syndrome is characterized by headache, lethargy and personality changes.

d. Post-concussion syndrome is characterized by headache, lethargy and personality changes.

Knowledge/Physiologic/Implementation

13. *Correct response: d*
Due to the magnetics in the AARI machine no metal may be introduced in the direction of the machine.

a. A lumbar puncture involves a spinal needle placed in the L4 and L5 subarachnoid space for CSF withdrawal.

b. A myelogram is an x-ray of the spinal cord after the injection of dye into the subarachnoid space.

c. An electromyelogram records brain activity to evaluate cerebral functioning.

Knowledge/Safe care/Assessment

14. *Correct response: b*
a, b, c. This pressure is moderately high; if stimulation is stopped the pressure may resume normal limits.

d. Continuing stimulation would elevate the pressure to dangerous limits.

Application/Physiologic/Implementation

15. *Correct response: d*
The symptoms associated with a subarachnoid hemorrhage include nuchal rigidity, headache, decreased LOC, and dilated ipsilateral pupil.

a. The pupil would most likely be dilated.

b. Quadriplegia is seen with spinal cord injuries.

c. Aphasia is not a common finding with a subarachnoid bleed.

Knowledge/Physiologic/Assessment

16. *Correct response: a*

    a. and **c.** Astereognosis is the inability to differentiate familiar objects by touch.

    b. Hemianopia is the disability to see objects with only one eye.

    d. PVD causes decreased hair growth on the lower extremities.

Knowledge/Physiologic/Assessment

17. *Correct response: d*

Common cause of a subdural hematoma is a tear in the bridging veins between the brain and the dura.

    a. Epidural hematoma is a collection of blood between the skull and the outer layer of the dura.

    b. A contusion is a bruising of the brain (without tearing).

    c. A hematoma is a collection of bleed within the cerebral tissue.

Knowledge/Physiologic/NA

18. *Correct response: d*

Carbon dioxide retention causes vasodilation with a subsequent increase in intracranial volume. This increased volume serves to increase the ICP.

    a, b, c. None of these increases ICP.

Comprehension/Physiologic/Assessment

19. *Correct response: d*

The risk factors for CVA stem from conditions that lead to the development of atherosclerosis.

Major risks include cardiac dysfunctions, hypertension, and diabetes mellitus.

Knowledge/Health promotion/Assessment

20. *Correct response: a*

The normal ICP reading is <10 mm Hg.

    b. 15–20 mm Hg is considered moderately high.

    c, d. >20 mm Hg is severely elevated.

Knowledge/Physiologic/Assessment

21. *Correct response: c*

Level of consciousness directly reflects level of neurologic functioning.

    a, b, d. May all be affected by dysfunctions not related to the neurologic system.

Comprehension/Physiologic/Evaluation

22. *Correct response: c*

A score of 7 or less indicates coma.

    a. The best possible score on the Glasgow coma scale is 15 and the lowest is 3.

    b. The Glasgow coma scale is a universal tool.

    d. The Glasgow coma scale measures LOC and is not a complete neurologic assessment tool.

Comprehension/Physiologic/Assessment

The Spinal Cord

I.   Anatomy and physiology
A.   Structure (Fig. 3-1)
1.   The vertebral column is composed of 33 vertebrae.
2.   Cervical (7) vertebrae support the head and neck muscles.
3.   The cervical vertebrae are the smallest of all vertebrae.
4.   Thoracic (12) vertebrae support the chest muscles.
5.   Lumbar (5) vertebrae support the back muscles.
6.   Sacral (5 fused) vertebral support the lower back muscles.
7.   Coccygeal (4 fused) vertebrae support the lower back muscles.
8.   The vertebrae are separated by disks. A disk has a covering, called an annulus, and the inner core, called the nucleus pulposus. Disks are the shock absorbers of the spine.
9.   The vertebrae protect the spinal cord.
10.   The vertebrae receives a vascular supply through the radicular, the posterior and anterior spinal arteries.
11.   The spinal cord contains cerebrospinal fluid (CSF) in the subarachnoid space and is covered by the meninges.
    a.   The spinal cord is composed of gray and white matter.
    b.   The descending tracts of the spinal cord are the corticospinal, ventral corticospinal, reticulospinal, and vestibulospinal.
    c.   The ascending tracts include the lateral and ventral spinothalamic and posterior column.

B.   Function

1.   **The overall function of the vertebral column is to provide support and protect the spinal cord.**
2.   The ascending and descending tracts transmit impulse for motor and sensory information.

II.   Peripheral nervous system
A.   Structure
1.   The peripheral nervous system is composed of the cranial nerves (see Chapter 2), as well as the spinal nerves.
2.   There are 31 pairs of spinal nerves that contain sensory, motor, and autonomic fibers.
3.   There are two types of motor fibers:
    a.   Somatic
    b.   Autonomic
4.   Autonomic fibers perform two functions when innervating smooth muscles and glands
    a.   Sympathetic (acceleration functions)
    b.   Parasympathetic (deceleration functions)

B.   Function

1.   **The spinal nerves transmit impulses from sensory and motor fibers**
2.   The motor fibers control skeletal muscle and glands

III.   Overview of spinal cord disorders
A.   Assessment (Table 3-1)
1.   Loss of muscle function is determined according to the level of spinal cord injury (SCI).
    a.   Cervical injury results in quadriplegia
    b.   Thoracic, lumbar, and sacral injury result in varying levels of paraplegia

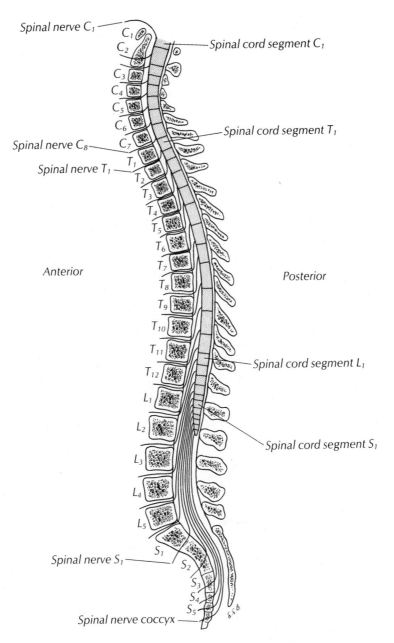

Spinal nerve C₁

C₁
C₂
C₃
C₄
C₅
C₆
C₇

Spinal cord segment C₁

Spinal cord segment T₁

Spinal nerve C₈

Spinal nerve T₁

T₁
T₂
T₃
T₄
T₅
T₆
T₇
T₈
T₉
T₁₀
T₁₁
T₁₂

Anterior

Posterior

L₁
L₂
L₃
L₄
L₅

Spinal cord segment L₁

Spinal cord segment S₁

Spinal nerve S₁

S₁
S₂
S₃
S₄
S₅

Spinal nerve coccyx

FIGURE 3-1.
The spinal cord, lateral view.

TABLE 3-1.
Consequences Related to Location of Spinal Cord Injury

LOCATION OF INJURY	CONSEQUENCES
C1–C4	Completely dependent for ADLs and ventilator for respiratory support; some sensory loss of the face and ears
C5	Dependent for ADLs; power wheelchair; brace for self-feeding; some respiratory distress
C6	Functional triceps; independent with hygiene; light housework; may drive with hand controls; remaining respiratory distress due to intestinal paralysis
C7–C8	Independent living
T1–T12	Independent living
L1–L5	Independent living
S1–S5	Independent living

2. **A complete lesion will cause the loss of all sensation and voluntary muscle control on both sides of the body below the level of injury.**
3. **An incomplete lesion causes some motor loss below the level of injury accompanied by spotty sensory loss.**
4. Some incomplete lesions cause specific patterns of dysfunction.
5. Mini neurologic exam:
    a. Estimate cord involvement.

 b. **Perform a baseline assessment so that future neurologic examinations can be compared to previous findings.**
    c. Evaluate for possible head injury.
    d. Evaluate adequacy of respiratory function.
    e. Focus on determining presence or absence of diminished sensory motor reflex systems function.
    f. Evaluate vital signs.
    g. Check for hypotension, bradycardia, and lowered body temperature.
B. Diagnostic testing
    1. Roentgenograms: anterior-posterior-lateral x-rays to assess for vertebral fracture.
    2. A computed tomography (CT) scan can assess for evidence of spinal cord edema.

3. Magnetic resonance imaging (MRI) is used to help determine degree and location of SCI and vertebral compression.
4. A lumbar puncture is used to ascertain the presence or absence of a spinal block.
5. A myelogram can be used to establish the presence of a spinal block.
6. Laboratory tests:
   a. Serum chemistry
   b. Hyper- or hypoglycemia
   c. Electrolyte imbalance
   d. Possibly decreased hemoglobin and hematocrit

C. Nutrition
1. The metabolic response to SCI has not been studied as extensively as head injury.
2. Some of the metabolic changes studied in this patient population include negative nitrogen balance, hypoalbuminemia, mineral alteration, and decreased energy expenditure.
3. Weight loss can also occur secondary to muscle loss and changes in body composition.
4. Considerations for medical nutrition therapy:
   a. The overall goal is to increase the nutrient intake to achieve caloric balance and meet intake needs.
   b. Increased urinary nitrogen loss can occur. The goal is to prevent nitrogen loss by providing nutrients and physical therapy.
   c. Altered mineral levels can be compensated for by providing nutrient supplementation and possible fluid restriction.

D. Psychosocial implications
1. Changes in body image/perception
2. Changes in physical mobility
3. Alterations in self care

E. Commonly used medications
1. Anti-anxiety agents
2. Corticosteroids to control cord edema: dexamethasone 5–10 mg qid PO
3. Anticoagulants: heparin 5000–7000 U SQ every 12 hours
4. Antihypertensives
   a. Diazoxide 1–3 mg/kg up to 150 mg IV repeated at intervals of 5–15 minutes until blood pressure is reduced
   b. Hydralazine 20 mg slow IV push
5. Muscle relaxants
   a. Baclofen 15–80 mg PO daily in divided doses
   b. Dantrolene 25 mg tid to 200 mg qid
6. Anti-infective agents: Sulfasoxazole 2–4 g initially, then 4–8 g daily in divided doses
7. Laxatives: Dulcolax rectal suppository
8. Antacids: Magnesium hydroxide and aluminum hydroxide 20 mL PO q4 hours

IV. Spinal cord injuries
A. Description: trauma resulting in damage to the spinal cord
1. Complete lesion: total loss of motor and sensory function below level of injury. Regardless of mechanism of injury, result is complete transection of spinal cord and its pathways.

    2.   Incomplete lesion: mixed loss of voluntary motor and sensation below lesion.

    3.   Brown–Sequard syndrome: transverse hemisection of cord. Injury to one side produces a loss of voluntary motor on that side with accompanying loss of pain and temperature sensation on the opposite side. The side of the body with best motor control has little or no sensation while the side with sensation has little or no motor control.

    4.   Central cord syndrome: contusion/compression, and/or hemorrhage on gray matter of cord. Associated with hyperextension/flexion injury. Produces motor and sensory deficit more pronounced in the upper extremities than in lower.

    5.   Anterior cord syndrome: associated with injury to anterior gray horn cells (motor), spino-thalmic track (pain), or cortico-spinal track (temperature). Loss of motor function, pain and temperature sensation below level of injury. Other sensations (touch, pressure, vibration) remain intact. Often caused by flexion injury or acute herniation or intravertebral disk.

    6.   Posterior cord syndrome: associated with cervical hypertension. Loss of light touch and proprioception below the level of injury.

B.   **Etiology**

    1.   Falls

    2.   Sports injuries

    3.   Motor vehicle accidents

    4.   Gunshot wounds

    5.   Diving accidents

    6.   Alcohol abuse (often a contributing factor)

C.   **Pathophysiology**

    1.   Spinal cord injury can come from stresses of flexion, extension, and rotation or compression.

    2.   Edema surrounding the injury causes pressure, resulting in diminished blood flow to area.

    3.   Nerves in the injured area may become ischemic and die.

    4.   Microhemorrhages in the gray matter within minutes of the injury.

    5.   Severe drop in blood pressure to the area, resulting in ischemia.

    6.   Within 4 hours the area is infarcted, followed by microhemorrhage and edema of the white area.

    7.   Hypoxia, ischemia, and elevated levels of norepinephrine, serotonin, and histamine along with a decrease in the dopamine levels are present at the site of the injury.

    8.   Permanent neurologic deficit results.

D.   **Assessment findings according to location (Table 3-2)**

    1.   Injury in the cervical area is caused by a violent impact to the back of the head, which can lead to shearing of ligaments and result in anterior dislocation. Findings can range from minimal to devastating due to damage of the nerves that innervate the diaphragm leading to respiratory paralysis.

    2.   Injury in the thoracic area is caused by a downward slamming force resulting in wedging and possible compression of the vertebrate. Cord damage may cause paraplegia but won't affect vital functions.

    3.   Injury of the lumbar area can cause lower limb paralysis.

    4.   Injury of the sacral area can cause bowel and bladder dysfunction.

TABLE 3-2.
Assessment Findings According to the Location of Spinal Cord Injury

LOCATION	ASSESSMENT
C1–C4	Diaphragm and intercostal muscles paralyzed No voluntary movement below the injury Sensory loss includes: occipital region, ear, and some areas of the face
C5	Initially the diaphragm is impaired due to edema Abdominal reflexes absent Upper extremities outwardly rotated and the shoulders raised Sensation present in the neck
C6	Initially the diaphragm is impaired due to edema Abdominal reflexes absent Shoulders elevated, arms abducted, and forearms flexed Sensation present in the lateral aspect of the arms and the dorsolateral aspect of the forearms
C7	Diaphragm and accessory muscles function Intercostal and abdominal muscles effected Shoulders elevated, arms abducted, and forearms flexed
C8	Normal upper body positioning (sitting upright is possible) Fingers appear in a clawed position Postural hypotension occurs if the patient is raised to a sitting position too quickly
T1–T5	Diaphragmatic breathing possible (the lower the injury, the better the inspiratory effort) Postural hypotension still a concern Sensory loss includes: touch, temperature, and pain

T6–T12	Spastic paralysis of the lower extremities
	Abdominal reflexes present at the T12 level and minimal at the T6 level
	Sensory loss secondary to area of lesion:
	    T2—upper body and inner side of upper arm
	    T3—axilla
	    T5—nipple
	    T6—xiphoid process
	    T7–T8—lower costal margin
	    T10—umbilicus
	    T12—groin, bowel/bladder function may return

L1–L5	Sensory loss secondary to lesion as follows:
	    L1—includes back of buttocks, groin, and lower extremities
	    L2—lower extremities up to but not including the upper third anterior thigh
	    L3—lower extremities and saddle area
	    L4—lower extremities and saddle area excluding the anterior thigh
	    L5—lower extremities, saddle area, and the outer aspects of the legs and ankles

S1–S3	Foot sensory displacement Sensory loss includes: scrotum, saddle area, anal area, glans penis, perineum, and upper third of the posterior thigh
S3–S5	No paralysis of the leg muscles

E. **Nursing diagnoses**
  1. Risk for Impaired Skin Integrity
  2. Impaired Breathing Pattern
  3. Body Image, Self-Esteem, and Personal Identity Disturbances
  4. Altered Urinary Elimination
  5. Altered Bowel Eliminations

6. Feeding, bathing/hygiene, dressing/grooming, and toileting self-care deficits
7. Alteration in role relationships

F.   Planning and implementation

1. Considerations in the acute phase include several factors:
   a. Stabilizing the patient.
   b. Preventing extension of injury.
   c. Supplementing oxygen as necessary.
   d. Providing ventilator support if the diaphragm is paralyzed or if the respiratory function is ineffective.
   e. Performing bronchial hygiene, which includes chest percussion, respiratory toilet, suctioning, and deep-breathing exercises.
   f. Consulting pulmonary physician as necessary.
   g. Treating life-threatening arrhythmias with antiarrhythmics as ordered and appropriate.
   h. Administering vasopressors as ordered and appropriate.
   i. Preparing the patient for a possible laminectomy to stabilize the fracture.
2. Provide halo care if applicable.
   a. Never use halo vest or bars to roll or move patient.
   b. Tape wrench to front of vest in case of need for immediate removal.
   c. Monitor pin sites for infection and clean sites as ordered by physician.
   d. Notify physician of any loose pins.
   e. Place protective covering over tips of pins.
   f. Monitor vest tightness around all edges, assessing for skin breakdown and edema.
   g. Check for breakdown beneath vest by sliding a pillowcase between vest and skin and assessing for any drainage.
   h. Use a rolled towel under the neck for support rather than a pillow.
   i. Notify physician if patient complains of difficulty swallowing. This may be due to neck overextension.
3. Use a specialty bed or a turning schedule of at least every 2 hours to provide skin pressure relief.
4. Provide passive range of motion to all extremities.
5. Consult a physiatrist or physical therapist to develop an individualized physical therapy program.
6. Insert a nasogastric tube to low intermittent suction for gastrointestinal (GI) decompression as ordered.
7. Maintain a gastric pH <5.0 by using antacids every 3 hours as ordered.
8. Administer H 2 blockers to decrease gastric secretions as ordered and appropriate.
9. Administer medication to facilitate a bowel program as ordered.
10. Insert an indwelling urinary catheter to decompress the bladder.
11. **Be aware that later treatment includes initiation of intermittent catheterization program every 8–10 hours.**

12. Maintain optimal nutrition:
    a. The method of providing nutrition will depend on the associated injuries, level of consciousness, and the presence or absence of peristalsis
    b. The body needs sufficient fluid, carbohydrates, and protein for energy and tissue repair.
13. Support the psychological/emotional needs of the patient and family
14. Allow the patient to ask questions when ready.
15. The family may require the most support as they begin to comprehend what has happened and what it means to the patient and to them.
16. Anticipate psychiatric evaluation and treatment for patient and family.

G. **Home health considerations**
    1. This client would be treated at a long-term rehabilitation center after discharge from the hospital. Teaching will focus on prevention of complications related to immobility.

V. Spinal shock

A. **Description: condition of unopposed parasympathetic response that follows an acute SCI and is related to the degree of spinal cord edema.**

B. **Etiology and incidence**
    1. Occurs in 50% of patients who are initially diagnosed with complete spinal cord injuries.
    2. The patient may regain some degree of function after spinal shock ends, due to resolution of cord edema.
    3. Actual permanent injury cannot be predicted because of the masking effects of spinal shock.
    4. It occurs immediately after injury in response to the acute SCI.
    5. Duration:
        a. Can last days to months
        b. Usual duration is 1–6 weeks
        c. Is characterized by gradual recovery

C. **Pathophysiology**
    1. Spinal cord injury results in impaired sympathetic pathways.

    2. **This results in complete loss of all reflex activity, sympathetic vasomotor tone, and reflex activity below the level of the lesion.**

D. **Assessment findings**
    1. Initial motor findings are of areflexia with flaccid paralysis immediately following an SCI.
    2. Systemic manifestations include hypotension, hypothermia, and bradycardia.
    3. Warm, dry, skin occurs secondary to peripheral vasodilation.
    4. Urinary retention and a paralytic ileus may also occur.

E. **Nursing diagnoses**
    1. Ineffective Thermoregulation
    2. Altered Bowel Elimination
    3. Altered Cardiac Output:Deficit
    4. Impaired Physical Mobility
    5. Impaired Gas Exchange
    6. Risk for Impaired Skin Integrity

       7.   Altered Tissue Perfusion (Cerebral, Renal, Gastrointestinal, Peripheral)

       8.   Urinary Retention

       9.   Anxiety

     10.   Fear

F. Planning and implementation

       1.   Assess respiratory status.

       2.   **Maintain patent airway and adequate ventilation.**

       3.   Monitor pulse oximetry and arterial blood gases (ABGs).

       4.   Monitor continuous ECG for bradycardia.

       5.   Administer atropine as ordered for bradycardia.

       6.   Assess vital signs and hemodynamic parameters.

       7.   Administer vasoactive medications to maintain adequate blood pressure.

       8.   Assess for flaccid paralysis and areflexia.

       9.   Assess for paralytic ileus and urinary retention.

     10.   Maintain optimal positioning, and apply antiembolitic stockings and compression boots.

     11.   **Venous pooling due to vasodilation increases the risk for deep vein thrombosis (DVT).**

     12.   Reposition every 2 hours or as tolerated by blood pressure or level of injury.

     13.   Monitor fluid balance by assessing UOP, CVP, PAP, PACWP, and CO measurements.

     14.   **Avoid overhydration with intravenous fluids. This may cause increased edema at SCI site.**

     15.   Monitor GI function and assess the need for nutritional supplementation.

     16.   Evaluate for presence of paralytic ileus.

     17.   Assess for manifestations of fear and anxiety.

     18.   Evaluate support systems available to the patient and family.

     19.   Administer medications as prescribed by physician:

          a.   Early administration of corticosteroids to decrease edema at injury site: bolus with methylprednisolone, IV 30 mg/kg/over 1 hour followed by continuous infusion of 5.4 mg/kg/hr over the next 23 hours.

          b.   Atropine as indicated for treatment of persistent bradycardia

          c.   Vasoactive drugs as indicated for hypotension

          d.   Anticoagulants to prevent the formation of DVT

          e.   Antacids to prevent the formation of gastric ulcers

          f. H_2-blocking agents to reduce stimulation of GI secretions and prevent stress ulceration

          g.   Anti-anxiety agents as indicated for anxiety

G. Evaluation

       1.   The client's hemodynamics will remain within an acceptable range.

       2.   The client will exhibit adequate oxygenation.

       3.   The client will be free of urinary retention.

       4.   The client will not develop a paralytic ileus.

       5.   The client will not experience skin breakdown.

       6.   The client will not acquire a DVT.

7. The client will show evidence of adequate hydration.
8. The client will experience optimal nutrition.
9. The client will verbalize coping strategies to manage anxiety and fear.

VI. Autonomic dysreflexia (AD)

A. Description: A life-threatening hypertensive condition in the post acute or rehabilitative phase of an SCI.

B. Etiology

1. Is frequently seen in SCIs at the level of T4–T6 or above.
2. In SCIs at T4–T6, most patients experience AD within 1 year of injury.
3. It can occur spontaneously for up to 6 years following acute SCI.
4. It may follow spinal shock.
5. It is triggered by any noxious stimuli below the level of injury such as a full bladder.

C. Pathophysiology

1. **An SCI at or above the T4–T6 level, which is where the thoracic-lumbar sympathetic outlet originates, creates a breakdown in the feedback between the sympathetic and the parasympathetic branches of the autonomic nervous system (ANS).**
2. An episodic trigger, which is generally a noxious stimuli, creates an exaggerated sympathetic response.
3. There is a mass reflex stimulation of the sympathetic nerves below the level of the injury, resulting in vasoconstriction below the lesion.

D. Assessment findings

1. Cardiovascular effects include bradycardia, sudden marked hypertension, and increased body temperature.
2. The patient may experience a pounding headache, flushing, and diaphoresis of the upper body and face.
3. Nausea may be experienced.
4. Nasal congestion may occur.
5. Piloerection or goosebumps may be seen.

E. Nursing diagnoses

1. Decreased Cardiac Output
2. Altered Tissue Perfusion: Cerebral
3. Ineffective Thermoregulation
4. Pain
5. Urinary Retention
6. Anxiety
7. Fear

F. Planning and implementation

1. Monitor continuous ECG and vital signs.
2. Administer antihypertensives and atropine as ordered.
3. **Assess for the presence of noxious stimuli. The goal is to resolve the trigger prior to the development of autonomic dysreflexia.**
4. The most common triggers are:
   a. Urinary tract infection, renal calculi
   b. Urinary retention/kinked catheter
   c. Bowel obstruction/constipation
   d. Pressure ulcer
   e. Object pressing into the skin

f. Rash/itching

g. Pain, ingrown toenail, DVT

h. Pregnancy, uterine contractions

i. Infection

5. Monitor for changes in mental status.

6. Evaluate for pain/anxiety.

7. Administer medications to relieve pain/anxiety.

8. Educate client and family to recognize AD and prevent/control it.

G. Evaluation

1. The patient will maintain vital signs within normal limits.

2. The patient will be free from urinary retention.

3. The patient will be free from constipation/fecal impaction.

4. The patient will be free of skin breakdown.

5. Autonomic dysreflexia will be recognized early and interventions implemented in a timely manner.

H. Home health considerations

1. The client and family members will verbalize knowledge of sympathetic trigger, response, and appropriate action.

VII. Guillain-Barré syndrome (GB)

A. Description: an acute inflammatory demyelinating disease of the peripheral nervous system.

B. Etiology and incidence

1. The etiology is unclear.

2. **It is believed to be associated with an infectious, febrile illness 1–4 weeks before the development of GB. The illness is believed to be viral in origin.**

3. **There is possible autoimmune phenomenon, with lymphocytes and macrophages destroying the myelin sheath.**

4. It is also believed that there is a possible humoral response, with production of antibodies which attack the myelin sheath.

5. The incidence in the general population is one in 100,000.

C. Pathophysiology

1. Schwann cells, which cover the nerve axons, form the myelin sheath. Degeneration of these cells occurs, causing a flaccid paralysis, which is usually in a ascending pattern.

2. It is primarily the motor neurons which are affected.

3. Sensory involvement is limited, and is usually confined to the hands and feet in what is termed the glove and stocking pattern.

4. **Spontaneous regeneration of the myelin sheath occurs, with complete recovery within 6 months to 1 year.**

5. **Management is aimed at supporting body functions and preventing complications associated with paralysis until recovery occurs.**

D. Assessment findings

1. Initial phase:

a. Bilateral muscle weakness in the lower extremities, with an ascending pattern progressing to potential involvement of the trunk, upper extremities, and cranial nerves except CN #1

b. **This may result in potential life-threatening respiratory compromise if the thoracic nerve roots and cranial nerves are affected**

2. Plateau phase:
   a. May last days to weeks
   b. Is an interim period in which no changes occur
3. Recovery phase
   a. Synonymous with re-myelination and axonal regeneration
   b. Paralysis resolves gradually in a descending symmetrical pattern
   c. Follows a proximal to distal pattern
4. **An autonomic component, if present, predisposes to cardiac dysrhythmias and/or postural hypotension. It may be manifested by:**
   a. Sinus tachycardia
   b. Hypo- or hypertension
   c. Atrioventricular block
   d. Asystole

E. Nursing diagnoses
1. Impaired Gas Exchange
2. Impaired Airway Clearance
3. Impaired Breathing Pattern
4. Pain
5. Risk for Infection
6. Impaired Physical Mobility
7. Altered Nutrition: Less than Body Requirements
8. Risk for Impaired Skin Integrity
9. Anxiety
10. Impaired Verbal Communication
11. Powerlessness
12. Altered Self Concept

F. Planning and implementation
1. Assess for respiratory compromise:
   a. Assess peak flow
   b. Assess negative inspiratory force
   c. Evaluate ABGs, and monitor continuous pulse oximetry
2. Be prepared to provide respiratory support.
3. Perform pulmonary toilet to prevent pneumonia:
   a. Suction as necessary
   b. Hyperoxygenate/hyperventilate before and after suctioning to prevent hypoxia
4. Monitor continuous ECG.
5. Administer antidysrhythmics as indicated and ordered.
6. Monitor vital signs.
7. Provide frequent assessment of level of muscle weakness and rate of ascension.
8. Assess for urinary retention and/or paralytic ileus.
9. Maintain optimal positioning:
   a. Elevate head of bed as tolerated to promote lung expansion and decrease risk for aspiration
   b. Turn and reposition every 2 hours
   c. Assist with active and passive ROM
10. Apply anti-embolitic stockings and compression boots to prevent the formation of DVT.

11. Assess for signs/symptoms of nosocomial infection, such as pneumonia or UTI.
12. Assess nutrition and hydration status by instituting a calorie count, and maintaining intake and output.
13. Administer medications as indicated and ordered, including:
    a. Analgesics
    b. Anti-anxiety agents
    c. Corticosteroids: methylprednisolone 125 mg IV every 6 hours for 1–3 days then taper down
    d. Antibiotics for prophylaxis or for pathogen specific use
    e. Antacids to control gastric irritation
    f. H_2 Blockers to reduce gastric acid secretion and prevent stress ulcers
    g. Anticoagulants to prevent formation of DVT
14. Administer and monitor the response to plasma pheresis. Plasmapheresis involves the mechanical separation of blood components, and subsequent discarding of the plasma which contains antibodies believed to contribute to neuronal degeneration. It involves 3–4 treatments, 1–2 days apart.
15. Replace plasma with fresh frozen plasma (FFP) or plasminogen as indicated and ordered by physician.

G. Evaluation
1. The patient will maintain vital signs within an acceptable range.
2. The patient will exhibit a patent airway and maintain adequate ventilation.
3. The patient will remain free of skin breakdown.
4. The patient will remain free from infection.
5. The patient will remain free from injury.
6. The patient will verbalize adequate control of pain and anxiety.
7. The patient will verbalize an understanding of the disease process.

H. Home health considerations
1. The client will improve gradually to a full recovery.
2. The client will not experience any complications of immobility.
3. The client and family will verbalize control over anxiety, disturbance in self concept, change in life-style

VIII. Multiple sclerosis
A. Description: a chronic, progressive, degenerative disease of the myelin sheath and conduction pathways of the central nervous system (CNS).
1. The disease process is characterized by episodes of remission and exacerbation.
2. These may be precipitated by infection, trauma, pregnancy, emotional stress, menstruation, cold or humid weather, overeating, or fatigue.
3. As the disease progresses, the duration and severity of episodes increases.

B. Etiology and incidence
1. The etiology is unknown, but theories revolve around viral infectious agents or autoimmune response.
2. The highest incidence occurs in the second to fourth decades of life.
3. Women have a slightly greater incidence than men.

    4.   There is evidence of a genetic component, with a 15 times greater incidence in persons with a first-degree relative with the disease.

C.   **Pathophysiology**

    1.   **Demyelination occurs throughout the white matter, and sometimes into the gray matter of the CNS. Remission and exacerbations occur.**

    2.   Permanent damage occurs after recurrent episodes cause scarring or plaque formation, preventing the regeneration of the myelin sheath in patchy areas.

    3.   Management is aimed at supporting body functions through the acute phase and preventing complications of immobility.

D.   **Assessment findings**

    1.   Symptoms vary widely, and are related to the areas of CNS affected by patchy demyelination and scarring plaques.

    2.   Sensory findings include numbness, parasthesia, pain, decreased proprioception, and sensation.

    3.   Motor findings include paresis, paralysis, spasticity, diplopia, bowel and bladder dysfunction (retention or incontinence).

    4.   Cerebellar findings include loss of balance and coordination, staggering gait, ataxia, nystagmus, speech disturbances, tremor, and vertigo.

    5.   Miscellaneous other findings include optic neuritis, impotence, altered mood state (depression or euphoria), and fatigue.

    6.   Laboratory findings:

        a.   Possible elevation of protein in CSF

        b.   CT scan may show areas of patchy demyelination

        c.   Presence of oligoclonal bands on electrophoresis in 80%–90% of patients

E.   **Nursing diagnoses**

    1.   Impaired Gas Exchange

    2.   Pain

    3.   Anxiety

    4.   Impaired Physical Mobility

    5.   Altered Bowel Elimination

    6.   Risk for Injury

    7.   Sensory Perceptual Alterations: Kinesthetic

    8.   Sleep Pattern Disturbance

    9.   Ineffective Individual Coping

    10.   Self Esteem Disturbance

    11.   Anticipatory Grieving

    12.   Hopelessness

    13.   Powerlessness

    14.   Ineffective Individual Coping

F.   **Planning and implementation**

    1.   Monitor respiratory status including breath sounds, continuous pulse oximetry, and ABGs.

    2.   Be prepared to support respiratory functions.

    3.   Perform pulmonary toilet as indicated.

    4.   Monitor vital signs and continuous ECG.

    5.   Assess motor function.

6. Maintain a safe environment.
7. Facilitate physical therapy to maximize independence in ADLs and assist with assistive devices as needed.
8. Assess sensory functions.
9. Minimize environmental triggers such as cold air and hot baths.
10. Allow for frequent rest periods.
11. Protect from infection.
12. Provide client/family education and support.
13. Administer medications as indicated and ordered by physician:
    a. Corticosteroids (controversial during exacerbations): ACTH 45–50 μ bid for 7–10 days
    b. Prednisone, 10 mg qid
    c. Anti-spasticity agents (baclofen, diazepam, dantrolene sodium)

     d. **Immunosuppressive protocols (azathioprine, cyclophosphamide)**

    ▸ Risk of bone marrow suppression and hemorrhagic cystitis

G. Evaluation
1. Vital signs will be maintained within normal limits.
2. The patient will remain free from infection.
3. The patient will remain free from injury.
4. The patient will be able to verbalize control over fear, anxiety, self-concept disturbance.
5. The patient will maximize independence.
6. The patient will verbalize an understanding of the disease process.

H. Home health considerations
1. The client will not experience any complications of immobility or decrease from previous functioning level.
2. The client and the family will verbalize control over anxiety, disturbance in self-concept, change in life-style

IX. Myasthenia gravis

A. Description: a progressive neuromuscular disorder which interferes with the impulses in voluntary muscles. It is characterized by muscular fatigability brought on by exertion and resolves with rest.

B. Etiology and incidence
1. The disease affects primarily women between ages 20 and 45. It is thought to be autoimmune.
2. Factors which can precipitate a crisis include colds and flu, changes in hormonal levels, fatigue, stress, anxiety, alcohol, and medication.

C. Pathophysiology
1. Acetylcholine (Ach) receptor antibodies interfere with the transmission of impulses across neuromuscular junctions.
2. The disease is characterized by periods of exacerbations and remissions. During an exacerbation period the client may suffer life-threatening respiratory distress or myasthenic crisis.

3. **The disease may exacerbate in two types of crisis:**
    a. **Myasthenic crisis occurs when there is not enough anticholinesterase.**

        b.   **Cholinergic crisis is precipitated by excessive anti-cholinesterase levels.**

D.   **Assessment**
1. The main symptoms is easy fatigability of specific muscle groups, characterized by weakness after exercise which improves with rest.
2. Ptosis, diplopia, and dysphagia may also occur.
3. Respiratory distress may present in severe cases.
4. Assess for a history of feeling tired or weak after exercise or late in the day.
5. Evaluate muscle strength by asking for a performance of repetitive movements of the same muscle group and observe for fatigability.
6. Diagnostic testing involves administration of an anticholinesterase such as edrophonium chloride (Tensilon). The client is injected with 2 mg IV and observed for an improvement in muscle strength it is repeated every 2 minutes until a response is seen.

E.   **Nursing diagnoses**
1. Impaired Gas Exchange
2. Fatigue
3. Ineffective Airway Clearance
4. Anxiety

F.   **Planning and implementation**
1. Provide for ongoing neuromuscular assessment.
2. Treat myasthenic crisis with pyridostigmine (Mestion) or neostigmine (Prostigmin).
3. Treat cholinergic crisis by withholding medications.
4. Support the client's respiratory status as needed.
5. Provide for a restful nonstimulating environment.
6. Maintain communication with the client.
7. Treat precipitating factors.
8. Provide for adequate nutrition and prevent complications due to dysphagia.
9. Prepare client for possible thymectomy. It is thought that the thymus is involved in the autoimmune process.
10. Prepare client for possible plasmapheresis which involves separating the client's blood components and removing the antibodies causing myasthenia gravis.
11. Prevent aspiration by offering semi-soft foods.
12. Provide client with reassurance.
13. Decrease anxiety.
14. Be aware of the following potential complications:
    a.   Respiratory insufficiency
    b.   Aspiration pneumonia
    c.   Myasthenic crisis
    d.   Cholinergic crisis

15. **Administer medications: Myasthenia gravis is an autoimmune disease, therefore, corticosteroids such as prednisone, azathioprine (Imuran), and cyclophosphamide (Cytoxan) may be used for immunosuppression.**

G.   **Evaluation**
1. The client will remain free of respiratory complications.

2. The client will be able to perform activities of daily living (ADLs).
3. The client will not suffer complications.
4. The client will not be in crisis.

H. Home health considerations

1. Instruct client and family on energy conservation techniques such as itinerary planning.
2. Rearrange household routine to decrease stress on the client.
3. Teach family members rescue breathing procedure in the event of respiratory compromise.
4. Instruct on the importance of avoiding crowds to decrease the risk of infection.
5. Teach client and family about the disease process in relationship to the client's abilities.
6. Refer client and family to the Myasthenia Gravis Foundation.

X. Neuromuscular blockade

A. Description

1. Neuromuscular paralysis is used most commonly as a type of treatment for patients with increased intracranial pressure to prevent increases in intrathoracic and venous pressure that may occur with coughing, straining and other activities.
2. Pancuronium is the most common drug of choice.

 3. **Sedation is necessary to decrease anxiety and fear, which are known to increase cerebral metabolism.**

B. Planning and implementation

1. When using these drugs, keep the following in mind:

 a. **These patients must be supported with a ventilator, as respiratory paralysis can occur.**
   b. Perform frequent assessment of respiratory status/oxygenation:

   ▸ Airway, breathing, circulation (ABCs)
   ▸ Continuous pulse oximetry

   c. Use extreme caution when turning these patients due to risk of accidental extubation
   d. Perform pulmonary toilet as necessary and tolerated by intracranial pressure (ICP).

2. Prevention and early recognition of complications:
   a. Monitor vital signs frequently (head injury may cause abnormal body temperature, blood pressure, and/or heart rate).
   b. Medicate as ordered by physician and appropriate.
   c. Monitor intake and output frequently.

3. Frequent assessment and monitoring of neurologic signs:

 a. **Neurologic exams will no longer be accurate as of 1 hour after loading dose is given.**
   b. Periodic assessment of level of paralysis as per hospital policy is necessary.

 c. **If the patient is moving, an increased dose is necessary.**

4. Supportive care of all body systems is required:
   a. Insert and monitor nasogastric tube (NGT).

   b. **Nutritional support may be given parenterally due to the presence of a paralytic ileus.**
   c. Position changes are required to prevent breakdown. These patients do not move spontaneously at all.

5. Provide emotional support to patient and family:
   a. The patient can hear everything that is said, but will not be able to respond.
   b. Reassure patient and try to anticipate and meet needs.
   c. Explain all procedures to patient before doing them.
   d. Allow patient to listen to favorite radio/television stations. Remove at night to maintain day/night orientation.

6. Paralytic agents are temporary and spontaneous movement occurs after withdrawal of the drug. However, permanent paralysis has been known to occur in rare cases.
   a. Benefits should clearly outweigh the risks.
   b. Administer the smallest possible dose for the shortest time necessary.

Bibliography

Bayley, E.W., & Turcke, S.A. (1992). *A comprehensive curriculum for trauma nursing.* Boston: Jones and Bartlett.

Chin, D.E., & Kearns, P. (1991). Nutrition in the spinal injured patient. *Nutr Clin Pract 6,* 213–222.

Kinney, M., Packa, D., & Dunbar, S. (1993). *AACN's clinical reference for critical-care nursing.* St. Louis: Mosby.

Marino, P.L. (1991). *The ICU book.* Malvern, PA: Lea & Febiger.

North American Nursing Diagnosis Association (NANDA). (1996). *Nursing diagnoses: Definitions & classification 1997–1998.* Philadelphia: Author.

Urden, L., Davie, J., & Thelan, L. (1992). *Essentials of critical care nursing.* St. Louis: Mosby.

Zaloga, G.P. (1994). *Nutrition in critical care.* St. Louis: Mosby.

STUDY QUESTIONS

1. The client has a partially transected spinal cord at the level of S2. The nurse's most appropriate response to the client's spouse who asks, "Will he be able to walk again?" is
   a. "It is to early to tell and the injury is below the majority of nerves that control the legs."
   b. "Sure, everyone with this type of injury walks."
   c. "You should ask the physician."
   d. "There is always hope."

2. Patients with Guillain-Barré syndrome frequently require
   a. psychological support
   b. mechanical ventilation
   c. rehabilitation during the acute phase
   d. all of the above

3. As a nurse caring for a patient with an acute L-3 injury, your assessment of the patient would include all except the following:
   a. inspection for skin breakdown on the sacrum, hips, and heels
   b. inspecting the area around the ETT for breakdown
   c. assessing the urinary output, assuring that the Foley catheter is not kinked or occluded
   d. assessing GI function for constipation or ileus

4. A patient with a T-3 incomplete lesion tells you that he can feel it when you lift his left heel. An appropriate response to this statement would be:
   a. "What you are experiencing is called 'phantom pain;' it is common after an injury like yours."
   b. "It is impossible for you feel your feet, you are paralyzed. You may be experiencing 'ICU psychosis,' but don't worry, it is only temporary."
   c. "That's great! You may have function returning to your legs."
   d. "Sometimes when you have an incomplete lesion you will have patchy areas of sensation."

5. A patient with a complete lesion of C-2 will experience which of the following disabilities?
   a. permanent ventilator dependency
   b. poor neck control; high-backed wheelchair necessary
   c. some sensory loss in the face and ears
   d. all of the above

6. The patient with C-7 injury can expect which of the following:
   a. independent living
   b. total and permanent ventilator dependency
   c. necessary assistance with ADLs
   d. to never again have to do light housework

7. Your patient is diagnosed with spinal shock. Which of the following would you expect to see?
   a. spastic paralysis
   b. tachycardia, hypertension, hyperthermia
   c. incontinent of diarrhea
   d. bradycardia, hypotension, hypothermia

Your patient is admitted with a T-4 complete lesion. Temperature 96.9 F, B/P 80/44, heart rate 44. Physical assessment shows a flaccid paralysis with no spontaneous respiratory function. CVP 4, PAP 26/12, PAWP 12, CI 2.0. Questions 8, 9, and 10 pertain to this scenario.

8. Which of the following actions would be appropriate?
   a. apply warming blankets
   b. atropine 1 amp, IVP
   c. NSS 5 liters over 2 hours
   d. dopamine at 2.5 µg/kg/min

9. His mother asks you if he will need "that breathing machine" for a long time. The correct response would be:
   a. "Yes, your son is paralyzed and will never breathe on his own."
   b. "No, we should have him stabilized

in the next 24–48 hours; he will be able to breathe on his own."

c. "Your son may need this breathing machine for a few days to a few months. Once he is stabilized, he should gradually improve."

d. "Yes, our social workers will be up to discuss advance directives with you."

10. This patient's cardiac index is:
a. normal for an adult weighing 180–250 lbs
b. very low; at least 4 liters of fluid replacement will be necessary
c. high; he is compensating for his brady cardia with vasoconstriction
d. borderline low for any patient, any size

11. Which of the following medications would you expect to administer to the patient with acute SCI?
a. methylprednisolone, 30 mg/kg over 1 hour, followed by 5.4 mg/kg over the next 23 hours
b. Coumadin 5–10 mg/day, dependent on daily PT level
c. Imodium 1 tab every 6 hours for 24 hours
d. Nipride 33 μg/min for 24 hours

A patient is admitted to your unit with a B/P of 220/115 and a heart rate of 50. Past medical history is positive for a T-5 SCI 7 months ago. The visiting nurse comments that the patient has experienced an unremarkable post-injury period. Questions 12 and 13 pertain to this scenario.

12. A priority in the assessment of this patient would be:
a. assessment of his urinary status
b. examining his back, feet, skin folds for breakdown
c. assessing for signs of infection
d. all of the above

13. During your assessment, you find that the patient's Foley catheter is kinked. After unkinking it, it drains 900 mL of yellow urine. The patient's blood pressure gradually comes down to 132/76. Patient/family teaching would include:
a. the signs and symptoms of a CVA
b. the signs and symptoms of AD (autonomic dysreflexia)
c. to routinely assess for signs if infection, skin breakdown, and distended bladder
d. all of the above

14. Your patient presents AAO × 3 with complaints of a progressive weakness in the legs and hands. Past medical history is significant for insulin-dependent diabetes mellitus and a recent "viral infection." Two days later, this patient is paralyzed in both lower extremities. The most probable cause of her paralysis is:
a. neurologic changes due to diabetic ketoacidosis secondary to a viral infection
b. brain abscess secondary untreated viral infection
c. Guillain-Barré syndrome
d. transient ischemic attack (TIA) progressing to CVA

ANSWER KEY

1. *Correct response: a*
   The S2 level of the cord innervates the lower legs but the cord is only partially transacted, therefore, it will take time to evaluate functioning. After the edema resolves functioning can be evaluated.
   b. Never offer a client or family false reassurance.
   c. The client's family is in need of an immediate response. The physician was not asked the question, the nurse was questioned.
   d. Stating there is always hope offers false reassurance.
   Comprehension/Physiologic/ Implementation

2. *Correct response: d*
   a. Patients may suffer from anxiety and impaired coping mechanism.
   b. Respiratory muscles may become temporarily paralyzed.
   c. In addition to supporting body functions, rehabilitation will be necessary to strengthen muscles, including respiratory muscles.
   Knowledge/Health promotion/Planning

3. *Correct response: b*
   Lumbar injuries do not impair respiratory function.
   a, d. All patients with limited mobility should be assessed for breakdown on bony areas and constipation or ileus.
   c. This is part of the basic assessment of a patient in the critical care setting. In the acute phase of an SCI the patient will probably have a Foley catheter inserted temporarily to prevent bladder distention.
   Application/Health promotion/ Assessment

4. *Correct response: d*
   Incomplete spinal cord lesions allow "spotty" sensation.
   a. Phantom pain occurs after the amputation of a limb.

   b. ICU psychosis is characterized by paranoia and disorientation. There is no evidence of either in this patient. It is however temporary.
   c. This statement is inaccurate and would offer the patient false hope.
   Comprehension/Physiologic/ Implementation

5. *Correct response: d*
   Injuries of the C-1, C-2, and C-3 cervical spine cause quadriplegia, respiratory paralysis, and spotty sensory loss of the face, occipital region, and ears.
   Knowledge/Physiologic/Assessment

6. *Correct response: a*
   a, c, d. The patient with the C-7 injury can expect to live independently after rehabilitation and occupational therapy, including light housework.
   b. The diaphragm and accessory muscles compensate for the abdominal and intercostal muscles; this patient will not be ventilator dependent.
   Application/Health promotion/Planning

7. *Correct response: d*
   b, d. Bradycardia, hypothermia, and hypotension are a triad of symptoms seen with spinal shock.
   a. Flaccid paralysis is evident in spinal shock
   c. Constipation and ileus are common in spinal shock
   Knowledge/Physiologic/Assessment

8. *Correct response: b*
   Atropine would be administered for the bradycardia which may be contributing to the hypotension.
   a. Although this person is mildly hypothermic, warming blankets at this time would cause further vasodilation and increase hypotension.

c. Volume replacement may be indicated due to the low hemodynamic values, but 5 liters would risk fluid overload and increase spinal edema.

d. < 2.5–3 µg/kg/min of dopamine is renal dose and would exacerbate the hypotension.

Application/Physiologic/Implementation

9. *Correct response: c*

This patient is in spinal shock which may last as long as a few months. His injury is lower than C-4 so he will be able to breathe on his own.

a, b. These statements are not true.

d. This response does not give the mother any accurate information or explanations.

Application/Psychosocial/Intervention

10. *Correct response: d*

a, d. Cardiac index takes into account the patient's BSA. The normals are 2–4.

b. It is borderline low, not extremely low. 4 liters of fluid may put this patient into fluid overload and increase spinal edema.

c. This is a low-normal CI, and this patient is in spinal shock and therefore vasodilated.

Knowledge/Physiologic/Evaluation

11. *Correct response: a*

Methylprednisolone would be administered to decrease edema at the injury site.

b. If bleeding is not a problem heparin would be initiated to prevent DVT. Coumadin would not be indicated.

c. This patient is at risk for an ileus or constipation, not diarrhea.

d. This patient is likely to be hypotensive rather than hypertensive.

Comprehension/Physiologic/Implementation

12. *Correct response: d*

This patient is at risk for autonomic dysreflexia, which is caused by any noxious stimuli below the level of injury. The goal is to identify and remove the trigger.

Comprehension/Health promotion/Assessment

13. *Correct response: d*

This patient experienced an episode of AD which puts him at risk for a CVA. The patient and family should be taught how to prevent AD and how to recognize it if it happens again. AD has been known to occur for up to 6 years after an SCI.

Application/Health promotion/Assessment

14. *Correct response: c*

Guillain-Barré syndrome usually presents with a progressive ascending weakness leading to paralysis. These patients often complain of a recent viral infection.

a. This patient did not experience any signs of DKA.

b. A patient with a brain abscess would probably experience a change in mental status.

d. TIAs resolve in less than 24 hours; both TIAs and CVAs are usually unilateral rather than ascending.

Application/Physiologic/Evaluation

The Cardiovascular System (Musculature and Vasculature)

I. Anatomy and physiology
  - **A.** Structure
  - **B.** Function

II. Overview of cardiovascular disorders
  - **A.** Assessment
  - **B.** Laboratory studies and diagnostic tests
  - **C.** Hemodynamic monitoring
  - **D.** Nutritional considerations
  - **E.** Psychosocial implications
  - **F.** Medications used to treat cardiovascular disorders

III. Acute myocardial infarction
  - **A.** Description
  - **B.** Etiology and incidence
  - **C.** Pathophysiology
  - **D.** Assessment findings
  - **E.** Nursing diagnoses
  - **F.** Planning and implementation
  - **G.** Evaluation
  - **H.** Potential complications
  - **I.** Home health considerations

IV. Heart failure
  - **A.** Description
  - **B.** Etiology and incidence
  - **C.** Pathophysiology
  - **D.** Assessment finding
  - **E.** Nursing diagnosis
  - **F.** Planning and implementation

  - **G.** Evaluation
  - **H.** Home health considerations

V. Angina
  - **A.** Description
  - **B.** Etiology and incidence
  - **C.** Pathophysiology
  - **D.** Assessment findings
  - **E.** Nursing diagnosis
  - **F.** Planning and implementation
  - **G.** Evaluation

VI. Cardiomyopathy
  - **A.** Description
  - **B.** Etiology and incidence
  - **C.** Pathophysiology and management: dilated (congestive) cardiomyopathy
  - **D.** Pathophysiology and management: hypertrophic cardiomyopathy (IHSS)
  - **E.** Pathophysiology and management: restrictive cardiomyopathy
  - **F.** Assessment findings
  - **G.** Nursing diagnosis
  - **H.** Planning and implementation
  - **I.** Evaluation

VII. Tricuspid stenosis
  - **A.** Description
  - **B.** Etiology and incidence
  - **C.** Pathophysiology
  - **D.** Assessment findings

VIII. Pulmonic stenosis
  A. Description
  B. Etiology and incidence
  C. Pathophysiology
  D. Assessment findings

IX. Mitral stenosis
  A. Description
  B. Etiology and incidence
  C. Pathophysiology
  D. Assessment findings

X. Aortic stenosis
  A. Description
  B. Etiology and incidence
  C. Pathophysiology
  D. Assessment findings
  E. Nursing diagnoses for stenotic valvular disease
  F. Planning and implementation for stenotic valvular disease
  G. Evaluation

XI. Tricuspid regurgitative disease
  A. Description
  B. Etiology and incidence
  C. Pathophysiology
  D. Assessment findings

XII. Pulmonic regurgitative disease
  A. Description
  B. Etiology and incidence
  C. Pathophysiology
  D. Assessment findings

XIII. Mitral regurgitative disease
  A. Description
  B. Etiology and incidence
  C. Pathophysiology
  D. Assessment findings

XIV. Aortic regurgitative disease
  A. Description
  B. Etiology and incidence
  C. Pathophysiology
  D. Assessment findings
  E. Nursing diagnoses for regurgitative valvular disease
  F. Planning and implementation for regurgitative valvular disease
  G. Evaluation

XV. Cardiac contusion
  A. Description
  B. Etiology and incidence
  C. Pathophysiology

  D. Assessment findings
  E. Nursing diagnosis
  F. Planning and implementation
  G. Evaluation

XVI. Cardiac tamponade
  A. Description
  B. Etiology and incidence
  C. Pathophysiology
  D. Assessment findings
  E. Nursing diagnosis
  F. Planning and implementation
  G. Evaluation

XVII. Dissecting aorta
  A. Description
  B. Etiology and incidence
  C. Pathophysiology
  D. Assessment findings
  E. Nursing diagnosis
  F. Planning and implementation
  G. Evaluation

XVIII. Cardiogenic shock
  A. Description
  B. Etiology and incidence
  C. Pathophysiology
  D. Assessment findings
  E. Nursing diagnosis
  F. Planning and implementation
  G. Evaluation

XIX. Thrombolytics
  A. Description
  B. Indications for administration in coronary patients
  C. Indications for administration in patients without coronary disease
  D. Assessment findings
  E. Nursing diagnosis
  F. Planning and implementation
  G. Evaluation

XX. Percutaneous transluminal angioplasty (PTCA)
  A. Description
  B. Indications
  C. Assessment findings
  D. Nursing diagnosis
  E. Planning and implementations
  F. Evaluation

XXI. Intracoronary stents
  A. Description
  B. Indications
  C. Assessment findings
  D. Nursing diagnosis
  E. Planning and imple-
       mentation
  F. Evaluation

XXII. Laser surgery
  A. Description
  B. Indications
  C. Planning and imple-
       mentation

XXIII. Endarterectomy
  A. Description
  B. Assessment findings
  C. Nursing diagnosis
  D. Planning and imple-
       mentation
  E. Evaluation

**XXIV. Intra-aortic balloon pump
          (IAP)**
  A. Description
  B. Indications
  C. Assessment findings
  D. Nursing diagnosis
  E. Planning and imple-
       mentation
  F. Evaluation

**XXV. Ventricular assist device
          (VAD)**
  A. Description
  B. Indications
  C. Assessment findings
  D. Nursing diagnosis
  E. Planning and imple-
       mentation
  F. Evaluation

XXVI. Myoplasty
  A. Description
  B. Indications
  C. Assessment findings
  D. Nursing diagnosis
  E. Planning and imple-
       mentation
  F. Evaluation

XXVII. Valvuloplasty
  A. Description
  B. Indications
  C. Assessment findings
  D. Nursing diagnosis
  E. Planning and imple-
       mentation

  F. Evaluation
  G. Potential complications

XXVIII. Coronary artery bypass graft
  A. Description
  B. Indications
  C. Assessment findings
  D. Nursing diagnosis
  E. Planning and imple-
       mentation
  F. Evaluation

XXIX. Femoral artery bypass graft
  A. Description
  B. Indications
  C. Assessment findings
  D. Nursing diagnosis
  E. Planning and imple-
       mentation
  F. Evaluation

XXX. Heart transplantation
  A. Description
  B. Indications
  C. Assessment findings
  D. Nursing diagnosis
  E. Planning and imple-
       mentation
  F. Evaluation

XXXI. Ventricular septal defect
  A. Description
  B. Etiology and incidence
  C. Pathophysiology
  D. Assessment findings
  E. Nursing diagnosis
  F. Planning and imple-
       mentation
  G. Evaluation

XXXII. Aneurysm
  A. Description
  B. Etiology and incidence
  C. Pathophysiology
  D. Assessment findings
  E. Nursing diagnosis
  F. Planning and imple-
       mentation
  G. Evaluation

XXXIII. Pericarditis
  A. Description
  B. Etiology and incidence
  C. Pathophysiology
  D. Assessment findings
  E. Nursing diagnosis
  F. Planning and imple-
       mentation
  G. Evaluation

I.   Anatomy and physiology

  A.   Structure

    1.   The heart is a muscle located in the mediastinum, situated between the two lungs, above the diaphragm and below the 2nd rib.

    2.   It is approximately the size of a person's fist.

    3.   The musculature of the heart is divided into three layers:

      a.   Endocardium: the inner lining of the heart; made up of endothelial cells, connective tissue and elastic fibers.

      b.   Myocardium: consists of muscle encompassing the right and left atria, the right and left ventricles, and the epicardium.

      c.   Epicardium: the outer covering of the heart.

      d.   Pericardial sac: a space between the parietal and visceral epicardium which contains 10–30 cc's of serous fluid.

    4.   There are four chambers of the heart, the right and left atria (upper chambers) and the right and left ventricles (lower chambers).

      a.   The right atrium is a low pressure chamber responsible for collecting the de-oxygenated blood from the system and sending it to the right ventricle.

      b.   The right ventricle sends the blood to the pulmonary artery through the respiratory circulation to pick up oxygen and drop off carbon dioxide.

      c.   The blood travels to the left atrium from the lung through the pulmonary veins.

      d.   From there blood flows to the left ventricle where oxygenated blood is pushed through the aorta into the body.

    5.   The four chambers of the heart are separated from each other by muscular walls known as septum.

    6.   Atria are connected to ventricles by valves:

      a.   The right atria opens into the right ventricle via the tricuspid valve.

    b.   The left atria opens into the left ventricle via the mitral valve.

    c.   The tricuspid and mitral valves are known collectively as the atrioventricular valves (A-V valves).

7.   The semilunar valves allow for blood to flow from the ventricles to the great vessels.

    a.   Pulmonic valve: allows the blood to flow from the right ventricle to the pulmonary artery.

    b.   Aortic valve: allows the blood to flow from the left ventricle to the aorta.

8.   The papillary muscles are muscles attached to each ventricular wall which extend into fibrous bands known as chordea tendenae.

9.   The chordae tendineae connect to the free edges of each of the leaflets preventing the leaflets from being pushed back into the atria during ventricular systole, maintaining unidirectional blood flow.

10.   Electrophysiology

    a.   Electrical impulses are produced by the cyclic exchange of ions across the myocardial cell membrane.

    b.   Ionic exchange results in a process of depolarization and re-polarization of cells. This is called the action potential.

    c.   This in turn results in muscle contraction or relaxation.

    d.   The electrocardiogram (ECG) is a record of the heart's electrical activity.

11.   Characteristics of cardiac cells

    a.   Automaticity is the ability to initiate an electrical impulse.

    b.   Excitability is the ability to respond to the electrical impulse.

    c.   Conductivity is the ability of a cell to transmit the impulse to other cells.

    d.   Contractility is the ability of a cell to contract in response to electrical stimulus.

12.   Types of cardiac cells

    a.   Pacemaker cells are responsible for initiating electrical impulses.

        ▸ Sinoatrial node (SAN) is located in the right atria and initiates impulses at a rate of 60–100 beats per minute

        ▸ Atrioventricular node (AVN) is located above the tricuspid valve and initiates impulses at a rate of 40–60 beats per minute.

    b.   The AVN functions as a pacemaker when failure of the SAN occurs.

    c.   Electrical conducting cells are long, thin cells that conduct impulses from the pacemaker cells to the myocardial cells.

        ▸ Bundle of His are fibers which emerge from the AVN conducting impulses from the node to the left and right ventricular cells.

> ► The left bundle branch (LBB) conducts impulses at a faster rate than the right bundle branch (RBB) allowing for adequate ventricular filling.
> ► Ventricular cells can serve as pacemaker cells if failure of the SA and AVN occurs. In this instance, impulses fire at a rate of 40 to 60 beats per minute.
> ► Purkinje fibers are small diffuse fibers which extend from the right and left bundle branches into the myocardial contractile tissue.

    d.   Myocardial contractile cells are large cells which respond to the electrical impulses and then contract in order to pump blood to the remainder of the body.

13.   The cardiac blood supply is provided via the coronary arteries. The heart receives its oxygen via the coronary arteries during ventricular diastole.

    a.   Sinuses of Valsalva are located behind the aortic valve and give root to the right and left coronary arteries.

    b.   The left main coronary artery (LMCA) arises from the left sinus of Valsalva and divides into the left anterior descending (LAD) artery and the left circumflex (LCA) artery. It is responsible for 60% of the blood supply.

    c.   The left anterior descending travels to the anterior portion of the heart ending in the posterior apex and supplies blood to the left ventricle, anterior papillary muscle, right bundle branch and anterior superior left bundle branch.

    d.   The left circumflex travels from the LMCA along the left heart margin, ending posteriorly and supplies the left atrium, posterior papillary muscle, SAN in 45% of the population, AV node in 10% of the population, and a large area of the left ventricle.

    e.   The right coronary artery (RCA) travels from the right sinus of Valsalva along the right atrium and supplies the right atrium, right anterior ventricle, posterior papillary muscle, SAN in 55% of the population, AVN in 90% of the population.

B. Function

1.   The heart has mechanical and electrical properties which function together to pump blood throughout the body.

2.   The chambers of the heart work together to coordinate direction and velocity of flow throughout the heart and into the systemic circulation.

3.   It is the function of the AV valves to open passively when the pressure in each of the atria exceeds that in each corresponding ventricle allowing the blood to flow from the atria into the ventricles.

4.   Conversely, it is also the function of the AV valves to remain tightly closed and impermeable to blood flow during times when the pressure ventricles is greater than that of the atria such as during ventricular systole.

5. The electrical system of the heart serves to initiate and conduct electrical impulses in order to initiate and control myocardial contraction and relaxation.
6. Systole, or ventricular pumping, occurs secondary to depolarization of cells.
7. Diastole, or ventricular filling, occurs when repolarization of cells takes place.
8. Preload is the volume of blood in the left ventricle prior to contraction and reflects maximal elasticity of the left ventricle.
9. Afterload is the pressure against which the left ventricle must work to eject blood. It is determined by the amount of resistance to outflow and the aortic distensibility.
10. Contractility refers to the stretch of the left ventricle. The greater the ability to stretch, the stronger the contraction.

II. Overview of cardiovascular disorders

A. Assessment

1. During the history the nurse should assess for significant past medical history including:
   a. concomitant disease processes such as hypertension, heart murmur, diabetes mellitus, coronary artery disease, angina and hyperlipidemia
   b. presence of varicosities or thrombophlebitis
   c. recent history of strep infection or rheumatic fever
2. Family history should also be ascertained as this may highlight cardiac risk factors.
   a. Family history of coronary artery disease, angina, myocardial infarction may indicate familial predisposition. Other familial risk factors include: hypertension, hyperlipidemia, cerebral vascular accidents and diabetes mellitus
3. Physical assessment should include the following:
   a. Assessment of patient's general appearance including cachexia, mottling or cyanosis of skin, diaphoresis, dyspnea with use of accessory muscles, anxiety, presence of edema (Display 4-1) or appearance of pain.
   b. Vital signs including temperature, respiratory rate, rhythm, and depth.
   c. Blood pressure, sitting and recumbent, should be taken in order to assess for orthostatic changes.

DISPLAY 4-1.
Etiology of Edema

Systemic edema may be caused by congestive heart failure, hypoalbuminemia, or salt and water retention.

Local edema may be caused by an occlusion or thrombophlebitis and may be accompanied by Homans' sign (pain in the affected calf with dorsiflexion), redness, and tenderness.

d. **Calculate pulse pressure, the difference between systolic and diastolic pressures which is normally between 30–40 mm Hg. A widened pulse pressure may indicate aortic regurgitation, whereas a narrowed pulse pressure may be associated with tachycardia, cardiac tamponade, pericardial effusion, or aortic stenosis.**

e. Assess heart rate and rhythm. Various pulse patterns may be indicative of disease processes.

   ▶ Pulsus alterans: a regular rhythm but amplitude varies from beat to beat which may indicate left heart failure.

   ▶ Bigeminal pulse: a normal beat alternating with premature contractions, every other beat having a decreased amplitude. This may indicate a cardiac dysrhythmia.

   ▶ Pulsus paradoxus: a regular rhythm with decreased amplitude resulting in a drop in systolic pressure on inspiration, and increased with expiration. It may be present with constrictive pericarditis, pericarditis, and severe chronic obstructive pulmonary disease.

   ▶ Absent, weak, normal, or bounding pulses: A bounding pulse may indicate increased cardiac output while a diminished or absent pulse may indicate decreased cardiac output or an occlusion.

   ▶ Carotid, radial, femoral, popliteal, post-tibial, and pedal pulses: commonly assessed by the critical care nurse. Carotid pulse: should be visualized for pulsations, palpated for thrills, and auscultated for bruits. While inspecting the neck assess for jugular venous distention.

f. Assess the heart by inspecting the chest for pulsations and palpate for thrills. The area for ausculation include: (Fig. 4-1)

   ▶ **Aortic: located right sternal border, 2nd intercostal space**

   ▶ **Pulmonary: located at the left sternal border, 2nd intercostal space**

   ▶ **Mitral: located at the left sternal border, 5th intercostal space**

   ▶ **Erbs Point: located at left sternal border, 3rd intercostal space**

   ▶ **Tricuspid: located at 4th intercostal space midclavicular line**

   ▶ **Apical: located at the 5th intercostal space midclavicular line**

g. Auscultate in all of the above areas for abnormal heart sounds (Display 4-2)

h. Auscultate for presence and type of murmurs (Display 4-3):

   ▶ Timing of the murmur, whether it occurs in systole or diastole. Systolic murmur is heard between S1 & S2. It may occur early, mid, or late in systole, or throughout

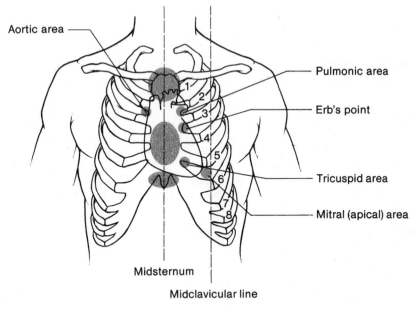

Aortic area

Pulmonic area

Erb's point

Tricuspid area

Mitral (apical) area

Midsternum

Midclavicular line

FIGURE 4-1.
Areas of the precordium to be assessed when evaluating heart function.

systole (pansystolic). Diastolic murmur is heard between S2 and S1 and may be early, mid, or late in diastole.
- ▶ Location of the murmur including the area where the murmur is heard the loudest
- ▶ Radiation of the murmur or the path that the sound of the murmur travels, (neck, axilla, sternal border)

B. Laboratory studies and diagnostic tests
1. Important laboratory data should include:
    a. Myocardial enzyme analysis including isoenzymes
    b. Complete blood count and sedimentation rate
    c. Arterial blood gases
    d. Serum electrolytes, myoglobin, lipid profile
    e. Coagulation studies
2. Noninvasive diagnostic testing for the cardiac patient allows for evaluation without invasive processing.
    a. An Echocardiogram uses ultrasonic sound waves transmitted to the heart via a transducer. Sound waves from cardiac structures are reflected back to the transducer and are converted to an electric signal and recorded on a strip recorder or a video tape.
    b. Magnetic resonance imaging (MRI) allows for visualization of cardiac structures and assesses tissue perfusion and blood flow in the proximal coronary arteries.
    c. Chest x-ray is indicated as a baseline assessment and in evaluating treatment.

DISPLAY 4-2.
HEART SOUNDS

Normal heart sounds

S1 = closure of the AV valves (tricuspid and mitral). Heard loudest over the tricuspid and mitral areas.

S2 = closure of the semilunar valves (pulmonic and aortic). Heard loudest over the aortic area.

Gallops

S3 = may be normal in young adults to age 40; over age 40 is considered pathological and may indicate ventricular overload as in mitral, aortic, or tricuspid regurgitation. It is heard just after S2, early in diastole and may sound similar to "Ken-tuck-y."

S4 = always abnormal, usually associated with increased resistance to ventricular filling, such as with congestive heart failure, coronary artery disease, and aortic stenosis. It is heard in late diastole, just before S1, and may sound similar to "Ten-ne-see."

Splitting

Physiologic: A slight delay of the closure of the right-sided valves. Heard on inspiration, usually due to increased blood return to the heart, causing prolonged ventricular ejection.

Wide splitting: Heard without relationship to the respiratory cycle. May signify pulmonary stenosis, right bundle branch block, right ventricular failure, or an atrial septal defect.

Paradoxical splitting: In contrast to physiological splitting, the paradoxical split is silent on inspiration and heard on expiration. It is usually present with left bundle branch block (due to a delay in the closure of the aortic valve).

Other

Ejection clicks: heard in early systole, may signify aortic valve dysfunction.

Opening snaps: Heard in early diastole, associated with stenosis of the AV valves.

Pericardial friction rub: A harsh, scraping sound heard when the layers of the heart rub together due to an inflammatory process. Easily heard throughout the cardiac cycle in the lower sternum and apical areas.

DISPLAY 4-3.
Etiology and Intensity of Murmurs

Etiology

- ► Stenosis: High pressure blood flow through a narrow opening
- ► Regurgitation: Backward blood flow due to incompetent valves
- ► Septal defects: Blood forced from high pressure area (left heart) to lower pressure area (right heart) due to an abnormal opening
- ► Increased force of blood flow through normal structures, such as with tachycardia

Classification of Intensity

- ► Grade I: Very difficult to hear, no thrill
- ► Grade II: Quiet but easily heard, no thrill
- ► Grade III: Fairly loud, no thrill
- ► Grade IV: Loud, possible thrill
- ► Grade V: Very loud even with stethoscope partly off chest, positive thrill
- ► Grade VI: Easily heard with stethoscope completely off chest, positive thrill

3. Invasive diagnostic testing may also be utilized for the cardiac patient but involves some risk secondary to the invasive nature.

    a. Transesophageal echocardiography (TEE) is an invasive technique where a miniature 2D transducer-tipped flexible endoscope is introduced into the esophagus to allow for visualization of the cardiac structures.

    b. Thallium imaging involves the IV administration of an isotope. Update is present in normal cardiac tissue, but is diminished in ischemic and/or infarcted cells. These are picked up by a gamma camera.

    c. Technetium-99m pyrophosphate (PYP) detects the accumulation of isotope in areas of necrotic tissue and not in normal myocardial tissue.

    d. **Indium-111 antimyson is a new diagnostic imaging test which is able to distinguish old from new infarcts. Indium-111 antimyson antibodies bind to necrotic myocytes making this test more sensitive in diagnosing Q wave versus non–Q wave MIs.**

    e. Positron emission tomography (PET) is a radionuclide imaging technique which quantifies metabolism and blood flow of the myocardium.

    f. **Multiple-gated acquisition scan (MUGA) or blood pool imaging is able to distinguish between anterior and inferior infarctions and determines multiple pathologic dysfunctions in cardiac performance.**

    g. Cardiac catheterization includes all processes whereby a catheter is threaded into the heart and a dye is introduced in order to identify the cause and severity of cardiac disease. These may include coronary angiography, ventriculography, and right and left catheterization.

C. Hemodynamic Monitoring

1. Swan Ganz catheters are invasive lines fed into a central vein, through the right of the heart and into the pulmonary artery (see Figures 4-2 and 4-3). Its placement allows for measuring pressures such as:

    a. Central venous pressure (CVP) is a measurement taken from the right atrium and represents the amount of blood return to the right atrium (preload). Readings may be used to guide volume replacement therapy.

       ▶ **Normal pressures range from 0–6 mm Hg.**

       ▶ Consists of three positive waves, A, C and V followed by three negative waves: X, X1, and Y (Fig. 4-4).

       ▶ The A wave represents atrial contraction, the C wave represents tricuspid valve closure, and the V wave indicates atrial filling.

       ▶ Common causes of elevated waveforms are ventricular failure, pulmonary hypertension or stenosis, tricuspid regurgitation, hypervolemia, cardiac tamponade, and constrictive pericarditis.

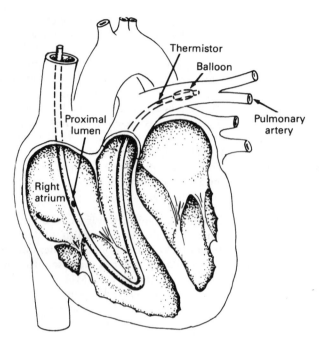

FIGURE 4-2.
Placement of the Swan Ganz catheter.

  b. **Right ventricular pressure (RVP) is measured directly only during the insertion of the Swan Ganz catheter.**

▶ Normal RV systolic is 20–30 mm Hg and RV diastolic is 0–5 mm Hg.

▶ In the absence of disease RV systolic and PA systolic pressures should be equal.

▶ Causes for RV pressure abnormalities include pulmonary hypertension, ventricular septal defects, pulmonic stenosis, right ventricular failure, cardiac tamponade, and constrictive pericarditis.

c. Pulmonary artery pressures (PAP) measure the pressure in the pulmonary artery and allow for interpretation of left-sided ventricular filling and function.

▶ Normal PA pressures are systolic of 20–30 mm Hg and diastolic of 8–12 mmg Hg. Mean PAP is 10–20 mmg Hg.

▶ Common causes of decreased PA pressures include hypovolemia. Causes of increased PA pressures include pulmonary disease, hypertension, mitral valve disease, left ventricular hypertrophy and tachycardia of greater than 120 bpm.

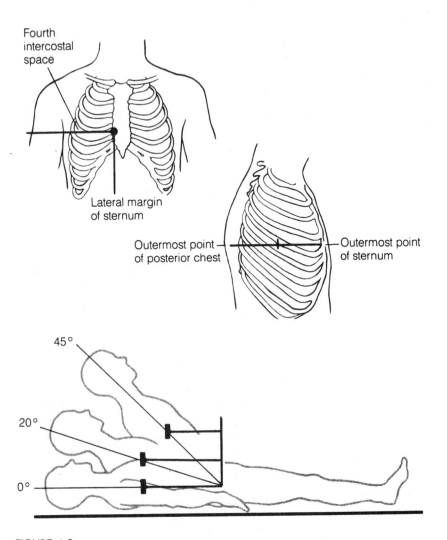

FIGURE 4-3.
To ensure accuracy with invasive lines, the zero mark on the transducer/manometer must be level with the phlebostatic axis. Wrap an imaginary line around the chest at the level where the fourth intercostal meets the sternum and fourth intercept it at the midaxillary line between the anterior and posterior chest walls to locate the phlebostatic axis.

    d.   Pulmonary artery capillary wedge pressures (PCWP)

        ▸ A balloon at the tip of the Swan Ganz catheter is inflated enough to occlude blood flow to a branch of the pulmonary artery. The pressures beyond the balloon are measured and represent retrograde pressures from the left atrium and the left ventricle at the end of diastole (LVEDP)—reflecting preload of the left side of the heart.

        ▸ **PCWP is an accurate indicator of the pump function of the left ventricle.**

Waveforms
Right Atrial Pressure

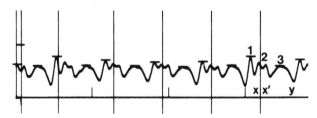

FIGURE 4-4.
Right atrial pressure waveform: 1) *a* wave, 2) *c* wave, 3) *v* wave.

- ► **Normal PCWP is 8–12 mm Hg**
- ► **Elevated PCWP pressures are usually indicative of pulmonary congestion. They may be falsely elevated if the patient is on PEEP or CPAP or if the catheter tip is not in the correct place.**
- ► Monitor tracing has three positive waves, A, C, and V. The A wave represents left atrial contraction and the C wave represents mitral valve closure. The V wave represents left atrial filling pressures (Fig. 4-5).
- ► Common causes of elevated PAWP waveforms: increased resistance to ventricular filling as with mitral stenosis of left ventricular failure, mitral valve regurgitation, and ruptured papillary muscle. May also be elevated with hypervolemia, cardiac tamponade, or constrictive pericarditis.

 e.   **Cardiac output (CO) is the volume of blood that is ejected from the left ventricle per minute. It is dependent on the amount of blood ejected with each beat (stroke volume) and the heart rate**

Pulmonary Artery Pressure

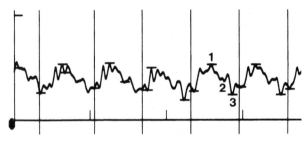

FIGURE 4-5.
Pulmonary artery pressure waveform: 1) systolic pressure, 2) dicrotic notch, 3) diastolic pressure.

▸ **Normal CO is 4–8 liters/minute**

- ▸ May be affected by preload, afterload, and contractility of the left ventricle.
- ▸ Cardiac output may be altered by a variety of factors including dysrhythmias, alterations in volume status, valvular stenosis, coronary artery disease, cardiomyopathy, cardiac tamponade, or pharmacologic intervention.

 f. **Cardiac index (CI) is a more accurate measure of cardiac output. It divides the cardiac output by the patient's BSA.**

- ▸ Normal CI for an adult is 2.5–4.0 L/min
- ▸ The formula for calculating CI = CO/BSA

g. Saturation of venous oxygenation (SVO_2) is a measurement of the percentage of oxygen in the blood returned from the pulmonary artery. This is the amount of oxygen remaining after the tissues have taken the oxygen they need.

- ▸ Normal SVO_2 is 60–80%
- ▸ SVO_2 gives information on tissue oxygenation and the balance between oxygen supply and tissue demand.
- ▸ SVO_2 is affected by Cardiac output, arterial oxygenation, and hemoglobin (HGB).
- ▸ Common causes of abnormal SVO_2 include altered cardiac output and altered tissue demand as in fevers, high or low metabolic states and sepsis.

2. Transvenous pacemaker (see Chapter 5)
3. Arterial lines (A-lines) are placed in peripheral arteries, usually the radial or brachial, for the purpose of a continuous, accurate blood pressure reading. They also allow for withdrawal of arterial blood for blood gases and laboratory testing.

 a. **Arterial systolic pressure is a reflection of the pressure created by the left ventricle vs. the compliance of the large arteries or peripheral vascular resistance (PVR).**

 b. **Diastolic pressure represents the pressure in the arterial system during the resting phase of the cardiac cycle. It is largely determined by compliance (elasticity) of the arterial system.**

c. Systole is indicated by a sloping positive wave on the arterial line tracing. The dicrotic notch signifies the beginning of diastole with closure of the aortic valve (Fig. 4-6).
d. Normal arterial pressures are systolic 100–140 mmg Hg, diastolic 60–80 mm Hg; mean (MAP) 60–90 mmg Hg.
e. Causes of low blood pressure (hypotension) include volume loss, increased heart rate, action of catecholamines, vasodilation, dysrhythmias sepsis, or pharmacologic effect.
f. Causes of elevated blood pressure (hypertension) include arteriosclerosis, volume overload, aortic regurgitation and essential hypertension.

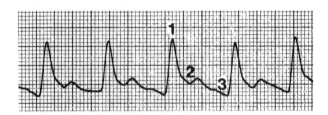

FIGURE 4-6.
A normal arterial waveform has three components: 1) systolic peak, 2) dicrotic notch, and 3) end-diastole.

     g.   Mean arterial blood pressure (MAP) is the average pressure in the arterial system. It is calculated by the following formula: $MAP = CO \times SVR$ or $MAP = SBP + 2(DBP)/3$

D.   Nutritional considerations
1. Prolonged heart failure can lead to a specific form of protein and calorie malnutrition known as cardiac cachexia.
2. It can be seen in patients with long-standing valvular heart disease or in patients with end-stage cardiomyopathy.
3. The pathogenesis has been described as secondary to congestive heart failure in conjunction with tissue hypoxia, anorexia, and hypermetabolism with resultant wasting of muscle protein and adipose tissue. Excessive protein requirements have been demonstrated with such patients.
4. Protein and calorie malnutrition can lead to both structural and functional myocardial impairment.
5. Malnutrition can lead to decreased baseline performance and the inability of the heart to respond to increased metabolic demands.
6. Blood pressure, heart rate, blood volume, and oxygen demand decrease in malnourished states and a hypoadrenergic state in the fasting individual can result in bradycardia.
7. Malnutrition has been demonstrated to be a significant risk for patients undergoing cardiac surgery.
8. Morbidity and mortality are greater in cachectic patients than in normally nourished patients.
9. Respiratory failure, pneumonia, renal failure and sternal wound complications are more frequent in malnourished patients.
10. Postoperative complications including ventricular arrhythmias and pulmonary infection further increase morbidity and mortality.
11. Considerations for medical nutrition therapy
    a.   The overall goal is to increase the nutrient intake to achieve caloric balance and meet intake needs.
    b.   Nutritional repletion to prevent loss of myocardial mass and function
    c.   Fluid intake is usually limited to 1 to 1.5 liters per day
    d.   When the patient is able to eat by mouth, advance the diet as tolerated to one that is limited in sodium, cholesterol, and fat.

E. **Psychosocial implications**

    1. Patients with cardiovascular disease often experience coping difficulties related to the disease process. They may experience:

        a. Anxiety related to stress, and present health status

        b. Altered coping related to pain and fear of illness

        c. Fear of death

    2. Patients may also experience altered health maintenance related to knowledge deficit of disease process, changes in lifestyle, treatment regimen, and cardiac rehabilitation

    3. There is a high risk for self-esteem disturbance related to perceived or actual role change,and loss of control of self-care activities

    4. There is also a high risk for grieving related to possible changes in family role and previous social lifestyle

F. **Medications used to treat cardiovascular disorders (Table 4-1)**

III. **Acute myocardial infarction (AMI)**

A. Description: a deficit in two oxygenation factors; supply and demand, which results in myocardial damage. The demand of oxygen by the myocardial tissue is not compensated by the perfusion of oxygenated blood necessary to sustain adequate coronary circulation to the tissue distal to the occlusion. There are various categories of AMI:

    1. Transmural (AKA Q-wave MI)

        a. **Entire thickness of all layers of the myocardium in a specific region is affected.**

        b. **These infarcts are also known as Q-wave infarcts because of the presence of Q-waves in specific leads on the ECG tracings. Because the majority of MIs affect the left ventricle, this type of infarct can compromise the efficacy of the pump.**

    2. Nontransmural (AKA non–Q wave, subendocardial)

        a. **Necrosis commonly affects the inner layers of the endocardium and are referred to as subendocardial infarcts.**

        b. On ECG tracings, there is a significant absence of a Q-wave.

        c. S-T segment elevation and or depression are characteristic findings.

        d. T-wave inversion may be seen.

        e. This type is known as non–Q wave infarcts.

    3. **Both types of infarcts can cause serious damage to the cardiac muscle and are treated aggressively. The location and size of both types dictate the degree of myocardial impairment.**

B. **Etiology and incidence**

    1. Most common cause of AMIs are deposits of atherosclerotic plaques in the coronary arteries.

    2. Atherosclerosis can trigger a coronary artery spasm with a resultant decrease in or complete blockage of blood flow.

text continued on page 103
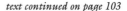

TABLE 4-1.
Medications Commonly Used in an ICU to Treat Cardiovascular Problems

DRUG CLASS	EXAMPLE	MECHANISM OF ACTION	COMMON CONTRAINDICATIONS	COMMON DRUG INTERACTIONS	NURSING IMPLICATIONS
Beta Adrenergic Blockers (Class II Antiarrhythmics)	**Nadolol:** 40–320 mg daily Maximum dose 640 mg/24 hours Propranolol: IV 1–3 mg, repeat in 2 minutes if necessary; PO 10–30 mg 3–4 times daily	↓Response to adrenergic stimuli by competitive inhibition = delayed impulse conduction through the sa and av nodes = ↓heart rate & ↓BP = ↓myocardial O_2 consumption.	Bradycardia, hypotension bronchial asthma	Antihypertensives, cardiac glycosides, epinephrine, indomethacin, hypoglycemic agents/insulin	If **apical rate** <60, hold drug and notify physician Monitor for hypotension **Abrupt withdrawal of drug may exacerbate angina** May mask symptoms of hypoglycemia
Beta Adrenergic Blockers (Class III Antiarrhythmics)	**Amiodarone** (Cordarone) For SVT and VT (refractory to other treatments) 5–10 mg/kg loading then 10 mg/kg/day for 3–5 days	↑Refractory period and ↓repolarization = ↓heart rate	Bradycardia, cardiomegaly, depressed ventricular function	Class I antiarrythmics, antihypertensives, Coumadin, dilantin, digitalis glycosides, calcium channel blockers, beta blockers	Monitor for pulmonary toxicity (dyspnea, dry cough, pleural chest pain), **CHF,** electrolyte imbalances, **thyroid function** and liver abnormalities. Patient must be on a continuous ECG. Monitor for hypotension and bradycardia.
Calcium Channel Blockers	**Verapamil:** For SVT: 5–10 mg IV push over 2 minutes, may repeat in 30 minutes Angina or A-FIB: 80 mg 3–4 times/day Maximum dose 480 mg over 24 hours **Nifedipine** Procardia: 10–20 mg TID	Inhibits calcium ions from crossing cell membranes into cardiovascular and smooth muscle cells = ↓contractility of cardiovascular and smooth muscle = ↓O_2 consumption. ↑Dilatation of systemic arteries = ↓blood pressure and afterload	Hypotension, **2nd or 3rd degree heart block, sick sinus syndrome,** bradycardia, caution with CHF	Digoxin, furosemide, beta blockers, cimetidine, cyclosporine, quinidine	If apical rate <60, systolic BP <90, or diastolic BP <60, hold dose and notify physician

	Action	Dosage	Contraindications/Cautions	Interactions	Nursing Considerations
Antiarrhythmic		Maximum daily dose 180 mg Diltiazem (Cardizem) For SVT/rapid A-FIB: 0.25 mg/kg over 2 min. then IV drip at 5–10 mg/hr. Max. 15 mg/hr. No longer than 24 hrs. For angina or HTN: 30 mg TID or QID Maximum dose 360 mg/day or 120–180 mg Dual release capsule. Maximum dose 480 mg/day			Continuous ECG, observe for heart block (may be transient), observe for shortness of breath and chest tightness monitor for hypotension
Antiarrhythmic	Acts directly on the AV node to ↓conduction and inhibit re-entry pathways, making it especially useful with treating Wolff-Parkinson-White Syndrome	Adenosine (Adenocard) For PSVT: 6 mg rapid IVP (1–2 seconds) If no response in 2 minutes, 12 mg rapid IVP If no response in 2 minutes, repeat 12 mg rapid IVP	A-Flutter, A-FIB, VT, 2nd or 3rd degree heart block. Sick sinus syndrome. Caution with asthma (causes bronchoconstriction)	Carbamazepine, dipyridamole, methylxanthines	
Antiarrhythmic Agents (Sodium Channel Blocking Agents) Class I.B.	↓Excitability of myocardial tissue by suppressing the influx of sodium during depolarization = stabilization of the myocardial cell membranes	**Lidocaine** *Loading dose:* 1–1.5 mg/kg IV (no faster than 25–50 mg/min.) q 3–5 min. until arrhythmia stops—no more than 300 mg in 1 hour. *Maintenance:* 20–50 mg/kg/min (1–4 mg/min). Maximum dose is 4 mg/min.	**2nd or 3rd degree heart block,** caution with bundle branch block, bradycardia, renal or hepatic insufficiency, CHF	Amiodarone, anticholinergics, cimetidine, neuromuscular blocking agents, anticholinesterase agents, other antiarrhythmic agents, digoxin	Infusion pump for IV use. **Monitor for prolonged Q-T intervals, widening QRS complex, heart blocks, and increased arrhythmias. If these occur, stop drip and notify physician.** Monitor for hypotension, dizziness, bradycardia, V-FIB, seizure activity.

(continued)

TABLE 4-1. (continued)

DRUG CLASS	EXAMPLE	MECHANISM OF ACTION	COMMON CONTRAINDICATIONS	COMMON DRUG INTERACTIONS	NURSING IMPLICATIONS
Class I.A.	**Procainamide** *Loading dose:* 100 mg every 5 min. IV (no faster than 25–50 mg/min) until arrhythmia converts, up to 1 g. *Maintenance:* 2–6 mg/min **Quinidine** Dose varies with brand. Maximum dose of quinidine sulfate is 3–4 g over 24 hours				Monitor electrolytes and renal function. Dizziness or seizure activity may be the first signs of lidocaine toxicity. **Normal levels of lidocaine are 2–5 mcg/mL. QUINIDINE TOXICITY OCCURS WITH LEVELS >8 mcg/mL.** Monitor NAPA levels for patients taking procainamide.
Anticoagulants	**Heparin** IV: Bolus 5000–7500 units followed by 8000–12,000 units/hr drip. Titrated according to ptt. SC: 5000 units every 12 hours	Prevents the conversion of fibrinogen to fibrin, thereby preventing the extension of an existing clot = ↓ size of infarct. Also used to prevent clotting in high-risk patients.	Active bleeding, intracranial hemorrhage, hemophilia, uncontrolled hypertension	Oral anticoagulants, salicylates, thrombolytics	*Antidote:* **Protamine sulfate** Monitor PTT and INR. PTT values are therapeutic at 1.5–2 times the control levels. **Inactivated by many antibiotics when given through same line.**
Anticoagulants	**Warfarin** (Coumadin) *Loading:* 10–15 mg daily PO for 3 days, based on PT. *Maintenance:* 2–10 mg daily PO based on PT	↓ Clotting factors by ↓ vitamin K in the liver through competitive inhibition. Largely used to prevent emboli associated with MI, prosthetic heart valves, atrial fibrillation, and rheumatic heart disease.	Vitamin K deficiency, bleeding disorders, uncontrolled hypertension	**Many drug interactions** including but not limited to acetaminophen, sulfonylureas, barbiturates, amiodarone, cimetidine, ciprofloxacin	*Antidote:* **Vitamin K** Monitor PT and INR; PT level is therapeutic when it is 1.5–2 times the control.
Antiplatelet Agents	**Aspirin:** 80–325 mg/day PO	Inhibition of platelet aggregation = prolonged bleed-	Active bleeding, bleeding disorders, GI ulcers, liver	Varies greatly with individual drug	Monitor bleeding time, CBC WBC, LFT's

Dipyridamole (Persantine): 75–100 mg PO QID (prosthetic heart valves) or 200–400 mg BID (TIAs) Ticlopidine hydrochloride (Ticlid): 250 mg PO BID	ing time. Used in cardiovascular patients at risk for clotting in patients at risk for strokes or developing emboli in the coronary arteries, valves of the heart, or heart chambers.	impairment, intracranial bleeding, ematopoietic disorders		Maintain bleeding precautions
Angiotensin-Converting Enzymes (ACE) Inhibitors Captopril (Capoten): 6.25–50 mg BID or TID. **Maximum dose 450 mg/day** Enalapril (Vasotec): PO: 10–40 mg/day IV: 1.25 mg given over 5 minutes every 6 hours	Inhibition of the angiotensin-converting enzyme = prevention of conversion of angiotensin I to angiotensin II = ↓ BP	Pregnancy. Caution with impaired renal disease and autoimmune disorders.	Digitalis glycosides, antacids, hypoglycemic agents/insulin, NSAIDs, potassium supplements, potassium-sparing diuretics, lithium	Monitor kidney function, WBC's, and electrolytes **Angioedema may occur even with 1st dose; watch for edema and difficulty breathing; have epinephrine at the bedside**
Catecholamines Epinephrine: Initial dose for cardiac arrest 0.5–1 mg IV or 1.5–3 mg via ETT. Maintain drip at 1–4 mcg/min. Titrate to BP.	Stimulation of alpha and beta adrenergic receptors = vasoconstriction and ↑ heart contractility and ↑ heart rate, and bronchodilation.	Hypertension, pheochromocytoma. Caution with heart failure, angina, and hyperthyroidism.	Digitalis glycosides, antacids, hypoglycemic agents/insulin, NSAIDs, potassium supplements, potassium-sparing diuretics, lithium	Monitor ECG, B/P, and heart rate. May cause **tachycardia,** nervousness tremors, palpitations, headache, hyperglycemia, **V-FIB,** CVA, **hypertension**
Catecholamines Norepinephrine (Levophed): Initial dose 8–12 mcg/min. Maintenance dose 2–4 mcg/min, titrated to BP	Stimulation of the alpha and B1-adrenergic receptors, but no effects on B2-adrenergic receptors = ↑ stroke volume and coronary artery blood flow but no ↑ cardiac output due to an in ↑ in peripheral resistance. ↑ BP = ↑ blood flow to the major organs including the kidneys = ↑ urine output.	Hypovolemic and cardiogenic shock (because potent vasoconstriction is already occurring) pregnancy, hypoxia, and hypovolemia secondary to fluid deficit. Caution with hypertension and hyperthyroidism.	MAO inhibitors, ergot alkaloids, alpha adrenergics, methyldopa, atropine, tricyclic antidepressants, guanethidine, and certain general anesthesics	Monitor for bradycardia, hypertension, **V-FIB,V-tach, complete heart block, and decreased cardiac output.** In case of tissue infiltration, phentolamine 5–10 mg/10–15 ml normal saline injected into affected tissue should prevent hypoxic necrosis. **Drip must be weaned**

(continued)

TABLE 4-1. (continued)

DRUG CLASS	EXAMPLE	MECHANISM OF ACTION	COMMON CONTRAINDICATIONS	COMMON DRUG INTERACTIONS	NURSING IMPLICATIONS
					down to prevent sudden drops in blood pressure.
Catecholamines	**Dobutamine** (Dobutrex): 2.5–10 mcg/kg/min titrated to BP. Maximum dose is 40 mcg/kg/min.	Stimulation of the B1-adrenergic receptors = ↑ cardiac contractility = ↑ stroke volume = ↑ cardiac output	Idiopathic hypertrophic subaortic stenosis	Beta blockers, general anesthesia	Monitor patient for hypertension, tachycardia, chest pain, premature ventricular contractions (PVCs). Monitor cardiac output, pulmonary artery pressures, ECG. **Correct hypovolemia before treating with Dobutrex.** Patients with atrial fibrillation should be digitalized before Dobutrex therapy to prevent ventricular tachycardia.
	Dopamine (the physiologic precursor of norepinephrine) 0.5–2.0 mcg/kg/min for renal dose >2.0 mcg/kg/min. titrated to BP. Maximum dose is 50 mcg/kg/min.	Stimulation of the dopaminergic B1-adrenergic receptors; in low doses (<2 mcg/kg/min), dilate the renal arteries = ↑ urine output In higher doses (2–10 mcg/kg/min) ↑ vasoconstriction = ↑ blood pressure and cardiac output	Tachyarrhythmias, V-FIB, pheochromocytoma. Caution with occlusive vascular disease, arterial embolism, diabetic endarteritis	Beta blockers, ergot alkaloids, MAO inhibitors, phenytoin, inhalational anesthetics, alkalotic solutions	Monitor ECG for ectopy, tachycardia, bradycardia, and widening of the QRS complex. Monitor IV site for tissue infiltration. **May cause necrosis.** A central line is recommended. If extravasation occurs injection of 5–10 mg. Phentolamine/10–15 mL normal saline into the area may be necessary. Do not discontinue suddenly, taper to prevent severe hypotension.

	Drug/Dose	Action	Contraindications/Cautions	Interactions	Nursing Considerations
Inotropic agents	**Digoxin:** *Loading dose* 0.5–1 mg IV or PO in divided doses over 24 hours. *Maintenance* 0.125–0.5 mg IV or PO daily. IV doses given over 5 minutes	↑ Influx of calcium across the myocardial cells = ↑ force of contraction = ↑ pumping efficiency of the heart = more complete emptying of the chambers = ↑ cardiac output = ↑ perfusion to all organs, including the kidneys = ↑ diuresis.	Digitalis toxicity, V-FIB, V-tach unless caused by CHF, incomplete AV block, bradycardia. Caution with renal insufficiency, hypothyroidism.	**Many drug interactions including but not limited to** quinidine, Verapamil, nifedipine, diltiazem, amiodarone, calcium, thiazides, anticholinergics, diuretics, amiloride, amphotericin B	**Do not give calcium salts to digitalized patients; it may cause serious arrhythmias.** Monitor for signs of toxicity including nausea, blurred vision, yellow-green halos around lights, fatigue, hallucinations. Hypokalemia and hypomagnesemia predispose to digoxin toxicity. Monitor electrolytes. If apical rate is <60, hold drug and notify physician. Normal digoxin levels are 0.5–2.0 ng/mL.
	Amrinone lactate (Inocor): *Initial dose* 0.75 mg/kg given over 2–3 min. IV. *Maintenance* 5–10 mcg/kg/min. Maximum dose 10 mg/kg/24 hours	↑Cellular levels of cyclic adenosine monophosphate = ↑contractility, also relaxes smooth vascular muscle, providing vasodilation = ↓BP	Severe aortic or pulmonic valvular disease. Caution with acute myocardial infarction.	Digitalis glycosides (additive effect), disopyramide. **Do not mix with furosimide, it causes a precipitate. Do not mix in dextrose, chemical reaction occurs.**	Monitor for arrhythmias, hypotension, thrombocytopenia, hepatotoxicity. Also monitor cardiac output, pulmonary artery pressures, and heart rate. Effects last up until 2 hours after drip is discontinued.
Diuretics	**Loop:** **Bumetanide** (Bumex): 0.5–2 mg, IV or PO 1–3 times a day. Maximum dose is 10 mg/24 hours. **Furosemide** (Lasix): 20–160 mg daily in two divided doses, when given IV, **give no more than 40 mg/min**	Inhibition of sodium and chloride reabsorption in the kidney = ↑excretion of water = ↓fluid volume returning to the heart (preload) = ↓fluid backup from the left ventricle to the lungs = ↓pulmonary edema	Anuria, caution with hepatic coma, electrolyte imbalances	Aminoglycosides, antihypertensives, chloral hydrate, NSAIDs, clofibrate, hypoglycemic agents, cholestyramine	Replace electrolyte losses (especially potassium) before giving diuretic. Monitor all electrolytes, I and O, hearing, and renal function. Do not give by rapid IV push. **1 mg of Bumex is equivalent to 40 mg of Lasix. ↑ Risk of digoxin toxicity may occur due**

(continued)

TABLE 4-1. (continued)

DRUG CLASS	EXAMPLE	MECHANISM OF ACTION	COMMON CONTRAINDICATIONS	COMMON DRUG INTERACTIONS	NURSING IMPLICATIONS
	Maximum daily dose 600 mg. **Hydrochlorothiazide** 25–100 mg PO daily according to BP				**to low potassium levels:** monitor patient for digoxin toxicity.
Nitrates	**Nitroglycerine** (NTG): IV drip is started at 5 mcg/min and increased by 5 mcg/min every 3–5 minutes.	Relaxation of vascular smooth muscle. Vasodilation = ↓ peripheral resistance for the heart to pump against and ↓ BP, = ↓ workload of heart and ↓ myocardial O₂ consumption = ↓ ischemia	Hypotension, head trauma	Antihypertensives	Headache may develop, relief with aspirin or acetaminophen. **When given IV mix in glass bottles, binds to plastic.** Do not suddenly discontinue IV drip; wean 5–10 mcg/min. every 15 minutes; effects will last up to 1 hour after drip is off.
Opiates	**Morphine sulfate** (MSO₄): Doses vary with route, solution, and purpose of drug	Pain relief by interfering with CNS receptors; **anxiety is also controlled = ↓ heart rate, blood pressure and O₂ consumption**	Respiratory rate <12, hypotension, concomitant CNS depressant or alcohol use, general anesthesia	Alcohol, CNS depressants	***Antidote: Narcan (Naloxone).*** Ambu bag at bedside.

3. Tissue damage from an injured vessel can trigger platelet aggregation which can cause a complete arterial occlusion.

4. Any profound disproportion between supply and demand of blood to the coronary arteries; eg, trauma, luminal narrowing, coronary emboli, coronary artery bypass graft, coronary arteriography, congenital anomalies, myocardial contusion, and cocaine abuse can contribute to an AMI.

5. Acute MI is the leading cause of death in America. One out of four deaths is caused by a myocardial infarction. Approximately one-half million fall victim to this cardiac crisis, with an increasing incidence in the female population.

C. **Pathophysiology**

1. Ischemic changes are reversible when normal blood flow is re-established.

2. Sustained regional ischemia beyond twenty minutes to several hours can cause irreversible cellular death and eventual necrosis to the myocardium distal to the cellular injury.

3. A result of decreased oxygenated blood to myocardial cell results in a decrease ATP (adenosine triphospate) and a rapid shift to anaerobic metabolism and lactic acid accumulation leads to acidosis. This acidotic state increases the vulnerability of the myocardium to conduction disorder, decreases contractility, and eventually decreases cardiac output.

4. To compensate for obstructed blood flow, endogenous vasoactive substances in the endothelium produce a vasodilation effect. In a diseased heart, this regulating mechanism is impaired and an opposite vasoconstricting effect occurs.

5. The concomitant tissue damage and necrosis arising in the endocardium can potentially extend to the epicardium.

6. The type and size of the infarct determines the contractual effectiveness of the cardiac muscle, thus affecting the efficiency of the pump.

D. **Assessment findings**

1. **Chest pain is the classic symptom presented by the majority of patients with an acute myocardial infarct. The pain is sudden, severe and may be intolerable to some patients. Pain assessment (PQRST) should include evaluation of the following factors:**
   a. P = Provocation/Palliative
   b. Q = Quality/Quantity
   c. R = Region/Radiation
   d. S = Severity/Scale
   e. T = Timing

2. Skin appears cold, clammy, diaphoretic with a pale or ashen color

3. Sensations of indigestion and/or bloating and nausea and vomiting may occur. Nausea and vomiting is mostly associated with an inferior MI.

4. **Dyspnea with or without crackles indicates AMI with left ventricular failure.**

5. Irregular heart rate with tachycardia and hypertension may be associated with an AMI. This results from sympathetic stimulation response or parasympathetic overactivity with resultant bradycardia and hypotension.

 6. **Syncope, or light-headedness, indicates decreased cardiac output in conjunction with a compromised cerebral circulation.**

7. Patients may feel confused, anxious, restless, weak, fatigued, apprehensive, and have a feeling of impending doom.

8. Jugular vein distention indicates right ventricular infarct with pulmonary congestion.

9. Abnormal heart sounds: S4 gallop, may include an S3 gallop, splitting of heart sounds, and a systolic murmur.

10. Vital signs
   a. Initially, there is often increased blood pressure and pulse, and irregular respirations resulting from the vasomotor response to pain.
   b. Later on, decreased cardiac output and vasodilatation results in hypotension, tachycardia with continued tachypnea, and shallow respirations

11. A delayed fever, an indirect measure of tissue necrosis, appears 24 to 48 hours after infarction, lasting approximately 1 week.

12. ECG changes are often indicative of AMI.
   a. ECG is the primary diagnostic criterion for acute and myocardial infarction diagnosis.
   b. The site of an MI corresponds with characteristic changes reflected by the leads facing the infarcted heart surface. Reciprocal changes occur in leads opposite the infarcted surface.

    c. **T-wave inversions = ischemia (temporarily decreased blood supply)**

   d. **Possible S-T segment depression/S-T segment elevation = injury (prolonged interruption of blood supply)**

   e. **Q-waves = infarction (perfusion failure causing necrosis)**

13. Laboratory data
   a. An elevated CK, CK-MB within eight hours after onset of symptoms is indicative of AMI. The ratio of MB 2 to MB 1 (subforms of CK-MB) is being studied as a more efficient and rapid diagnosis of AMI.
   b. The LDH, LDH1/LDH2 ratio, "flipped LDH," rises within 48 hours after onset.

   c. **Cardiac troponin-T (cTNT) and cardiac troponin-I (cTNI) levels are detected in the serum within six hours of AMI. The subforms of the protein troponin are specific to cardiac muscle.**

   d. White blood cell count is normal at onset of chest pain. Leukocytosis occurs within approximately two hours in response to a high fever from myocardial necrosis.

      e. Sedimentation rate is normal at onset of chest pain, rises within one week and remains elevated for a month or longer after infarct.

      f. Hematocrit is elevated due to hemoconcentration. Normal values are seen within one week.

      g. Arterial blood gases show a rise in pH in response to stress.

       h. **Serum electrolytes, especially potassium level, should be assessed.**

      i. An elevation in myoglobin reflects tissue breakdown. Recent studies indicate usefulness as an indicator of reperfusion post–thrombolytic therapy with a return to normal within 24 hours.

E. Nursing Diagnoses

    1. Pain

    2. Decreased Cardiac Output

    3. Impaired Gas Exchange

    4. Risk for Activity Intolerance

    5. Altered Tissue Perfusion: Cardiopulmonary

    6. Constipation

F. Planning and implementation

    1. Assess presence and degree of pain and chest discomfort

      a. Instruct patient to immediately notify the staff of any chest pain.

      b. Observe for nonverbal cues of pain.

      c. Assess pain history using the PQRST assessment parameter.

      d. Assess and record the degree of pain relief using the scale of 1 to 10.

     2. **Promote interventions toward relief of pain.**

      a. Administer pain medication per physician's order.

      b. Remain with patient until discomfort/pain is relieved.

      c. Administer opiate analgesics as ordered. Morphine sulfate is the drug of choice for acute cardiac pain relief. It is usually given IV and may lower blood pressure and heart rate.

      d. Administer nitrates as ordered.

        ▸ Nitroglycerine may be the initial therapeutic treatment in an AMI.

        ▸ This drug is administered by many routes, but in the acute phase intravenous administration produces a more rapid preload and afterload reducing affect with resultant decreased myocardial oxygen consumption.

      e. Notify physician if pain is not relieved.

    3. Auscultate heart and lung sounds; monitor heart rate and rhythm, respirations, blood pressure with each episode of chest pain and after administration of medication.

     4. **Promote measures to maintain cardiac parameters within normal limits and maintain an effective cardiac rhythm.**

      a. Place the patient on a cardiac monitor and continuously monitor cardiac rate and rhythm in lead II.

    b.   Document rhythm strip each shift and any rhythm changes that occur during a shift.

    c.   Monitor rhythm at least every 2 hours and PRN.

    d.   Report any changes in mental status, level of consciousness (LOC), heart and lung sounds, vital signs, peripheral pulses and edema, jugular vein distention, skin color and temperature, capillary refill, urinary output, and decreased activity level.

    e.   If accessible, monitor hemodynamic parameters: PAP, PCWP, CO, CI.

    f.   Administer and monitor oxygen as ordered; continuous oximetry.

    g.   Closely monitor arterial blood gas, cardiac enzymes, electrolytes, and complete blood cell count as ordered.

    h.   Maintain IV flow rate and assess insertion site.

    i.   Administer medications as ordered and monitor therapeutic and/or nontherapeutic effects of nitrates, beta blockers, calcium channel blocker, inotropic agents, antiarrhythmics, and diuretics.

    j.   Obtain a 12-lead ECG, as ordered.

    k.   Assume position as tolerated by patient: semi- to high-Fowler's position.

    l.   Schedule adequate rest periods and limit visiting time and visitors.

    m.   Instruct patient which activities create a Valsalva response and to avoid these activities.

    n.   Administer stool softeners, as ordered.

5. Assess anxiety level of patient and family and explain equipment, tests, and visiting restrictions.

6. If needed, prepare for intubation and mechanical ventilation and/or IABP (intra-aortic balloon pump).

7. **Promote measures to maintain adequate oxygen and carbon dioxide exchange.**

    a.   **Monitor and report any changes in mental status, LOC, respiratory effort, color of skin and mucous membranes, heart and lung sounds, capillary refill, and vital signs.**

    b.   Observe nature of secretions with coughing or via suctioning.

    c.   Administer oxygen and monitor continuous oximetry as ordered, and report any significant changes.

    d.   Report abnormal blood gas results.

    e.   Monitor patient before and after respiratory treatments and document any changes.

    f.   If patient's respiratory system becomes compromised, prepare for intubation and mechanical ventilation.

8. Administer anticoagulants as ordered.

    a.   **Administer anticoagulants as ordered. The two major anticoagulants are heparin and warfarin (Coumadin).**

- ▸ The administration of intravenous heparin in the treatment of AMI is thought to inhibit formation of new thrombus and prevent extension and propagation of existing thrombus.
- ▸ The use of warfarin as a therapy to prevent or reduce reinfarction is inconclusive. Current literature revealed AMI is an indication for concomitant use of warfarin and low-dose aspirin.

b. Administer beta-adrenergic blockers as ordered

- ▸ The beneficial effects in AMI are a result of the decreased heart rate, blood pressure, conduction, and myocardial oxygen consumption.
- ▸ These drugs reduce the size of the infarct.

c. Administer calcium channel blockers as ordered: Verapamil, nifedipine, and diltiazem are the most commonly used drugs in this class with the latter being most effective inpatients with non–Q wave MIs.

d. Administer angiotensin-converting enzyme (ACE) inhibitors as ordered. The prevention of left ventricular thinning after myocardial infarction is the most recent therapeutic use for this classification of drugs.

e. Administer antiplatelet agents as ordered.

- ▸ The most common agents are aspirin, dipyridamole, and ticlopidine with aspirin being the original and most effective drug in this category.
- ▸ The remaining agents affect platelet aggregation but are not effective in the treatment of AMI.

f. Administer antidysrhythmic drugs as ordered.

- ▸ Ventricular dysrhythmias are life-threatening complications associated with AMI.

𝑛 ▸ **Intravenous lidocaine is the most common drug administered in the treatment of these dysrhythmias.**

g. Administer thrombolytic agents as ordered.

9. Prepare patient for percutaneous transluminal coronary angioplasty (PTCA). Special balloon-tipped catheters are used to dilate obstructed segments of coronary arteries thereby returning blood flow distal to the occlusion. (See Section XX for nursing care.)

10. Prepare patient for intracoronary stents which are balloon expandable, spring-loaded, and thermal memory stents which are placed in coronary arteries during PTCA procedure. These new investigative devices are designed to prevent closure or restenosis of the coronary vessels.

11. Prepare patient for laser angioplasty, which is an investigational procedure designed to dilate blocked vessels due to the interaction of laser light with the obstructive material.

12. Prepare patient for directional coronary atherectomy (DCA). this procedure is associated with PTCA and is currently being investi-

gated. The procedure involves excising and extracting plaque by using rotary cutting and extraction devices.

13.   Invasive coronary artery bypass graft (CABG) is a surgical procedure performed to increase flood flow distal to the blocked vessel(s). (See Coronary Artery Bypass Graft.)

G.   Evaluation

1.   The patient offers no complaints of pain with activities.
2.   The patient identifies and implements coping strategies.
3.   The patient demonstrates a reduction in anxiety.
4.   The patient exhibits an effective cardiac rate and rhythm.
5.   The patient maintains cardiac parameters within normal limits.
6.   The patient does not exhibit any compromise in respiratory status.
7.   The patient and significant other verbalize and demonstrate an understanding of the information imparted at teaching sessions.

H.   Potential complications

1.   **Dysrhythmias are the most common complication of AMI. Most dysrhythmias result from failure of the left ventricle causing life threatening ventricular dysrhythmias.**
     a.   Fib is the most common dysrhythmia.
     b.   See Display 4-4 for a summary of ECG findings and complications associated with each location of infarct.
     c.   See Chapter 5 for further discussion on dysrhythmias.
2.   Heart failure occurs in the majority of patients with AMI. Some degree of left ventricular compliance is exhibited. Immediate aggressive treatment is necessary to prevent pulmonary and circulatory involvement.

DISPLAY 4-4.
Summary of ECG Findings and Complications
Associated With Infarcts by Location

Anterior Infarct

S-T elevation in leads VI and VII

Complete heart block, right bundle branch block, B/L bundle branch block, ventricular septal defect

Inferior Infarct

S-T elevation in leads II, III, and AVF

Mitral valve damage, papillary muscle damage, transient sinus bradycardia (due to sinus node ischemia)

Lateral Infarct

S-T elevation in leads I and AVL

Mitral valve damage and papillary muscle damage

Posterior Infarct

S-T depression in leads VI and VII

Transient sinus bradycardia (due to sinus node ischemia)

3. Cardiogenic shock: this shock state occurs as a result of inadequate coronary and systemic tissue perfusion due to massive left ventricular failure. (See Cardiogenic Shock.)
4. Ventricular aneurysm:
   a. Fibrosis and scar formation formed by a healing necrotic myocardium can cause thinning and weakening of the left ventricular wall.
   b. These events cause a protrusion in wall of the left ventricle during systole and a diversion of blood into the protruded portion of the wall.
   c. The distention of the wall results in increased workload of the heart, ineffective muscle contraction, cardiac enlargement, and eventual failure.
   d. This complication is seen with a transmural (Q wave) MI.5. Post-infarct chest pain with ECG changes and recurring cardiac enzyme elevation may suggest extension of the infarct. Usually seen in nontransmural (non–Q wave) MIs.
6. Pericarditis
   a. This inflammatory response to myocardial damage may be difficult to differentiate between early pericarditis and AMI especially if the patient is seen on the second or third day of the evolving infarct.
   b. Chest pain that intensifies with inspiration and a friction rub are common signs of this complication.
7. Dressler's syndrome (AKA post–myocardial infarction syndrome): a late pericarditis can occur from weeks to months post-AMI. In addition to precordial pain and friction rub, a fever, pleuritis, and/or pleural effusion may occur.
8. Pulmonary embolism: a mural thrombi in the left ventricle or a thrombus from atrial dysrhythmias, immobility, may occur in acute or in convalescent phase of AMI.
9. Interventricular septal rupture: worsening of left ventricular function may result in this complication. Left-to-right shunting and a higher oxygen concentration in the pulmonary artery confirms the diagnosis of this serious complication. Surgical repair is necessary to reduce the high mortality rate.
10. Papillary muscle rupture: worsening of left ventricular function may also cause this complication.
    a. Rupture of this muscle results in dysfunction of the mitral valve.
    b. Valvular replacement is necessary to prevent heart failure and pulmonary complications.

I. **Home health considerations**
   1. Institute cardiac rehabilitation plan based on client/family understanding of disease process and client needs.
   2. Cardiac rehabilitation education should include specifics as to reporting signs and symptoms, identification of ways to change his/her life-style such as diet, alcohol, smoking, weight loss, and stress reduction.
   3. Gradual increase of exercise program including activities of daily living (ADLs).

IV. Heart failure

A. Description: the inability of the heart to pump sufficient blood to meet the needs of the tissues for oxygen and nutrients. There are various classifications of heart failure.

1. Right- vs. left-sided failure.

    a. **Right-sided failure: failure of right side resulting in high oncotic pressures that push fluid into tissues**

    b. **Left-sided failure: failure of left side resulting in high oncotic pressures that push fluid into alveoli of lungs**

2. High output failure vs. low output failure

    a. High output failure is characterized by disease processes that result in high cardiac output, with high volumes (high preload) such as anemia, hyperthyroidism, sepsis, pregnancy

    b. Low output failure is characterized by insufficient volume such as several days of vomiting or diarrhea with insufficient PO fluid intake and impaired contractility resulting in low cardiac output

3. Systolic dysfunction vs diastolic dysfunction

    a. Systolic dysfunction is the impaired ability of the LV to contract; after myocardial damage.

    b. Diastolic dysfunction is the impaired ability of the LV to relax, as in hypertrophy, hypertension, ischemia, or amyloidosis;

4. New York Heart Association Classification of Severity (Display 4-5)

B. Etiology and incidence

1. The cardiac causes of CHF include myocardial infarction, hypertension, fluid overload, and valve disease.

2. Can also occur with normal changes of aging, and with inflammatory diseases (lupus erythematosus).

3. Seen with other conditions such as chemotoxicity (adriamycin), alcohol abuse, and vitamin B1 deficiency.

4. Heart failure accounts for 10%–15% of all hospital admissions with 400,000 new diagnoses each year in U.S.

C. Pathophysiology

1. CHF occurs secondary to the inability of the ventricle to adequately pump blood to the systemic circulation.

DISPLAY 4-5.
NYHA Classification of Severity

Stage I: No S and S

Stage II: Fine rales, shortness of breath with exercise, requires occasional Lasix

Stage III: Moderate rales, shortness of breath at rest, requires Lasix and digoxin

Stage IV: Loud rales, shock (hypotension), gallop rhythm, requires technological support and IV vasoactive drugs

      2. Congestion and backup of fluid can result, leading to pulmonary or systemic congestion.

      3. Consequently, blood flow to vital organs decreases, potentially resulting in end organ damage.

D. **Assessment findings**

    1. Symptoms of left-sided failure include:

        a. Crackles, HR, SOB, RR, DOE, PND, cough

        b. Chest pain, 1–3 pillow orthopnea (inability to lie flat)

        c. S and S pulmonary edema (frothy/bloody sputum, cyanosis, pallor, severe dyspnea, diaphoresis), PCWP >12 mm Hg

        d. Cerebral hypoxia, anxiety, clubbing of nailbeds

        e. Lateral displacement of the PMI secondary ventricular enlargement, and gallop rhythm

        f. Decrease in UOP, peripheral vasoconstriction

    2. Symptoms of right-sided failure include:

        a. Edema, easy fatigability, liver enlargement

        b. increased hepatojugular reflux, JVD, anorexia

        c. Blue nail beds, ascites, S3

        d. Chest pain, CVP >10 cm H_2O

E. **Nursing diagnoses**

    1. Activity Intolerance

    2. Anxiety

    3. Colonic Constipation

    4. Decreased Cardiac Output

    5. Altered Family Processes

    6. Fluid Volume Excess

    7. Impaired Gas Exchange

    8. Altered Tissue Perfusion

F. **Planning and implementation**

    1. Administer medications to reduce HR (beta blockers, Ca++ channel blockers) and increase cardiac output (digoxin, sedatives)

    2. Administer medications to increase stroke volume by reducing preload: ACE inhibitors, diuretics, nitrates, and hydralazine. Other interventions such as low-salt diet, fluid restriction, and rotating tourniquets (seldom used) may also be used.

    3. Administer medications to increase stroke volume by decreasing afterload. These include ACE inhibitors, beta blockers, Ca++ channel blockers, and hydralazine. Use caution with beta blockers and Ca++ channel blockers as these may worsen CHF due to negative inotrope action.

    4. Administer medications to increase stroke volume by increasing contractility. These include digoxin, amrinone, milrinone, and O_2.

    5. Administer medications to reduce oxygen demand. These include beta blockers and calcium channel blockers. Other interventions include rest/sedatives, visit with family, positioning, stool softeners, and correcting any infections.

G. **Evaluation**

    1. The patient demonstrates a patent airway, and is free of frothy, bloody sputum (as with pulmonary edema).

    2. The patient demonstrates normal breathing pattern as evidenced by a respiratory rate of 12–24 breaths/min, no retractions (use of accessory muscles), no crackles or rhonchi, pulse oximetry >94%, color pink with no nailbed cyanosis, no SOB, DOE, or orthopnea, no PND or cough.

3. The patient demonstrates adequate circulation as evidenced by a heart rate of 60–100, skin warm and dry, increasing pulse quality, improved UOP >30 mL/hr, diminishing edema, no JVD or hepatojugular reflux, no gallop rhythm.

H.   Home health considerations

1. Ensure client is educated regarding disease process and need for dietary changes, including sodium restriction and fluid restriction if ordered.

2. Ensure rest periods, elevation of feet, and instructions on home oxygen therapy.

V.   Angina

A.   Description: a transient ischemic attack resulting from decreased blood supply through partially occluded coronary arteries.

1. **Stable (chronic) angina: has a predictable symptomatic onset.**

    a. Physical exertion, emotional stress, or cold weather may precipitate an anginal attack.

    b. The pain or discomfort varies from mild to severe and usually lasts 1 to 5 minutes.

    c. Often the patient may take sublingual nitroglycerin (NTG) before exertional activities to ward off any attacks.

2. **Unstable (pre-infarct) angina, crescendo angina, and acute coronary insufficiency are unpredictable and may be a progression from stable angina.**

    a. Often described as progressive, prolonged, or frequent angina with increasing severity that may occur at rest and with minimal exertion.

    b. Unlike the pain or discomfort of stable angina, it is more intense, lasting up to 30 minutes, and often arouses the patient from sleep.

    c. The pain is not completely relieved with NTG and the patient may require narcotic administration (morphine sulfate) for complete relief.

    d. Without significant ECG changes, the patient's history and present clinical condition may be the basis for diagnosis and hospitalization.

    e. Unstable angina can be associated with deterioration or rupture of a stable atherosclerotic plaque.

3. **Printzmetal's or variant angina is quite the opposite of stable angina. It occurs with rest and not with exertional or emotional stress.**

    a. The episode of angina usually occurs the same time every day, in the early morning hours, in a patient with no evidence of coronary atherosclerosis.

    b. A spasm of a major coronary artery is usually the cause.

    c. NTG generally yields quick relief. An AMI may coexist with variant angina.

d.   **Nitrates and calcium channel blockers are most effective because of their vasodilating properties and reducing myocardial oxygen demands.**

B.   Etiology and incidence

1.   Coronary artery obstruction caused by atherosclerosis is the most common cause. Secondary causes include thrombosis, spasms, or coronary arteritis.

2.   Predisposing clinical conditions may include valvular dysfunctions, congenital anomalies, left ventricular; hypertrophy, anemia, tachydysrhythmias, hypertension, or pharmacologic effects.

3.   AMIs, PTCA, coronary artery bypass graft (CABG), or certain types of diagnostic testing (stress test) may cause angina.

4.   Precipitating factors may include:
   a.   Extreme changes in temperature
   b.   Physical exercise
   c.   Emotional factors
   d.   Eating a heavy meal
   e.   Sexual intercourse
   f.   Valsalva maneuver
   g.   Cigarette smoking
   h.   Stimulants

5.   Approximately 5 million of annual hospital admissions represent patient's with unstable angina. Prognosis depends on life-style changes.

C.   Pathophysiology

   1.   **When myocardial ischemia occurs, the coronary arteries respond by vasodilating, thereby increasing coronary artery blood flow.**

2.   Compromised coronary arteries lose the ability to vasodilate when metabolic demands of myocardial cells increase with a resultant decrease in oxygenated blood flow.

3.   Myocardial cells that are denied oxygen for a short period of time convert from aerobic to anaerobic metabolism.

4.   Lactic acid buildup from anaerobic metabolism irritates myocardial muscle fibers, causing the cardinal symptom of chest pain.

5.   Although coronary artery spasms are associated with atherosclerotic plaques, spontaneous narrowing of the coronary arteries induced by spasms can be experienced in normal coronary arteries and have an unknown underlying pathology.

6.   The duration of a spasm determines the life or death of myocardial cells.

D.   Assessment findings

   1.   **The cardinal symptom of angina is substernal or retrosternal chest pain, sometimes referred to as chest discomfort, varying from mild to severe in intensity. It may be described as pressure, tightness, squeezing, crushing, aching, suffocating, or burning. The pain may or may not radiate to the neck, jaw, back, left shoulder, or down inner aspect of one or both arms.**

2.   **Pain assessment (PQRST); see AMI. The pain is not relieved or exacerbated with position changes but is relieved with medication or rest.**

3.   The patient may experience all or one of these symptoms or only epigastric discomfort.

4.   Systemic manifestations reveal cold, clammy, pale skin with diaphoresis, nausea, dyspnea, anxiety, apprehension, feeling of impending doom, tachycardia and hypertension, bradycardia, hypotension, and S4 gallop.

5.   Absence of pain or chest discomfort are atypical signs and symptoms. This is typically known as a silent myocardial infarction and is usually documented on ECG, radionuclide, or stress test.

6.   Diagnostic evaluation includes:

   a.   **Patient's health history. In all patients complaining of chest pain, always assume an AMI until a different diagnosis has been made.**

b.   **ECG findings: ST segment depression and T-wave inversion occur with chest pain and return to normal when episode subsides; hyperacute upright T-waves denote transmural ischemia and may be a precursor to patterns typical of an AMI; ST segment elevation typically seen in Prinzmetal's (variant) angina with a normal ECG when spasm subsides.**

c.   Diagnostic procedures

▶ See AMI.

▶ Rapid atrial pacing: an invasive test involves inserting one end of a pacing wire into the patient's right atrium and attaching the other to a pulse generator. The pacing starts @ 100 beats per minute, with a maximum of 160 BPM. After each 20-beat increase an ECG is performed. The test is abated with the detection of chest pain or ST segment depression.

E.   Nursing diagnoses
1.   Activity Intolerance
2.   Decreased Cardiac Output
3.   Impaired Gas Exchange
4.   Anxiety

F.   Planning and implementation
1.   Assess for potential complications such as dysrhythmias or an AMI.
2.   General nursing care is the same as for the patient with an AMI.
3.   Treatment options reflect the type of angina. The therapeutic options include pharmacologic agents, CABG, stent placement, PTCA, atherectomy, laser angioplasty, and possible intra-aortic balloon counterpulsation (IABP).

G.   Evaluation
1.   The patient demonstrates relief of pain without evidence of myocardial compromise.

2. The patient demonstrates adequate oxygenation.
3. Anxiety is relieved.

VI.   Cardiomyopathy

A.   Description: a primary or secondary disorder of the heart muscle that effects the structure and function of the myocardium, and is classified into three distinct functional types: dilated, hypertrophic, and restrictive.

B.   Etiology and incidence

1. The cardiomyopathies are secondary to other disease processes and the etiology of the primary disorder is unknown.
2. Dilated or congestive cardiomyopathy follows a course of progressive deterioration generally seen in the third to fourth decade, with a five year survival rate in 75% of the population after diagnosis. Associated factors may include alcohol abuse, myocarditis, inflammation, hypertension, metabolic disorders, pregnancy, viral infections, and multiple MIs.
3. Genetic transmission and hypertension are thought to be the secondary cause of hypertrophic cardiomyopathy, formerly known as idiopathic hypertrophic subaortic stenosis (IHSS).
4. Incidence is greater in men than women and is most often detected in active, athletic young adults.
5. Restrictive cardiomyopathy is the less common of the disorders. The pathologic processes associated with this disorder include endocardial fibrosis, amyloidosis, neoplastic tumor, and post-radiation. The severity of heart failure and possibility of an embolism dictates the prognosis of the disorder.

C.   Pathophysiology and management: dilated (congestive) cardiomyopathy

1. This form of cardiomyopathy impairs the size and function of the heart.

2. **With dilatation of the heart chambers, mainly the ventricles, the contraction is decreased, thus impairing systolic function, decreasing stroke volume, and reducing ejection fraction.**
3. The impaired systolic function stimulates several compensatory mechanisms, the first being an increased end-diastolic volume (EDV).
4. Other mechanisms include increased circulation of catecholamines, sodium and water retention, and activation of the renin-angiotension mechanism. With failure of these mechanisms biventricular failure frequently occurs with heart failure as the primary consequence.
5. Other characteristics of cardiomyopathy are atrial enlargement and stasis of the blood resulting from increased blood volume and reduction of the ejection fraction. The possibility of thrombus formation is a direct result of stasis of the blood.
6. Management includes diuretics, digoxin, and vasodilators. Other therapies may include steroids for inflammation and anticoagulants to prevent embolism.

D. **Pathophysiology and management: hypertrophic cardiomyopathy (IHSS)**

1. **The abnormalities associated with this disease are ventricular dysfunction, mitral valve dysfunction, systolic pressure gradients, and impaired relaxation.**
2. Hypertrophy of the free muscle wall, and upper portion of the interventricular septum encroaches on the left ventricular chamber.
3. This increased thickness leads to left ventricular rigidity during diastole, thus interfering with the relaxation and adequate filling.
4. This abnormality causes an elevation of left ventricular end-diastolic pressure, pulmonary venous and pulmonary capillary wedge pressures, and high atrial pressure.
5. The systolic pressure gradient effects the functioning of the mitral valve with eventual incompetency. Mitral insufficiency together with the hypertrophic anterior septum obstructs the outflow tract with subsequent decreased cardiac output.
6. This muscle disease causes pronounced hypertrophy of the ventricular muscle mass without ventricular dilatation.
7. The basic goal of treatment is to enhance ventricular filling and alleviate outflow obstruction of the left ventricle. Beta blockers, most commonly propranolol (Inderal), and in some cases calcium channel blockers (verapamil), constitute the drug therapy.
8. Implantable defibrillators have been more beneficial than antidysrhythmics for the treatment of dysrhythmias.
9. Surgery such as a ventriculomyotomy and myectomy are usually reserved for patients whose symptoms are refractory to therapy.
10. Terminal end-stage cardiomyopathy may require cardiac transplantation. Approximately 50% of heart transplants are performed for treatment of cardiomyopathic conditions. Many patients with dilated (congestive) cardiomyopathy die awaiting heart transplantation.

E. **Pathophysiology and management: restrictive cardiomyopathy**

1. Least common form of cardiomyopathy
2. Muscle stiffness of the ventricular walls affects only the diastolic function by impairing its filling during relaxation.
3. Increased preload, elevated end-diastolic pressure, and impaired filling lead to decreased cardiac output and eventually right- and left-sided heart failure.
4. Management is similar to dilated cardiomyopathy.

F. **Assessment findings**

1. Symptoms of dilated right- and left-sided heart failure (left sided more predominate) include:
   a. Fatigue and weakness, dyspnea, paroxysmal nocturnal dyspnea (PND)
   b. Systemic vascular congestion, systemic or pulmonary emboli, cardiomegaly (moderate to severe)
   c. S3 and S4 gallop, mitral regurgitation, dysrhythmias (atrial and ventricular)
2. Symptoms of hypertrophic cardiomyopathy include:
   a. Exertional dyspnea, PND, orthopnea
   b. Angina pectoris, IHSS palpitations, syncope

    c.   Dysrhythmias (especially ventricular), apical systolic thrill and heave, mild cardiomegaly

    d.   S4, systolic murmur heard at the left sternal boarder and apex, sudden death.

3.   Symptoms of restrictive cardiomyopathy include:

    a.   Dyspnea, exercise intolerance, fatigue, right-sided failure

    b.   Mild-to-moderate cardiomegaly, atrioventricular valve regurgitation, S3 and S4

    c.   Dysrhythmias

    d.   Kussmaul's sign (bulging of jugular neck veins on inspiration)

4.   Diagnostic studies reveal:

    a.   Chest x-ray: Cardiomegaly on chest x-ray depending on severity of the disease; more severe in dilated cardiomyopathy (CMP).

    b.   ECG: Atrial and ventricular dysrhythmias, S-T segment and T-wave abnormalities seen in dilated and hypertrophic CMP.

        ▸ Dilated: intraventricular conduction defects.

        ▸ Hypertrophic: Q-wave and T-wave inversion.

        ▸ Restrictive: intraventricular and atrioventricular (AV) conduction defects.

    c.   Echocardiogram: Dilated CMP: dilatation and dysfunction of the left ventricle; abnormal compliance and filling pressures causing abnormal mitral valve motion.

        ▸ Hypertrophic: asymmetrical septal hypertrophy; narrowing left ventricle outflow; left ventricle is small or normal size

        ▸ Restrictive: increased thickness and mass of the left ventricle; ventricular cavity may be normal or small in size; pleural effusion.

    d.   Radionuclide studies:

        ▸ Dilated: dilatation and dysfunction of the left ventricle.

        ▸ Hypertrophic: hypertrophy of the septum is asymmetrical; left ventricle is normal to small in size.

        ▸ Restricted: left ventricle is normal to small in size; infiltration of the myocardium; normal systolic function.

    e.   Cardiac catheterization:

        ▸ Dilated: diminished cardiac output; enlargement and dysfunction of the left ventricle; regurgitation of the mitral and/or tricuspid valves; elevated filling pressure in the left and right sides of the heart (especially the left side).

        ▸ Hypertrophic: Left ventricular compliance is diminished; mitral regurgitation murmur; vigorous systolic function.

        ▸ Restrictive: elevated filling pressures in the left and right side of the heart; diminished left ventricular compliance.

G. **Nursing diagnoses**

  1.   Decreased Cardiac Output

  2.   Activity Intolerance

        3. Anxiety

        4. Ineffective Breathing Pattern

        5. Risk for Infection

H. Planning and implementation

1. Provide frequent rest periods; conserving energy is the main goal.
2. Monitor pulse, respirations, and cardiac monitor for dysrhythmias with ADLs.
3. Discontinue activity if chest, dyspnea, hypotension, sustained tachycardia, or dysrhythmias develop.
4. Administer supplemental oxygen.
5. Monitor IV site for signs and symptoms of infection.
6. Monitor vital signs q4hr or PRN and after activity.
7. Observe cardiac monitor for rate and rhythm and administer antidysrhythmic drugs per protocol.
8. Monitor I and O and daily weights: weight gain >2 lb in 1 week and urine output <30 mL/hr is clinically significant.
9. Provide a sodium-restricted diet as prescribed.
10. Monitor laboratory values, especially electrolytes, and report abnormal. Decreased potassium and magnesium increase the risk for ventricular dysrhythmias.
11. Monitor arterial blood gas (ABG) values as prescribed
12. Perform appropriate physical assessment for signs and symptoms of heart failure.
13. Perform hemodynamic monitoring: CVP, PAP, PCWP, CO, CI, and arterial pressure if A-line and Swan-Ganz catheters are in place.
14. Maintain adequate circulation by administering medication specific to the type of CMP (see Table 4-1).
15. Digoxin and nitrates are not usually used in the treatment of hypertrophic CMP.
16. Instruct the patient that calcium and beta blockers are taken to prevent angina attracts and that NTG will not relieve angina.
17. Counsel athletic patients regarding danger of strenuous exercise.
18. Recommend screening and genetic counseling for family members.
19. Provide adequate calories and protein and a decreased sodium diet.
20. Be aware of potential complications such as heart failure, dysrhythmias, pulmonary embolus, and pulmonary edema.

I. Evaluation

1. The patient demonstrates increased tolerance for activities.
2. The patient and family members verbalize their fears and anxieties and received emotional support.
3. The patient displays an effective cardiac rate and rhythm.
4. The patient verbalizes an understanding of his disease process, medications, and follow-up care.

VII. Tricuspid stenosis

A. Description: a reduction in the size of the valvular orifice obstructing right ventricular filling during diastole.

B. Etiology and incidence

1. Rare as a primary disease
2. Accompanies mitral stenosis caused by rheumatic fever.

      3.   Increased risk with IV drug abusers.

      4.   More common in females than males.

C. **Pathophysiology**

      1.   The valvular orifice is narrowed by fibrotic cusps impeding complete closure

      2.   A pressure increase in the right atrium results in enlargement of the chamber.

      3.   Backward pressure forces the blood into the systemic circulation resulting in increasing venous pressure, decreased right ventricular filling and blood volume to pulmonary vasculature and left side of the heart, and eventually reducing cardiac output, stroke volume, and tissue perfusion.

D. **Assessment findings**

      1.   Clinical manifestations are usually associated with right-sided heart failure

      2.   Major signs and symptoms include fatigue, dyspnea, weakness, mitral murmur (low pitched, rumbling murmur, intensity increased with inspiration) auscultated at the fourth intercostal space, left sternal border.

      3.   Diagnostic findings:

          a.   ECG reveals peaked P waves and atrial dysrhythmias.

          b.   Chest x-ray shows enlargement of the right atrium.

          c.   Echocardiography reveals abnormal motion and obstructions causing fibrosis and/or calcification.

          d.   Cardiac catheterization confirms increased pressure of the right atrium.

VIII. Pulmonic stenosis

A. **Description: narrowing of the pulmonary valve with resultant blood flow obstruction.**

B. **Etiology and incidence**

      1.   The major cause is congenital.

      2.   Acquired causes are associated with rheumatic fever, endocarditis, tuberculosis, syphilis, cancerous valvular lesions.

C. **Pathophysiology**

      1.   A decreased valvular orifice is attributed to thickened leaflets caused by inflammatory changes from infected endocarditis and rheumatic heart disease

      2.   Hypertrophy of the right ventricle occurs from increased pressure needed to pump blood through a stenotic valve.

      3.   Hypertrophy of the right atrium occurs from the increased valvular pressure of the right ventricle

      4.   As the right heart fails, venous engorgement and decreased cardiac output follow.

D. **Assessment findings**

      1.   Typical asymptomatic patient presents with dyspnea on exertion, fatigue and syncope as early signs of severe disease.

      2.   Also peripheral edema, ascites, hepatomegaly, increased venous pressures, harsh (medium pitched) murmur at second intercostal space, left sternal border and a widely split S2 (present or absent).

3. Diagnostic findings:
    a. ECG is normal or shows right axis deviation in the presence of pulmonary hypertension; P wave changes indicate right atrial enlargement.
    b. Chest x-ray reveals right ventricular hypertrophy, pulmonary artery prominence.
    c. Echocardiography is the most valuable diagnostic tool. Stenotic severity is ascertained by the echodoppler.

IX.   Mitral stenosis

A.   Description: a reduction in the size of the valvular orifice obstructing left ventricular filling during diastole.

B.   Etiology and incidence
1. The most common cause is rheumatic heart disease.
2. The least common causes are congenital mitral stenosis, rheumatoid arthritis, and systemic lupus erythematosus.
3. It is more common in females than males and can be fatal with pregnancy.

C.   Pathophysiology
1. The structures of the mitral valve are thickened and shortened, creating a narrow conduit for the natural emptying of blood from one chamber to another.
2. The narrowing of the valve creates an increase in volume, pressure in the left atrium, and eventually atrial dilatation.

3. **Backward pressure is reflected in the pulmonary vasculature, resulting in pulmonary edema and pulmonary hypertension.**
4. Pressure in the pulmonary system increases the workload of the heart.

5. **The resultant effects from the pulmonary system are increased workload, dilatation, hypertrophy of the right ventricle, and eventually right-sided heart failure.**
6. Diuretics, low-sodium diet, anticoagulation drugs, and avoidance of exertion are usually prescribed for symptoms of heart failure.
7. Quinidine and digoxin are given for atrial fibrillation. Cardioversion should be used with caution because of possibility of atrial thrombi.
8. Antibiotic therapy is prescribed before and after dental visits or other invasive procedures.
9. Balloon valvuloplasty is recommended for patients at operative risk.
10. Valve repair or replacement are recommended for reducing obstruction from a stenotic valve.

D.   Assessment findings
1. Most frequent symptoms are dyspnea on exertion (DOE), fatigue, palpations, cough, hemoptysis.
2. Less common symptoms are orthopnea, dysphasia, hoarseness, PND, chest pain, embolism, seizures, cerebral vascular accident (CVA)
3. Physical exam reveals:
    a. Low-pitched rumbling murmur best heard with the bell of

the stethoscope at the apex with the patient in the left lateral recumbent position.

b. A palpable thrill may be felt at the apex.

c. A loud S1, a split S2, and an opening snap (heard with the diaphragm of a stethoscope)

d. Atrial fibrillation, JVD

e. Ascites, hepatomegaly

f. Peripheral edema, narrow pulse pressure

g. With severe disease, cyanosis of the face and extremities may be seen.

4. Diagnostic findings:

a. ECG reveals atrial fibrillation, notched P waves.

b. Chest x-ray reveals enlargement of the left atrium and ventricle, pulmonary congestion, and calcification of mitral leaflets.

c. Echocardiography shows mitral valve thickening, diminished or restrictive leaflet movement, and possible thrombi in the atrium.

d. Cardiac catheterization shows a decrease in cardiac output, an increase in left atrial pressure, LVEDP, PAWP, peripheral vascular resistance, and an increase pressure gradient across the mitral valve.

X. Aortic stenosis

A. Description: a reduction in the size of the aortic orifice obstructing the left ventricular blood flow during systole and increasing the afterload.

B. Etiology and incidence

1. The causes are congenital aberrations, rheumatic fever (acquired), and idiopathic calcification.

2. Most common in men; constitutes 25% of all persons with valvular heart disease.

3. Increase incidence in correlation with longevity.

C. Pathophysiology

1. Progressive narrowing of the aortic valve causes left ventricular hypertrophy.

2. **Myocardial oxygen demands increase and coronary perfusion decreases due to the pressure of the left ventricle on the coronary arteries precipitating cardiac ischemia.**

3. Pressure from the left ventricle increases and the left atrium enlarges to compensate.

4. Back pressure from the left atrium produces increased pulmonary pressure and congestion and right-sided heart failure will ensue.

5. Mitral valve involvement often accompanies aortic stenosis.

6. Management options are antibiotic therapy before and after dental visits, and close observation for disease progression and manifestations of the disease process.

7. Symptomatic treatment of complications or surgical interventions are necessary to control the disease and to relieve mechanical obstruction.

D.   Assessment findings
1.   Characteristic symptoms: DOE, exertional syncope, angina, fatigue
2.   Symptoms occurring in the late stages:
     a.   Weakness, cough, orthopnea, PND, pulmonary edema, dysrhythmias
     b.   S3 and S4 heart sounds indicating heart failure and left ventricular hypertrophy.
     c.   Harsh midsystolic murmur and thrill over the aortic area auscultated at the second intercostal space, right sternal border.
     d.   Sustained, forceful apical impulse
     e.   Paradoxical split S2
     f.   Narrow pulse pressure
3.   Diagnostic findings
     a.   Swan-Ganz measurements reveal an increased pulmonary artery wedge pressure and left atrial pressure.
     b.   ECG changes include first degree AV block, left bundle branch block, and left atrial and ventricular hypertrophy.
     c.   Chest x-ray reveals left ventricular enlargement, aortic valve calcification, and possible enlargement of the left atrium, pulmonary artery, and right ventricle and atrium.
     d.   Echocardiography reveals thickened mitral valve, left atrial enlargement, and decreased valve mobility.
     e.   Cardiac catheterization reveals increased valvular pressure, left atrial pressure, PCWP, right heart pressure, and decreased cardiac output.

E.   Nursing diagnoses for stenotic valvular disease (of the aortic, tricuspid, mitral, and pulmonic valves):
1.   Anxiety
2.   Decreased Cardiac Output
3.   Decreased Activity Tolerance
4.   Fluid Volume Excess
5.   Impaired Gas Exchange
6.   Knowledge Deficit
7.   Risk for Infection

F.   Planning and implementation for stenotic valvular disease
1.   Provide supplemental oxygen or mechanical ventilation as prescribed.
2.   Provide time with patient and focus attention on the patient; use relaxation techniques and therapeutic touch as needed.
3.   Explain disease process to the patient and clarify misconceptions and answer the patient's questions.
4.   Monitor vital signs and auscultate heart sound q4hr or PRN and record severity and quality of murmurs.
5.   Motor heart rate and rhythm for dysrhythmias as indicated, document abnormal ECG, and administer antidysrhythmic medications per protocol.
6.   Prepare the patient for cardioversion for atrial fibrillation, balloon valvuloplasty, or surgical procedure as ordered.
7.   Assess pain (PQRST) and administer NTG for chest pain; document pain relief.

8. Administer diuretics and NTG (especially the first dose) with caution to prevent depletion of blood volume.

9. Administer vasodilators and inotropic agents to decrease preload and afterload and increase contractility and cardiac output.

10. In patients with aortic stenosis NTG should be used with caution because of the resultant severe hypotension from decreased cardiac output.

11. Monitor intake and output, daily weights and laboratory values for electrolyte imbalances especially potassium.

12. Maintain restricted sodium and fluid intake as prescribed.

13. Auscultate breath sounds for crackles, wheezing, or diminished sounds, and assess for JVD q4hr or PRN.

14. Maintain patient in semi- or high-Fowler's or a position comfortable for the patient and monitor for dyspnea or fatigue with ADLs.

15. Monitor arterial blood gases, electrolytes, hemoglobin and hematocrit, and blood chemistry values.

16. Monitor hemodynamic status: CVP, PCWP, PAP, CO, CI as prescribed or PRN.

17. Monitor all invasive sites (IV, etc.) and wounds for signs and symptoms of infection.

18. Maintain sterile technique with all dressing changes.

19. Administer antibiotics as prescribed.

20. Administer heparin or Coumadin as prescribed and monitor PTT and PT.

21. Provide explanations of compliance with medication regimen, bleeding precautions for anticoagulation therapy adhering to scheduled medical appointments, reporting to the physician any abnormalities, alternate periods of activity with rest, refrain from contact sports, minimize strenuous exercise.

22. Be aware of potential complications such as dysrhythmias, heart failure, thromboembolic sequelae, rupture of the papillary muscle and infective endocarditis.

G. Evaluation

1. The patient and family members verbalize their fears and anxieties and received emotional support.

2. The patient demonstrates increased tolerance for activities.

3. The patient exhibits no difficulty in breathing as evidenced by lungs clear to auscultation.

4. The patient exhibits normal fluid and electrolyte balance as evidenced by normal laboratory values and no edema.

5. The patient displays an effective cardiac rate and rhythm.

6. The patient verbalizes an understanding of disease process, medications, and follow-up care.

XI. Tricuspid regurgitative disease

A. Description: during systole the right ventricular blood volume inversely flows into the right atrium.

B. Etiology and incidence

1. Sequelae to left ventricular failure and/or pulmonary hypertension.

  2. Leaflet closure impeded by dilated valvular orifice and/or annulus enlargement.

  3. Ineffective endocarditis

  4. Rheumatic heart disease

  5. Chest trauma

  6. Myocardial infarction

  7. Right atrial myxoma

  8. Cancer

  9. Tricuspid valve prolapse

 C. **Pathophysiology**

  1. The backward flow of blood during ventricular systole is reflected in the elevation of the right atrial and systemic venous pressures.

  2. Increased right atrial pressure results in systemic venous congestion, decreased right ventricular volume, decreased blood flow to the left side of the heart and reduction in cardiac output.

  3. The resultant factor is right ventricular dilatation and hypertrophy which further complicates the tricuspid regurgitation.

  4. Management options include administration of vaso-dilators, digitalis, diuretics, dopamine, dobutamine, and a low-sodium diet to treat right-sided failure and pulmonary hypertension, if present.

  5. Surgical interventions depend on the involvement of mitral valvular disease.

  6. Valvuloplasty or annuloplasty is preferred to valvular replacement.

 D. **Assessment findings**

  1. Clinical manifestations include:

   a. High-pitched, blowing, pansystolic murmur increased on inspiration, heard at the fourth or fifth intercostal space at the left sternal boarder.

   b. Dyspnea, orthopnea

   c. Pulmonary edema

   d. Fatigue, atrial fibrillation

   e. Hepatomegaly, anorexia

   f. Peripheral cyanosis

  2. Diagnostic findings:

   a. ECG reveals atrial fibrillation, right bundle branch block, and peaked P waves

   b. Chest x-ray shows right atrial and ventricular enlargement.

   c. Echocardiography shows vegetative lesions on valve leaflets, abnormal valvular movement, rupture of the papillary muscles and chordae tendineae.

   d. Cardiac catheterization reveals regurgitation of contrast medium into the right atrium.

XII. **Pulmonic regurgitative disease**

 A. **Description: the regurgitation of blood through the pulmonic valve back into the right ventricle during diastole.**

 B. **Etiology and incidence**

  1. Congenital defect, main

  2. Acquired, mainly from pulmonary hypertension.

  3. Pulmonary artery aneurysm

  4. Infective endocarditis

  5. Syphilis

C. Pathophysiology
1. Scarring and thickening of the leaflets causing valvular contraction and permitting backflow of blood with ensuing right ventricular hypertrophy

2. **Increased right atrial volume and pressure eventually causes hypertrophy of the right atrium and right-sided heart failure.**
3. Symptomatic treatment with digoxin, diuretics, and a low-sodium diet.

D. Assessment findings
1. Clinical manifestations include:
   a. High-pitched, blowing murmur with concurrent pulmonary hypertension, moderate-pitched without pulmonary hypertension, both sounds are heard at the fourth or fifth intercostal space, left sternal boarder. Murmur can be heard at Erb's point.
   b. May be asymptomatic unless concurrent pulmonary hypertension exists.
2. Diagnostic findings:
   a. ECG, chest x-ray, and echocardiography findings are similar to pulmonary stenosis.

XIII. Mitral regurgitative disease

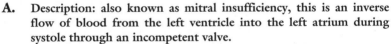

A. Description: also known as mitral insufficiency, this is an inverse flow of blood from the left ventricle into the left atrium during systole through an incompetent valve.

B. Etiology and incidence
1. The most common causes are:
   a. Rheumatic fever
   b. Mitral valve prolapse
   c. Coronary artery disease
   d. Infective endocarditis
2. Less common causes are:
   a. Acquired mitral regurgitation
   b. Calcification of mitral annulus
   c. Myocardial infarction
   d. Papillary muscle dysfunction
   e. Chordae tendenae rupture
   f. Congenital
3. Mitral regurgitation is more common in men than women.

C. Pathophysiology
1. The incompetent mitral valve is the result of inflammatory changes and scarring from such conditions as rheumatic heart disease.
2. The normal motion of the posterior leaflet is affected by the enlargement of the left atrium to compensate for the increased blood volume
3. Dilatation and hypertrophy of the left ventricle ensues in an attempt to accommodate the increased volume (preload) and decreased cardiac output.

4. This compensatory mechanism is ineffective and a backflow of blood from the left ventricle into the left atrium and into the pulmonary system occurs. In time this creates pulmonary edema, pulmonary hypertension and eventually right sided heart failure.

 5. Management is symptomatic and includes administration of digoxin, diuretics, vasodilators, anticoagulants, and a low-sodium diet. Surgical intervention is similar to that for mitral stenosis.

D. Assessment findings
   1. Clinical symptoms include:
      a. Fatigue, weakness, exhaustion
      b. Cachexia, palpations, atypical chest pain
      c. Dysphagia, symptoms of mitral stenosis
      d. Tachypnea, hypotension, pulmonary edema

       e. **DOE, fulminating pulmonary edema and a rapidly developing shock state in the acute stage**

   2. Clinical signs include:
      a. High-pitched, blowing, systolic murmur heard at the apex, radiating to the mid-axillary.
      b. Diminished S1, split S2, S3 gallop may be heard.
      c. Atrial pulsations may be felt at the third intercostal space at the left sternal boarder.
      d. Atrial fibrillation
      e. JVD
      f. Hepatomegaly
      g. PMI is displaced downward and to the left

   3. Diagnostic findings:
      a. ECG reveals atrial fibrillation, abnormal P waves, non-specific S-T segment changes.
      b. Chest x-ray reveals enlargement of the left atrium and ventricle, congestion in the pulmonary vasculature.
      c. Echocardiography visualizes abnormal wall and leaflet motion, left atrial and ventricle enlargement, hyperdynamic left ventricle usually seen with shock.
      d. Cardiac catheterization shows the amount of regurgitation, increased left atrial pressure, PAWP, LVEDP (preload), abnormal wall motion, and decreased cardiac output.

XIV. Aortic regurgitative disease
  A. Description: also known as aortic insufficiency, this is an inverse flow of blood from the ascending aorta into the left ventricle during diastole resulting in increased preload secondary to aortic valvular incompetence.
  B. Etiology and incidence
    1. Acute causes include:
      a. Ascending aortic dissection
      b. Infective endocarditis
      c. Trauma

2. Chronic aortic regurgitation may result from:
   a. Rheumatic heart disease
   b. Syphilis
   c. Prolonged severe hypertension
   d. Congenital heart disease (tetralogy of Fallot, coarctation of the aorta, and ventricular septal defect).
   e. Connective tissue disorders (rheumatoid arthritis, Marfan syndrome)
   f. Unsuccessful valvular surgery.
3. Commonly associated with mitral valve disease.

C. Pathophysiology
1. Abnormal accumulation of blood in the left ventricle occurs secondary to the incompetent aortic valve.

2. **Over a period this backflow of additional blood causes volume overload by increasing the end-diastolic volume of the left ventricle and consequently the workload of the heart.**
3. The resultant effects are left ventricular hypertrophy and dilatation in an attempt to maintain adequate cardiac output.
4. With acute aortic regurgitation there is an overwhelming increase in end-diastolic pressure of the left ventricle. The consequence is backward pressure being reflected to the left atrium and pulmonary vasculature. As the blood pressure drops an increase in the systemic vascular resistance (SVR) occurs to maintain cardiac output.
5. Depending on the severity of the incompetent valve, the compensatory mechanism is tolerated by the left ventricle for a long period of time.
6. Management options include prophylactic antibiotics and medications to reduce preload and afterload are prescribed. Emergency surgical treatment is necessary for acute aortic regurgitation.

D. Assessment findings
1. Acute manifestations include:
   a. Profound dyspnea, chest pain, tachycardia, shock state
   b. Signs and symptoms of acute pulmonary edema such as S3 may be noted.
2. Chronic manifestations include:
   a. Water-hammer pulse (hallmark sign)
   b. High-pitched, blowing diastolic murmur heard at the second intercostal space radiating to the left sternal boarder at the third or fourth intercostal space.
   c. Precordial thrill
   d. PMI downward and to the left
   e. Widened pulse pressure
   f. Head nods with pulse (deMusset's sign)
   g. Fatigue, weakness, syncope
   h. Palpitations

   i. **Angina pectoris with diaphoresis is usually nocturnal and responsive to conventional treatment.**
   j. Orthopnea, PND, dyspnea on exertion, cough

        k.   Neurologic status varies depending on cerebral blood flow.

   3.   Diagnostic evaluations include:

        a.   ECG reveals left ventricular hypertrophy, prolonged AV conduction, sinus tachycardia, and premature ventricular contractions (PVCs)

        b.   Chest x-ray reveals inferior and posterior elongation of the apex. Valve leaflets may show calcifications and annular openings. Depending on the stage of the disease, pulmonary vasculature congestion, ascending aortic dilatation and enlargement of the cardiac silhouette may be visible.

        c.   Echocardiography visualizes leaflet vegetation and annular opening of the aortic valve, left ventricular enlargement, and abnormal movement of mitral valve. If an ascending aortic dissection is a suspected cause, the dissection can be visualized with this diagnostic test.

        d.   Cardiac catheterization is used to determine pressure elevation within the heart chambers and aortic valve reflux with dye injection.

E.   **Nursing diagnoses for regurgitative valvular disease**

   1.   Altered Tissue Perfusion

   2.   Impaired Individual Coping

   3.   See Stenosis for additional nursing diagnoses

F.   **Planning and implementation for regurgitative valvular disease**

   1.   **Monitor heart rate and rhythm for tachycardia, blood pressure for hypotension and respiratory rate for tachypnea and arterial blood gases for abnormal values.**

   2.   Monitor extremities for cyanosis, coldness, pallor, rubor, absent or diminished pulses, and assess for calf pain or tenderness.

   3.   Monitor neurological status q4hr or PRN for changes in mentation, dysphagia, weakness, paralysis, and parasthenia.

   4.   Assess left upper quadrant pain with radiation to the left shoulder for splenic emboli.

   5.   Assess for flank pain, hematuria, oliguria, renal emboli; monitor BUN and creatinine.

   6.   Administer anticoagulants as prescribed and monitor coagulation studies as appropriate.

   7.   Reinforce patient's and/or family members' coping mechanisms or assist in establishing new coping strategies.

   8.   Be aware of potential complications: Same as indicated in Stenosis.

G.   Evaluation (see Stenosis)

XV.   **Cardiac contusion**

A.   **Description: an injury resulting in a bruised myocardium, commonly affecting the right ventricle due to the chamber's location in the chest cavity.**

B.   **Etiology and incidence**

   1.   Any type of trauma resulting from a blow to the anterior chest wall or compression of the heart between the sternum and spine.

   2.   The most common cause of contusion occurs during a motor vehicle accident (MVA) when the steering wheel or dashboard impacts against the chest wall.

        3.   Approximately 15%–20% of cardiac injuries result from blunt chest trauma.

C. **Pathophysiology**

        1.   Increased intravascular pressure from a sudden compression may result in damage or bleeding of the cardiac vasculature.

        2.   Bruising of the myocardium is usually localized and may cause edema, hemorrhage or necrosis.

        3.   These consequences of the contusion may further result in compression of the myocardial circulation with resultant decrease in blood supply leading to ischemia and possible necrosis.

        4.   **Myocardial infarctions and cardiac contusions have similar presentations, such as depressed contractility and myocardial dysfunction, which makes diagnosis difficult.**

        5.   Cardiac monitoring, serial ECGs and specific tests are ordered for differential diagnosis.

        6.   Nonsteroidal anti-inflammatory drugs (NSAIDs) are administered for pain.

D. **Assessment findings**

        1.   Clinical manifestations include:

            a.   History of appropriate mechanism of injury

            b.   Shortness of breath

            c.   Decreased blood pressure

            d.   Chest wall ecchymosis

            e.   Chest pain

            f.   Tachycardia

            g.   Pericardial friction rub

            h.   Signs and symptoms similar to an AMI

        2.   Laboratory values and diagnostic findings:

            a.   Elevated cardiac enzymes and isoenzymes

            b.   Echocardiography may reveal abnormalities in ventricular wall movement and decreased ejection fraction.

            c.   ECG may reveal nonspecific ST segment and T wave changes, PVCs, PACs, ventricular or atrial tachycardia. Most dysrhythmias occur within 24 hours post-injury.

E. **Nursing diagnoses**

        1.   Pain

        2.   Activity Intolerance

        3.   Decreased Cardiac Output

F. **Planning and implementation**

        1.   **Observe cardiac monitor for rate and dysrhythmias and treat according to hospital protocol.**

        2.   Monitor IV fluids, site, amount of infusion, and urinary output to prevent overload.

        3.   Administer supplemental oxygen via nasal cannula, 2 L/min or as ordered.

        4.   Closely monitor pulse oximetry.

        5.   Administer inotropic medications to increase cardiac output.

        6.   Monitor electrolytes, hemoglobin and hematocrit, serial cardiac enzymes, and arterial blood gases (ABGs).

7.   Perform a pain assessment (PQRST) and administer pain medications as ordered.
8.   Auscultate the heart for murmurs and the lungs for adventitious sounds.

 9.   **Assume the patient is having an AMI until proven otherwise.**
10.   Prepare the patient for diagnostic studies to determine the extent of injury.
11.   Prepare the patient for a pericardiocentesis if cardiac tamponade is suspected.
12.   Prepare the patient for insertion of chest tubes if a pneumothorax or hemothorax is suspected.
13.   Be aware of potential complications including:
    a.   Cardiac tamponade
    b.   Dysrhythmias
    c.   Pericarditis, which is an acute or chronic fibrotic thickening and inflammatory process in the pericardial sac. It is characterized by chest pain that intensifies with respiration, pericardial friction rub, and fatigue.
    d.   Cardiogenic shock
    e.   Myocardial rupture which occurs when the continuity of the myocardium is interrupted as a result of the initial injury to the chest wall.
    f.   Pneumothorax
    g.   Hemothorax
    h.   Flail chest
    i.   AMI
    j.   Lacerated aorta, which is a tear in one or all of the layers lining the aortic wall.
    k.   Fractured ribs can be associated with blunt chest trauma. Interruption in the continuity in a bone of the thoracic cage results from trauma.
    l.   Cardiac arrest, a cessation of the heart, can also occur.

G.   **Evaluation**
    1.   The patient displays improved cardiac output.
    2.   The patient exhibits no evidence of dysrhythmias.
    3.   The patient verbalizes only minimal pain.
    4.   The patient exhibits no evidence of respiratory difficulties.

XVI.   **Cardiac tamponade**

A.   **Description: elevation in intracardiac pressure from rapid accumulation of fluid in the pericardial cavity impeding diastolic filling and cardiac output. This is an emergency situation that must be treated or cardiogenic shock and arrest will ensue.**
B.   **Etiology and incidence**
    1.   Causes include:
        a.   Pericardial effusion
        b.   Hemorrhage
        c.   Trauma
        d.   Cardiac rupture
        e.   Pericarditis
        f.   AMI

      g.   Recent cardiac catheterization or surgery

      h.   Pacemaker insertion

      i.   Bacterial infection

      j.   Chronic renal failure

      k.   Cancer

C.   Pathophysiology

   1.   Accumulation of fluid in the pericardial cavity can be rapid or insidious. It is the rate in which the fluid rises that determines the pressure between the pericardial cavity and the intracardial structures.

   2.   As fluid increases, intrapericardial pressure rises and equals intracardial pressure during diastole. The first structures to be compromised are the right atrium and ventricle which have the lowest diastolic pressures.

   3.   Venous pressure then rises, resulting in elevated diastolic pressures, bilaterally.

   4.   This interferes with filling and pumping of both ventricles, thereby decreasing diastolic filling, stroke volume, and cardiac output with eventual circulatory collapse.

D.   Assessment findings

   1.   Rapid onset manifestations include:

      a.   Beck's triad: hypotension, increased CVP, and muffled or distant heart sounds.

      b.   Tachycardia

      c.   Dyspnea, agitation and restlessness

      d.   Narrow pulse pressure

      e.   Pulsus paradoxus (inspiratory drop in blood pressure >10 mm Hg).

      f.   Distention of neck veins (Kussmaul's sign: distended neck veins with inspiration).

      g.   Increased PAP

      h.   Chest pain (mid-thoracic)

      i.   Sudden decrease in chest tube drainage

   2.   Slow onset manifestations are similar to the signs and symptoms of heart failure.

   3.   Diagnostic findings:

      a.   ECG reveals decreased QRS voltage or flat or inverted T waves. May have nonspecific changes.

      b.   Echocardiography is the most helpful diagnostic tool. It may reveal fluid in pericardial sac, increase in the size of the right ventricle and tricuspid valve flow, and a decrease in the size of the left ventricle and mitral valve flow during inspiration.

      c.   Chest x-ray reveals widening of the mediastinum.

E.   Nursing diagnoses

   1.   Decreased Cardiac Output

   2.   Ineffective Breathing Pattern

   3.   Altered Tissue Perfusion

   4.   Risk for Fluid Volume Deficit

   5.   Impaired Gas Exchange

F. Planning and implementation

1. Monitor continuously for heart rate and rhythm, blood pressure, respiratory rate and depth, and level of consciousness (LOC).

2. Monitor continuously for dysrhythmias and treat according to hospital protocol.

3. Monitor pulse oximetry and prepare for possible mechanical ventilation if not already in place.

4. Administer parenteral fluids for hemodynamic stability.

5. Monitor for increasing CVP, PAP, and PCWP

6. Monitor for signs and symptoms of cardiogenic shock.

7. **Administration of inotropic therapy (dopamine) is ineffective and may be harmful. Impeded diastolic filling and adequate systolic functioning is the cause of hemodynamic instability. Therapy may be instituted after fluid evacuation.**

8. Monitor laboratory values and ABGs.

9. Monitor peripheral pulses, skin color and temperature, and capillary refill.

10. **Prepare the patient for a pericardiocentesis which involves evacuation of fluid from the pericardial cavity with an 18g or larger needle that inserted at the subxiphoid region.**

11. Prepare the patient for drainage catheter insertion during pericardiocentesis, if recurrent effusion is anticipated.

12. Depending on cause, antineoplastic agents, or corticosteroids may be instilled.

13. Prepare the patient for possible pericardectomy or opening of the chest at the bedside or in the operating room.

14. Monitor CVP during and after pericardiocentesis for decreasing CVP and increasing blood pressure as pressure released.

15. Continuously monitor vital signs and cardiac rhythm q15min × 1 hr, q30min × 1 hr, and q1hr × 24 hr.

16. Auscultate heart and breath sounds for abnormalities.

17. Be aware of potential complications:
    a. Cardiogenic shock
    b. Cardiac arrest

G. Evaluation

1. The patient maintains adequate cardiac output as evidenced by normal CVP, pulse pressure, heart rate and rhythm.

2. The patient maintains adequate tissue perfusion as evidenced by a normal respiratory pattern, palpable peripheral pulses, warm and pink skin, and no mentation changes from normal baseline.

XVII. Dissecting aorta

A. Description: an abrupt disruption of the intimal layer of the aorta resulting in a medial hemorrhage and the abnormal flow of blood between the intima and adventitia.

B. Etiology and incidence

1. The exact cause is unknown.

2. Normal aging, disease processes, congenital defects, pregnancy, sheering stress from arterial pulse waves, trauma from deceleration injury, special procedures, surgery, or the IABP are thought to be risk factors for dissection.

3. Between the fifth and seventh decade of life men are two to three times more prone to dissections than women.

C. **Pathophysiology**

1. A sudden tear in the intimal layer of the aorta permits blood to enter the media creating a dissection within the wall of the aorta.

2. **Pressure from the contraction of the heart forces blood through the tear creating a hemorrhage in the medial layer and forming a false lumen between the intima and adventitia.**

3. With each pulsation, expansion of the dissecting hematoma is increased either proximal of distally and may vary in distance.

4. The origin of the dissection has led to the following classification:

   a. Type I is most common, originates in the proximal ascending aorta and through the aortic arch and may extend distally to the bifurcation of the aorta.

   b. Type II is restrained within the ascending aorta.

   c. Type III originates immediately distal to the left subclavian artery and may remain in the thoracic aorta or extend down the descending aorta to the aortic bifurcation or beyond.

   d. Types I and II (proximal dissections) are proximal to the aortic valve and may cause aortic insufficiency and has a high mortality rate. Surgical intervention is necessary for survival with continual medical treatment.

   e. Type III is termed a distal dissection and is treated medically with anti-hypertensives and surgery is not necessary in most cases.

5. Proximal or distal dissection effect the organs in its path by decreasing their blood supply, ie, the brain, spinal cord, abdominal organs and extremities.

6. The longitudinal dissection may rupture at any point along its course or develop a distal tear in the intima and re-enter the true circulation.

D. **Assessment findings**

1. Clinical manifestations include:

   a. Sudden severe chest, epigastric or back pain with radiation to the neck, jaw, throat, or back.

    b. **The above signs and symptoms may be confused with AMI.**

   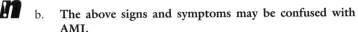 c. **The pain is usually described as a ripping, tearing, or throbbing sensation in the chest. The ripping or tearing description coincides with dissection as it extends down the aorta.**

   d. Unequal, weakened, or absent pulses, including carotid and temporal.

   e. Blood pressure variance from right to left side may occur. Hypertension or hypotension may be seen if rupture is in progress.

   f. Decreased LOC with possible syncope, apprehension, dizziness.

      g.   Heart sounds reveal aortic insufficiency.

      h.   Dyspnea, orthopnea, and bilateral crackles with left ventricular failure and pulmonary edema.

      i.   Hypoactive or absent bowel sounds and abdominal distention, nausea and vomiting.

  2. Laboratory studies reveal:

      a.   Decreased hemoglobin and hematocrit

      b.   Increased WBC

  3. Diagnostic studies include:

      a.   Chest x-ray may reveal abnormal widening of the aorta and left pleural effusion.

      b.   ECG reveals nonspecific S-T–T wave changes.

      c.   Aortography or supravalvular angiography can assess the site and extent of the dissection.

      d.   CT scan with an echocardiography can aid in distinguishing the dissection.

      e.   TEE can visualize a dissecting aneurysm.

E. **Nursing diagnoses**

  1. Pain

  2. Altered Tissue Perfusion

  3. Decreased Cardiac Output

  4. Anxiety

F. **Planning and implementation**

  1. Assess pain parameters (PQRST); obtain an ECG with pain experience.

  2. Continuous cardiac monitoring for dysrhythmias and treat according to hospital protocol.

  3. Administer pain medication as prescribed.

      a.   Narcotics/morphine sulfate are usually given to relieve pain, and diazepam (Valium) may be administered for anxiety.

      b.   Nitroprusside may be given for hypertension and dopamine may be given for hypotension. Nitrates and beta blockers (Inderal) are usually given to decrease myocardial contractility and afterload.

  4. Obtain a chest x-ray per protocol.

  5. **Closely monitor heart rate and rhythm, blood pressure, respirations, and peripheral pulses; auscultate heart, lung, and bowel sounds; palpate abdomen; and assess neurologic and motor function q1hr or PRN.**

  6. Monitor volume replacement: IV fluids, blood, fresh frozen plasma (FFP), albumin.

  7. Monitor PAP, PCWP, CVP, CO, CI q1hr or PRN.

  8. Monitor hemoglobin, hematocrit, electrolytes, BUN, creatine, coagulation studies, cardiac enzymes and isoenzymes, and ABGs.

  9. Monitor for possible mechanical ventilation or apply supplemental oxygen as prescribed.

  10. Keep environment as quiet as possible and maintain patient on bed rest in semi-Fowler's position preferable, unless contraindicated.

  11. Explain all procedures to the patient if possible.

        12. Be aware of potential complications:

            a. Fatal hemorrhage (cardiac arrest as a result of exsanguination can occur)

            b. Cardiac tamponade

            c. Organ failure especially kidneys, spinal cord, and gastrointestinal (GI) tract

G. **Evaluation**

    1. The patient verbalizes relief of pain.

    2. The patient exhibits a calm demeanor.

    3. The patient displays adequate cardiac output as evidenced by blood pressure within normal range, pulses present bilaterally, hourly urinary output >30 mL/hr.

XVIII. **Cardiogenic shock**

    A. **Description: a life-threatening condition in which the heart loses its ability to effectively pump blood throughout the body to meet the metabolic demands of the tissues and bodily organs.**

    B. **Etiology and incidence**

        1. Causes include:

            a. **AMI (this is the major cause resulting in extensive myocardial necrosis)**

            b. Cardiac tamponade

            c. Cardiomyopathy

            d. Restrictive pericarditis

            e. Cardiac arrest

            f. Cardiac dysrhythmias

            g. Heart failure

            h. Tension pneumothorax

            i. Ventricular septal defect

            j. Rupture of ventricular wall, papillary muscle or chordae tendineae

            k. Valvular rupture

            l. Pulmonary embolism

        2. AMI is the major cause with approximately 15%–20% resulting in cardiogenic shock.

        3. Cardiogenic shock resulting from an AMI reflects approximately an 80% mortality rate.

    C. **Pathophysiology**

        1. Cardiogenic shock is precipitated by decreased cardiac output, coronary artery perfusion and oxygenation. The dynamic effect on the myocardium and its tissue can be a result of necrosis or the inability of the heart to adequately maintain its blood flow.

        2. Presents with vasoconstriction, a compensatory mechanism which is a direct result of decreased myocardial contractility.

        3. In an attempt at compensation, the body attempts to supply vital organs, ie, brain, heart and kidneys with sufficient blood to maintain their functions.

        4. The second clinical picture arises from the failed compensatory mechanism. Decreased cardiac output, hypotension and hypoperfusion leads to cellular hypoxia and metabolic acidosis.

        5. If shock cannot be reversed, the third phase of cardiogenic shock is circulatory failure, cellular injury, organ failure, and death.

D.   Assessment findings
1.   Clinical manifestations include:
    a.   Hypotension
    b.   Pulse that is rapid, irregular, and thready. Faint heart sounds, S3 and S4 may also be heard.
    c.   Respirations are rapid, shallow, and labored. Crackles and wheezes may be heard on auscultation.
    d.   Skin is cold, pale, clammy, diaphoretic, and cyanotic with dry, pale mucous membranes.
    e.   Bowel sounds are hypoactive.
    f.   Neurologic findings include diminished deep-tendon reflexes.
    g.   Mental status may be manifested by anxiousness, restlessness, apathy, and lethargy with possible progression to a comatose state.
    h.   Urine shows oliguria progressing to anuria.
    i.   Dysrhythmias may occur.
    j.   Dependent edema and increased JVD.
    k.   Elevated CVP, PCWP, and decreased CO, CI, and increased SVO_2.
2.   Laboratory values may include:
    a.   Cardiac enzymes and isoenzymes to determine AMI.
    b.   BUN and creatinine increased indicating impaired kidney function.
    c.   Hemoglobin and hematocrit decreased secondary to volume loss.
    d.   WBC with differential may show leukocytosis with increased neutrophils.
    e.   Erythrocyte sedimentation rate (ESR) is increased as a result of tissue injury.
    f.   Glucose is increased in early shock in response to catecholamines.
    g.   Sodium is increased with acute tubular necrosis. Potassium is increased following cellular death.
3.   Diagnostic studies:
    a.   ECG to evaluate for AMI, dysrhythmias, and ischemic changes.
    b.   Chest x-ray may reveal pulmonary edema.
    c.   Echocardiography reveals altered ventricular function and pericardial tamponade.
    d.   Ventriculography will reveal a decreased ejection fraction.

E.   Nursing diagnoses
1.   Decreased Cardiac Output
2.   Altered Tissue Perfusion
3.   Anxiety
4.   Ineffective Breathing Pattern
5.   Impaired Gas Exchange
6.   Altered Thought Processes
7.   Fluid Volume Deficit
8.   Powerlessness

F.   Planning and implementation

1. Monitor strict intake and output q1hr and monitor BUN and creatinine.
2. Strict monitoring of vital signs, neurologic assessment, and peripheral pulses q1–2hr or PRN (especially in acute phase).
3. Continuous cardiac monitoring for dysrhythmias and ECG changes indicative of AMI. Treat per protocol.
4. Monitor CVP, PAP, PCWP, CO, and CI.
5. Closely monitor administration of parenteral fluids and volume expanders with PCWP and PAP readings.
6. Calculate SVR, CO, and CI.
7. Administer inotropic agents as ordered.
8. IABP is frequently instituted in the management of cardiogenic shock to prevent cardiovascular collapse, reduce afterload, reduce the workload of the heart and improve coronary blood flow and cardiac output.
9. A ventricular assist device (VAD) is another method employed to assist the failing ventricle. This device is a temporary measure to maintain coronary and systemic circulation until transplantation or surgery can be performed.
10. Drug therapy includes:
    a. Low-dose dopamine for renal perfusion and dobutamine to increase stroke volume, contractility, cardiac output and decrease systemic vascular resistance
    b. **Dopamine at higher doses is used in conjunction with vasodilators to maintain an adequate blood pressure.**
    c. Dobutamine decreases preload and systemic vascular resistance, increases contractility, cardiac output, stoke volume, and renal perfusion (low dose).
    d. **Dopamine and dobutamine increase myocardial oxygen demand rendering the patient at risk for infarct extension.**
    e. **Amrinone decreases systemic resistance, myocardial oxygen consumption, pulmonary capillary wedge pressure, and blood pressure**
    f. Vasodilators such as nitroprusside and nitroglycerin are used to decrease preload, afterload and myocardial oxygen consumption
         ▸ **Nitroglycerin (vasodilator) may be used to decrease peripheral vascular resistance and preload and improve cardiac output.**
        ▸ If nipride is used, serum thiocyanate levels should be obtained q24hr.
        ▸ Long term use may cause cyanide toxicity.
        ▸ **Norepinephrine (Levophed), a potent vasoconstrictor, may be used for severe hypotension, at a dose of 2–6 mg/kg/min. It causes arterial constriction increasing PVR, cardiac output and improves coronary artery blood flow.**

n ▶ The major disadvantage is that it increases oxygen consumption.

    g.   Digitalis may be used for its positive inotropic affects but it increases the oxygen demand of the myocardium.

11.   The treatment goal of cardiogenic shock is to increase myocardial contractility and maintain renal blood flow. Patients are treated according to clinical and hemodynamic presentation.

12.   Administer and monitor sodium bicarbonate infusion if acidosis is present.

13.   Apply a non-rebreather mask or prepare for intubation and mechanical ventilation as indicated.

14.   Monitor serial ABGs, respiratory pattern, auscultate breath sounds q1–2hr or PRN, and suction PRN.

15.   Monitor electrolytes, especially potassium, BUN, creatinine, hemoglobin, hematocrit, and urinalysis, especially specific gravity.

16.   Administer tube feedings, TPN, and/or lipids as prescribed.

17.   Prepare for and monitor IABP as indicated.

18.   Explain treatment and procedures in a soft calm voice to the patient and family members and encourage expression of feelings; stay with the patient for reassurance.

19.   Be aware of potential complications such as AMI, multiple system organ failure, cardiac arrest, DIC, and adult respiratory distress syndrome.

G. **Evaluation**

1.   The patient demonstrates an adequate rise in blood pressure and hemodynamic monitoring values; warm and dry skin, palpable pulses, and increased urinary output.

2.   The patient exhibits normal a breathing pattern and ABGs return to normal values.

3.   The patient experiences a reduction in anxiety as evidenced by verbalizing fears and asking questions.

XIX. **Thrombolytics**

A. **Description: these agents cause lysis of the pathogenic clot and a hypocoagulable state in the entire circulatory system.**

1.   When employed as a lytic agent in coronary artery thrombi, treatment should be initiated within 4–6 hr of onset of symptoms.

2.   Currently there four are thrombolytic agents in use: streptokinase (SK), urokinase, anisoylated plasminogen-streptokinase activator complex (APSAC), and tissue plasminogen activator (t-PA) or recombinant tissue-type plasminogen activator (rt-PA).

3.   t-Pa and rt-PA are clot specific in that they attack the fibrin. The fibrin is broken down by the plasmin and the clot dissolves.

4.   Streptokinase and urokinase are proteolytic enzymes which covert plasminogen to plasmin promoting a systemic thrombolytic state. These agents are also effective in the treatment of deep vein thrombosis (DVT) and pulmonary embolism. Urokinase works best on newly formed clots and is useful in clearing occluded catheters.

     5.   Streptokinase is derived from streptococcus organisms thereby producing an antigen–antibody reaction in a patient who previously received this agent. Severe hypersensitivity reactions or anaphylaxis may result.

B.   Indications for administration in coronary patients
1.   Signs and symptoms consistent with AMI.
2.   Persistent chest pain 4–6 hours from onset of symptoms.
3.   S-T segment elevation of 1 mm or >1 mm in a minimum of two contiguous limb leads.
4.   S-T segment elevation of 2 mm or >2 mm in a minimum of two contiguous precordial leads.

C.   Indications for administration in patients without coronary disease
1.   Pulmonary embolism
    a.   Streptokinase started within 7 days after development of embolism; maximum effects are 24 hours after administration; continue 24 hours after drug completion.
    b.   Urokinase is most effective when started within 5 days of onset of symptoms; works best on newly formed clots.
2.   Acute ischemic strokes:
    a.   t-PA when used within first few hours after stroke decreases the risk of bleeding.
    b.   Research is currently being done regarding efficacy, safety, optimal dose, and timing.
3.   Arterial thrombosis or embolism:
    a.   No presence of tissue necrosis
    b.   Treatment with thrombolytic agents such as streptokinase, urokinase, t-PA
    c.   Lysis is approximately 50%–80% of cases.
    d.   Recent surgery, uncontrolled bleeding, hypertension, or pregnancy are contraindications to administration.
4.   Venous thrombosis
    a.   Streptokinase, urokinase, alteplase, and anistreplase have been shown to destroy venous emboli that are < 72 hours old more rapidly and efficiently then heparin therapy without additional damage to venous valves.
    b.   Not used in instances of intracranial disease, recent stoke, active bleeding or bleeding disorder, pregnancy, severe hypertension, recent surgery or trauma.
    c.   No invasive procedures are to be performed.

D.   Assessment findings
1.   Obtain a patient history to elicit contraindications to thrombolytic therapy such as:
    a.   Recent surgery (10 days to 2 weeks)
    b.   Bleeding disorders
    c.   Active or recent internal bleeding
    d.   Intracranial bleed or disease
    e.   Diabetic hemorrhagic retinopathy
    f.   Uncontrolled hypertension
    g.   Recent cerebral vascular accident (CVA)
    h.   Malignancy
    i.   Acute pericarditis or endocarditis

    j. Pregnancy

    k. Active peptic ulcer disease

    l. Significant liver or kidney dysfunction

    m. Oral anti-coagulants

    n. Previous streptokinase or APSAC therapy (<1 year)

    o. Streptococcal infection within the last six months

  2. During therapy assess the patient for indications of therapeutic success such as:

    a. Sudden relief or reduction of chest pain

    b. Resolution of ECG abnormalities

    c. Reperfusion dysrhythmias

    d. CK-MB isoenzymes peak within 12 hours

  3. Laboratory values pertinent to thrombolytic therapy:

    a. Prothrombin time (PT)

    b. Activated partial thromboplastic time (APTT)

    c. Hemoglobin and hematocrit (H and H)

    d. Cardiac enzymes and isoenzymes (CK-MB)

E. Nursing diagnoses

  1. Altered Tissue Perfusion: Cardiopulmonary

  2. Altered Protection

  3. Risk for Fluid Volume Deficit

  4. Ineffective Breathing Pattern

  5. Anxiety

F. Planning and implementation

  1. Reinforce physician's explanation of thrombolytic therapy.

  2. **Before administration of thrombolytic agent, establish necessary IV accesses and obtain pertinent blood specimens.**

  3. Prepare and administer thrombolytic agent as ordered.

  4. Administer supplemental oxygen; 2–4 L/min via nasal cannula.

  5. Monitor IV infusion rate and sites for bleeding.

  6. Assess patient for chest pain.

  7. Observe cardiac monitor for heart rate, regression of ECG abnormalities, and reperfusion dysrhythmias.

  8. Avoid IM injections for approximately 24 hr.

  9. Assess urine, feces, nasogastric tube (NGT) aspirate, or vomitus for evidence of bleeding.

  10. Monitor laboratory values, PT, APTT, H and H, WBC.

  11. Assess neurologic status for evidence of increased intracranial pressure and changes in LOC and restlessness.

  12. Monitor vital signs and blood pressure for hypotension and tachycardia.

  13. Handle patient as little as possible to avoid bruising.

  14. Apply direct pressure to all puncture sites for 30 min.

  15. **Monitor for signs and symptoms of reocclusion and reinfarction such as chest pain, nausea, diaphoresis, shortness of breath, S-T segment elevation, dysrhythmias, and hemodynamic instability.**

  16. Assess heart and breath sounds, abdomen, and peripheral pulses.

  17. Prepare the patient for possible subsequent interventions such as PTCA, CABG, or possible repeat thrombolytic therapy.

18. Inspect skin for bruises or ecchymosis and gums and nose for bleeding.
19. Support the patient and family members during therapy.
20. Monitor continuous heparin and nitroglycerin infusions.
21. Apply sterile dressings to all puncture sites.
22. Be aware of potential complications such as hemorrhage; reperfusion dysrhythmias, such as PVCs and ventricular dysrhythmias; and allergic reactions (particularly with streptokinase).

G. Evaluation
1. The patient maintains hemodynamic stability during therapy.
2. The patient exhibits no evidence of bleeding.
3. The patient verbalizes a reduction in chest pain.
4. The patient verbalizes a reduction of fears and concerns.

XX. Percutaneous transluminal angioplasty (PTCA)

A. Description: a nonsurgical procedure, performed under fluoroscopy, that uses a pressurized balloon catheter with an independent moveable guidewire located within the catheter. The purpose of the procedure is to expand stenotic coronary arteries.
1. The dilation catheter is inserted through a previously inserted guiding catheter and slowly advanced over its internal guidewire into the area of stenosis and inflated.
2. Radio-opaque markers on the balloon determine the position of the dilation catheter.
3. Contrast media is injected to access luminal diameter and blood flow through the stenosed coronary artery.

B. Indications
1. AMI with or without thrombolytic therapy.
2. Asymptomatic angina with severe underlying stenosis.
3. Stable/unstable angina unresponsive to medical treatment.
4. High risk surgical patient.
5. Possible progression of coronary artery disease in a young adult.
6. Stenosis equal to or >50%.
7. Distal and proximal lesions.
8. Multivessel and single vessel disease.
9. Lesions located at bifurcations.
10. Coronary arteries that are totally occluded.
11. CABG patients with stenosis or graft closure or progression of coronary artery disease.
12. Rescue PTCA after thrombolytic therapy in patients with persistent occlusion of a diseased artery.
13. Stenosis that is single, proximal, noncalcific, and concentric.

C. Assessment findings
1. Physical assessment should include heart rate and rhythm, breath sounds, peripheral pulses, neurologic status, urinary function, and body weight.
2. Pertinent laboratory values:
   a. Cardiac enzymes
   b. Coagulation profile
   c. Serum electrolytes (K, BUN, and creatinine are particular important) and hemoglobin and hematocrit.
   d. Type and cross for potential blood replacement.

D.   **Nursing diagnoses**
1.   Decreased Cardiac Output
2.   Altered Tissue Perfusion: Peripheral, Cerebral
3.   Activity Intolerance
4.   Pain
5.   Fluid Volume Excess
6.   Knowledge Deficit
7.   Anxiety
8.   Altered Protection

E.   **Planning and implementations**
1.   Explain all procedures to the patient and family members
2.   Initiate rehabilitation education to include pathophysiology of disease process, risk factors, diet, medications, importance of medical follow-up care.
3.   Monitor and record vital signs q15min × 4, q30min × 4, q1hr × 4 then q4hr × 24 hr post-procedure.
4.   Monitor CVP, PAP, and PCWP q1hr and continuously assess cardiac monitor for dysrhythmias and administer antidysrhythmics per protocol.
5.   Auscultate, breath sounds for crackles and heart sounds for S3 gallop.
6.   Maintain bed rest for 6 to 8 hours and assist with ADLs.
7.   Monitor IV site for infection and/or bleeding and maintain infusion rate as prescribed.
8.   Monitor and record intake and output and report < 30 mL/hr.
9.   Head of bed should be raised 30–45 degrees for the first 8 hr only.
10.   Instruct the patient to verbalize recurrence of angina and administer vasodilators, NTG, isordil, or narcotics as ordered and assess for pain relief. Calcium channel blockers, nifedipine, or diltiazem may be used for coronary spasms.
11.   Administer diuretics, digoxin, nitrates or vasopressors, levophed/norepinephrine, dopamine, as ordered.
12.   Monitor laboratory values, cardiac enzymes, coagulation studies, serum electrolytes, and ABGs.
13.   Assess neurologic status.
14.   Prepare the patient for repeat PTCA or CABG as necessary and alert the operating room if indicated.
15.   **Have temporary pacemaker of external pacemaker on standby and access to IABP.**
16.   **Be prepared for cardiac arrest and endotracheal intubation.**
17.   Elevate extremities and observe site for hematoma, ecchymosis, warmth, tenderness, and drainage.
18.   Maintain sterile pressure dressings to arterial puncture site.
19.   Apply 5-lb sandbag over puncture site if prescribed.
20.   Maintain involved leg in a straight position.
21.   Assess for restenosing as manifested by signs and symptoms of AMI.
22.   Observe for allergic complications of contrast media.
23.   Administer anticoagulants, aspirin, persantine, heparin as ordered.

24. Be aware of potential complications:
   a. Reocclusion: reblockage of the diseased artery.
   b. Coronary artery spasm: a sudden onset of a transient constriction of the diseased vessel or any other coronary artery.
   c. Perforation: a piercing of the entire thickness of the involved coronary artery.
   d. Rupture: a sudden break in the continuity of the diseased coronary artery.
   e. AMI
   f. Hemorrhage
   g. Hematoma: a trapping of blood in the tissues of the skin or organ resulting from trauma.
   h. Dye reaction: an antigen–antibody response to the contract media.
   i. Cerebral vascular accident
   j. Sinus bradycardia: a myocardial contraction rate of <60 beats per minute.
   k. Embolism: an embolus that travels through the circulatory system and lodges in a blood vessel.

F. Evaluation
   1. The patient maintains hemodynamic stability and optimal systemic perfusion.
   2. The patient exhibits no evidence of infection or bleeding at cannulation site.
   3. The patient offers no complaints of chest pain.
   4. The patient does not exhibit any compromise in respiratory or neurologic status.
   5. The patient demonstrates a reduction in anxiety.
   6. The patient verbalizes an understanding of the information imparted at teaching sessions.

XXI. Intracoronary stents
   A. Description: self-expanding or balloon expandable, tubular mesh, or coilspring devices that are placed in the lumen of diseased coronary arteries during the PTCA procedure.
   1. These new investigative devices are designed to reduce the rate of restenosis by maintaining an adequate artificial lumen.
   2. Another investigative device is a heat-sensitive stent that expands after placement by reacting to the temperature of the blood
   B. Indications: Restenosis or acute closure of a coronary artery after PTCA.
   C. Assessment findings (see PTCA)
   D. Nursing diagnosis (see PTCA)
   E. Planning and implementation
   1. Administer anticoagulant therapy; heparin and warfarin (Coumadin) to prevent thrombus formation and antiplatelet agent.
   2. Explain to the patient and family members that hospitalization may be extended to establish anticoagulant level.
   3. Teach the patient and family members the importance of drug therapy, medical follow-up care, and seeking medical care if signs and symptoms of AMI recur.

4.   **Monitor heart rate and rhythm, respiratory rate, blood pressure and observe the cannulation site for signs of bleeding.**

    5.   Be aware of potential complications such as hemorrhage, embolism, reocclusion, and rupture.

    6.   For additional planning and interventions see PTCA.

F.   Evaluation (see PTCA)

XXII.   **Laser surgery**

    A.   **Description: an investigative procedure designed to dilate coronary arteries through the interaction of a pulsed-wave laser energy with atheromatous plaques and thrombi.**

        1.   **A catheter containing a laser is threaded through a coronary artery to the area of occlusion. At this point, the physician activates the laser and rapid bursts of laser energy are emitted. The plaque is vaporized increasing the lumen size and coronary artery blood flow.**

        2.   A balloon catheter is used to widen the artery further and an angiography may be done to document patency.

    B.   **Indications**

        1.   Totally or partially blocked coronary arteries and/or restenosed arteries.

        2.   Useful in removing fibrous, calcified, or fatty plaques.

        3.   Best results with thrombotic occlusions have been documented.

    C.   **Planning and implementation (see PTCA)**

XXIII.   **Endarterectomy**

    A.   **Description: a surgical procedure removing the intimal lining of an artery.**

        1.   It is performed to remove atherosclerotic plaques from the aortic arch or common carotid bifurcation.

        2.   A carotid endarterectomy may be required before a CABG to alleviate the possibility of plaques dislodging and obstructing coronary artery blood flow.

    B.   **Assessment findings**

        1.   Patient history of a transient ischemic attack (TIA)

        2.   Physical exam should include:

            a.   Auscultation for presence of a carotid bruit

            b.   Thorough neurologic exam

            c.   Vital signs, blood pressure, heart sounds, and peripheral pulses

        3.   Diagnostic tests may include:

            a.   Carotid Doppler studies and CT scans are performed to rule out a CVA.

            b.   ECG may reveal a mural thrombosis.

            c.   An angiogram may reveal areas in the carotid plaque that have broken free. These areas are called niches.

        4.   A 70% occlusion is considered significant.

    C.   **Nursing diagnoses**

        1.   Alterations in Tissue Perfusion: Cerebral

        2.   Ineffective Breathing Pattern

        3.   Altered Protection

D. **Planning and implementation**
1. Maintain the head in a straight position.
2. Monitor post-operative vital signs per protocol and elevate head of bed when the vital signs are stable.
3. Monitor blood pressure frequently to ensure cerebral perfusion.
4. Assess operative site q1hr or PRN for excessive swelling or formation of a hematoma.

5. **Monitor neurologic functions including pupillary reactions, LOC, sensory and motor function, and pay particular attention to cranial nerves VII (facial), X (vagus), XI (spinal accessory, and XII (hypoglossal).**
6. Administer pain medication as prescribed.
7. Auscultate lung fields for adventitious breath sounds.
8. Be aware of potential complications
   a. Hemorrhage
   b. Hematoma
   c. Embolism
   d. CVA
   e. TIA
   f. Increased intracranial pressure

E. **Evaluation**
1. The patient verbalizes relief of pain after administration of pain medication.
2. The patient exhibits normal neurological functions.
3. The patient exhibits normal respiratory functioning.

XXIV. **Intra-aortic balloon pump (IABP)**

A. **Description: a circulatory support device that increases coronary artery blood flow and perfusion, decreases oxygen demand and workload of the left ventricle, and increases oxygen supply to the heart and vital organs by mechanical counterpulsation.**
1. The balloon catheter is inserted into the femoral artery via a percutaneous incision in the groin. The catheter is advanced and the balloon is positioned in the thoracic aorta above the renal arteries and distal to the origin of the left subclavian artery (Fig. 4-7).
2. After proper placement of the balloon, the end of the catheter is connected to a console. A triggering mechanism within the console determines the inflation and deflation of the balloon.
3. The inflation and deflation cycles are regulated according to the arterial waveform and the ECG.
   a. Balloon inflation during diastole is triggered on the downslope of the T wave or an interval after the R wave, and is represented by the dicrotic notch on the arterial waveform.
   b. With inflation aortic diastolic pressure and coronary perfusion pressure are increased, thus improving coronary and systemic blood flow and oxygen supply.
4. Deflation occurs during systole and is triggered by the R wave on the ECG and begins on the upstroke of the arterial waveform. This counterpulsation decreases the afterload, allowing lower aortic pressure when ejecting blood from the left ventricle, thus decreasing the workload and oxygen demand of the left ventricle.

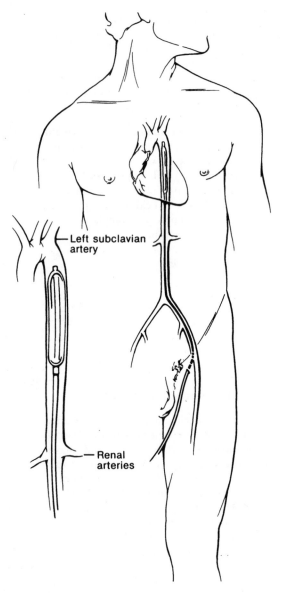

FIGURE 4-7.
Location of IABP.

B.   Indications

1.   Cardiogenic shock
2.   Left ventricular failure
3.   Unstable angina
4.   Post-infarct ventricular septal defect or mitral regurgitation
5.   Septic shock
6.   Pre-operative, intra-operative, and post-operative open heart surgery

       7.   May be used to wean from cardiopulmonary bypass

       8.   May be used as a circulatory assist before heart transplantation

C.   Assessment findings

       1.   Physical assessment should include heart rate and rhythm, auscultation of lung fields for adventitious sounds and heart for murmurs, palpation of peripheral pulses, and assessment of neurological and renal status.

       2.   Assess hemodynamic pressures: PAP, PCWP, CO, CI, and MAP.

D.   Nursing diagnoses

       1.   Decreased Cardiac Output

       2.   Altered Tissue Perfusion

       3.   Impaired Gas Exchange

       4.   Risk for Impaired Skin Integrity

       5.   Risk for Infection

       6.   Sensory-Perceptual Alterations: Visual, Auditory, Tactile

       7.   Sleep Pattern Disturbance

E.   Planning and implementation

       1.   **Verify correct IABP timing q1hr and document settings. Re-evaluate timing for increased or decreased heart rate >10 BPM. Variations may affect the performance of the pump.**

       2.   Maintain good arterial waveform to monitor timing. Notify physician if A-line if not functioning properly.

       3.   **Assess vital signs q1hr and observe cardiac monitor for dysrhythmias; irregular dysrhythmias may inhibit effective pumping.**

       4.   Assess neurologic and cardiovascular status hourly and document. Notify physician of change in mental status, edema, and decreased peripheral pulses, especially of the cannulated extremity.

       5.   **Maintain heparin infusion and additional parenteral fluids at prescribed rates.**

       6.   Maintain head of bed at 15 degrees or lower and cannulated leg in a straight position to avoid hip flexion.

       7.   Active and passive range of motion of ankles q1hr and evaluate pulses with complaints of leg and/or foot pain.

       8.   Maintain motion of balloon to prevent thrombus formation on balloon.

       9.   Auscultate breath sounds at least q2–4hr and if intubated, suction PRN.

      10.   Observe pulse oximetry and obtain ABGs as indicated.

      11.   Talk with patient and inform him or her of date and time and respond to any personal inquiries regarding his progress.

      12.   Explain all procedures, activities and minimize unnecessary noises in the room.

      13.   Turn q2hr and assess skin integrity.

      14.   Maintain TPN and/or nasogastric feedings.

      15.   Administer sedation as prescribed.

      16.   Observe all insertion sites and incisions for signs and symptoms of infection and perform sterile dressing changes.

17. Change all infusion tubings as per protocol.
18. Administered antibiotics as prescribed.
19. Monitor CVP, PAP, PCWP, CO, CI q1–2hr or PRN.
20. Be aware of potential complications such as:
    a. Hemorrhage
    b. Infection
     c. **Thromboembolism causing the blockage of a blood vessel. An embolus travels through the circulatory system from its point of origin to the involved vessel and obstructs flow.**
    d. Arterial insufficiency occurs when blood flow in the arteries is inadequate.
     e. **Compartment syndrome is a pathologic condition resulting from decreased blood supply and compression of the arteries.**
    f. Balloon leakage and/or rupture occurs when disruption in the surface of the balloon occurs because of a large tear or small pinhole. Gas embolism may be a result of this complication.

F. **Evaluation**
  1. The patient maintains hemodynamic stability and optimal systemic perfusion.
  2. The patient exhibits no evidence of infection or bleeding at cannulation or incisional sites.
  3. The patient displays no evidence of cardiovascular, respiratory, or neurologic compromise.
  4. The patient and family members verbalizes an understanding of condition and activities in the intensive care or coronary care unit.

XXV.   Ventricular assist device (VAD)
  A. **Description: mechanical devices that temporarily provide partial or complete control of left ventricular function.**
    1. Three types of VADs are currently in use: IABP (see IABP), centrifugal pump, and the pulsatile pump.
    2. The centrifugal pump, located outside the body, collects blood from a cannulated left atrium.
       a. Linear blood flow controlled by a centrifugal force within the pump propels blood forward to the ascending aorta via a separate cannula.
       b. The left ventricle is bypassed and is given time to recover and resume normal functioning.
    3. Implanted in the abdomen or located outside the body, a pulsatile pump can assume the workload of the left ventricle.
       a. The blood enters the pump via the cannulated right or left ventricle.
       b. When the pump is filled the blood is forced out by a pneumatic or electrical mechanism and the blood is returned via a cannula inserted into the ascending aorta.

c. **The pumping action is synchronized with the R wave of the ECG or controlled by a sensing mechanism within the pump.**
    d. This device can maintain a patient awaiting a heart transplant or assist the ventricle in its recovery process.

B. **Indications**
    1. Ventricular failure caused by an MI.
    2. Failure to wean from cardiopulmonary bypass after open heart surgery.
    3. Patients awaiting cardiac transplantation.

C. **Assessment findings**
    1. Assessment of cardiac history including medications should be attained;
    2. A pulmonary and cardiac assessment should be performed on all patients;
    3. Patient's and family members' knowledge level, and psychological state and role/relationship pattern should be ascertained.

D. **Nursing diagnoses**
    1. Decreased Cardiac Output
    2. Pain
    3. Impaired Gas Exchange
    4. Risk for Infection
    5. Anxiety

E. **Planning and implementation**

 1. **Maintain strict aseptic technique with dressing changes at incisional sites, and observe for drainage and signs and symptoms of infection.**
    2. Monitor for signs and symptoms of right-sided heart failure.
    3. Administer pain medication as prescribed including narcotic analgesics, such as morphine sulfate.
    4. Continuous cardiac monitoring for pacemaker capture if wires are connected and for dysrhythmias. Administer antidysrhythmics per protocol.
    5. Monitor for signs and symptoms of decreased cardiac output.

 6. **Monitor cardiovascular, peripheral vascular, pulmonary and neurologic status for changes, document, and report changes from baseline.**
    7. Monitor PCWP, CVP, CO and CI q1–4hr or PRN.

 8. **Monitor and evaluate chest tube drainage q1hr, if applicable. Notify physician if >200 mL/hr.**
    9. Monitor laboratory values including electrolytes, WBC, hemoglobin and hematocrit, and coagulation studies.
    10. Maintain parenteral fluids infusion rate, and observe site for signs and symptoms of infection.
    11. Monitor blood pressure and temperature and administer inotropic agents (dopamine, dobutamine) and an antipyretic (Tylenol), as prescribed.
    12. Maintain heparin infusion as prescribed and monitor PTT.

13. Observe pulse oximetry and obtain ABGs as indicated.
14. Administer antibiotics as prescribed.
15. If intubated, suction PRN and auscultate breath sounds q1–2hr or PRN.
16. Teach the patient and family members the mechanisms of VAD, performing sterile dressing changes, monitoring for complications, administration of medications, and use of emergency medical personnel.
17. Provide emotional support and encourage verbalization of fears and anxieties.
18. Be aware of potential complications such as:
    a. Infection
    b. Thromboembolism
    c. Cardiac tamponade
    d. Hemorrhage

F. Evaluation
1. The patient exhibits decreased anxiety and verbally expressed feelings.
2. The patient displays stabilization of hemodynamic parameters, cardiac rhythm, and vital signs.
3. The patient and family members verbalize an understanding of teaching associated with VAD.
4. The patient remains free of infection at incisional and IV sites.

XXVI. Myoplasty

A. Description: a grafting together of a patient's latissimus dorsi with the left ventricle and implanting a pacemaker to stimulate contractions thereby augmenting the pumping action of a failing left ventricle.

B. Indications
1. Heart failure refractory to medical management.
2. Cardiomyopathy.

C. Assessment findings: Complete physical assessment including review of systems (see Heart transplantation).

D. Nursing diagnosis (see Heart transplantation)

E. Planning and implementation
1. Continuous cardiac monitoring postoperatively because the transplanted muscle does not immediately support the failing heart.
2. Be aware of potential complications such as:
    a. Heart failure
    b. Cardiac tamponade
    c. Infection
    d. Dysrhythmias
    e. Pacemaker failure: failure of the stimulus to depolarize the myocardium.
    f. Loss of pacemaker sensing: failure of the pacemaker to sense intracardiac signals.
3. For additional interventions, see Heart transplantation

F. Evaluation (see Heart transplantation)

XXVII. **Valvuloplasty**

    A. Description: an open surgical procedure to repair or reconstruct cardiac valves (valvuloplasty) or a nonsurgical invasive procedure to dilate stenotic valves (percutaneous balloon valvuloplasty [PBV]).

        1. A valvuloplasty is similar to a CABG in that a cardio-pulmonary bypass is necessary for the surgical procedure.

        2. The PBV procedure is similar to a PTCA. A major difference is the catheter shaft and balloon diameter is larger in the PBV than ones used for the PTCA.

    B. Indications

        1. Valvuloplasty:

           a. Mitral and tricuspid regurgitation

           b. Mitral valve prolapse

           c. Aortic stenosis

        2. PBV:

           a. Patients who refuse surgery

           b. High risk for surgery

           c. Moderate to severe valvular narrowing or calcification

           d. Mild valvular regurgitation

    C. Assessment findings (see PTCA)

    D. Nursing Diagnosis (see PTCA)

    E. Planning and Implementation (see PTCA)

    F. Evaluation (see PTCA)

    G. Potential complications:

        1. Hemorrhage at the arterial puncture site due to the large diameter of the catheter

        2. Embolism

        3. Valvular restenosis

        4. Aortic dissection

        5. Aortic rupture: a sudden break or tear in the continuity of the wall of the aorta

        6. Cardiac tamponade

        7. Chordae tendineae rupture: a sudden break in the continuity of the strands of tendon that secure the cusps of the valves (mitral and tricuspid) to the papillary muscles.

        8. Valvular regurgitation

        9. Hypotension

        10. Left-to-right atrial shunt. The blood is shunted from the left side to the right side of the heart through a transseptal puncture that was created during a mitral valvuloplasty procedure.

        11. Left ventricular perforation: a hole through the entire thickness of the ventricle.

XXVIII. **Coronary artery bypass graft**

    A. Description: diversion of blood flow around an occluded coronary artery.

        1. This conduit is accomplished through anastomosing of the saphenous vein or internal mammary artery to the vessel distal to the obstruction or to the aorta.

2.   Intraoperatively, a cardiopulmonary bypass pump is used to arrest the heart during surgery and provide adequate perfusion and oxygenation throughout the body.

B.   Indications
1.   Unstable angina refractory to medical management.
2.   Chronic stable angina unresponsive to medical management.
3.   Significant stenosis of the left main coronary artery (stenosis >50).
4.   Severe coronary artery disease in three vessels.
5.   Continued angina after an MI.
6.   AMI.
7.   Unsuccessful PTCA.

C.   Assessment findings
1.   Health history should include:
   a.   Cardiac history, including prescribed and over-the-counter medications.
   b.   Pulmonary history, including medications.
   c.   Review of systems, focusing on respiratory and renal status, including family history.
   d.   Patient's and family members knowledge level, psychological status and role/relationship pattern.
   e.   Physical assessment: see PTCA.
2.   Pertinent laboratory values should include:
   a.   Cardiac enzymes
   b.   CBC
   c.   Coagulation profile
   d.   Serum electrolytes (potassium, BUN, and creatinine are particularly important) and hemoglobin and hematocrit
   e.   Urinalysis
   f.   Type and cross for potential blood replacement; if elective surgery, autologous blood may be available.
3.   Diagnostic testing
   a.   ECG
   b.   Chest x-ray

D.   Nursing diagnoses
1.   Decreased Cardiac Output
2.   Pain
3.   Ineffective Thermoregulation
4.   Impaired Gas Exchange
5.   Anxiety
6.   Knowledge Deficit
7.   Risk for Infection
8.   Altered Tissue Perfusion: Cardiopulmonary

E.   Planning and implementation
1.   Preoperative
   a.   Reinforce teaching and information on the procedure provided by the surgeon and anesthesiologist; reinforce preoperative routine.
   b.   Inform the patient of anticipated postoperative care and equipment.

    c.   Encourage patient and family members to express positive and negative feelings and concerns; be nonjudgmental and respect their feelings.

    d.   Obtain preoperative blood studies and urine analysis as ordered.

    e.   Demonstrate postoperative techniques that the patient will perform (eg, deep breathing and coughing).

    f.   Verify patient's signature and witnessed signature of informed consent.

    g.   Administer sedative as prescribed.

2.   Postoperative

    a.   Monitor vital signs and hemodynamic parameters; PAP, PCWP, CVP, LAP, CO, CI, A-line, and oxygen saturation.

    b.   Auscultate heart and breath sounds, peripheral pulses, and level of consciousness (LOC).

    c.   **Monitor and record chest tube drainage and report >200 mL/hr.**

    d.   Administer parenteral fluids and assess rate of infusion and insertion site for signs and symptoms of infection.

    e.   Administer medications as ordered: inotopic medications, dopamine, dobutamine, digoxin, and vasodilators: nitroprusside and nitroglycerin and antiarrhythmics as per protocol.

    f.   **Temporary pacer box should be at the bedside and initiate pacing as indicated.**

    g.   Assess for signs of cardiac tamponade and notify physician immediately.

    h.   Institute rewarming if temperature is <96.8°F. Administer medications for shivering as prescribed: meperidine, morphine sulfate, thorazine, or diazapam.

    i.   Instruct the patient and family to immediately report any pain.

    j.   Assess pain parameters (PQRST) and administer analgesics for pain and assess for relief. (Analgesics may be administered on a scheduled basis for the first 24–48 hr post-surgery.)

    k.   Secure endotracheal tube, suction PRN, and monitor ventilator settings as ordered. Continuous or q1hr pulse oximetry and obtain and monitor ABGs.

    l.   Prepare the patient for weaning and extubation as appropriate.

    m.   Assess incisions, especially sternal, every shift and record appearance and/or drainage of any signs of infection.

    n.   Maintain strict sterile technique with all dressing changes.

    o.   Continuously monitor cardiac rate and rhythm and document every shift.

    p.   Monitor serum electrolytes, hemoglobin and hematocrit, WBC, coagulation studies, and urinalysis.

    q.   Frequently orient the patient after anesthesia and involve family members with patient orientation.

   r. Perform neurologic assessment every shift.

   s. Report hallucinations, agitation, and secure all invasive tubes and catheters.

   t. Monitor Foley catheter for patency and color, odor, consistency, and amount and maintain strict intake and output.

   u. Assess bowel sounds and monitor nasogastric tube drainage.

   v. Keep open communication with the patient and family members to address positive and negative concerns and relieve anxieties and fears regarding daily progression and offer encouragement.

   w. Patient may be maintained on an IABP. See IABP section for nursing care.

  3. Be aware of potential complications:

   a. Hemorrhage

   b. Pulmonary embolism

   c. Atelectasis: collapse of lung tissue thereby preventing proper gas exchange within the respiratory system

   d. Dysrhythmias

   e. Cardiac tamponade

   f. Infection

   g. Cardiac arrestt

F. **Evaluation**

 1. The patient maintains hemodynamic stability as evidenced by stable vital signs, normal sinus rhythm, and palpable peripheral pulses.

 2. The patient verbalizes decreased pain after administration of pain medication.

 3. The patient and family members experience a reduction in fears and anxiety as evidenced by verbalization of feeling less fearful and anxious.

 4. The patient does not exhibit any compromise in respiratory status.

 5. The patient displays normal responses to neurologic assessment.

 6. The patient does not exhibit any signs and symptoms of infection around incisional and/or drainage sites.

XXIX. **Femoral artery bypass graft**

 A. **Description: an occluded artery is bypassed by an autogenous or synthetic graft. The most common site of occlusion is in the lower extremities**

 B. **Indications**

  1. An ischemic limb with pain at rest

  2. Severe ulceration or gangrene of the limb

  3. Incapacitating intermittent claudication

 C. **Assessment findings**

  1. Obtain health history to include any of the following:

   a. Hypertension

   b. Diabetes mellitus

   c. Obesity

   d. Smoking (pack/years)

   e. Diet: fat intake
   f. Activity intolerance
   g. Family history of vascular disease
  2. Physical assessment should include evaluation of:
   a. Heart rate and rhythm, breath sounds, peripheral pulses, and presence of bruits
   b. Neurologic and integumentary status.
  3. Diagnostic studies may include:
   a. Doppler pressures
   b. Angiography
   c. Plethysmography

D. **Nursing diagnoses**
  1. Altered Tissue Perfusion
  2. Pain
  3. Impaired Skin Integrity
  4. Risk for Fluid Volume Deficit

E. **Planning and implementation**

  1. **Monitor operative extremity q15min × 1 hr then q1hr for pedal and posterior tibial pulses distal to operative site, for color, temperature and capillary refill, numbness and tingling of affected extremity.**
  2. Report absent or diminished pulses STAT.
  3. Monitor vital signs, oxygen saturation, neurologic status, wound drainage q15min × 4, q30min × 4, q1hr × 4, then every shift.
  4. Administer supplemental oxygen via nasal cannula as ordered or maintain endotracheal tube if indicated.
  5. Avoid knee-flexed position and keep heel of affected extremity off the bed.

  6. **Do not use knee gatch of bed.**
  7. Assess pulmonary arterial pressures and cardiac output if available.
  8. Monitor cardiac rate and rhythm.
  9. Monitor for increased pulse, blood pressure, anxiety, restlessness, pallor, cyanosis, clammy skin, oliguria, and LOC.
  10. Monitor laboratory values especially hemoglobin and hematocrit, albumin and coagulation studies and notify physician if abnormal.
  11. Monitor extremity for edema, hematoma, sensory and motor function.
  12. Pain management via patient-controlled analgesic (PCA), epidural or PRN medications.
  13. Assess bowel sounds for resumption of diet for nutrition and wound healing.

  14. **Strict aseptic technique with dressing changes and observe for signs and symptoms of infection.**
  15. Perform incentive spirometry q2hr.
  16. Assess coping status and provide ongoing emotional support to the patient and family members.
  17. Administer IV antibiotics as prescribed.

18.   Monitor parenteral fluids: prescribed type and amount, rate of infusion and insertion site for signs and symptoms of infection.
19.   Be aware of potential complications:
      a.   Hemorrhage
      b.   Compartment syndrome
      c.   Thromboembolism
      d.   Deep vein thrombosis (DVT): a thrombus in one of the deep veins of the body, can be a life-threatening complication

F.   Evaluation
   1.   The patient maintains adequate circulation to affected extremity.
   2.   The patient verbalizes control of incisional pain with prescribed medications.
   3.   The patient is free of infection as evidenced by a normal temperature, stable vital signs and a clean dry and intact incision.
   4.   The patient exhibits hemodynamic stability, stable vital signs, hemoglobin and hematocrit, urine output, and no covert signs of hemorrhagic shock.
   5.   The patient demonstrates and verbalizes ability to cope with stress.

XXX.   Heart transplantation
   A.   Description: open heart surgery with cardiopulmonary bypass to replace a diseased human heart by a human donor heart, referred to as an orthotopic transplantation or a heterotopic transplantation, connecting the native heart and donor heart together.
      1.   A orthotopic is the most common type of transplantation.
         a.   This procedure consists of excising the recipient's heart leaving in place the posterior and lateral walls of the atria and the atrial septum as well as the inferior and superior vena cavae, pulmonary veins and the SA node.
         b.   These remnants act as support anchors to the donor heart. As a result of the intact recipient and donor SA nodes, double P-wave tracings at independent rates will appear on the patient's ECG tracings.
      2.   The heterotopic procedure is a technique whereby the donor heart is attached to the recipient heart.
         a.   The donor heart is placed in the right thoracic cavity and attached to the recipient heart by parallel anastomosing, via a synthetic graft of the right atria, pulmonary arteries, and aortas.
         b.   Indications for this procedure would include patient's with pulmonary hypertension and in a lifesaving situation when a donor heart is too small.
         c.   When using this method of transplantation, the ECG tracings show an additional QRS complex at an independent rate.

   B.   Indications
      1.   Severe coronary artery disease
      2.   End stage heart disease related to congestive CMP
      3.   Valvular heart disease
      4.   Myocarditis

     5. Congenital heart disease
C. **Assessment findings**
    1. Health history should be obtained to include the following:
       a. Primary cardiovascular problems
       b. Pulmonary history
       c. Current medication regime including oxygen administration.
       d. History of coping abilities, support systems, ability to follow rigorous follow-up care, and compliance with lifelong immunosuppressive therapy.
       e. Complete physical assessment, including review of systems, with emphasis on cardiac status, respiratory evaluation for adventitious breath sounds, and renal function.
    2. Preoperative laboratory values should include:
       a. CBC
       b. Urine analysis, urine culture and sensitivity, and creatinine clearance.
       c. Cardiac enzymes and isoenzymes
       d. Serum electrolytes, BUN and creatinine, fasting cholesterol, and lipid profile and ABGs. Coagulation studies and type and crossmatch of blood
    3. Diagnostic studies should include:
       a. Pulmonary function tests
       b. Ventilation and perfusion lung scans
       c. MRI
       d. CT scan
       e. ECG for cardiac status
       f. Phonocardiogram
       g. Two-dimensional echocardiogram
       h. Chest x-ray
       i. Cardiac catheterization
D. **Nursing diagnoses**
    1. Risk for Injury (Rejection)
    2. See CABG
E. **Planning and implementation**
    1. Monitor for signs and symptoms of right ventricular failure.
    2. Administer mannitol, Lasix, or other diuretics as prescribed.
    3. Monitor ventilator settings and maintain patent airway and integrity of endotracheal tube.
    4. Apply PEEP as ordered and monitor for decreased blood pressure and cardiac output as a result of PEEP.
    5. Administer platelets, fresh frozen plasma, crystalloids, colloids as prescribed.
    6. Administer beta blockers, calcium channel blockers, or cardioversion as ordered for supraventricular tachycardia (SVT).
    7. Administer and maintain TPN infusion as prescribed.
    8. Maintain isolation practices per protocol of institution.
    9. Administer prophylactic antibiotics for 48 hr postoperatively.
    10. Remove vascular assess, monitoring devices, Foley catheter, and chest tubes within 24 hr postoperatively, if possible.
    11. Maintain strict aseptic technique with all dressing changes and removal of all invasive devices.

12.   **Monitor for signs and symptoms of rejection and administer cyclosporine, azathioprine, okt3, and fk506 as prescribed for rejection.**

13.   Be aware of potential complications:

a.   Rejection: a humoral or cellular reaction of the body to foreign substances. Types of rejection include:

▶ *Hyperacute* occurs immediately after transplant in the operating room.

▶ *Acute* usually occurs within the first 3 months after transplantation and is the major cause of death.

b.   *Chronic* can occur any time after 3 months to years after transplantation.

c.   Infection

d.   Cardiac tamponade

e.   Heart failure

f.   Pulmonary hypertension: abnormally high pressure within the pulmonary circulation

g.   Hemorrhage

14.   See CABG for additional planning and implementation.

F.   Evaluation

1.   The patient remains free of infection as evidenced by normal temperature and leukocyte count.

2.   The patient exhibits no signs of rejection.

XXXI.   Ventricular septal defect

A.   Description: an acquired or congenital left-to-right shunting of blood through an abnormal membranous or muscular opening between the right and left ventricle.

B.   Etiology and incidence

1.   Although VSD is the most common congenital cardiac birth anomaly, the defect affects approximately less than 1% of 1000 live births annually.

2.   Acquired VSD occurs as a complication of a pre-existing condition.

3.   This serious complication occurs in approximately 2% of AMI patients within 7 days of infarct.

C.   Pathophysiology

  1.   **Because of decreased oxygen distal to the infarcted myocardium the tissue in this area becomes necrotic.**

2.   As a result of this dynamic occurrence, the friable necrotic tissues become vulnerable to this life-threatening complication.

3.   The defect or rupture of the septal wall results in left-to-right shunting of blood.

4.   The size of the defect determines the mix of oxygenated and unoxygenated blood and volume of blood in the right ventricle and lungs.

5.   The consequence of this shunting is the reduction in cardiac output and increased pulmonary blood flow and congestion and heart failure.

6. Congenitally, this abnormality is due to a malfusion of the membranous or muscular tissues that occurs during the fourth to eight week of gestation.
7. Surgery within 48 hours after diagnosis decreases mortality to approximately 50%.

D. **Assessment findings**
1. Clinical manifestations:
   a. Sudden, harsh, blowing, pansystolic, or holosystolic murmur auscultated on either side of the sternum between the fourth and sixth intercostal space.
   b. S2 split on expiration with widening on inspiration.
   c. Palpable thrill felt at the left sternal border.
   d. Chest pain, dyspnea, tachycardia, hypotension.
   e. Rapid onset of heart failure.
   f. Impending cardiogenic shock.
2. Diagnostic tests:
   a. Cardiac catheterization confirms diagnosis, and reveals systolic pressure in right ventricle and pulmonary artery.
   b. Blood samples during cardiac catheterization reveal a higher PO_2 in the right ventricle than right atrium.
   c. Echocardiography reveals a left-to-right shunt and enlarged left atrium.
   d. Doppler echocardiogram with color locates site and estimates pressure crop across defect.

E. **Nursing diagnoses**
1. Decreased Cardiac Output
2. Anxiety
3. Impaired Gas Exchange

F. **Planning and implementation**
1. **Prepare for IABP insertion.**
2. Administer nitroprusside to reduce afterload and diuretics as ordered.
3. Monitor for chest pain (PQRST) and administer pain medication, nitroglycerin, as ordered.
4. Maintain patent IV.
5. Administer oxygen at 2–4 L/min via nasal cannula or prepare for intubation and mechanical ventilation if not previously instituted.
6. **Continuous cardiac monitoring for dysrhythmias.**
7. Monitor PAP, PAWP, CO, CI and systemic vascular resistance (SVR).
8. Prepare patient for surgery per order.
9. Assess anxiety level, encourage expression of feelings, and explain procedures in a calm, soft voice.
10. **Monitor for impending shock.**
11. Be aware of potential complications:
    a. Heart failure
    b. Cardiogenic shock
    c. **Rupture of the interventricular septum**

G.   Evaluation

1.   The patient verbalizes fears and concerns.

2.   The patient demonstrates an adequate rise in blood pressure, skin warm and dry, palpable pulses, adequate urine output, and hemodynamic monitoring values returning to normal limits.

3.   The patient exhibits normal breathing pattern and ABGs return to normal values.

XXXII.   Aneurysm

A.   Description: a localized dilatation, protrusion, or disruption involving all three layers of the arterial wall.

B.   Etiology and incidence

1.   Risk factors associated with aortic aneurysm include:

    a.   Atherosclerosis: more predominant in abdominal aortic aneurysms.

    b.   Marfan's syndrome

    c.   Cystic medial necrosis

    d.   Hypertension

    e.   Aging process

    f.   Pregnancy

    g.   Congenital weakening of vessel wall

    h.   Infection

    i.   Trauma

    j.   Injury from surgery or procedures.

2.   Aneurysms occur in the fifth decade of life and are more common in men than women

3.   Abdominal aortic aneurysms (infrarenal) are more common than thoracic aneurysms.

4.   **When an aneurysm is not surgically repaired and continues to enlarge, rupture and death result.**

5.   Progress is improved with elective surgery.

C.   Pathophysiology

1.   The common thread in the formation of an aneurysm is a damaged or degenerating tunica media.

2.   Once the media loses its elasticity, the aortic wall weakens and pressure increases from mechanical stress and hemodynamic forces.

3.   These stressors cause the lumen to dilate and protrude with eventual rupture or dissection as the vessel enlarges and weakens.

4.   Aneurysms are categorized according to their structure:

    a.   Saccular: a true aneurysm, with the appearance of a balloon; a round unilateral protrusion with a narrow neck.

    b.   Fusiform: a true aneurysm, is a uniform, circumferential, spindle-shaped dilatation of the arterial wall.

    c.   Pseudoaneurysm: a false aneurysm, is a hematoma formed by a rupture or tear of all three layers of the aortic wall.

    d.   Aortic dissection: formerly called a dissecting aneurysm.

D.   Assessment findings

1.   Clinical manifestations associated with thoracic aneurysms vary according to location and size.

DISPLAY 4-6.
Manifestation of Aneurysms According to Location

Ascending aorta (thoracic aorta)

Substernal chest pain radiating to the aortic arch neck, throat, back, shoulder, or abdomen.

Sudden tearing, ripping scapular or chest pain may indicate rupture or dissection.

Dyspnea, hoarseness.

Superior vena cava

Cyanosis, edema of neck, face, and upper extremities.

Jugular venous distention.

Abdominal aorta

Periumbilical palpable, pulsatile abdominal mass.

Abdominal bruit on auscultation.

Abdominal pain, distention, and sensation of fullness.

Intense back pain.

Sudden excruciating back and abdominal pain with rupture.

Severe back pain and possible flank pain and ecchymosis (Turner's sign) with tamponade.

Signs and symptoms of hypovolemic shock with dissection.

Hematuria, testicular pain, and/or flank pain.

Possible claudication; hip, groin, and leg pain.

Diminished or Doppler pedal pulses with mottling of the feet and toes.

Possible nausea and vomiting.

---

    2. In the early stage patients are usually asymptomatic with rupture being the first sign (Display 4-6).

    3. Abdominal aneurysms are usually discovered on a routine evaluation of another problem.

    4. Diagnostic findings determine the size and are specific to the location of the aneurysm (Display 4-7).

E. **Nursing diagnoses**

    1. Anxiety

    2. Pain

    3. Altered Tissue Perfusion

    4. Decreased Cardiac Output

    5. Risk for Fluid Volume Deficit

F. **Planning and implementation**

    1. Abdominal aneurysms <5 cm are medically treated with antihypertensives and are reevaluated every 6 months.

    2. Abdominal aneurysms >6 cm and thoracic aneurysms are surgically repaired.

    3. The surgical procedure involves proximal and distal cross-clamping of the aorta. The aorta is incised, a synthetic graft is inserted to replace the diseased segment, the diseased lumen is stripped of all clots, and the native aorta is sutured around the graft.

DISPLAY 4-7.
Diagnostic Findings According to Aneurism Location

Thoracic
Chest x-ray will visualize a widening of the mediastinum.
ECG will rule out an AMI.
Echocardiography identifies aortic insufficiency associated with dilatation of the ascending aorta.
Transesophageal echocardiogram (TEE) visually locates and assesses the extent of the thoracic aneurysm.
CT scan accurately determines the anterior–posterior and cross-sectional dimensions of the aneurysm.
MRI is useful in measuring the size of the aneurysm.

Abdominal
Abdominal x-ray reveals calcification of the aneurysm wall.
Ultrasound is diagnostic in tracking the growth of an abdominal aneurysm. Not a useful tool in diagnosing thoracic aneurysms.
CT scan determines the size and location and identifies the severity and unsuspected complication of aneurisms.
MRI determines the size and identifies the effect of the aneurysm on associated arteries (iliac and renal).
Aortography aids in the diagnosis by identifying the location and size of the aneurysm and determines patency and perfusion distal to the affected portion of the aorta.

4. When clamping above the renal arteries in an abdominal aneurysm, postoperative renal complications are greatly increased.
5. With thoracic aneurysms cardiopulmonary bypass is used and an IABP may be inserted prior to surgery.
6. Offer patient realistic assurance.
7. Maintain patient in supine position.
 8. **Monitor CVP, PAP, PCWP, and arterial pressure if appropriate lines are inserted.**
 9. **Closely monitor vital signs, JVD, quality of peripheral pulses, skin color and temperature, and aortic insufficiency qlhr or PRN and immediately report any changes.**
10. Administer supplemental oxygen or prepare the patient for possible mechanical ventilation.
11. Assess flank for ecchymosis and abdomen for an increase in size.
12. Maintain patent IV and monitor accurate intake and output qlhr or PRN and report output <30 mL/hr.
13. Calculate CO, CI, and SVR.
14. Monitor for changes in mentation.
15. Observe cardiac monitor for rate and rhythm.
16. Monitor hemoglobin and hematocrit, BUN, creatinine, and cardiac enzymes and isoenzymes.
17. Closely monitor pain parameters.
18. Administer nitroprusside (for hypertension), or dopamine (for hypotension), morphine sulfate for pain, Valium (diazepam) for anxiety, diuretics, and blood products as ordered by physician.

19. Prepare patient and family for possible surgery.
20. Be aware of potential complications:

𝖓 a. **Rupture/dissection with potential fatal hemorrhage**
b. Vascular insufficiency
c. Distal embolization
d. Death

G. **Evaluation**
1. The patient exhibits a calm demeanor and verbalizes fears and concerns.
2. The patient displays hemodynamic parameters within normal limits and urine output >30 mL/hr.
3. The patient demonstrates adequate tissue perfusion as evidenced by pink, warm skin, palpable peripheral pulses with no decreased character or quality.

XXXIII. Pericarditis

A. **Description: an acute or chronic fibrotic thickening and inflammatory process in the pericardial sac.**
B. **Etiology and incidence**
1. Acute pericarditis may be idiopathic, infectious, or noninfectious
2. Infectious causes include viral, bacterial, fungal and parasitic infection
3. Noninfectious causes include:
a. AMI, Dressler's syndrome
b. Post cardiac injury, trauma or surgery
c. Radiation therapy and neoplasms
d. Uremia, myxedema, rheumatologic diseases
e. Dissecting aortic aneurysm
f. Drug reactions (procainamide, hydralazine)
C. **Pathophysiology**
1. The acute phase of the disease may be present as either a fibrinous (dry) or exudative (hemorrhagic, purulent or serous) process.
2. Chronic constrictive pericarditis results from scar tissue forming between the pericardial layer causing progressive thickening and eventually adherence of the pericardium.
3. Symptomatic treatment of the underlying disease may include thoracotomy for open drainage of fluid with possible instillation of chemotherapeutic agents to prevent recurrence.
a. Pericardiocentesis is an emergency treatment if cardiac tamponade is the cause,
b. Palliative surgical resection of fibrous tissue is indicated in fibrotic thickening.
D. **Assessment findings**
1. Clinical manifestations (acute and chronic)
a. Chest pain mimicking angina exacerbated with respirations and truck movement and lessening by an upright position and leaning forward.
b. Pericardial friction rub auscultated at the lower left sternal border while patient is holding his/her breath; may be constant or transient, does not radiate, and may be timed with the pulse.
c. Dyspnea

        d.   Dysrhythmias

        e.   Fever

        f.   Chronic pericarditis mimics heart failure and cor pulmonale findings as well as a diastolic pericardial knock auscultated at the left sternal boarder.

  2.   Diagnostic studies and laboratory findings: acute and chronic

        a.   **ECG changes evolving from hours to weeks: S-T elevation that is diffuse and present in majority leads, T-wave changes range from flattening, inversion to normal with Q waves.**

        b.   Atrial dysrhythmias may occur but usually accompany underlying cardiac pathology.

        c.   Atrial fibrillation and nonspecific T-wave inversion or flattening are seen in chronic constrictive pericarditis.

        d.   Echocardiography is useful to identify a thickened pericardium in chronic constrictive pericarditis, pericardial effusion, and cardiac tamponade.

        e.   Chest x-ray

        f.   Computed tomography (CT scan) or magnetic resonance imaging (MRI) is helpful in identifying the characteristic pericardial thickening of chronic constrictive pericarditis and pericardial effusions.

        g.   Cardiac catheterization: the pulmonary artery and wedge pressures in conjunction with the right and left ventricular pressures are more specific tools for diagnosing chronic constrictive pericarditis.

        h.   Normal or slightly elevated cardiac enzymes.

        i.   Elevated white blood count and erythrocyte sedimentation rate (ESR).

        j.   Antibody titers, serologic studies, pericardial fluid, and tissue biopsy identify causative organism.

E. **Nursing diagnoses**

    1.   Pain

    2.   Ineffective Breathing Pattern

    3.   Decreased Cardiac Output

    4.   Activity Intolerance

F. **Planning and implementation**

    1.   Assess complaints of chest pain on a scale of 1 to 10, and PQRST method of pain evaluation before and after treatment (see AMI.)

    2.   Administer pain medication as ordered.

        a.   NSAIDS, analgesics, or narcotics may be prescribed.

        b.   **NSAIDS are the drugs of choice to resolve the inflammation and control pain.**

        c.   NSAIDS should be administered with food to control GI side effects, and avoid aspirin because of interference with their activity.

    3.   Maintain the patient on bed rest in high Fowler's position or resting in a chair.

4. Medications are prescribed specific to causative organism. Corticosteroids are usually prescribed for patients not responding to NSAIDS or patients who are presently taking the drug for another disease process or cases with severe infection.

5. Corticosteroid doses are tapered.

6. Monitor and document respiratory rate, effort, and depth q4hr or PRN.

7. Auscultate the lungs q4hr or PRN and document and report adventitious and or diminished breath sounds.

8. Administer oxygen as ordered for optimal gas exchange and tissue oxygenation and perfusion.

9. Administer pain medication 30 minutes before prescribed incentive spirometry treatments and deep-breathing exercises to promote patient participation.

10. Encourage independent performance of ADLs to enhance patient's self-esteem, self-image, and sense of control.

11. Assess skin color and temperature and measure vital signs before and after activity. Document abnormal findings and adjust activity accordingly.

12. Explain all procedures to decrease anxiety and promote reassurance and cooperation.

13. **Monitor for signs and symptoms of the two major complications of acute pericarditis:**
    a. Pericardial effusion: muffled or distant heart sounds, sign of venous congestion
    b. Cardiac tamponade: pulses paradoxus, distant or muffled heart sounds, tachycardia, decreased blood pressure, JVD, narrowing pulse pressure, change in LOC.

14. Prepare the patient for pericardiocentesis procedure as ordered; explain procedure to patient and family.

15. Prepare the patient for pericardectomy as ordered for patients with chronic constrictive pericarditis; explain the procedure to patient and family.

16. Be aware of potential complications:
    a. Pericardial effusion
    b. Cardiac tamponade

G. **Evaluation**
    1. The patient exhibits relief of pain, increased activity tolerance, reduced anxiety, and no signs or symptoms of complications.
    2. The patient maintains normal vital signs, heart and breath sounds.
    3. The patient and family members verbalize an understanding of the disease process, the importance of reporting recurring manifestations, and the continuation of prescribed treatments.

XXXIV. **Myocarditis**
    A. **Description: an invasion of organisms into the myocardial wall resulting in an acute or subacute inflammatory disorder of the myocardium.**
    B. **Etiology**
        1. Viral (coxsackie A and B, poliomyelitis, varicella, rubella, rubeola, adenovirus, echovirus, mumps, hepatitis, cytomegalovirus, influenza A and B, Epstein-Barr)

2. Parasitic (trichinosis, trypanosomiasis, schistosomiasis).
3. Mycotic (candida, toxoplasmosis, histoplasmosis)
4. Rickettsial (typhus)
5. Bacteria (pneumococcus, diphtheria)
6. Idiopathic
7. Predisposing factors:
    a. Acute rheumatic fever
    b. Pericarditis
    c. Drugs
    d. Specific metabolic diseases
    e. Chronic diseases of unknown causes associated with cardiomyopathy
    f. Immunosuppressive therapy
    g. Radiation and burns
    h. Stress and advanced age

C.   Pathophysiology

1. **In the acute phase there is an infiltration of causative organism into the interstitial tissues of the myocardium.**
2. This leads to an inflammatory process damaging the myocardial cells. Cardiomegaly may ensue as the result of the unaffected myocardial fibers of both ventricles taking on the workload of the heart.
3. The severity can be mild, moderate, or severe, with a local or diffuse distribution.
4. An immunologic response may be a factor in the subacute or chronic phase.
5. This infective process is a contributing factor in dilated (congestive) cardiomyopathy.

D.   Assessment findings

1. Clinical manifestations include:
    a. Fever, fatigue, and dyspnea
    b. Palpitations and tachycardia disproportionate to temperature elevation, pericardial friction rub
    c. Heart failure and chest pain
    d. Syncope
    e. GI disturbances
2. Diagnostic evaluation:
    a. Chest x-ray shows mild to moderate cardiomegaly.
    b. ECG changes include S-T segment elevation, T-wave inversion or flat, prolonged QT interval, supraventricular tachycardia, ventricular dysrhythmias.
    c. Echocardiography reveals ventricular dilatation and abnormalities of the regional wall.
3. Laboratory findings are often inconclusive:
    a. Mild-to-moderate leukocytosis and atypical lymphocytes.
    b. Elevated viral titers in initial 10 days of illness.
    c. Elevated LDH, CPK, and transaminases.
    d. Histologic confirmation via an endomyocardial biopsy (EMB) study.
    e. Biopsy specimen from the right ventricle should be obtained within 6 weeks of acute onset of illness.

      f.   Evidence of lymphacytic infiltration and myocyte damage is present within 6 weeks of acute illness.

E.   **Nursing diagnoses**
1. Hyperthermia
2. Decreased Cardiac Output
3. Anxiety
4. Activity Intolerance
5. Pain
6. Fluid Volume Excess
7. Altered Tissue Perfusion

F.   **Planning and implementation**
1. Monitor temperature q4hr or PRN and administer antipyretics as prescribed.
2. Encourage patient to verbalize his or her fears, feelings, and concerns about the illness, hospitalization, and course of treatment.
3. Explain all procedures and treatments relevant to the illness.
4. Assess for pain (PQRST) and administer analgesics as prescribed.
5. Elevate head of bed; place patient in position of comfort to help alleviate pain.
6. Provide supplemental oxygen as prescribed.
7. Observe cardiac monitor for evidence of dysrhythmias administer antidysrhythmics as per protocol.
8. Monitor vital signs q4hr or PRN for decreased cardiac output and auscultate heart and breath sounds.
9. Administer antimicrobial therapy relevant to infective organism.
10. Administer digoxin if heart failure is present.
11. **Continual assessment for digoxin toxicity due to sensitivity of digoxin in patients with myocarditis.**
12. **Immunosuppressant therapy may include azathioprine or cyclosporine and corticosteroids. This therapy inhibits the body's normal mechanism to fight infection; therefore, monitor CBC, WBC, platelet count, and for signs and symptoms of infection.**
13. **Corticosteroids effect the function of the adrenal gland and should never by abruptly discontinued but gradually reduced in dose increments.**
14. Administer diuretic (Lasix) and medication that decrease preload and afterload as prescribed.
15. Monitor IV for exact rate of administration and site for signs and symptoms of infection.
16. Maintain adequate nutrition by adhering to prescribed diet of increased proteins and carbohydrates if fever is present and decreased sodium if signs of heart failure are present.
17. Administer anticoagulant therapy (heparin or coumadin) to prevent emboli.
18. Monitor laboratory values as ordered by physician.
19. Be aware of potential complications:
    a.   Heart failure
    b.   Dysrhythmias
    c.   Cardiac tamponade

      d.   Infection

      e.   Pulmonary emboli

      f.   Thrombophlebitis

G. **Evaluation**

    1. The patient exhibits relief of pain, increased activity tolerance, reduced anxiety, and no signs or symptoms of complications.

    2. The patient maintains normal vital signs and heart and breath sounds.

    3. The patient and family members verbalize an understanding of the disease process, the importance of reporting recurring manifestations, and the continuation of prescribed treatments.

XXXV. Endocarditis

A. **Description: an infection of the endothelial lining of the heart, most frequently involving the leaflets of heart; may be classified as acute or subacute. This disorder was previously referred to a subacute bacterial endocarditis (SBE).**

B. **Etiology and incidence**

    1. Causative bacteria include *Staphylococcus spp.* (most common virulent organism in acute endocarditis), and *Streptococcus viridens* (most often causative organisms of low virulence in SBE).

    2. Fungi

    3. Yeasts

    4. Rickettsiae

    5. Other gram-negative and positive bacilli

    6. Predisposing conditions:

      a. Pre-existing valvular disease

      b. Mechanical or tissue valve replacement

      c. Acquired or congenital heart disease

      d. Invasive procedures and devices

      e. Dental procedures

      f. IV drug abuse

      g. Prolonged IV therapy

      h. Debilitation

      i. Cardiac surgery

      j. Immunosuppression resulting from drugs or a disease process.

      k. An increase in endocarditis is attributed to the growing elderly population, an increase of IV drug abuse, patients with prosthetic valves, and the proportionate number of cases caused by less-common–causing microbes.

C. **Pathophysiology**

    1. Microorganisms enter the circulation and begin to colonize on healthy valves as in the acute form or pre-existing damaged valvular and/or endothelial surfaces seen in the subacute form.

    2. Colonization of the infective organism stimulates aggregation of sterile platelet-fibrin thrombi.

    3. The body's defense mechanism against the specific organism cannot penetrate existing platelet-fibrin thrombi. Thrombi provide growth medium for the infective organism.

    4. The growing organisms adhere to the thrombotic lesions and are called vegetations.

5. These vegetations are friable and easily shear off or tear away from the edges of the involved valve and travel via the bloodstream to other organs with possible subsequent dysfunction of the affected organ.

6. Eventually the vegetation causes scarring and deformity of the valves, which compromise the functions of the valve. This causes erosion, necrosis, and rupture of the valve leaflets, chordae tendinae, and papillary muscles.

7. Heart valves on the left side are the most common site of involvement. Infections stemming from IV drug use most often affect the right side, particularly the tricuspid valve.

8. **Management** includes identifying the infective organism and appropriate microbial treatment is instituted.

D. Assessment findings

1. Common acute and subacute clinical manifestations

   a. Sudden spiking fever and chills are the hallmark symptoms of acute endocarditis.

   b. Gradual onset of a low-grade fever with flulike symptoms is classic symptom of SBE.

   c. Cough or shortness of breath

   d. Malaise, fatigue, and arthralgias

   e. Abdominal pain and splenomegaly

   f. Murmurs (new or a change in quality and intensity of existing murmurs)

   g. Anorexia, weight loss

   h. Petechiae on the trunk, conjunctiva, and mucous membranes

   i. Splinter hemorrhages under the fingernails and toenails

   j. Janeway lesions: lesions on the palms and soles

   k. Osler's nodes: painful nodules on the pads of the extremities

   l. Roth's spots: hemorrhagic areas with white centers seen on the retina

2. Laboratory data and diagnostic findings:

   a. Elevated WBC in acute endocarditis; a normal WBC and differential with anemia in SBE.

   b. Positive blood cultures confirm involved organism.

   c. Urinalysis is positive for proteinuria and/or hematuria which may indicate renal damage.

   d. Serologic immune testing may reveal a positive rheumatoid factor.

   e. Two-dimensional echocardiography identifies valvular vegetations and is helpful in determining the necessity of surgical intervention.

   f. Transesophageal echocardiography is a more sensitive tool for diagnosing infective endocarditis.

   g. Chest x-ray is useful for detecting heart failure.

   h. ECGs indicate conduction abnormalities, dysrhythmias, ischemia, or cardiomegaly.

   i. Cardiac catheterization may be performed if surgery is indicated.

E. Nursing diagnoses
1. Activity Intolerance
2. Altered Nutrition: Less than Body Requirements
3. Decreased Cardiac Output
4. Ineffective Thermoregulation
5. Altered Tissue Perfusion: Cardiopulmonary

F. Planning and implementation

1. **Monitor and document patient's temperature q2hr or PRN and notify physician if temperature >101° F.**
2. Provide light blankets for covering the patient to prevent shivering which could contribute to a temperature rise.
3. Administer anti-inflammatory or antipyretic (aspirin or Tylenol) medications as prescribed.
4. Administer IV antibiotics as prescribed and observe for allergic reactions, especially anaphylaxis. Obtain blood samples for a peak and trough levels to ascertain therapeutic blood levels.
5. Obtain blood cultures before administration of first dose and follow-up cultures to monitor therapeutic response.
6. Monitor and document any symptoms of decreased perfusion to the brain, kidneys, cardiovascular, or pulmonary system.
7. Observe and report any integumentary and peripheral vascular abnormalities.
8. Provide a high-protein, high CO diet.
9. Observe cardiac monitor for dysrhythmias.

10. **Monitor the apical pulse for rate and rhythm and auscultate for new murmurs or a change in a present murmur.**
11. Administer supplemental oxygen as ordered or prepare for mechanical ventilation if necessary.
12. Provide frequent rest periods to decrease workload of the heart.
13. Administer medications as ordered (eg, inotropic and diuretic therapy for past or present cardiac involvement).
14. Monitor for signs and symptoms of heart failure.
15. Surgical preparation of the patient is necessary if valve replacement is ordered.

G. Evaluation
1. The patient exhibits increased activity tolerance, reduced anxiety, and no signs and symptoms of complications.
2. The patient exhibits no chills, fever, or flulike symptoms.
3. The patient demonstrates adequate cardiac output.
4. The patient and significant others verbalizes knowledge of disease, its process, rationale for treatment, and procedures requiring prophylactic antibiotic therapy.

Bibliography

Apple, S. (1995). Advances for diagnosing acute myocardial infarction. *Heartbeat* 6(2), 1–7.

Black, J. M. & Matassarin-Jacobs, E. (1993). *Luckman and Sorenson's medical-surgical nursing: A psychophysiologic approach* (4th ed.). Philadelphia: W. B. Saunders.

Carpenito, L. J. (1995). *Nursing care plans and documentation* (2nd ed.). Philadelphia: J. B. Lippincott.

Clem, J. R. (1995). Pharmacotherapy of ischemic heart disease. *AACN Clin Issues* 6(3), 404–417.

Coombs, V. J. & Brinker, J. A. (1995). Primary angioplasty in the acute myocardial infarction setting. *AACN Clin Issues* 6(3), 387–395.

Corley, M. C. & Sneed, G. (1994). Criteria in the selection of organ transplant recipients. *Heart Lung* 23(6), 446–455.

Cox, H. C. (1993). *Clinical applications of nursing diagnosis: Adult, child, women's, psychiatric, gerontologic and home health considerations* (2nd ed.). Philadelphia: F. A. Davis.

Creel, C. A. (1994). Silent myocardial ischemia and nursing implications. *Heart Lung* 23(3), 218–226.

Cronin, L. A. (1993). Beat the clock: Saving the heart with thrombolytic drugs. *Nursing 92* 23(8), 34–42.

Effat, M. A. (1995). Pathophysiology of ischemic heart disease: An overview. *AACN Clin Issues* 6(3), 369–374.

Goran, S. F. (1996). From counterpulsation to paralysis: A case presentation. *Crit Care Nurse* 16(2), 54–57.

Grady, K. L. (1989). Myocarditis: Review of clinical enigma. *Heart Lung* 18(4), 347–352.

Herreros, J., De Oca, J., & Sanchez, R., (1985). Etat nutritionnel et immunologique des patients operes de chirurgie cardiaque valvulaire. *J Chir (Paris)* 122, 707–710.

Hudak, C. M. & Gallo, B. M. (1994). *Critical care nursing: A holistic approach* (6th ed.). Philadelphia: J. B. Lippincott.

Keller, G. B. & Lemberg. L. (1994). Q and non–Q wave myocardial infarctions. *Am J Crit Care* 3(2), 158–161.

Kinney, M. R. & Packa, D. R. (1996). *Comprehensive cardiac care* (8th ed.). St Louis: Mosby-Year Book.

Kyger, E. R., Block, W. J., & Roach, G., (1978). Adverse effects of protein malnutrition on myocardial function. *Surgery* 84, 147–156.

Lewis, S. M., Collier, I. C., & Heitkemper, M. M. (1996). *Medical-surgical nursing: Assessment and management of clinical problems* (4th ed.). St. Louis: Mosby-Year Book.

North American Nursing Diagnosis Association (NANDA). (1996). *Nursing diagnoses: Definitions & classification 1997–1998*. Philadelphia: Author.

Owen, A. (1995). Tracking the rise and fall of cardiac enzymes. *Nursing 95* 25(5), 35–38.

Phipps, W. J. & Cassmeyer, V. L. (1995). *Medical-surgical nursing: Concepts and clinical practice* (5th ed.). St. Louis: Mosby-Year Book.

Shannon, M. T., Wilson, B. A., & Stank, C. L. (1992). *Govoni and Hayes' drugs and nursing implications* (7th ed.). Norwalk, CT: Appleton and Lange.

Sokolow, M. T. (1990). *Clinical cardiology* (5th ed.). Norwalk, CT: Appleton and Lange.

Springhouse Corporation. (1991). *Cardiopulmonary emergencies*. Springhouse, PA: Author.

Springhouse Corporation. (1996). *Handbook of critical care nursing*. Springhouse, PA: Author.

Thelan, L. A. (1994). *Critical care nursing* (2nd ed.). St. Louis: Mosby-Year Book.

Williams, K. & Marton, P. G. (1995). Diagnosis and treatment of acute myocardial infarction. *AACN Clin Issues* 6(3), 375–386.

Zaloga, G. P. (1994). *Nutrition in critical care*. St. Louis: Mosby.

STUDY QUESTIONS

1. On your initial assessment of a patient with an AMI you would expect the vital signs to be:
   a. hypotension, tachycardia
   b. hypertension, irregular heart rhythm
   c. fever, tachycardia
   d. hypotension, tachypnea

2. Which is the most important finding when assessing chest pain? The pain:
   a. increases with inspiration
   b. lasts longer than 30 minutes
   c. is relieved with one nitroglycerin tablet
   d. is relieved with rest

3. Your patient is 1 hour post–endomycar-dial biopsy (EMB) surgery. Which of the following assessment findings is the most important?
   a. pericardial friction rub and dys-rhythmia
   b. muffled heart sounds and decreased blood pressure
   c. sudden spiking fever, chills, and ab-dominal pain
   d. angina exacerbated with movement

4. A priority nursing intervention for a pa-tient with an aneurysm of the superior vena cava would be to:
   a. increase nitroprusside infusion rate
   b. administer an extra dose of Valium
   c. assess flank for pain and ecchymosis
   d. assess respiratory status and prepare for possible intubation

5. In a patient with hypertrophic cardio-myopathy, which of the following drugs would be contraindicated?
   a. digoxin, positive inotropic
   b. Inderal, negative inotropic
   c. heparin, anticoagulant
   d. verapamil, calcium channel blocker

6. Which of the following discharge in-structions should you stress to a patient with stable angina?
   a. Take the sublingual nitroglycerin (NTG) before exertional activities.
   b. Only take your NTG tablet when anginal attacks occur.

c. The NTG tablet should only be taken in the morning.
   d. Take as many NTG tablets as needed to relieve the pain.

7. A patient involved in an motor vehicle accident is admitted with a diagnosis of cardiac contusion. The patient is com-plaining of chest pain and the cardiac monitor shows frequent premature ven-tricular contractions (PVCs). Which of the following nursing interventions would you NOT anticipate?
   a. administration of an analgesic for pain
   b. nitroglycerin infusion and titrate to pain
   c. lidocaine infusion for dysrhythmia
   d. oxygen at 2 L/min via nasal cannula

8. When discussing postoperative care with a patient undergoing a coronary artery bypass graft (CABG), what infor-mation should be a priority?
   a. Inform the patient that he will have one or two chest tubes.
   b. Encourage the patient to express their fears and concerns.
   c. Inform the patient that he will un-able to talk while a breathing ma-chine is breathing for him.
   d. Deep-breathing and coughing exer-cises will be performed to prevent pneumonia.

9. Which of the following would not be included in the nursing care of a post–percutaneous translumenal coro-nary angioplasty (PTCA) patient?
   a. Monitor the patient for chest pain.
   b. Ambulate the patient within 2 hours post-procedure.
   c. Maintain intravenous heparin.
   d. Maintain intravenous fluids.

10. Your patient is being prepared for ad-ministration of streptokinase for an acute myocardial infarction. Which as-sessment parameter would indicate a change in the thrombolytic agent?

a. history of diabetes mellitus
b. history of a urinary tract infection
c. streptococcal infection 2 months ago
d. 1 year post–abdominal surgery

11. An intra-aortic balloon pump (IABP) is inserted as an intervention for a patient experiencing chest pain unrelieved by IV NTG. Your nursing intervention would include monitoring for which of the following complications?
   a. decubitus ulcer
   b. reperfusion dysrhythmias
   c. pneumonia
   d. thromboembolism

12. Your patient with a history of rheumatic fever is admitted with shortness of breath and weight loss. Your admission assessment findings reveal dyspneic on exertion, fatigue, and a blowing diastolic murmur auscultated at the second intercostal space. Your assessment data and patient history indicates:
   a. aortic regurgitation
   b. tricuspid stenosis
   c. pulmonic regurgitation
   d. mitral stenosis

13. When caring for a patient in cardiogenic shock your nursing priority would be to:
   a. Prepare for insertion of an IABP.
   b. Administer IV fluids and inotropic agents.
   c. Monitor intake and output.
   d. Perform a neurologic assessment.

ANSWER KEY

1. **Correct response: b**
   Increased blood pressure with irregular heart rate is due to the vasomotor response to pain.
   a and d. Decreased blood pressure and increased heart rate is due to decreased cardiac output and vasodilatation.
   c. fever is a delayed reaction and results from necrosis of affected myocardial tissue. It is an inflammatory response.
   Comprehension/Physiologic/Assessment

2. **Correct response: b**
   Chest pain greater than 30 minutes is indicative of an AMI.
   a. Increased chest pain with respirations indicates pericarditis pneumonia, costrochondritis.
   c and d. These findings indicate angina pectoris.
   Comprehension/Physiologic/Assessment

3. **Correct response: b**
   These are signs and symptoms of cardiac tamponade which is a possible complication of an EMB.
   a. These are clinical manifestations of myocarditis.
   c. These are clinical manifestations of endocarditis.
   d. These are clinical manifestations of pericarditis
   Comprehension/Safe care/Assessment

4. **Correct response: d**
   Clinical manifestations include edema of the neck and face, which could compromise respiratory status and would be a priority.
   a. Nitroprusside could be administered to lower the blood pressure if ordered by the physician.
   b. Valium would decrease anxiety and must be order by a physician.
   c. Pain and ecchymosis of the flank are seen in a ruptured abdominal aortic aneurysm.
   Application/Physiologic/Implementation

5. **Correct response: a**
   The upper portion of the interventricular septum encroaches on the left ventricular chamber. This effects the functioning of the mitral valve and adequate filling of the left ventricle. These abnormalities cause an obstruction in ventricular outflow. A positive inotrope increases myocardial contractility and exaggerates the already obstructed ventricular outflow.
   b. Beta blockers decrease myocardial contractility relieving the outflow obstruction.
   c. Anticoagulants may be prescribed to prevent systemic embolization.
   d. Calcium channel blockers promote relaxation and decrease myocardial contractions.
   Application/Physiologic/Implementation

6. **Correct response: a**
   With stable angina nitroglycerin should be taken before exertional activities and before any circumstances that may precipitate an attack.
   b. Patients with angina should take nitroglycerin when attacks occur, however stable angina can be anticipated and medication should be taken before anticipated attacks.
   c. Anginal attacks occurring in the morning are generally associated with Printzmetal's angina.
   d. Only three sublingual nitroglycerin tablets should be taken for pain relief. If the pain is not relieved after three tablets the patient should contact his physician or be transported to an emergency room via an ambulance.
   Comprehension/Health promotion/ Implementation

7. **Correct response: b**
   Nitroglycerin is not a treatment for patient's with a cardiac contusion.

a. Analgesics are the treatment of choice until test results reveal a myocardial infarction.

c. Lidocaine is indicated for ventricular dysrhythmias.

d. Oxygen is administered to increase oxygen supply to a damaged myocardium.

Application/Physiologic/Planning

8. *Correct response: c*

Informing the patient that he will be ventilated and unable to speak is a priority. This action will decrease the patient's fears and anxieties and help the patient to understand the reason why he is unable to talk.

a, b, and d. These interventions are also necessary preoperative instructions.

Comprehension/Psychosocial/Planning

9. *Correct response: b*

The patient should be maintained on bed rest for 6–8 hours post-procedure.

a. Chest pain could indicate occlusion or restenosis, coronary artery spasm or pulmonary embolism.

c. Intravenous heparin is continued up to 24 hours post-PTCA to decrease the risk of arterial reocclusion.

d. Fluids facilitate excretion of contrast dye.

Application/Physiologic/Planning

10. *Correct response: c*

A history of a streptococcal infection would produce an antigen–antibody reaction resulting in a severe hypersensitivity reaction or possible anaphylaxis.

a, b, and d. These are not contraindications to thrombolytic therapy.

Knowledge/Safe care/Assessment

11. *Correct response: d*

Thromboembolism in the blockage of a blood vessel by an embolus traveling through the circulatory system, and is directly associated with the IABP as a result of blood clots forming on the tip of the catheter

a and c. These are complications of bed rest.

b. This could be a complication of thrombolytic therapy, PTCA, and laser surgery.

Knowledge/Safe care/Assessment

12. *Correct response: a*

The most important assessment finding associated with aortic regurgitation is high-pitched, blowing diastolic murmur heard at the second intercostal space. The murmur radiates to the left sternal boarder at the third or fourth intercostal space.

b. In tricuspid stenosis a harsh medium pitched murmur is heard at the second intercostal space, left sternal boarder.

c. In pulmonic regurgitation a high-pitched blowing murmur with concurrent pulmonary hypertension or moderate-pitched murmur without pulmonary hypertension is heard. Both sounds are heard at the fourth or fifth intercostal space, left sternal boarder. The murmur can be heard at Erb's point.

d. In mitral stenosis a low-pitched rumbling murmur best heard with the bell of the stethoscope at the apex with the patient in the left lateral recumbent position.

Analysis/Physiologic/Assessment

13. *Correct response: b*

Intravenous fluids and vasopressors are administered to increased blood volume and blood pressure.

a. This action is necessary if the patient does not respond to initial therapy.

c and d. These nursing evaluations are not the first priorities.

Application/Physiologic/Planning

Cardiac Dysrhythmias

5

I.   Cardiac conduction cycle (Fig. 5-1)

    A.   P wave

        1.   Represents atrial depolarization.
        2.   Precedes the QRS complex.
        3.   Amplitude of <3 mm, duration of 0.06–0.11 sec.
        4.   Significance: indicates atrial depolarization has occurred.

    B.   PR Interval

        1.   Represents AV conduction time, from atrial depolarization to ventricular depolarization.
        2.   From beginning of P wave to beginning of QRS complex.
        3.   Duration 0.12–0.20 sec.
        4.   Significance: can show evidence of non SA node generated impulse (junctional rhythm) or impulse delay (AV block).

    C.   The Q wave

        1.   First negative deflection on the strip; may not be seen in all leads.

        2.   Represents septal depolarization and normally lasts 0.03 seconds or less.

    D.   QRS complex

        1.   Represents ventricular depolarization.
        2.   Follows P wave.

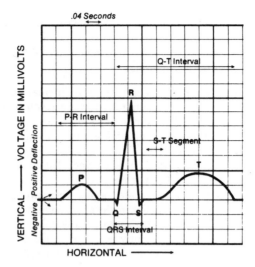

FIGURE 5-1.
ECG waveforms.

3. Duration: 0.06–0.10 sec.

4. **Significance: important indicator of ventricular myocardial cell activity.**

E. **ST segment**

1. **Represents the beginning of ventricular repolarization.**
2. Extends from end of S wave to beginning of T wave.
3. Most important characteristic is the deflection, ie, positive or negative.

4. **Significance: crucial in evaluating myocardial ischemia and injury.**

F. **T wave**

1. **Represents ventricular repolarization.**
2. Follows the S wave.
3. Amplitude and deflection are the most important characteristics evaluated.

4. **Significance: a critical relative refractory period during which myocardial cells are vulnerable to extra stimuli.**

G. **QT interval**

1. **Represents ventricular depolarization and repolarization.**
2. From beginning of the QRS complex to the end of the T wave.
3. Duration: <0.44 sec.

4. **Significance: indicator of the time the heart needs for the depolarization–repolarization cycle. An abnormal duration may indicate myocardial problem.**

II. **Overview of cardiovascular dysrhythmias**

A. Description

1. A dysrhythmia can occur with any disturbance in the origin, rate, or conduction of the electrical impulses of the heart.

2.   These disturbances generally fall into two broad categories:
  a.   problems with the generation of the impulses
  b.   problems with conduction of the impulses

B.   Causes of dysrhythmias

1.   **Altered automaticity is an increase or decrease in the pacemaker cell firing rate that can result in a dysrhythmia.**
2.   An accelerated firing rate can cause premature beats or tachycardia, while a decreased firing rate can result in bradycardias or escape rhythms.
3.   Reentry occurs when myocardial tissue is stimulated more than once by the same impulse.
  a.   Circus reentry occurs when an impulse is delayed by a slow conduction pathway, remains active, and reenters the tissue producing another impulse.
  b.   Focal reentry occurs when repolarizing cells restimulate cells that are already stimulated, creating a second impulse.

C.   Monitoring techniques

1.   Holter monitoring
  a.   An ECG which is continuously recorded on tape over a 24-hour period.
  b.   Patient wears a recorder with leads II and V_5.
  c.   Used to document suspected dysrhythmias not found in short testing periods, silent ischemia, and pacemaker function.
  d.   Patient keeps a diary to record symptoms, activity, and time of occurrence that are compared with the Holter tape to evaluate correlation of symptoms with ECG changes.
2.   Bedside cardiac monitoring.
  a.   Monitors that continuously monitor ECG pattern, and other measurements such as non-invasive blood pressure, arterial pressure, pulmonary artery pressure, oxygen saturation, and respiratory rate.
  b.   Monitors have adjustable alarms, lead selection and gain control capability, and a recorder that allows a printout of the rate and rhythm.
  c.   Can be hard wired to monitor or use telemetry with a small radio transmitter that allows patient mobility.

  d.   **Commonly use five leads: lead I, lead II, lead III, lead MCL1, lead MCL6**

III.   Normal sinus rhythm

A.   Definition: normal impulses initiated by the SA node

B.   ECG criteria

1.   Rate
  a.   atrial rate: 60–100 beats per minute (BPM)
  b.   ventricular rate: 60–100 BPM
2.   Rhythm
  a.   P:P interval: P waves are present and occur at regular intervals.2
  b.   R:R interval: R waves are present and occur at regular intervals.

       3. Duration
          a.   PR interval: lasts 0.12–0.20 seconds
          b.   QRS complex: lasts 0.12 seconds or less

C.   **Clinical significance**
       1.   **Signifies a functioning SA node conduction system.**
       2.   **Signifies a normal functioning electrical system.**

IV.   **Sinus bradycardia**

    A.   **Definition: impulses initiated by the SA node but at a slower rate.**

    B.   **ECG criteria**
       1.   Rate
          a.   Atrial rate: less than 60 BPM
          b.   ventricular rate: less than 60 BPM
       2.   Rhythm
          a.   P:P interval: regular
          b.   R:R interval: regular
       3.   Duration
          a.   PR interval: within normal limits
          b.   QRS interval: within normal limits

    C.   **Clinical significance**
       1.   Sinus bradycardia may be normal in certain individuals, eg, athletes.
       2.   Monitor patient for signs and symptoms of hypotension, lethargy, or complaints of syncope.

    D.   **Treatment**
       1.   The treatment of choice is atropine 0.5 mg IV push, up to a total of 3.0 mg. Pacing is also another treatment option.

V.   **Premature atrial contraction (PAC)**

    A.   **Definition: impulses initiated by atrial tissue that occur before the next anticipated sinus beat.**

    B.   **ECG criteria**
       1.   Rate: underlying rate is 60–100 BPM
       2.   Rhythm
          a.   R:R interval: irregular
          b.   P:P interval: irregular
       3.   Duration
          a.   PR interval: normal
          b.   QRS interval: normal

    C.   **Clinical significance**
       1.   PACs are caused by some irritation to the atrial tissue.
       2.   They may be caused by emotional stress, tobacco, alcohol, caffeine, or in some disease states, eg, heart failure.
       3.   PACs originate from foci in the atrium other than the SA node.

    D.   **Treatment**
       1.   Continue to monitor the patient and treat the underlying cause.

VI.   **Sinus tachycardia**

    A.   **Definition: impulses arising out of the sinus node but at an accelerated rate.**

    B.   **ECG criteria**
       1.   Rate: A/V rates are both >100 BPM
       2.   Rhythm
          a.   R:R interval: regular
          b.   P:P interval: regular

      3.   Duration
         a.   PR interval: normal
         b.   QRS interval: normal

C.   **Clinical significance**
      1.   Tachycardia is usually a secondary response to sympathetic stimulation.
      2.   It may be caused by fever, caffeine, stress, pain, decreased cardiac output.

D.   **Treatment**
      1.   Treatment involves monitoring the patient and treating the underlying cause.

VII.   Paroxysmal atrial tachycardia

A.   **Definition: impulses arising out of atrial tissue at a rapid rate, which suppress normal sinus impulses.**

B.   **ECG criteria**
      1.   Rate: AV rates are 150–250 BPM
      2.   Rhythm
         a.   R:R interval: regular
         b.   P:P interval: regular
      3.   Duration
         a.   PR interval: normal
         b.   QRS interval: normal

C.   **Clinical significance**
      1.   PAT is usually of abrupt onset and termination.
      2.   It originates in the right atrium above the bundle of His.
      3.   Causes vary from rheumatic heart disease and pulmonary edema to stress, overexertion, and other stimulants.

D.   **Treatment**
      1.   Continue to monitor and treat underlying cause if possible.
      2.   Other treatments include Valsalva maneuver, digitalis, calcium channel blockers, beta blockers, and if sustained, electrical cardioversion.

VIII.   Supraventricular tachycardia

A.   **Definition: a rhythm that arises out of atrial or nodal tissue and conducts impulses at a rapid rate.**

B.   **ECG criteria**
      1.   Criteria vary depending on the origin of the tachycardia.
      2.   If the origin is atrial, rates tend to be greater than if the origin is nodal.

C.   **Clinical significance**
      1.   SVT is any tachycardia originating above the ventricles, eg, PAT and paroxysmal junctional tachycardia.
      2.   Causes tend to vary.

D.   **Treatment: varies according to cause.**

IX.   Atrial flutter

A.   **Definition: impulses arising out of the atrium, resulting in variable conduction to the ventricle.**

B.   **ECG criteria**
      1.   Rate
         a.   A: variable but may be as fast as 350 BPM
         b.   V: depends on the degree of block but slower than atrial

2. Rhythm
   a. P:P interval: absent
   b. R:R interval: may be regular or irregular
3. Duration
   a. PR interval: absent secondary to flutter waves
   b. QRS interval: normal
   c. There is an appearance of "saw-tooth" waves.

C. Clinical significance
1. The AV node does not conduct every impulse, so there may be two or more flutter waves to every ventricular response.
2. Cardiac output may be decreased.
3. The patient also is at risk for thrombus formation in the atrium secondary to decreased emptying of the atrium.

D. Treatment
1. Attempts to convert the patient to normal sinus rhythm are done to control the ventricular response.
2. Treatments include digoxin, calcium channel blockers, and/or electrical cardioversion.

X. Atrial fibrillation

A. Definition: irregularly irregular rhythm occurring secondary to atrial irritability.

B. ECKG criteria
1. Rate
   a. A: >350 BPM
   b. V: ≤ 100 BPM is considered a controlled rhythm; >100 BPM is uncontrolled.
2. Rhythm
   a. P:P interval: absent secondary to absence of discernible P waves
   b. R:R interval: irregular
3. Duration
   a. PR interval: absent secondary to fibrillation waves
   b. QRS interval: normal

C. Clinical significance (same as for atrial flutter)

D. Treatment (same as atrial flutter)

XI. Inherent junctional rate

A. Description: impulses arising out of the AV node.

B. ECKG criteria
1. Waves may or may not be present depending on where in the AV node the electrical impulse is coming from.
2. The inherent rate of the AV node is 40–60 BPM.
3. Proximal AV impulses will show an inverted P wave before the QRS.
4. Mid-AV impulses will have no identifiable P wave.
5. Distal AV impulses will show P waves occurring after the QRS.
6. Rate
   a. Atria: if visible may be ≤ the ventricular rate.
   b. V: 40–60 BPM.
7. Rhythm
   a. P:P interval: cannot be determined
   b. R:R interval: regular

8. Duration
   a. PR interval: <0.12 if present
   b. QRS interval: normal

C. Clinical significance
1. This rhythm may occur in healthy individuals. However, it may be caused by excessive slowing of the SA node, in which the AV node takes over as primary pacemaker.
2. Signs and symptoms may be present depending on the cardiac history of the patient.

D. Treatment: atropine and/or pacing are the treatments of choice if the patient becomes symptomatic.

XII.   Premature junctional contractions

A. Definition: impulses arising out of the AV node before the next anticipated sinus beat.

B. ECG criteria
1. Rate (same as for junctional rhythm)
2. Rhythm
   a. P:P interval: irregular, if present
   b. R:R interval: irregular
3. Duration
   a. PR interval (same as junctional rhythm)
   b. QRS interval: normal

C. Clinical significance
1. Caused by irritation to the AV node tissue, but may occur in healthy persons.
2. Occur post-MI (inferior wall), digitalis toxicity, and post-cardiac surgery.

D. Treatment: if any is indicated, deals with alleviating underlying causes (ie, digitalis toxicity)

XIII.   Junctional tachycardia

A. Definition: impulses arising out of the AV node at a rate faster than the inherent nodal rate.

B. ECG criteria
1. Rate
   a. A: >60 BPM, if visible
   b. V: >60 BPM
2. Rhythm
   a. P:P interval: same as junctional rhythm
   b. R:R interval: regular
3. Duration
   a. PR interval: <0.12, if present
   b. QRS interval: normal

C. Clinical significance
1. Junctional tachycardia is usually seen in patients post-AMI (acute myocardial infarction) or those with digitalis toxicity.
2. It also occurs whenever the SA node has failed

D. Treatment: involves alleviating the underlying cause

XIV.   Inherent ventricular rate

A. Definition: rhythm arising out of the ventricles

B. ECG criteria

1. The inherent rate of the ventricles is 20–40 BPM.
2. Rate
   a. Atrial activity: absent
   b. V: 20–40 BPM
3. Rhythm
   a. P:P interval: absent
   b. R:R interval: regular
4. Duration
   a. PR interval: absent
   b. QRS interval: >0.20, widened and bizarre

C. **Clinical significance: this is a lethal rhythm and usually precedes asystole.**
D. **Treatment: treatment involves pacing, atropine, dopamine, or inotropic/chronotropic support.**

XV. Premature ventricular contractions (PVCs)
   A. **Definition: impulses arising out of the ventricles, which occur before the next anticipated sinus beat.**
   B. **ECG criteria**
      1. Rate
         a. Atrial rate of normal complexes: 60–100 BPM
         b. Ventricular rate of normal complexes: 60–100 BPM
      2. Rhythm
         a. R:R interval: irregular secondary to the PVC
         b. P:P interval: irregular secondary to the PVC
      3. Duration
         a. PR interval: absent with the PVC but otherwise within normal limits
         b. QRS interval: >0.20 sec with PVC, but otherwise normal

         c. **Clinical significance: PVCs may occur during any rhythm and originate from an irritable focus within the ventricle. PVCs may be warning signs of an impending lethal rhythm if:**

            ► there are >5–6/min. and originate from one primary focus (unifocal or uniformed)
            ► They originate from multiple foci (multifocal or multiformed)
            ► R on T phenomena occurs (the R wave of the PVC falls on the T wave of the previous beat, causing ventricular tachycardia).

         d. Patterns of PVCs include:

            ► Bigeminy: every other beat is a PVC.
            ► Trigeminy: every third beat is a PVC.
            ► Quadrigeminy: every fourth beat is a PVC.

   D. **Treatment**
      1. Treatment depends on the underlying cause.
      2. Some causes for PVCs are hypoxia, hypokalemia, hypomagnesemia, digoxin toxicity, and ischemia.

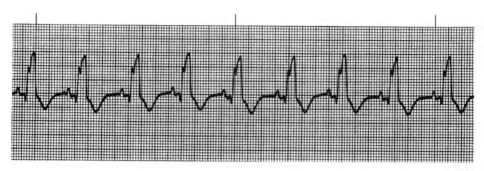

FIGURE 5-2.
A bundle branch block.

3. Lidocaine is the treatment of choice if pharmacologic means are necessary to alleviate PVCs.

XVI. Bundle branch blocks

A. Definition:
1. Ventricular depolarization occurs in two phases.
   a. The first phase is septal depolarization.
   b. The second phase is ventricular depolarization.
2. A bundle branch block occurs when there is a blocking of electrical impulses along either the left or right bundle branches during septal depolarization.
3. This results in a bizarre ventricular configuration without interruption of normal rhythm and rate (Fig. 5-2).

B. ECG criteria
1. Rate
   a. If underlying rhythm is NSR, then rate is 60–100 BPM
   b. If underlying rhythm is atrial or nodal, then rate varies accordingly
2. Rhythm
   a. P:P interval: normal
   b. R:R interval: normal
3. Duration
   a. In an incomplete block, QRS is greater than .10 mm.
   b. In a complete block, QRS is greater than .12 mm.
   c. In an RBBB, an RSR configuration is present.

C. Clinical significance

1. **Left BBB is a much more ominous sign and could be due to acute hypoxia, ischemia, or myocardial damage.**
2. Right BBB can be found in normal adults and usually presents without signs or symptoms.

D. Treatment
1. Left BBBs are treated with pacing after treating the underlying cause, if possible.
2. Right BBB are usually not treated.

XVII. **Ventricular tachycardia**
- **A.** Definition: a rapid rhythm arising out of the ventricles.
- **B.** ECG criteria
    - 1. Rate
        - a. A: absent
        - b. V: >150 BPM
    - 2. Rhythm
        - a. P:P interval: absent
        - b. R:R interval: regular
    - 3. Duration
        - a. PR interval: absent
        - b. QRS interval: widened and bizarre, >0.20 seconds
- **C.** Clinical significance
    - 1. VT may be self-limiting or sustained.
    - **2.** **It can be caused by hypoxia, ischemia, catheters, pacer wires, drug toxicity, or electrolyte imbalances.**
    - 3. Most patients are symptomatic with cerebral unresponsiveness, but some patients are able to maintain enough perfusion to remain awake.
- **D.** Treatment
    - 1. Treatment requires early and rapid electrical defibrillation.
    - 2. Refer to AHA's Advanced Cardiac Life Support algorithm for VT.

XVIII. **Ventricular fibrillation (VF)**
- **A.** Definition: chaotic electrical activity arising from multiple foci in the ventricles.
- **B.** ECG criteria
    - 1. Rate
        - a. A: cannot be determined
        - b. V: cannot be determined
    - 2. Rhythm
        - a. R:R interval: cannot be determined
        - b. P:P interval: cannot be determined
    - 3. Duration
        - a. PR interval: none
        - b. QRS interval: coarse or fine fibrillating waves
- **C.** Clinical significance
    - 1. VF results in a complete loss of cardiac output and death occurs within 3–4 minutes unless quick, immediate action is taken.
    - 2. This rhythm is usually preceded by VT.
- **D.** Treatment: refer to ACLS protocol for VF/VT

XIX. **Torsades de pointes**
- **A.** Definition: a ventricular dysrhythmia that is considered to be intermediate between ventricular tachycardia and fibrillation.
- **B.** ECG criteria
    - 1. Rate
        - a. Cannot be determined.
        - b. Estimated to be 100–350 BPM.
    - 2. Rhythm
        - a. R:R interval: irregular
        - b. P:P interval: none

3. Duration
    a. PR interval: none
    b. QRS interval: >0.12 seconds
    c. Oscillations in waveform present

C. **Clinical significance**
    1. Causes and symptoms of torsades de pointes are the same as VT. The difference between the two is the morphology.
    2. Torsades is a multiform VT. The stimulation is coming from multiple areas in the ventricles.
    3. Torsades has a helical, irregular shape rather than the regular shape of VT.

D. **Treatment: follow ACLS protocol for VF/VT but instead of lidocaine, magnesium is usually used.**

XX. **Heart blocks**

A. **Definition: heart block refers to an interruption in the conduction of an electrical impulse somewhere along the conduction system of the heart.**

B. **First-degree heart block**
    1. Definition: impulses originate out of the SA node, but there is a delay in conduction through the AV node, resulting in a prolonged PR interval.
    2. ECG criteria
        a. Rate: A/V rates are both within normal limits
        b. Rhythm

            ▶ P:P interval: regular
            ▶ R:R interval: regular

    3. Duration
        ▶ PR interval: prolonged; >0.20 seconds
        ▶ QRS interval: normal

    4. Clinical significance
        a. This type of heart block is usually insignificant and less dangerous than other types of block.
        b. Possible causes include drug therapy (quinidine, propanolol, procainimide), rheumatic fever, hypothyroidism, and inferior wall ischemia or infarction.
        c. The patient may experience symptomatic bradycardia but is usually otherwise asymptomatic.
    5. Treatment: treat underlying cause and monitor patient for any progression in heart block.

C. **Second-degree type 1**
    1. Definition: Progressive prolongation in conduction of sinus impulses through the AV node resulting in occasional non-conducted beats.
    2. ECG criteria
        a. Rate: A>V but both normal
        b. Rhythm

            ▶ P:P interval: regular
            ▶ R:R interval: irregular

c. Duration

> ▶ PR interval lengthens with each beat until a P wave appears without a QRS complex, then cycle begins again.
> ▶ QRS is normal, but is dropped periodically.

3. Clinical significance
    a. Causes include post-MI, dysrhythmia, and CAD with ischemia.
    b. Signs and symptoms, if any, are secondary to a slow ventricular response rate.
4. Treatment focuses on the underlying rate, rather than the block. Treatment is therefore administration of atropine or pacing.

D. Second-degree type 2

1. Definition: delay in conduction through the AV node resulting in constant prolongation of the PR interval with non-conducted beats.
2. ECG criteria
    a. Rate: A>V
    b. Rhythm

    > ▶ P:P interval: regular
    > ▶ R:R interval: may be regular or irregular

    c. Duration

    > ▶ PRI: normal for the conducted beats
    > ▶ QRS: may be normal or widened depending on where the block occurs

3. Clinical significance
    a. In this block, only a certain number of impulses are conducted from the SA node to the ventricles.
    b. The resulting rhythm will show two or more P waves for every QRS.
    c. The block may be intermittent or constant, thus the rhythm may be regular or irregular.
    d. This block is more serious and frequently progresses to complete or third-degree heart block.
    e. Possible causes include severe CAD, acute anterior wall MI, acute myocarditis, and digoxin toxicity.
    f. Signs and symptoms include hypotension and bradycardia.
4. Treatment depends on the signs and symptoms exhibited. Pacemakers are the treatment of choice.

E. Third-degree heart block

1. Definition: this block is characterized by the atria and ventricles beating independently of each other.
2. ECG criteria
    a. Rate: A>V, ventricular rate: usually <45
    b. Rhythm

    > ▶ P:P interval: regular (P waves appear to be "marching" through the rhythm)
    > ▶ R:R interval: regular (R waves also appear to be "marching" through)

        c.   Duration

            ▸ PR interval: not applicable because there is no relation between the P and R waves.

            ▸ QRS interval: may be narrow or wide depending on where the block occurs.

    3. Clinical significance

        a.   **Third-degree heart blocks with slow ventricular rates impair cardiac output and pose a danger to the patient.**

        b.   **If the ventricular pacemaker fails, cardiac arrest can occur.**

        c.   Possible causes include digoxin toxicity, hypoxia, post–cardiac surgery complications, congenital abnormalities, and infections such as rheumatic fever.

        d.   Signs and symptoms depend on ventricular response and the patient's ability to adapt to a slower ventricular rate.

        e.   Symptoms include fatigue, hypotension, and congestive heart failure.

        f.   If block is congenital the patient may be asymptomatic.

    4. Treatment

        a.   Treatment is the same as for bradycardia.

        b.   The patient usually requires pacemaker insertion.

XXI. **Cardiac arrest—asystole**

    A. **Definition: total absence of ventricular activity although some atrial activity may be present.**

    B. **ECG criteria**

        1. Rate is indiscernible because there is no electrical activity.

        2. Rhythm

            a.   P:P interval: usually indiscernible

            b.   R:R interval: indiscernible

        3. Duration

            a.   PR interval: not measurable

            b.   QRS interval: absent

    C. **Clinical significance: life threatening**

    D. **Treatment: begin CPR and follow ACLS protocol for asystole.**

XXII. **Pulseless electrical activity (PEA)**

    A. **Definition**

        1. Electromechanical dissociation (EMD), pseudo-EMD, idioventricular, bradyasystolic, and post-defibrillation idioventricular rhythms are included under the heading of PEA.

        2. PEA is defined as the absence of a detectable pulse and the presence of some form of electrical activity.

        3. **These arrhythmias are often associated with specific causes and can be reversed when detected and treated early.**

    B. **ECG criteria**

        1. ECG criteria varies depending on the underlying rhythm.

        2. The rhythm strip will show electrical activity normally associated with a pulse, but no pulse will be palpated.

    C. **Clinical significance**

        1. When the specific cause is properly identified and treated the rhythm is reversed.

2. Possible causes include hypovolemia, hypoxia, cardiac tamponade, tension pneumothorax, hypothermia, pulmonary embolism, and hyperkalemia, among others.

D. Treatment
    1. Treatment involves treating underlying cause.
    2. Refer to ACLS protocol for PEA.

XXIII. **Twelve lead ECG concepts**

A. General information
    1. The heart is a three-dimensional organ and must be evaluated in three dimensions.

 2. **The standard twelve lead placement allows viewing the heart at various angles of orientation. It enhances sensitivity of particular regions of the heart.**

    3. There are six frontal or limb leads and six horizontal or precordial leads.

B. Lead placement
    1. Bipolar leads measure the frontal plane using the difference between the two limb leads. QRS complexes normally appear upright.
       a. Lead I: right arm is negative, left arm is positive.
       b. Lead II: right arm is negative, left leg is positive.
       c. Lead III: left arm is negative, left leg is positive.
    2. Unipolar leads are augmented leads which use only one electrode as positive, with the negative computed by the ECG.
       a. AVR: right arm positive with negative deflection.
       b. AVL: left arm positive with a biphasic deflection.
       c. AVF: left leg positive with a positive deflection.

 3. **Precordial (chest) leads measure the horizontal plane. The R wave gets progressively larger from leads V1 through V6, while the S wave gets progressively smaller.**

    a. **V_1: 4th intercostal space (ICS) at the right sternal border.**
       b. **V_2: 4th ICS at the left sternal border.**
       c. **V_3: between V_2 and V_4.**
       d. **V_4: 5th ICS at the mid clavicular line.**
       e. **V_5: 5th ICS at the anterior axillary line.**
       f. **V_6: 5th ICS at the mid axillary line.**

C. Myocardial ischemia
    1. A temporary disruption of myocardial blood flow causes ischemia to the surrounding tissue.
    2. The resulting altered repolarization is represented on an ECG as:
       a. T-wave inversion
       b. ST-segment depression
       c. May be seen in all leads

D. Myocardial injury
    1. A prolonged myocardial blood flow disruption that causes reversible damage to the surrounding tissue.

2. Represented on an ECG as:
   a. T-wave inversion.
   b. ST-segment elevation

E. Myocardial infarct
   1. A prolonged absence of myocardial blood flow that causes necrosis of the tissue.
   2. Leads to abnormal or absent depolarization in the damaged tissue.
   3. ECG changes include:

   a. Pathologic Q wave with duration >0.04 sec and an amplitude more than one-third of the QRS height.
   b. ST-segment elevation over infarcted area
   c. ST depression in the reciprocal or opposite leads.

   4. Common ECG changes
      a. Anterior MI

         ► Occlusion of the LAD
         ► Changes seen in leads V_1 through V_4, I, AVL
         ► Reciprocal changes in leads II, III, AVF
         ► Pathologic Q wave
         ► ST-segment elevation
         ► T-wave inversion
         ► Loss of R-wave progression

      b. Posterior MI

         ► Occlusion of RCA or left circumflex
         ► Changes seen in leads V_1 and V_2
         ► R waves taller than S waves
         ► ST depression
         ► Tall T waves

      c. Lateral MI

         ► Occlusion of circumflex, branch of LAD
         ► Changes in leads I, AVL, V_5, V_6
         ► Reciprocal changes in leads II, III, AVF
         ► Pathologic Q wave
         ► ST depression
         ► T-wave inversion

      d. Inferior MI

         ► Occlusion of the RCA
         ► Changes in leads II, III, AVF
         ► Reciprocal changes in leads I, AVL
         ► Pathologic Q wave
         ► ST depression
         ► T-wave inversion

      e. Hyperkalemia: Elevation in serum potassium level (>5.5 mEq/L) slows electrical impulse conduction and can progressively evolve into ventricular fibrillation. ECG changes with increasing potassium levels:

- ▶ Peaked T waves.
- ▶ Prolonged PR interval with P wave flattening.
- ▶ QRS widens, merges with the T wave.
- ▶ Can lead to a sine wave and ventricular fibrillation.

 f. **Hypokalemia: Low levels of potassium (<3.0) can cause an increase in electrical current across cell membranes and trigger spontaneous ectopic impulses. ECG changes with decreasing potassium levels:**

- ▶ Prominent U wave.
- ▶ Flattened T wave, may become inverted with severe hypokalemia.
- ▶ ST-segment depression.
- ▶ Prolonged PR interval.
- ▶ Atrial and ventricular dysrhythmias, commonly atrial tachycardia, PVCs, and heart blocks.

g. Pericarditis: an acute inflammation of the pericardial sac, usually caused by a general disease process. ECG changes with pericarditis:

- ▶ **ST elevation in leads I, II, AVF and V_4 through V_6**
- ▶ **ST depression in leads V_1, and AVR**
- ▶ **No Q wave formation**
- ▶ **With time, as ST segment returns to baseline, the T wave flattens, then inverts**

XXIV. Interventions of cardiac dysrhythmias
A. Electrophysiologic obliteration
1. Patient is taken to the lab and electrical activity of his heart is mapped out by giving medications that should elicit a rapid conduction.
2. If an accessory pathway is found it is obliterated at that time.

B. Pacemaker
1. A pacemaker is a mechanical device that stimulates the heart to depolarize when the heart is unable to pace itself.
2. Indications
   a. Third-degree heart block
   b. Lesser heart blocks with patient symptoms
   c. AV block with an MI
   d. Recurrent tachycardias
3. Types
   a. Temporary pacemakers pace with an external generator that has external controls. The leads can be inserted into the right ventricle transvenously, transthoracically, or into the pulmonary artery with a catheter (Fig. 5-3).
   b. A transcutaneous temporary pacemaker can be used in an emergency. The type of pacemaker stimulates the heart through external electrodes placed on the chest and back of the patient. Patients can feel this shock.
   c. Permanent pacemakers are implanted subcutaneously under the patient's clavicle or under the abdominal wall.

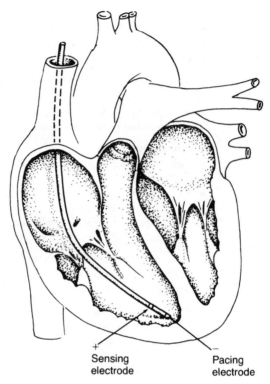

FIGURE 5-3.
Placement of a pacing electrode.

    d.   **Pacemakers can be asynchronous or fixed rate, with a predetermined rate set, or synchronous, demand pacemakers that fire only when the patient's own intrinsic heart rate falls below a predetermined threshold (Display 5-1).**

4.   Pacemaker waveforms (Fig. 5-4):
   a.   A pacemaker spike appears before every P wave that is stimulated by the pacemaker.
   b.   The P wave may be inverted or have a shape different from the patient's baseline wave.
   c.   With the electrode in the ventricle, a spike appears before each QRS complex that is stimulated by the pacemaker.
   d.   These QRS complexes are usually taller and wider than the patient's baseline complex.
   e.   With electrodes in both the atrium and ventricle, a spike is seen before each P wave and QRS complex stimulated by the pacemaker.

DISPLAY 5-1.
ICHD Code for Differentiation of Pacemaker Functional Capabilities

Paced Chamber	Sensing Chamber	Response to Sensing	Programmable Function	Special Antitachycardia Functions
V = Ventricle	V = Ventricle	I = Inhibited	P = Program (rate and/or output)	P = Standard pacer technology
A = Atrium	A = Atrium	T = Triggered	M = Multiprogrammable	S = Shock
D = Dual chambers	D = Dual	D = Dual	C = Communicating	D = Paces and shocks
0 = None	0 = None	0 = None	R = Rate modulation	
			0 = None	

5. Nursing considerations
   a. Assess ECG rhythm for rate and regularity.
   b. Assess the pacemaker settings for set rate and existence of atrial or ventricular pacing
   c. Analyze whether pacemaker is sensing and pacing or is solely pacing at 100%.
   d. Evaluate pacemaker sensing capability, eg, appropriateness of pacing spike, and response of the myocardium.
   e. Does the heart rate match the set rate; is it lower or higher than the set rate?

C. **Automatic implantable cardioverter defibrillator (AICD): a surgically implanted device that monitors heart activity and produces counter-shocks when dysrhythmias occur.**
   1. Used to treat patients with recurrent tachydysrhythmias, and those who have survived at least one cardiac arrest without an MI. Many times these arrests are caused by unstable tachycardias.
   2. The AICD continuously monitors the heart for a predetermined heart rate and amount of time that the ECG stays on baseline, called the probability density function (PDF).

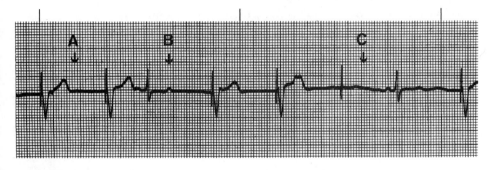

FIGURE 5-4.
A) ventricular paced beats, B) patient beat, C) loss of capture.

3. Ventricular fibrillation and tachycardia rhythms tend to stay on baseline for much shorter time periods than sinus rhythms do. After the heart rate and PDF reach a predetermined limit, the AICD will deliver a first shock of 25 joules.

4. If the patient's rhythm does not return to normal, then subsequent shocks of 30 joules for three cycles are delivered. The patient's rhythm must return to baseline before the AICD can reset for a new four shock cycle.

5. The number of joules programmed varies with each patient.

6. ECG characteristics of AICD show a tall spike that is followed by a long downward sloping line that is followed by a normal ECG wave.

7. Nursing considerations:
   a. Monitor heart rhythm.
   b. Assess rhythm strip for episodes of ventricular tachycardia.
   c. Assess AICD response to episode.
   d. Assess patient response to AICD.
   e. Document all episodes and patient response.

Bibliography

Apple. S. (1995). Advances for diagnosing acute myocardial infarction. *Heartbeat* 6(2), 1–7.

Creel, C. A. (1994). Silent myocardial ischemia and nursing implications. *Heart Lung* 23(3), 218–226.

Hudak, C. M. & Gallo, B. M. (1994). *Critical care nursing: A holistic approach* (6th ed.). Philadelphia: J. B. Lippincott.

Keller, G. B. & Lemberg. L. (1994). Q and non-Q wave myocardial infarctions. *Am J Crit Care* 3(2), 158–161.

Kinney, M. R. & Packa, D. R. (1996). *Comprehensive cardiac care* (8th ed.). St Louis: Mosby-Year Book.

North American Nursing Diagnosis Association (NANDA). (1996). *Nursing diagnoses: Definitions & classification 1997–1998.* Philadelphia: Author.

Sokolow, M. T. (1990). *Clinical cardiology* (5th ed.). Norwalk, CT: Appleton and Lange.

Thelan, L. A. (1994). *Critical care nursing* (2nd ed.). St. Louis: Mosby-Year Book.

Williams, K. & Marton, P. G. (1995). Diagnosis and treatment of acute myocardial infarction. *AACN Clin Issues* 6(3), 375–386.

Zaloga, G. P. (1994). *Nutrition in Critical Care.* St. Louis: Mosby.

STUDY QUESTIONS

1. Which of the following is not a characteristic of the myocardial cells?
   a. automaticity
   b. conductivity
   c. contractility
   d. myomaticity

2. The normal rate of the SA node is
   a. 60–100 BPM
   b. 80–120 BPM
   c. 20–40 BPM
   d. 50–70 BPM

3. The natural pacemaker of the heart is the
   a. ventricle
   b. SA node
   c. AV node
   d. atria

4. Which of the following may cause a resting heart rate of 76 BPM?
   a. hypovolemia
   b. an idioventricular rhythm
   c. a temperature of 102.8° F
   d. the SA node pacing the heart

5. Which of the following is the natural electrical pathway of the cardiac cells?
   a. AV node, SA node, bundle of His, Purkinje fibers
   b. SA node, AV node, Purkinje fibers, bundle of His
   c. AV node, SA node, left bundle, right bundle
   d. SA node, AV node, bundle of His, Purkinje fibers

6. The pattern of waves on an ECG is as follows:
   a. P, Q, R, S, T
   b. A, C, V
   c. P, A, C, W, P
   d. P, A, P

7. Which of the following does not describe the normal P wave on an ECG?
   a. represents ventricular contraction
   b. <3 mm amplitude
   c. 0.06–0.11 second duration
   d. indicates atrial depolarization

8. Which of the following indicates a normal PR interval?
   a. duration of 0.15 seconds
   b. duration of 0.02 seconds
   c. duration of 0.5 seconds
   d. duration of 0.32 seconds

9. Your patient has a heart rate of 80–100 BPM with no visible P waves. Your first response is to:
   a. Shock! Shock! Shock!
   b. Call the physician and ask for an order for atropine.
   c. Call the physician and ask for an order for nipride.
   d. Perform 12-lead ECG to determine rhythm.

10. Which of the following is true concerning the T wave on an ECG?
    a. It precedes the QRS complex.
    b. It extends from the R wave to the S wave.
    c. A peaked T wave may indicate hyperkalemia.
    d. It represents atrial depolarization.

11. Identify the following strip.
    a. normal sinus rhythm (NSR)

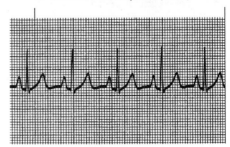

    b. sinus tachycardia
    c. atrial fibrillation
    d. ventricularly paced rhythm

12. Identify the following strip.

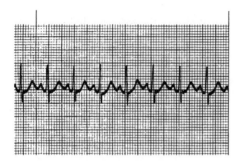

    a. normal sinus rhythm (NSR)
    b. sinus tachycardia
    c. atrial fibrillation
    d. ventricularly paced rhythm

13. Identify the following strip.

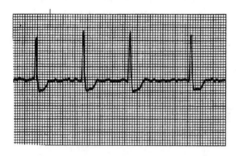

    a. normal sinus rhythm (NSR)
    b. sinus tachycardia
    c. atrial fibrillation
    d. ventricularly paced rhythm

14. Identify the following strip.

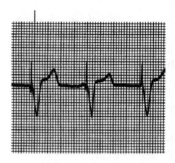

    a. normal sinus rhythm
    b. sinus tachycardia
    c. atrial fibrillation
    d. ventricularly paced rhythm

ANSWER KEY

1. *Correct response: d*
The term myomaticity is the result of far too many hours of sitting at this computer!
a, b, and c. The characteristics of myocardial cells are automaticity, conductivity, contractility, and contractility.
Knowledge/Physiologic/NA

2. *Correct response: a*
The normal rate of the SA node is 60–100 BPM.
Knowledge/Physiologic/NA

3. *Correct response: b*
The SA node is the natural pacemaker of the heart.
a. The ventricles will initiate a rhythm only if the SA or the AV nodes fail to do so.
c. The AV node will initiate conduction if the SA node fails to do so.
d. If the SA node fails to initiate conduction another area of the atria may fire, but the natural pacemaker is the SA node.
Knowledge/Physiologic/NA

4. *Correct response: d*
The normal resting heart rate is 60–100 BPM. The SA node is the natural pacemaker.
a and c. A febrile state and hypovolemia would both cause tachycardia.
b. A normal idioventricular rate would be 20–40 BPM.
Knowledge/Physiologic/NA

5. *Correct response: d*
The natural conduction pathway of the heart is SA node, AV node, bundle of His, Purkinje fibers
c. The bundles are conducted simultaneously.
Knowledge/Physiologic/NA

6. *Correct response: a*
The waves seen on an ECG are P, Q, R, S, T.
b. These are CVP waveforms.
c and d. These are not waves.
Knowledge/Physiologic/NA

7. *Correct response:*
a. The QRS complex represents ventricular contraction.
b, c, and d. All are true of the P wave.
Knowledge/Physiologic/NA

8. *Correct response: a*
The normal PR interval is 0.12–0.20 seconds
Knowledge/Physiologic/NA

9. *Correct response: d*
The patient's heart rate is within normal limits; the next step is to determine what the rhythm is.
a. This would be the correct intervention for ventricular tachycardia.
b. This patient is not bradycardic.
c. There is no mention of hypertension in the question.
Comprehension/Physiologic/ Implementation

10. *Correct response: c*
A peaked T wave may indicate hyperkalemia.
a, b. The T wave follows the QRS complex.
d. The T wave represents ventricular repolarization.
Knowledge/Physiologic/NA

11. *Correct response: a*
Normal sinus rhythm has a P wave, followed by a QRS, at a rate of 60–100 BPM.
b. Sinus tachycardia has a P wave followed by a QRS at a rate of 100–150 BPM.

   c. Atrial fibrillation contains no visible P waves, the QRSs may be regular but are usually irregular. The rate may be within normal limits or "a-fib with a rapid ventricular response" >100 BPM.

   d. V-paced rhythm will show a ventricular rate at a set rate (usually 60–80) BPM.

Application/Physiologic/NA

12. *Correct response: b*

Sinus tachycardia has a P wave followed by a QRS at a rate of 100–150 BPM.

   a. Normal sinus rhythm has a P wave, followed by a QRS at a rate of 60–100 BPM.

   c. A-fib contains no visible P waves, the QRSs may be regular but are usually irregular. The rate may be within normal limits or "a-fib with a rapid ventricular response" >100 BPM.

   d. V-paced rhythm will show a ventricular rate at a set rate (usually 60–80) BPM.

Application/Physiologic/NA

13. *Correct response: c*

A-fib contains no visible P waves, the QRSs may be regular but are usually irregular. The rate may be within normal limits or "a-fib with a rapid ventricular response" >100 BPM.

   a. Normal sinus rhythm has a P wave, followed by a QRS at a rate of 60–100 BPM.

   b. Sinus tachycardia has a P wave followed by a QRS at a rate of 100–150 BPM.

   d. V-paced rhythm will show a ventricular rate at a set rate (usually 60–80) BPM.

Application/Physiologic/NA

14. *Correct response: d*

V-paced rhythm will show a ventricular rate at a set rate (usually 60–80) BPM.

   a. Normal sinus rhythm has a P wave, followed by a QRS at a rate of 60–100 BPM.

   b. Sinus tachycardia has a P wave followed by a QRS at a rate of 100–150 BPM.

   c. Atrial fibrillation contains no visible P waves, the QRSs may be regular but are usually irregular. The rate may be within normal limits or "a-fib with a rapid ventricular response" >100 BPM.

Application/Physiologic/NA

The Respiratory System

I. **Anatomy and physiology**
   A. Structures
   B. Functions
   C. Respiratory regulation
   D. Factors affecting oxygenation
   E. Oxyhemoglobin dissociation curve

II. **Overview of respiratory pathology**
   A. Assessment
   B. Arterial blood gas (ABG)
   C. Diagnostic testing
   D. Nutritional considerations
   E. Psychosocial implications
   F. Commonly used medications

III. **Status asthmaticus**
   A. Description
   B. Etiology and incidence
   C. Pathophysiology
   D. Assessment findings
   E. Nursing diagnosis
   F. Planning and implementation
   G. Evaluation

IV. **Chronic obstructive pulmonary disease (COPD)**
   A. Description
   B. Etiology and incidence
   C. Pathophysiology
   D. Assessment findings
   E. Nursing diagnosis
   F. Planning and implementation
   G. Evaluation
   H. Home health considerations

V. **Acute respiratory failure**
   A. Description
   B. Etiology and incidence
   C. Pathophysiology
   D. Assessment findings

   E. Nursing diagnosis
   F. Planning and implementation
   G. Evaluation

VI. **Adult respiratory distress syndrome (ARDS)**

VII. **Pulmonary embolism**
   A. Description
   B. Etiology and incidence
   C. Pathophysiology
   D. Assessment findings
   E. Nursing diagnosis
   F. Planning and implementation
   G. Evaluation

VIII. **Lung cancer**
   A. Description
   B. Etiology and incidence
   C. Pathophysiology
   D. Assessment findings
   E. Nursing diagnosis
   F. Planning and implementation
   G. Evaluation

IX. **Laryngeal cancer**
   A. Description
   B. Etiology and incidence
   C. Pathophysiology
   D. Assessment findings
   E. Nursing diagnosis
   F. Planning and implementation
   G. Evaluation
   H. Home health considerations

X. **Lobectomy**
   A. Description
   B. Types of pulmonary resection
   C. Assessment
   D. Nursing diagnosis
   E. Planning and implementation
   F. Evaluation

I. Anatomy and physiology

A. Structures:

1. Main function is to supply oxygen to body cells and to remove carbon dioxide from cells.
2. There are 12 pairs of ribs, which attach to the vertebral column posteriorly:
   a. Ribs 1–7 are attached to the sternum anteriorly.
   b. Ribs 8–10 are attached to the 7th rib cartilage anteriorly
   c. Ribs 11–12 are "floating"
3. The chest wall includes the sternum and manubrium. The manubrium is the attachment site of second rib.
4. The angle of Louis marks the attachment of the manubrium and sternum.
5. There are 3 right lobes and 2 left lobes in the lungs.
6. Surrounding the lung is the parietal and visceral pleurae, with pleural space between the two.
7. The bronchi, consisting of right and left mainstem, divide at the carina, which is located beneath the angle of Louis.
8. They then divide into bronchioles, which continue to divide until alveoli appear.
9. Alveoli consist of:
   a. Type I: gas exchange units
   b. Type II: surfactant production
10. The alveolocapillary membrane allows for rapid gas diffusion.
11. Pulmonary circulation consists of:
    a. Bronchial vessels, which supply oxygenated blood to the trachea, bronchi, nerves, and supporting tissue of the lungs, arteries, and veins.
    b. Pulmonary vessels, which supply oxygenated blood to the left side of the heart and therefore to the rest of the body.

12.   Accessory muscles associated with the pulmonary system are the sternocleidomastoid, scalene, intercostals, and abdominals.

B.   Functions

1.   Ventilation involves gas exchange between the person and environment as well as air movement between the atmosphere and alveoli and distribution of air within the lungs.

2.   Ventilation consists of active inspiration and passive expiration.

3.   Measurements of ventilation are either:

a.   Static or constant, which is affected by age and body size.

b.   Dynamic or changing.

c.   Measurements include:

- ▶ F = frequency (respiratory rate)
- ▶ dead space (VD)—part of tidal volume not involved with alveolar gas exchange
- ▶ compliance—measures lung expandability and alveolar wall elasticity
- ▶ resistance—measures patency of airway diameter and promotes return to original shape (Table 6-1)

4.   Diffusion of gases—carbon dioxide and oxygen diffuse across the alveolar capillary membrane and pulmonary capillary beds from greater to lesser partial pressures (Table 6-2). This allows for gas exchange.

5.   Transport of O_2 and CO_2

a.   97% of oxygen is attached to hemoglobin. The remainder is dissolved in plasma.

b.   **1.34 mL O_2 is the maximum amount that can combine with each gram of hemoglobin.**

c.   Decreased hemoglobin results in less oxygen-carrying capacity of blood.

d.   70% of CO_2 combines with HCO_3 in RBCs, 25% is bound to Hgb in RBCs, and 5% or less is dissolved in plasma.

C.   Respiratory regulation

1.   Types of regulation are:

a.   autonomic: involving the medulla and pons

b.   voluntary: involving the cortex

2.   Cerebral control of respiration

a.   Respiratory center is located in the medulla.

TABLE 6-1.
Disorders Contributing to Dynamic Disorders

FACTORS	DISORDERS
Decreased compliance	Atelactasis, pulmonary edema, fibrosis, pneumonia
Increased resistance	Bronchospasm, emphysema excessive secretions

TABLE 6-2.
Factors Affecting Diffusion and O_2/CO_2 Transport

FACTORS AFFECTING DIFFUSION	FACTORS AFFECTING O_2/CO_2 TRANSPORT
Surface area	Ventilation
Oxygen entering lungs	Amount of perfusion
H and H	Blood flow to lungs and diffusion
Membrane integrity	Efficiency of flow capacity
Diffusion coefficient of gas	Amount of oxygen that can be carried in the blood
Nitrogen	

      b.   Apneustic center is located in the lower pons.

      c.   Pneumotaxic center is located in the upper pons.

  3. Chemoreceptors are receptors that assist with respiratory control.

      a.   Central receptors are located below the surface of the medulla.

      b.   Peripheral receptors are located in carotid bodies in the neck and aortic arch.

  4. **CO_2 is normally the most powerful stimulus to affect respirations.**

D. **Factors affecting oxygenation**

  1. Level of wellness

  2. Oxygen-carrying capacity of blood

  3. Inspired oxygen

  4. Cardiac output

  5. Fluid volume

  6. Metabolic rate

  7. Chest expansion (rate, rhythm, depth)

  8. Presence of chronic diseases

  9. Age

  10. Life-style and/or occupation

E. **Oxyhemoglobin dissociation curve: shows affinity of Hgb for oxygen at various oxygen tensions.**

  1. Indicates how easily Hgb will give up O_2 for tissue use.

  2. Shift to right: decreased affinity of Hgb for oxygen; less oxygen can be picked up in lungs but that oxygen is more easily released to the capillary tissues.

  3. Shift to left: increased affinity of Hgb for oxygen; more oxygen can be picked up in lungs but oxygen is not as easily released to the capillary tissues, which could result in tissue hypoxia even with adequate PaO_2 (Fig. 6-1).

  4. Oxygen is carried in blood:

      a.   Dissolved in plasma: 0.3 mL/100 mL blood

      b.   Combined with Hgb: 19.4 mL/100 mL blood

      c.   Total in whole blood: 19.7 mL/100 mL blood

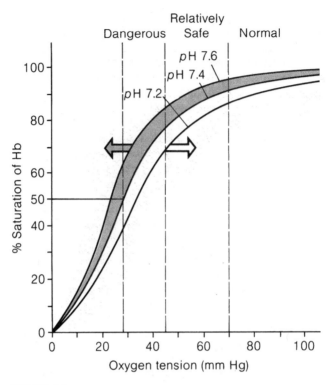

FIGURE 6-1.
Oxygen–hemoglobin dissociation curve. The oxygen can attach to the hemoglobin more easily (higher oxygen saturation per PO_2) but has trouble coming off the hemoglobin at the tissues, resulting in less tissue oxygenation. Decreased oxygen affinity (shift to the right) means that it is more difficult for the oxygen to attach to the hemoglobin (there is lower oxygen saturation per PO_2), but it can come off at the tissues more easily. The P_{50} is normally 27 mm Hg. A shift to the right gives a higher P_{50}; a shift to the left gives a lower P_{50}.

II.   Overview of respiratory pathology
A.   Assessment
1.   Obtain history of current illness including:
   a.   Duration of symptoms
   b.   Associated cardiopulmonary history
   c.   Cough/sputum production: color, odor, consistency, amount
   d.   Presence of dyspnea/discomfort
   e.   Precipitating and relieving factors
2.   Obtain history of risk factors for pulmonary disease:
   a.   Life-style/occupation
   b.   Environment, ie, exposure to secondary smoke
   c.   Smoking history
3.   Obtain medical history including:
   a.   Last chest x-ray (CXR)

b. General health status (immunizations for influenza, pneumonia)

c. Developmental status (compare with chronologic age)

4. Physical examination should include evaluation for signs and symptoms of oxygen deficit including:

a. Tachypnea

b. Tachycardia

c. Neurologic changes

d. Cyanosis (late sign)

e. Inspect for general appearance, skin color, level of consciousness

f. Evaluate breathing patterns, chest wall movement, and use of accessory muscles

g. Palpate for areas of tenderness

h. Percuss for resonance, hyperresonance, hyporesonance, and measure diaphragmatic excursion.

i. Auscultate breath sounds and compare bilaterally

- ▶ Bronchial: loud sounds mainly heard over sternum and between scapulae; longer time spent on expiration than inspiration.
- ▶ Bronchovesicular: medium sounds heard over mainstem bronchi at level of 1st and 2nd intercostal spaces anteriorly and posteriorly between scapulae. Inspiration is longer than expiration.
- ▶ Vesicular: soft, low, mainly inspiratory sounds heard over most of lung fields.
- ▶ Adventitious breath sounds are always considered abnormal: note pattern of adventitious sounds and location, and timing (ie, whether they are heard on inspiration or expiration; Display 6-1).

5. Altered respiratory patterns

a. Cheyne-Stokes: "waxing and waning" respirations

b. Apneusis: prolonged inspiration with a pause

c. Central neurogenic hyperventilation (CNH): fast, deep breathing

d. Cluster: irregular with apneic periods

e. Ataxic: totally irregular

DISPLAY 6-1.
Etiology of Adventitious Breath Sounds

Rhonchi (low-pitched rhales): Partial large airway and snoring obstruction

Wheezes: Bronchiolar narrowing, musical, high-pitched

Crackles: Airway fluid, alveoli bursting open during inspiration, atelectasis

Decreased basilar: Alveolar hypoventilation

B. **Arterial blood gas (ABG)**

1. Measures partial pressure each gas exerts on blood.

2. **pH—indicates the concentration of hydrogen ions in the blood (H+)**

   a. **pH under 7.35: acidosis that is secondary to excessive amount of acid or decrease in alkaline substances.**

   b. **pH over 7.45: alkalosis that is due to a low concentration of H+. Caused by either too many alkaline substances or not enough acid substances.**

3. **$PaCO_2$: = respiratory parameter; combines with water in the blood to form carbonic acid; CO_2 considered an acid**

4. **HCO_3: = metabolic parameter; considered a base**

5. Steps in analysis of ABGs:

   a. Determine the underlying pH disorder, if any.

   b. Does the pH show acidosis or alkalosis?

   c. Is the cause of the pH imbalance respiratory or metabolic?

   d. Assess $PaCO_2$ and HCO_3- for acidosis, alkalosis, or WNL.

   e. Note attempted compensation if both $PaCO_2$ and HCO_3 are abnormal.

   f. **If the pH is normal, the blood gas is considered to be compensated; if the pH is abnormal, the blood gas is not compensated.**

   g. Assess for oxygenation: PaO_2.

   h. Evaluate oxygen saturation = amount of O_2 combined with Hgb × 100.

6. Pulse oximetry: SpO_2 = 95%–100%

   a. Indicates percentage of capillary saturation.

   b. **Not specific for oxygen. SpO_2 cannot differentiate between types of saturated hemoglobin (ie, patients who are smokers, CO_2 poisoned, anemic may show normal saturation). See Table 6-3.**

C. **Diagnostic testing: Some diagnostic tests used in the assessment of pulmonary diseases include:**

1. CXR

2. VQ scan

3. Bronchoscopy

4. Continuous monitoring

   a. SaO_2: Measured via intra-arterial line

TABLE 6-3.
Correlation of Pulse Oximetry With PaO_2 From Arterial Blood

SpO_2, %	PAO_2, %
98	100
95	80
90	60
75	40

   b. $ETCO_2$: Actual measurements of exhaled gas allow for an estimation of arterial PCO_2 for clients with artificial airways.

D. Nutritional considerations

 1. Malnutrition can cause or worsen respiratory failure by decreasing respiratory muscle function and ventilatory drive.

 2. Pulmonary defense mechanisms could also be compromised.

 3. During critical illness, with inadequate calorie intake, the body will convert energy from muscle protein; the diaphragm and intercostal muscles are also susceptible to this catabolic effect.

 4. Hypermetabolism creates additional increases in caloric demands. The malnourished patient must sacrifice body mass to supply energy to decrease oxygen consumption (VO_2) and lessen metabolic demands. Consequently, weight loss will result.

 5. Isolated mineral and electrolyte deficiencies can also impair respiratory muscle function.

 6. Hypophosphatemia reduces diaphragmatic contractile strength and has been shown to precipitate acute renal failure.

 7. Hypomagnesemia and hypokalemia can also cause a decrease in respiratory muscle strength.

 8. Considerations for medical nutrition therapy:

   a. The overall goal is to increase the nutrient intake to achieve caloric balance and meet intake needs.

   b. There is some controversy as to the proportion of nutritional support given in the form of carbohydrate vs. fat.

   c. Some believe carbohydrates require higher oxygen consumption. Once the required amount of protein is given, the remaining carbohydrate and fat calories are usually delivered in equal proportions, plus or minus 20%.

   d. Obtain daily weights; prevent weight loss and maintain lean body mass.

   e. Control fluid intake to avoid unsuspected fluid loading.

   f. Monitor electrolytes, particularly phosphorus, calcium, and magnesium.

   g. When the patient is able to eat by mouth, a high-calorie, high-protein diet is the therapy of choice. Small, frequent meals and liquids are often better tolerated. The foods should be nutritionally dense so as to minimize the volume of food.

E. Psychosocial implications

 1. The patient with pulmonary disease must face the knowledge that this is often a chronic illness with possible long-term disability.

 2. Life-style changes necessitating a decrease in daily activities often occur.

 3. Possible guilt about life-style risk factors such as smoking may be experienced.

 4. Fear/anxiety about medical management may occur.

 5. Change in self-image if using oxygen devices in public may be experienced.

 6. Chronic medical problems often result in decreased financial resources.

F. Commonly used medications (Table 6-4)

text continues on page 212

TABLE 6-4.
Respiratory Medications

CATEGORY	ACTION	USES	ROUTES	SIDE EFFECTS/ADVERSE REACTIONS	EXAMPLES	NURSING CONSIDERATIONS
Steroids	Decrease number and activity of respiratory tract inflammatory cells while inhibiting bronchoconstriction	Chronic asthma; in conjunction with other drugs for status asthmaticus	Inhalation, IV, PO	Sore throat, candida infection, GI irritation, systemic effects	Beclomethasone (Vanceril) triamcinalone (Azmacort), flunisolide (AeroBid), prednisone, dexamethasone (Decadron)	Mouth hygiene for maintenance and prevention, not for acute attacks; assess for systemic effects give bronchodilators before steroids during concomitant use
Sympathomimetic bronchodilators	Decrease muscular bronchospasm and increase mucociliary clearance; direct stimulation of cyclic AMP production	Bronchospasm; bronchial asthma; emphysema	Inhalation IV, PO, IM, PR, SQ	"Fight-or-flight": palpitations, tachycardia, headache, flushing, nausea, vomiting, insomnia, cardiac ischemia, angina	Epinephrine; isoproterenol (Isuprel), isoetharine (Bronkosol), metaproterenol (Alupent), terbutaline (Brethine), albuterol (Ventolin, Proventil)	Caution with MAO inhibitors as well as with tricyclic antidepressants, thyroxin, antihistamines, and other nervous system stimulants; note increased metabolic rate, must differentiate between B1 and B2 stimulants; give ASAP in the morning

	Action	Use	Route	Side effects	Examples	Nursing considerations
Xanthine bronchodilators	decrease muscular bronchospasm and increase mucociliary clearance; indirect decrease of cyclic AMP production by phosphodiesterase	bronchospasm; bronchial asthma; emphysema	PO, IV, PR	"fight-or-flight"	caffeine, theophylline (Theo-Dur, Aminophylline), theobromine, oxytriphylline	use with caution with non-cardioselective beta blockers (may cause severe bronchospasm); caution with peptic ulcer disease note increased metabolic rate therapeutic blood level is 10–20 mcg/mL; give with food/milk for GI irritation smoking decreases half-life
mucolytics	disrupt chemical bonds that hold segments of mucoproteins together	adjunct for treatment of tenacious mucous secretions due to bronchopulmonary disease, cystic fibrosis, atelectasis, etc.	inhalation, intratracheal	bronchospasm, stomatitis, nausea, epistaxis, rhinorrhea, insomnia, tachycardia	acetylcysteine (Mucomyst)	discontinue with bronchospasm oral hygiene after use use only glass, plastic, aluminum, or stainless steel to mix lasts 96 hours (store in refrigerator with date, time, and initials) promote compliance

III.   Status asthmaticus

    A.   Description: acute episode of airway obstruction characterized by airway hyperreactivity to various stimuli that results in recurrent wheezing caused by edema and bronchospasm.

    B.   Etiology and incidence

        1.   May be precipitated by antigen–antibody reactions, respiratory infection, dust/pollutants, certain foods.

        2.   Exacerbated by cold weather, physical exertion, emotions, some medications.

    C.   Pathophysiology

        1.   **The major physical abnormality is expiratory airflow obstruction, resulting in accumulation of large amounts of mucus in bronchial tubes and alveolar hyperinflation.**

        2.   Bronchospasm leads to both airway obstruction and air trapping.

        3.   Inspired air cannot be exhaled in time before the next inspiration, causing retention of air and alveolar hyperventilation.

    D.   Assessment findings

        1.   Pulmonary symptoms may include severe dyspnea, chest tightness, absent breath sounds.

        2.   Use of accessory muscles, cough, and wheezing may be pronounced.

        3.   Inspection may reveal inspiratory retractions and changes in speech.

        4.   A prolonged I:E ratio may be noted.

        5.   Cardiovascular symptoms include tachycardia, ECG changes, hypertension, decreased cardiac contractility, and pulsus paradoxus.

        6.   Neurologic findings include anxiety, restlessness, fear, and disorientation.

        7.   Decreased urine output and decreased gastrointestinal (GI) motility may present.

        8.   ABG analysis reveals alkalosis progressing to acidosis and hypoxia.

    E.   Nursing diagnoses

        1.   Impaired Gas Exchange

        2.   Fluid Volume Excess

        3.   Ineffective Breathing Patterns

        4.   Ineffective Airway Clearance

        5.   Anxiety

    F.   Planning and implementation

        1.   Assess respiratory status: rate, rhythm, depth, breath sounds, work of breathing, use of accessory muscles, ABGs, pulse oximetry.

        2.   Increase head of bed to high-Fowler's position to improve respiratory status and patient comfort.

        3.   Maintain humidification and oxygen therapies.

        4.   Anticipate and prepare for possible intubation.

        5.   Assess for changes in neurologic status.

        6.   **Assess for hypoxemia: tachycardia, tachypnea, restlessness, diaphoresis, headache, lethargy, confusion, pallor.**

        7.   Administer all medications and respiratory treatments as ordered.

        8.   Pace activities to conserve oxygen and energy.

9. Monitor for dysrhythmias.
10. Assess anxiety level and intervene appropriately.
11. Explain all care activities using simple explanations.
12. Administer analgesics/antianxiety agents as necessary.
13. Be aware of potential complications:
    a. Respiratory failure
    b. Need for temporary mechanical ventilation

G. **Evaluation**
1. Client experiences reduced anxiety/fear as evidenced by calm and trusting appearance and verbalization of fears and concerns.
2. Gas exchange and oxygen balance are restored, as evidenced by PaO_2 over 80, SaO_2 over 90%, absence of cyanosis, absence of restlessness, confusion, irritability, heart rate 60–100 BPM, airways clear of mucus.
3. Adequate breathing pattern is restored, as evidenced by increased FEV; resting respiratory rate 12–20 BPM; $PaCO_2$ return to baseline; PaO_2 over 60 mm Hg.
4. Maintains effective airway clearance.
5. Verbalizes basic understanding of pathophysiology of disease, necessary life-style adjustments, methods to decrease incidence of attack, correct use of medications.

IV. **Chronic obstructive pulmonary disease (COPD)**
A. **Description: a group of persistent, irreversible, chronic pulmonary disorders that develop as responses to various noxious stimuli and lead to slowly progressive airway obstruction.**

1. **Emphysema: progressive and irreversible alveolocapillary destruction with abnormal alveolar enlargement causing alveolar wall destruction, which leads to increased lung compliance, decreased diffusion, and increased airway resistance.**
2. **Bronchitis: disorder characterized by excessive mucus secretions in the bronchial airways, leading to chronic and recurrent productive coughing for at least 3 consecutive months for 2 consecutive years.**

B. **Etiology and incidence**
1. Cigarette smoking is the number one risk factor for the development of COPD.
2. Incidence greater in men than in women, possibly because of smoking history and occupation.
3. Hypertrophy of mucus-producing cells leads to narrowing of small airway causing alveolar inflammation.

C. **Pathophysiology**
1. Emphysema: main defect is dysfunction of lung elastase, which normally fuses with bacteria that reach the alveolar level. Amount of elastase is equally balanced with an equal amount of the protease inhibitor, alpha-1-antitrypsin.
2. Cigarette smoking, recurrent infections, environmental irritants, and alpha-1-antitrypsin deficiency probably cause elastase breakdown.
3. There is evidence that smoking decreases alpha-1-antitrypsin function.

4. The imbalance in this system results in elastin destruction in distal airways and alveoli, promoting emphysema development.
5. Emphysematous lungs appear large, hyperinflated, and pale. Bronchiole destruction may result in bullae formation.
6. Two major effects of emphysema are air trapping and decreased gas exchange.
    a. Air is trapped due to loss of elastic recoil, which results in decreased ventilation and increased bronchiolar collapse.
    b. Decreased gas exchange causes pulmonary diffusion and perfusion abnormalities due to less alveolar surface area.
    c. Resulting hypoxemia causes pulmonary artery constriction, shunting blood away from even normal lung areas and resulting in increased FRC, increased compliance, and hypoxia.
7. Chronic bronchitis: early in the disease there is an increased size and number of secretory glands, which results in increased amounts of sputum, bronchial congestion, and narrowing of bronchioles and small bronchi.
8. Over time, the normally sterile lower respiratory tract is colonized by bacteria.
9. Fibrotic cells replace normal bronchial cells with disease progression.

D. Assessment findings
1. Obtain history of the following:
    a. Cigarette/marijuana smoking
    b. Exposure to respiratory irritants and length of exposure
    c. Prior respiratory diseases, infections, allergies
    d. Presence of chronic cough and characteristics
2. Obtain family history of pulmonary disease.
3. Assess degree of activity tolerance including fatigue and dyspnea.
4. Assess current medications, including those obtained over-the-counter.
5. Assess oxygen use and use of IPPB or respiratory assistive devices, including amount, frequency, duration, and therapeutic response of each.
6. Physical exam should include assessment of dyspnea, cough, and prolonged expiration.
7. Perform auscultation for presence of audible expiratory wheeze or decreased breath sounds over diseased area.
8. Evaluate level of anxiety and impact on bronchospasm.
9. Assess for presence of sputum-producing cough.
10. Assess for hyperresonance and barrel chest development.
11. Assess nailbed and mucous membranes for cyanosis.
12. Evaluate posturing and use of accessory muscles.
13. Evaluate for restlessness, tachycardia, confusion, and hypotension.
14. ABGs may show elevated $PaCO_2$ and decreased PaO_2.

E. Nursing diagnoses
1. Impaired Gas Exchange
2. Activity Intolerance
3. Ineffective Breathing Patterns
4. Ineffective Airway Clearance
5. Anxiety
6. Fatigue

F. Planning and implementation

    1. Assess respiratory status including rate, rhythm, depth, breath sounds, work of breathing, use of accessory muscles, ABGs, and pulse oximetry.

    2. Maintain humidification and oxygen therapies.

    3. **Assess for hypoxemia. Symptoms include tachycardia, tachypnea, restlessness, diaphoresis, headache, lethargy, confusion, and pallor.**

    4. Anticipate and prepare for possible intubation.

    5. Assess anxiety level and intervene appropriately.

    6. Explain all care activities and keep explanations simple.

    7. Provide adequate rest for patient by grouping activities and encourage conservation of energy.

    8. Administer analgesics/antianxiety agents and respiratory treatments as necessary.

    9. Refer to social service or chaplaincy as needed.

    10. Teach diaphragmatic and "pursed-lip" breathing to prolong expiration, reducing air-trapping and resistance.

    11. Teach measures to decrease viscosity of secretions, eg, fluid intake to 2000 L/d.

    12. Explain activities and factors that increase oxygen demand, eg, smoking and stress.

    13. Avoid extremes in temperature and excessive weight.

    14. Assess for problems associated with eating such as breathing competing with eating.

    15. Administer a diet that is high in lipid/proteins and low in carbohydrates to reduce CO_2 build-up during metabolism.

    16. Avoid milk, chocolates, and other foods that increase viscosity of secretions.

    17. Avoid caffeine and alcohol.

    18. Teach chest physiotherapy (CPT) techniques.

    19. Avoid sedation if possible.

    20. Elevate head of bed for comfort.

    21. Be aware of potential complications:

        a. Respiratory failure

        b. Oxygen toxicity

G. Evaluation

    1. Client will demonstrate effective coughing and increased air exchange in lungs.

    2. Patient will demonstrate strategies to decrease tenacious secretions.

    3. Patient will demonstrate ways to conserve energy, and identify a realistic activity level to achieve or maintain.

    4. Patient will be able to identify adjustments needed in order to maintain self care.

    5. Patient will be able to state how to prevent further pulmonary deterioration.

    6. Patient will be able to state signs and symptoms to report.

    7. Patient will be able to identify community resources.

    8. Patient will experience reduced anxiety/fear as evidenced by calm and trusting appearance, and verbalize fears and concerns.

9.   Patient will maintain effective airway clearance.
10.   Patient will verbalize basic understanding of pathophysiology of disease, necessary life-style adjustments, methods to decrease incidence of attack, and correct use of medications.

H.   Home health considerations

1.   **Teach importance of not smoking and of avoiding dust-producing items and substances (feathers, animal dander, cleaning equipment) and powders and aerosols that may cause bronchospasm.**
2.   Teach food and eating modifications.
3.   Provide information about care, cleaning, and maintenance of inhalation or oxygen equipment being used.
4.   Provide information such as regarding pollution indexes, secondary infection exposure, and community support groups.

V.   Acute respiratory failure

A.   Description: life-threatening event that occurs when cardiopulmonary system is unable to maintain adequate oxygenation and CO_2 elimination.

B.   Etiology and incidence

1.   Obstructive disease (emphysema, chronic bronchitis, asthma)
2.   Restrictive disease (atelectasis, ARDS, pneumonia)
3.   Multiple rib fractures, postoperative abdominal/chest surgery, central nervous system (CNS) depression
4.   V/Q abnormalities (PE)

C.   Pathophysiology

1.   A possible cause is oxygenation failure.
2.   Lungs are unable to oxygenate arterial blood and do not move air sufficiently, owing to alveolar congestion.
3.   **This decreased lung function results in decreased compliance, as occurs with left ventricular failure, fluid overload, ARDS, and inhalation injury.**
4.   Another possible cause is ventilation and oxygen failure; this occurs in abnormal lungs with decreased alveolar oxygenation and frequently leads to hypoxemia.
5.   **COPD is the number one cause of respiratory failure.**
6.   Ventilatory system failure occurs when CNS dysfunction results in decreased cerebral respiratory drive leading to alveolar hypoventilation, such as in medication reactions, drug overdose, and increased intracranial pressure.

D.   Assessment findings

1.   The first signs of respiratory compromise may include headache, agitation, and confusion.
2.   This may be followed by tachycardia, hypertension, vasoconstriction, and palpitations.
3.   Other symptoms include dysrhythmias, chest pain, and hypotension.
4.   Tachypnea and dyspnea also are commonly noted.

5. **Crackles are rarely heard in acute respiratory failure because alveoli are closing and not reopening.**

6. Volume compromise is manifested by decreased urine output; edema; cool, clammy skin; and diminished capillary refill.

7. GI symptoms include hypoactive/absent bowel sounds, abdominal distention, nausea, and vomiting.

8. Diagnostic findings include:
   a. ABGs: early respiratory alkalosis leading to hypoxemia, resulting in acidosis
   b. CXR and pulmonary function tests (PFTs)

E. **Nursing diagnoses**
   1. Impaired Gas Exchange
   2. Ineffective Breathing Patterns
   3. Ineffective Airway Clearance
   4. Pain
   5. Ineffective Individual/Family Coping
   6. Fear
   7. Alteration in Communication
   8. Inability to Sustain Spontaneous Ventilation
   9. Dysfunctional Ventilatory Weaning Response

F. **Planning and implementation**
   1. Assess respiratory status: rate, rhythm, depth, breath sounds, work of breathing, use of accessory muscles, ABGs, and pulse oximetry.
   2. Maintain oxygenation and ventilation and effective airway clearance.
   3. Suction clients who are unable to clear secretions independently.
   4. Check for adventitious sounds.
   5. Monitor hemodynamics, tachycardia, and dysrhythmias.
   6. Monitor for respiratory changes, intercostal retractions, and increased use of accessory muscles.
   7. Assess for cough, evidence of hypoxia, dyspnea, and tachypnea.

   8. **Cyanosis is a late sign because 5 g of Hgb must desaturate for cyanosis to occur (if Hgb is under 5, there will be no cyanosis).**

   9. Provide pain relief, comfort, adequate rest, and emotional support.
   10. Maintain adequate hemodynamic and fluid status and provide nutritional support.
   11. Promote bowel management.
   12. Administer analgesics/antianxiety agents as necessary.
   13. Be aware of potential complications:
       a. Oxygen toxicity
       b. Failure to wean
       c. Recurrent episodes of respiratory failure

G. **Evaluation**
   1. Patient experiences reduced anxiety/fear as evidenced by calm and trusting appearance, and verbalized fears and concerns.
   2. Patient effectively communicates needs and concerns.
   3. Patient verbalizes basic understanding of pathophysiology of disease, necessary life-style adjustments, methods to decrease incidence of attack, and correct use of medications.

4.   Ventilatory demand is decreased as evidenced by no increased use of accessory muscles and ABGs within normal limits for client.

5.   Airway is clear of secretions and breath sounds are clear.

VI.   Adult respiratory distress syndrome (ARDS) (see Chapter 13)

VII.   Pulmonary embolism

A.   Description: obstruction in pulmonary vascular bed caused by thrombus/thrombi; sometimes defined as obstruction of more than 50% of the major pulmonary arteries.

B.   Etiology and incidence

1.   **One of the most common causes of mortality in critically ill persons, due to stasis of blood flow.**

2.   Risk factors include postoperative status, use of oral contraceptives, immobility, trauma to vessels, obesity, diabetes mellitus, infection, venous stasis, postpartum, circulatory disorders, and orthopedic trauma.

3.   Most result from a deep vein thrombosis (DVT) that dislodges and follows venous circulation to heart and into pulmonary circulation

4.   **Pulmonary embolism is characterized by Virchow's triad: venous stasis, hypercoagulability, and vascular wall damage.**

5.   Sites of embolization include calf, femoral, popliteal, and iliac veins.

C.   Pathophysiology

1.   Gas exchange is absent. Alveoli receive no perfusion, although ventilation is maintained.

2.   Hypoxia leads to decreased surfactant and alveolar collapse.

3.   Intrapulmonary shunting ("silent units") occurs.

4.   Resolution occurs through absorption and fibrosis.

5.   **Patients who have had orthopedic or major abdominal surgery are at risk, as is anyone on bed rest or suffering from cellulitis, severe peripheral edema, sepsis, or cancer.**

D.   Assessment findings

1.   Respiratory symptoms include:

   a.   Dyspnea, tachypnea, wheezing to diminished breath sounds to crackles and wheezes

   b.   Cough/hemoptysis

   c.   Chest pain that intensifies with inspiration and is non-radiating

2.   Other symptoms include:

   a.   Tachycardia

   b.   Apprehension/restlessness/anxiety

   c.   Friction rub

3.   Diagnostic tests include:

   a.   Elevated cardiac enzymes

   b.   Chest x-ray may reveal a pleural effusion

   c.   Ventilation/perfusion scan: perfusion defect with normal ventilation indicates high probability for PE

   d.   Pulmonary angiography: invasive; reserved for those for whom surgery seems imminent

E. **Nursing diagnoses**
1. Impaired gas exchange
2. Alteration in fluid volume
3. Ineffective breathing patterns
4. Ineffective airway clearance
5. Alteration in comfort
6. Fear/anxiety/powerlessness

F. **Planning and implementation**
1. Successful treatment depends on rapid diagnosis and initiation of anticoagulant/other therapies.
2. Assess respiratory rate, rhythm, depth, breath sounds, and use of accessory muscles.
3. Assess ABGs and pulse oximetry.
4. Elevate head of bed.
5. Prepare for intubation PRN.
6. Maintain O_2 delivery systems, humidification and oxygen therapies.

 7. **Assess for hypoxemia: tachycardia, tachypnea, restlessness, diaphoresis, headache, lethargy, confusion, and pallor.**
8. Administer anticoagulant therapy.
9. Once anticoagulant therapy has been initiated, perform bleeding assessment:
   a. Monitor for bruises, epistaxis, gingival bleeding, hematuria, severe headaches, tarry stools; petechiae, hematoma, bleeding from catheter insertion sites, hematuria, GI bleeding, and decreased Hgb/Hct
   b. Reduce hematomas at injection sites: use small-gauge needle; do not massage site; rotate sites; use subcutaneous route; apply steady pressure for 1–2 minutes
   c. Test stools for occult blood
   d. Assess for high-risk bleeding conditions (hepatic disease, renal disease, hypertension)

    e. **If actual bleeding occurs, stop infusion, recheck PTT, and administer protamine sulfate, which is the antidote for heparin overdose.**

    f. **Monitor laboratory studies to ensure dosage and delivery of anticoagulation (therapeutic anticoagulant blood levels should be 1 1/2–2 times the normal control value)**
   g. Foods high in vitamin K: see Display 6-2
10. Administer appropriate medications:
   a. Heparin: administered IV at a high dose for 7–10 days

    b. **Heparin has no direct effect on existing emboli; it prevents additional fibrin deposits and thrombus extension.**
   c. Low molecular weight heparin (LMWH)
   d. Hirudin: obtained from bats
   e. Oral (maintenance) warfarin: action takes 3–5 days, so must wean off heparin slowly until therapeutic effects attained
   f. Lovenox: synthetic heparin

DISPLAY 6-2.
Foods High in Vitamin K

collard greens	asparagus
broccoli	watercress
cauliflower	beef liver
turnip greens	green tea
cabbage	coffee
lettuce	high-fat foods

     g.   **Vitamin K is the antidote for warfarin (Coumadin) overdose**

     h.   Thrombolytic agents: t-PA, streptokinase, urokinase (Display 6-3)

11.   Provide reassurance to decrease anxiety from air hunger.

12.   Administer analgesics/antianxiety agents as necessary.

13.   Recommend bedrest to decrease oxygen demand and lessen risk of dislodging additional emboli.

14.   Use antiembolic stockings/compression boots.

15.   Initiate isometric and active range-of-motion (ROM) exercises.

16.   Advise patient to:
     a.   avoid aspirin/salicylates
     b.   do leg exercises to minimize recurrence
     c.   use a soft toothbrush

17.   Be aware of potential complications:
     a.   pulmonary artery occlusion
     b.   dislodgment of additional emboli
     c.   may need vena cava filter or embolectomy

G.   **Evaluation**

1.   Breathing pattern is maintained as evidenced by regular rate, depth, and rhythm of respirations and normal skin color.

2.   Patient maintains optimal gas exchange as evidenced by normal ABG and return to pre-illness neurologic state.

DISPLAY 6-3.
Contraindications to Thrombolytic Therapy

Active internal bleeding history of intracranial neoplasm
Hemorrhagic stroke
Arteriovenous malformation
Intracranial or severe uncontrolled hypertension
Intraspinal trauma
Aneurysm in past 2 months

3. Patient achieves adequate cardiac output: strong peripheral pulses; normal vital signs; and warm, dry skin.

4. Patient experiences reduced anxiety/fear as evidenced by verbalized fears and concerns.

5. Risk of bleeding is decreased via continuous assessment and early interventions.

6. Patient understands importance of medications, signs of excessive anticoagulation, and means to decrease risk of bleeding and recurrence of emboli.

VIII. Lung cancer

A. **Description: most common lethal cancer in the U.S.**

1. Squamous cell lung cancers account for about 45% of cases, adenocarcinoma for about 25%, small cell undifferentiated for about 25%. Large cell undifferentiated is least common type of cancer.

2. Diagnosis and staging are crucial for determination of appropriate treatment.

3. Most lung tumors are malignant and have a continuous, progressive course with an ultimately poor prognosis.

4. Small cell anaplastic carcinoma (oat cell) is most sensitive to chemotherapy and radiation therapy.

5. Non-small cell carcinoma (squamous cell) tends to arise in the central areas of the lung, making diagnosis more difficult.

6. Adenocarcinoma is highly metastatic.

B. **Etiology and incidence**

1. **Smoking prevention remains the key to reducing deaths and is a major focus for nursing intervention; latency period between initiation of smoking and development of lung cancer is about 15–20 years.**

2. Air pollution has a questionable correlation.

3. Other risk factors include industrial hazards such as mustard gas, radon, asbestos, radiation, hydrocarbons (present in crude petroleum, tars, coal, combustion products of most organic materials), certain metals (nickel, chromium, iron ore), halo ethers, and wood dust.

C. **Pathophysiology**

1. Appearance is one of three types:
    a. Hilar, infiltrating form: causes large tumor that compresses bronchi
    b. Peripheral or nodular form: may appear as a single tumor or multiple nodular masses through the lung
    c. Diffuse type: may be difficult to diagnose due to radiologic resemblance to pneumonia

2. Common cancers include:

    a. **Squamous cell carcinoma, the most common type, causing 45%–60% of lung malignancies.**

      ▶ Has a very high correlation with heavy cigarette smoking.
      ▶ Has the best survival rates, perhaps due to earlier diagnosis and because of slower growth and metastatic rates.

  b. Small-cell (oat cell) carcinoma produces large, obstructive growths in the main bronchi that often secrete substances normally found the body, including adrenocorticotropic hormone (ACTH) and antidiuretic hormone (ADH).

   ▶ ACTH secretion results in Cushing's syndrome, which may lead to obesity, osteoporosis, hypokalemia, and alkalosis.

   ▶ ADH secretion leads to water retention, hyponatremia, renal sodium loss, anorexia, nausea, and lethargy.

   ▶ Surgery is the treatment of choice; pneumonectomy for early stages, although some wedge or segmental resections may be done, but at least lobectomy with regional lymph node dissection.

  c. Large-cell undifferentiated (giant-cell) carcinoma is large and anaplastic, often located in lung periphery.

  d. Adenocarcinoma is one of the few lung cancers without a known relationship to smoking. Occurs in peripheral lung areas and is associated with rapid growth rate with early metastasis to bloodstream.

 3. **The majority of persons with lung carcinoma initially present with metastasis at the time of diagnosis. The spread commonly occurs to other lung areas, mediastinum, lymph nodes, liver, bone, brain, and adrenal glands.**

D. **Assessment findings**

 1. Most common symptoms of the primary tumor are cough and expectoration of bloody sputum, which may be severe.

 2. Lymphadenopathy may compress the superior vena cava, resulting in obstruction and rapid deterioration in clinical status.

 3. Chest pain, dyspnea, and hoarseness may be present.

 4. X-ray evidence on routine film is often the first sign.

 5. Sputum cytology and bronchoscopy are used to confirm diagnosis.

 6. Diagnostic tests include chest x-ray, bronchoscopy, needle aspiration/biopsy, mediastinoscopy, PFTs, CT, MRI, bone marrow aspiration, and biopsy.

E. **Nursing diagnoses**

 1. Impaired Gas Exchange

 2. Pain

 3. Ineffective Breathing Patterns

 4. Ineffective Airway Clearance

 5. Altered Nutrition: Less than Body Requirements

 6. Anxiety

 7. Ineffective Individual/Family Coping

 8. Fear/Powerlessness

F. **Planning and implementation**

 1. **Assess respiratory status: rate, rhythm, depth, breath sounds, work of breathing, use of accessory muscles, ABGs, and pulse oximetry.**

2. **Assess for hypoxemia as manifested by tachycardia, tachypnea, restlessness, diaphoresis, headache, lethargy, confusion, and pallor.**

3. Maintain humidification and oxygen therapies; anticipate and prepare for possible intubation.

4. Monitor for dysrhythmias.

5. Assess and encourage progression through grief stages and encourage verbalization of feelings.

6. Administer the following medications:
   a. analgesics/antianxiety agents as necessary
   b. chemotherapy: single agents, combination therapy

7. Be aware of potential complications:
   a. sepsis
   b. hemorrhage
   c. cardiac dysrhythmias, congestive heart failure, fluid overload
   d. airway obstruction, dyspnea, hypoxemia, respiratory failure
   e. pneumothorax, pulmonary embolism, pneumonia
   f. pleural effusions

G. Evaluation

1. The patient will maintain effective airway clearance.

2. The patient will effectively communicate needs and concerns.

3. The patient will progress through grieving stages toward acceptance of altered body image.

4. The patient will be able to discuss stop-smoking strategies (nicotine patch, nicotine gum, behavior modification, support groups).

5. The patient will have an understanding of cancer, treatments, risk for metastasis, and emergency situations.

6. The patient will verbalize relief of or ability to tolerate discomfort.

IX. Laryngeal cancer

A. **Description: accounts for only 2%–3% of all malignancies, but this disease is especially challenging, due to the cosmetic and functional changes that often occur as a result of treatment.**

 1. **At times the operation may render client unable to speak, breathe through the nose or mouth, or eat normally.**

2. There is significant deformity and a need for more than one operation to restore appearance.

B. Etiology and incidence

1. Cigarette smoking is the major cause.

2. Increased risk in clients who smoke and abuse alcohol.

C. Pathophysiology

1. Most often this is a squamous cell carcinoma.

2. It commonly occurs on the glottis (true vocal cords), the supraglottic structures (above the vocal cords), or the subglottic structures (below the vocal cords).

3. Laryngeal cancer is classified and treated by anatomic site.
   a. Supraglottic tumors occur on the posterior surface of epiglottis to the vocal cords, including the false vocal cords.
   b. Glottic tumors are tumors of the true vocal cords.

DISPLAY 6-4.
Clinical Warning Signs of Cancer

Change in voice quality
Lump anywhere in neck or body
Persistent cough, sore throat, or earache
Hemoptysis
Sores within the throat that do not heal
Difficulty swallowing or breathing

     c.   Subglottic tumors occur on the undersurface of the true vocal cords

D.   **Assessment findings**
    1.   Clinical warning signs (Display 6-4)
    2.   Site-specific symptoms include:
       a.   Glottis tumors prevent glottis from closing during speech, resulting in hoarseness or a voice change.
       b.   Supraglottic tumors cause pain in the throat, particularly during swallowing, a sensation of a "something in the throat," neck masses, and pain radiating to the ear due to glossopharyngeal and vagus nerve effects. It may be treated with radiation therapy or partial laryngectomy with or without lymph node dissection.
       c.   Subglottic tumors have no early symptoms. Airway obstruction is usually the presenting symptom. Because of this, metastasis is common. Treatment requires total laryngectomy with or without radical neck dissection. The surgical site may require reconstruction with pectoralis myocutaneous flaps.
    3.   Diagnostic testing may include:
       a.   Direct or indirect laryngoscopy
       b.   CXR
       c.   Barium swallow or esophagram is performed once the tumor is located and biopsy done.
       d.   Staging is by use of the TNM classification (tumor, nodes, metastasis):

         ▶ Measure size of the primary tumor.
         ▶ Determine presence of enlarged lymphatic nodes.
         ▶ Determine the presence of distant metastasis.

E.   **Nursing diagnoses**
    1.   Impaired Gas Exchange
    2.   Ineffective Airway Clearance
    3.   Ineffective Breathing Patterns
    4.   Pain
    5.   Altered Nutrition: Less than Body Requirements

6. Ineffective Individual/Family Coping
7. Impaired Verbal Communication
8. Fear/Anxiety/Powerlessness
9. Risk for Aspiration
10. Inability to Sustain Spontaneous Ventilation
11. Risk for Infection (Respiratory)

F. Planning and implementation

1. Ensure adequate pain relief.
2. Evaluate nutritional status. Most patients have malnutrition from not being able to eat, as well as from the effects of the cancer, so nutritional needs may be varied.
3. Administer medications as prescribed.

4. **Because the airway is permanently altered after surgery it is essential to perform a comprehensive respiratory assessment to identify possible preexisting pulmonary disorders that could affect breathing (Table 6-5).**
5. Ensure that wound care is provided.
6. Ensure that oral hygiene needs are met.
7. Assist patient with accepting altered body image. Counseling may be necessary.
8. Support clients who still actively drink and smoke through the withdrawal process.
9. Provide alternative methods of communication and family support networks such as having the patient communicate on a pad or point to statement.
   a. Artificial larynx may be used as early as 3–4 days postoperatively. The speech quality is monotonous and artificial.

TABLE 6-5.
Care of the Laryngectomy Patient

SURGICAL PROCEDURE	PURPOSE/PROCEDURE	NURSING IMPLICATIONS
Partial Laryngectomy	Cancer of one true vocal cord; part of cord is removed	Mild difficulty swallowed, altered but adequate voice
Supraglottic	Removal of the superior part of larynx; may extend upward to remove part of base of tongue. Lymph node dissection also possible. Major postoperative problem is risk of aspiration because epiglottis is removed.	True vocal cords are preserved so voice quality is excellent. Tracheostomy after surgery; can usually be removed when edema subsides. Patient must be taught how to swallow to avoid aspiration
Total Laryngectomy	When removed, permanent opening made into trachea for breathing and voice is lost. Because trachea and pharynx are permanently separated, no risk of aspiration unless tracheoesophageal fistula forms.	Loss of sense of smell due to no air entering nose. Care is same as for partial laryngectomy except for feeding and permanent stoma care.

b.   **Esophageal speech: technique that requires the client to swallow and hold air in the upper esophagus. By controlling the air flow, the client can pronounce as many as 6–10 words before stopping to reswallow air. Voice quality is deep but loud and clear when the technique is mastered.**

10.   Be aware of potential complications:

   a.   **Airway obstruction due to edema in the surgical site, bleeding into the airway, or loss of airway from a plugged tracheostomy tube.**

b.   Hemorrhage as the result of an inadequate tracheostomy during surgery. Some blood-tinged sputum is normally expected in tracheal secretions in the first 48 hours. Other symptoms include hematoma, unilateral swelling, tachycardia, hypotension, and changes in respiratory patterns.

G.   Evaluation

1.   The patient maintains effective airway clearance.
2.   Patient effectively communicates needs and concerns.
3.   Patient progresses through grieving stages toward acceptance of altered body image.
4.   Patient verbalizes basic understanding of pathophysiology of disease, necessary life-style adjustments, methods to decrease incidence of attack, and correct use of medications.
5.   Patient participates in stop-smoking strategies.
6.   Patient experiences reduced anxiety/fear as evidenced by calm and trusting appearance, and verbalized fears and concerns.

H.   Home health considerations

1.   Tracheo-esophageal (T-E) puncture: surgical technique used to restore speech. A small one-way valve is inserted (voice button) that can be occluded by a person, which shunts air into the esophagus, producing speech.
2.   Requires maintenance, so only highly motivated and self-care clients are eligible (also need good manual dexterity).
3.   Speech therapy should be instituted after discharge.
4.   Support groups include Lost Cord Club, International Association of Laryngectomees. Family should be encouraged to give client enough time to form words and not to speak for the person.

X.   Lobectomy

A.   Description: surgical resection of one or more lung lobes to remove a tumor or other mass while damaging as little of the surrounding lung tissue as possible.

B.   Types of pulmonary resection

1.   Wedge resection: removal of small, localized area of tissue near lung surface to maintain stable pulmonary structure and function after healing.
2.   Segmental resection: removal of one or more lung segments (bronchiole and its alveoli). The remaining lung tissue expands to fill space.

3. Lobectomy: removal of entire lung lobe, resulting in some compensatory emphysema as remaining lung tissue overexpands to fill the area previously occupied by the removed lobe.

4. Pneumonectomy: removal of entire lung, with phrenic nerve severed on the affected side to reduce the size of the empty cavity postoperatively by paralyzing the diaphragm in an elevated position. Closed chest drainage usually not used, due to postoperative serous fluid accumulation that prevents extreme mediastinal shift of heart and remaining lung.

C. Assessment

1. Preoperatively, prepare patient to decrease anxiety/guilt about need for surgery.
2. Assess baseline respiratory parameters and monitor appropriately.

D. Nursing diagnoses

1. Impaired Gas Exchange
2. Ineffective Breathing Pattern
3. Ineffective Airway Clearance
4. Pain
5. Ineffective Individual/Family Coping
6. Fear/Anxiety/Powerlessness

E. Planning and implementation

1. **Assess respiratory status and monitor for development of hypoxemia.**
2. Maintain humidification and oxygen therapies.
3. Ensure adequate nutrition.

4. **Promote optimal oxygenation by positioning the patient with "good lung DOWN" in unilateral disease.**
5. Maintain pulmonary toilet.
6. Ensure adequate fluid balance and provide wound care.
7. Administer analgesics/antianxiety agents as necessary.

F. Evaluation

1. The patient is able to maintain effective airway clearance.
2. The patient is able to effectively communicate needs and concerns.
3. The patient progresses through grieving stages toward acceptance of altered body image.
4. The patient experiences reduced anxiety/fear as evidenced by calm and trusting appearance, and verbalized fears and concerns.

XI. Radical neck surgery

A. Description: surgical removal of specific cervical lymph node groups and anatomic structures in the treatment of head and neck cancer.

B. Indications

1. Metastasis to cervical lymph nodes common with tumors of upper respiratory/GI tracts, which necessitates removal of lymph systems, sternocleidomastoid muscle, spinal accessory nerve, jugular vein, and submandibular area.
2. Modified radical neck dissection leaves various structures in the neck to decrease deformity.

C. Assessment

1. Most clients report minimal postoperative pain because of sensory nerve fiber resection.

2. En bloc dissection results in shoulder dysfunction due to forward rotation and dropping of the shoulder.
3. Spinal accessory nerve resection will result in loss of upper trapezius muscle innervation.

D.   Nursing diagnoses
1. Ineffective Airway Clearance
2. Impaired Verbal Communication
3. Self Esteem Disturbance
4. Impaired Physical Mobility
5. Anxiety

E.   Planning and implementation

1. **Provide ROM to shoulder. To increase ROM and muscle strength and to prevent frozen shoulder and restore full movement, ROM exercises should be performed.**
2. Monitor pectoralis myocutaneous flap and surrounding tissue. Maximum redness should occur within the first 12 hours postoperatively. Area should be pink and warm, with minimal edema, and recover color slowly after blanching.
3. Monitor drainage tubes for air, odor, appearance of drainage.
4. Maintain alignment of body, keeping head of bed elevated 30–45 degrees. Use pillows/sandbags and do not allow patient to lay on operative side.
5. Monitor for external flap pressure from IV lines, drainage or feeding tubes, tracheostomy/laryngectomy ties.

6. **Assess carotid artery for signs of rupture: change in color (redness, pallor, blackness), bleeding/pulsations at site.**
7. Assess for hypoxemia.
8. Explain all care activities and keep explanations simple.
9. Provide adequate rest by organizing care and decreasing sensory stimulation.
10. Administer analgesics/antianxiety agents as necessary.
11. Refer to other support systems: social service, chaplaincy.
12. Assess myocutaneous flap for arterial inflow and venous outflow. Assess temperature, color, and blanching.
13. Ensure that appropriate therapies, eg, speech, respiratory, physical, and social work are available.
14. Be aware of potential complications: facial and CNS edema, flap rejection, fistula formation hemorrhage, and carotid artery rupture.

F.   Evaluation
1. Patient experiences reduced anxiety/fear as evidenced by calm and trusting appearance, and verbalized fears and concerns.
2. Patient maintains effective airway clearance.
3. Patient effectively communicates needs and concerns.
4. Patient and family progress through grieving stages toward acceptance of altered body image.
5. Patient and family are able to demonstrate tracheostomy care using clean technique.

XII. **Pneumonia**

A. Description: pneumonia is an inflammation of the lung parenchyma, usually associated with the filling of the alveoli with fluid.

B. Etiology and incidence: depends on the etiologic agent

    1. Causes include various infectious agents, chemical irritants, radiation therapy, and hypersensitivity.

    2. Types of pneumonias are infectious, lobar, bronchial, aspiration, chemical, and traumatic.

C. Pathophysiology

    1. Bacterial pneumonia is marked by an intra-alveolar exudate with consolidation.

    2. Lobar pneumonia causes consolidation of the entire lobe.

    3. Bronchopneumonia causes patchy distribution of infectious areas around and involving the bronchi, which show patchy segmental infiltration in one or more dependent lobes.

    4. Mycoplasmal and viral pneumonias produce interstitial inflammation with accumulation of an infiltrate in the alveolar walls. There is no consolidation or exudate.

    5. Fungal and mycobacterial pneumonia are marked by patchy distribution of granulomas that may undergo necrosis with the development of cavities.

    6. Aspiration pneumonia presents a still different physiologic response, which is based on the pH of the aspirated substance. If the pH is below 2.5, atelectasis occurs, followed by pulmonary edema, hemorrhage, and type II cell necrosis. The alveolar capillary membrane may be damaged, leading to exudation and, in severe cases, adult respiratory distress syndrome (ARDS).

D. Assessment findings

    1. Dullness on percussion of chest on the side with consolidation may be heard.

    2. Bronchial breath sounds may be auscultated over consolidated lung fields, diminished over involved areas, with crackles and pleural friction rub.

    3. Sudden onset of fever over 100°F.

    4. Chills and malaise (especially with bacterial pneumonia).

    5. Chest pain and dyspnea.

    6. Productive cough with sputum that is viscous and tenacious. Color of sputum ranges from rusty to yellow.

    7. Sputum cultures may be positive for causative microorganism.

E. Nursing diagnoses

    1. Impaired Gas Exchange

    2. Ineffective Airway Clearance

    3. Ineffective Breathing Pattern

    4. Fluid Volume Balance

    5. Pain

    6. Knowledge Deficit

    7. Altered Nutrition: Less than Body Requirements

    8. Fear/Anxiety/Powerlessness

F.   Planning and implementation

1.   **Encourage adequate fluid intake with IV fluid administration and oral hydration as appropriate.**
2.   Humidify inspired air and encourage effective coughing.
3.   Analyze and evaluate ABG values to determine need for oxygen and client response to oxygen therapy.
4.   Administer treatments or medications to relieve discomfort.
5.   Enhance patient ability to rest between specific activities.
6.   Administer medications as prescribed:
   a.   Antibiotic therapy for specific bacterial pneumonia
   b.   Antipyretics
   c.   Expectorants/cough syrup
   d.   Inhalers
   e.   Oxygen

7.   **Assess respiratory status: rate, rhythm, depth, breath sounds, work of breathing, use of accessory muscles, ABGs, pulse oximetry.**
8.   Assist with coughing, deep breathing, and splinting.
9.   Monitor sputum gram stain/culture/sensitivity.
10. Provide chest PT as needed.
11. Assess for hypoxemia as evidenced by tachycardia, tachypnea, restlessness, diaphoresis, headache, lethargy, confusion, and pallor.
12. Monitor for dysrhythmias.
13. Be aware of potential complications caused by gram-negative bacteria:
   a.   Pleurisy: fever, pleural friction rub, shallow, rapid breathing, dullness to percussion, hemoptysis with coughing
   b.   Atelectasis: pleuritic pain, tachypnea, dyspnea, absence of breath sounds over affected area, anxiety, cyanosis, flat percussion tone over area, mediastinal shift toward affected area
   c.   Empyema: persistent fever despite antibiotics, foul-smelling sputum, localized chest pain, dullness to percussion, decreased breath sounds at lung bases

G.   Evaluation

1.   Patient maintains optimal gas exchange/airway and is free of secretions as evidenced by adequate air movement and clear breath sounds after coughing/suctioning.
2.   Patient is normothermic, has a normal WBC, and negative sputum culture on repeat culture.
3.   Patient maintains effective airway clearance.
4.   Patient verbalizes basic understanding of pathophysiology of disease and correct use of medications.

H.   Home health considerations: Client and family have sufficient discharge information to maintain wellness.

1.   Client continues deep-breathing exercises at home with effective coughing for productive cough.
2.   Client knows schedule of medications and action and side effects of all medications.
3.   Client maintains resistance to infection: nutrition, rest, exercise.
4.   Client avoids contact with those with upper respiratory infections.

     5.   Client takes pneumococcal vaccine as indicated (the elderly; those with chronic disease, COPD, sickle cell anemia, splenectomy, pneumonectomy, immunosuppression; health care workers).

XIII.   **Pulmonary tuberculosis (TB)**

    A.   **Description: contagious lung disease caused by the tubercle bacillus (*Mycobacterium tuberculosis*).**

    B.   **Etiology and incidence**

        1.   The bacillus is an acid-fast rod spread by airborne droplets when an infected person coughs, sneezes, or otherwise transmits droplets.

        2.   Pulmonary TB can develop into a clinical disease characterized by inflammatory infiltrations, formation of tubercles, caseation necrosis, fibrosis, abscesses, and calcification.

        3.   Pulmonary TB has increased in incidence since 1985, owing to AIDS, immigration, homelessness, IVDA, overcrowding, immunosuppression, increases in multi-drug resistant TB (MDR-TB) outbreaks, and decreased funding for research.

    C.   **Pathophysiology**

        1.   Characteristics of *Mycobacterium tuberculosis*:

            a.   Resembles a fungus

            b.   Acid-fast bacillus (AFB)

            c.   Slow-growing and often dormant, which results in chronic disease

             d.   **Aerobic: requires oxygen to survive**

            e.   Destroyed by heat, sunshine, ultraviolet light, drying

             f.   **Not highly infectious unless recipient is immunocompromised**

            g.   Transmission is via air droplets

        2.   Lung is almost always the portal of entry.

        3.   Aerosol droplets dry out, leaving bacilli. Some stay in the air to be inhaled.

        4.   Bacilli are acquired by inhalation, but spread via lymph channels and bloodstream to other organs.

        5.   When tubercles are sealed off, bacilli become dormant but do not die.

        6.   Uninhibited growth period occurs, after which bacilli are ingested by phagocytes, forming small masses (tubercles) to "wall off" infection.

        7.   Phagocytes then process bacillus antigens, which are then presented to T-lymphocytes.

            a.   T-lymphocytes proliferate, tubercles are sealed off, and bacilli die. Tubercles become fibrosed and calcified.

             b.   **Bacilli survive. The tissues in tubercle center become necrotic and cheeselike (can also liquefy and spread elsewhere; called liquefaction).**

        8.   May enter latent/dormant period in persons producing effective immune responses, but disease activation can occur later in those with decreased resistance, concomitant diseases, and/or immunosuppression.

D.   Assessment findings

1.   History may reveal known exposure to TB or patient may belong to a high-risk group

2.   Constitutional symptoms include low-grade temperature, "night sweats," malaise, fatigue, weakness, weight loss, and anorexia.

3.   Pulmonary symptoms include cough, hemoptysis, pleuritic chest pain, shortness of breath, and possible crackles.

4.   Tuberculin skin test tests exposure to TB and *not* the presence of bacillus.

    a.   Procedure involves the injection of the material, which normally should cause a delayed hypersensitivity reaction.

    b.   Positive results occur because of the restimulation of previous antibodies to the bacillus.

    c.   Positive result is presence of induration. Induration is caused by cellular infiltration mediated by sensitized lymphocytes.

5.   Mantoux skin test involves intradermal injection with purified protein derivative (PPD) of TB bacillus. It is the most definitive test.

6.   Induration is determined by touch, not redness, and is indicated by hardness of tissue. Size of the induration is also significant.

7.   If positive, this indicates that the body has activated immune defenses against TB (48–72 hours; see Display 6-5).

8.   Tine test is less sensitive but good for broad screening:

    a.   pointed tines puncture the skin

    b.   results read at 48–72 hours

    c.   considered positive if papules form

9.   BCG (bacillus Calmette-Guerin) given in the past, generally outside the United States; is being given more frequently. Current Centers for Disease Control and Prevention (CDC) recommendations are against routine administration.

10.   Sputum testing is indicated for the diagnosis of active TB. It is the most reliable indicator.

    a.   Smear results can be obtained within 24 hours.

    b.   It takes 12–21 days for culture results.

    c.   Best to use 5–10 mL morning sputum specimen.

11.   Chest x-ray may help wih diagnosis as certain patterns are highly suspicious of TB.

DISPLAY 6-5.
Assessment of Mantoux Test

Size of induration
Under 5 mm negative
5–9 mm doubtful
Over 10 mm positive exposure only
Anergic results (no response) may be positive if immunosuppressed
If client is immunocompromised, 5 mm or greater is considered a positive response

E. **Nursing diagnoses**
1. Knowledge Deficit
2. Impaired Adjustment
3. Altered Protection
4. Social Isolation
5. Ineffective Airway Clearance
6. Sleep Pattern Disturbance
7. Ineffective Individual Coping

F. **Planning and implementation**

1. **Medications are number one factor, thus compliance is a major nursing focus.**
2. Administer antimycobacterial medications as ordered and appropriate.
3. Patients are always treated with multi-drug regimen to prevent resistance. The CDC recommends at least a four-drug regimen.
   a. "First-line" drugs include isoniazid (INH), rifampin, ethambutol, pyrazinamide, and streptomycin.
   b. Various "second-line" drugs include para-aminosalicylic acid, capriomycin, kanamycin, ethionamide, viomycin.
   c. Therapy begins with intense treatment to kill large numbers of bacilli, then maintenance treatment is implemented.
   d. Treatment procedure is long-term, taking 6 months to 2 years; average is 9 to 12 months. (See Table 6-6 for TB medications.)

4. **Noncompliance is a major problem.**
5. Six months of drug therapy is relatively inexpensive and can cure many clients, but one problem is that patients stop treatment once they feel better.
6. Partial treatment is worse than none because it promotes the cultivation of resistant strains.
7. The major side effect of antitubercular medications is hepatotoxicity.
8. After 2 weeks of intensive treatment, the TB bacillus will no longer be isolated in the sputum, so it is not considered communicable.

9. **Assessment of respiratory status includes evaluation of rate, rhythm, depth, breath sounds, work of breathing, use of accessory muscles, ABGs, and pulse oximetry.**
10. Ensure respiratory isolation as indicated and maintain good hygiene.
11. Administer analgesics/anti-anxiety agents as necessary.
12. Be aware of potential complications:
    a. resistant TB: resistance to two or more first-line antimycobacterial medications used to treat TB
    b. death

G. **Evaluation**
1. Patient experiences reduced anxiety/fear as evidenced by calm and trusting appearance, and verbalized fears and concerns.
2. Patient maintains effective airway clearance.
3. Patient effectively communicates needs and concerns.

TABLE 6-6.
Medications used in the Treatment of TB

MEDICATION	ACTION	SIDE EFFECTS/ ADVERSE REACTIONS	NURSING CONSIDERATIONS	MISCELLANEOUS
Isoniazid (INH)	Tuberculostatic and tuberculocidal	Peripheral neuritis; fever; rash; anemia; blood dyscrasias; arthritis; hepatitis; resistance	Metabolized by liver; cleared by kidneys; renal insufficiency does not usually affect drug accumulation *B6 supplements to prevent peripheral neuritis liver studies needed	Experimenting with slow-release forms; does not enter CSF
Rifampin	Bacteriocidal against TB, most gram-positive and some gram-negative organisms (interferes with RNA synthesis)	GI problems: nausea, vomiting, diarrhea resistance	Eliminated by bile excretion; turns urine orange-red; may discolor contact lenses; may be given with renal failure; ASA decreases absorption (give 8–12 hrs. apart); increases metabolism of liver-metabolized meds	Product of *Streptomyces*; present in body fluids (eg, CSF)
Pyrazinamide (PZI)	Bacteriocidal ONLY against *intracellular* organisms in an acid pH	Hepatotoxicity (must stop drug if this occurs) resistance	GI absorption; excreted by kidneys (caution with renal insufficiency)	Used during first 2 months of treatment
Ethambutol	Bacteriostatic	Blurred vision/loss of green perception; optic neuritis; resistance	Excreted by kidneys (caution with renal insufficiency); ototoxicity; nephrotoxicity	Must use for time prescribed to minimize chance of resistance
Streptomycin	Bacteriocidal in alkaline environment against extracellular organisms	8th cranial nerve damage (ototoxicity); nephrotoxicity; resistance	Renal excretion; increased chance of optic side effects with concurrent renal problems; give with food	Given parenterally due to no GI absorption; enters CSF only with meningeal irritation

    4.   Patient verbalizes basic understanding of pathophysiology of disease, necessary life-style adjustments, methods to decrease spread, and correct use of medications.

    5.   Patient maintains hygiene measures.

H. **Home health considerations**

    1.   General goal is to prevent transmission.

       a.   Respiratory isolation: mask must be worn at all times by either the client, health care team member, or anyone entering the client's room.

       b.   Hygiene practices such as mouth care and clean disposal of tissues are important.

    2.   Ensure client education regarding signs and symptoms, transmission, and treatment.

    3.   Education minimizes noncompliance. Noncompliance can result in a 20%–50% failure to cure.

XIV. **Carbon monoxide (CO) poisoning**

A. **Description: CO is a colorless, tasteless, odorless gas that is nonirritating to mucous membranes.**

B. **Etiology and incidence**

    1.   Common sources of CO are automobile exhaust fumes, burning charcoal, poorly ventilated wood or coal stoves, and malfunctioning furnaces.

    2.   CO also is present in all fires and may be a hazard to firefighters.

    3.   Natural gas does not contain CO, but it may be produced if the gas is burned without sufficient oxygen.

    4.   Methylene chloride is metabolized to CO.

    5.   **Toxicity accounts for over half of fatal inhalation injuries. It is the most common cause of death by poisoning in the United States.**

    6.   Many patients with major burns have inhalation injuries. Smoke inhalation is the leading cause of death among burn patients.

C. **Pathophysiology**

    1.   Hgb normally carries 98% of the available oxygen to the tissues.

    2.   When inhaled, CO readily diffuses across the alveolar membrane where it competes with oxygen for the same binding sites on the Hgb molecule.

    3.   CO has an affinity for Hgb that is up to 250 times greater than that of O_2.

    4.   Decreased oxygen delivered to the tissues reduces the ability of Hgb to transport oxygen.

    5.   CO combines with Hgb to form carboxyhemoglobin (COHgB), which causes a shift to the left in the oxygen dissociation curve.

    6.   Tissue hypoxia results from the decreased oxygen-carrying capacity of Hgb and not from change in partial pressure of oxygen, which remains normal.

D. **Assessment findings**

    1.   Severity depends on the percentage of CO inspired, length of exposure, ventilatory rate, and general health of the individual.

    2.   **Signs and symptoms are mainly related to cerebral hypoxia, although cherry red skin is commonly noted.**

3. Carboxyhemoglobin levels are normally under 5%; however, levels in smokers are often around 5%, and in urban dwellers may be as high as 10% (Display 6-6).

4. Metabolic acidosis may develop, due to impaired oxygen transport and delivery to the cells.

m 5. **In severe CO poisoning, serum lactate may be a more reliable indicator than carboxyhemoglobin with respect to the level of CO poisoning.**

6. Diagnosis is based on history of enclosed space injury. Enclosed space increases the likelihood of inhalation injury due to decreased available O_2 in enclosed spaces.

E. Nursing diagnoses
1. Impaired Gas Exchange
2. Ineffective Breathing Patterns
3. Ineffective Airway Clearance
4. Ineffective Individual/Family Coping
5. Fear/Anxiety/Powerlessness

F. Planning and implementation

m 1. **Prompt administration of 100% high flow oxygen is indicated. Treatment is based on the half-life of COHgB.**

2. Administer parenteral fluids at two-thirds to three-fourths normal maintenance for the patient's weight.

3. Grief counseling for family members of victims of house fires may be necessary.

4. For intentional exposures, mental health counseling should be arranged.

5. Assess respiratory status.

6. Maintain humidification and oxygen therapies.

m 7. **Assess for hypoxemia and anticipate and prepare for possible intubation.**

8. In some cases hyperbaric chamber therapy may be indicated.

9. Potential complications include neuropsychiatric problems such as parkinsonism, gait disturbances, hearing disturbances, disorientation, speech disturbances, and personality changes such as depression, moodiness, irritability, aggressiveness, impulsiveness, and signs of increased intracranial pressure. It may be necessary to hyperventilate with 100% FIO_2 via ETT to keep PCO_2 at 25–30 mm Hg.

DISPLAY 6-6.
Comparison of CO Levels and Expected Findings

10% hyperventilation (may be within normal limits in smokers)
15%–20% headache, disorientation
20–40% fatigue, dizziness, visual disturbances, chest pain
40%–60% ataxia, hallucinations, combativeness, coma
over 60% usually fatal

G. Evaluation
   1. Patient maintains effective airway clearance
   2. Patient and family verbalize basic understanding of pathophysiology of disease and treatment modalities.
   3. Adequate oxygenation is maintained.

XV. Steam inhalation injuries

A. Description: inhalation of air that is hot enough to prevent sufficient cooling by upper airways; results in damage to the mucosa of the respiratory tree.

B. Etiology and incidence: most often occurs in persons working around steam pipes. May also occur from microwave oven injuries.

C. Pathophysiology
   1. Inhaled hot air may immediately damage upper airway mucosa, but not necessarily lung tissue, because upper airways can cool air significantly before it reaches major airways.
   2. This causes capillary leak by changing microvascular permeability of protein.
   3. Due to the inflammatory response of the WBC, proteins move interstitially, followed by plasma, resulting in upper airway edema.
   4. Problems are increased, due to copious mucous production that develops in response to airway mucosa irritation.
   5. Heat injury causes laryngeal edema, laryngospasm, airway ulcers, and erythema, which are compounded by concurrent surface burn.
   6. **Edema is further increased due to massive fluid resuscitation and resulting protein loss, as well as by vasoactive substances that are released from damaged tissues.**
   7. This interferes with clearance of secretions.
   8. The length of time to heal a steam injury depends on the complications that develop. Within 4–5 days after injury, local tissue edema and superficial mucosal burns will have returned to pre-damaged status.

D. Assessment findings
   1. Extent of injury is determined by direct visualization via laryngoscopy.
   2. Symptoms are representative of airway obstruction and include stridor, tachypnea, and dyspnea.

E. Nursing diagnoses
   1. Impaired Gas Exchange
   2. Ineffective Breathing Patterns
   3. Ineffective Airway Clearance
   4. Ineffective Individual/Family Coping
   5. Fear/Anxiety/Powerlessness

F. Planning and implementation
   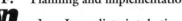 1. **Immediate intubation for laryngoscopic evidence of erythema, edema, and ulcers at vocal cord levels is indicated.**
   2. Less severe injuries may be treated with racemic epinephrine, humidified oxygen, and elevation of head of bed.
    3. **Assess respiratory status and maintain humidification and oxygen therapies.**

ffl   4.   **Assess for hypoxemia and prepare for intubation.**

G.   Evaluation

    1.   Patient will maintain adequate airway and optimal oxygenation.

    2.   Patient and family will show appropriate coping skills.

XVI.   **Smoke inhalation**

  A.   **Description: the most serious of the inhalation injuries and the most difficult to diagnose and treat**

  B.   **Etiology and incidence**

    1.   Most frequently occurs in conjunction with flame fire events.

    2.   More persons succumb to smoke inhalation than to an actual burn.

  C.   **Pathophysiology**

    1.   After inhalation of smoke, mucosal irritation causes increased fluid in the airways and possible surfactant inactivation, with resulting alveolar collapse.

    2.   Normal ciliary action is hampered, which additionally increases the likelihood of infection to occur 2–3 days after injury.

    3.   The denuding of tracheobronchial tree also creates pseudomembranes that occlude smaller airways.

  D.   **Assessment**

    1.   True severity may not be fully apparent until 24–48 hours post-injury.

    2.   Respiratory symptoms include tachypnea, bronchospasm, wheezing, dyspnea, crackles, and hoarseness.

ffl   3.   **Diagnostic testing involves fiberoptic bronchoscopy, which provides visualization of mucosa including presence of edema, inflammation, necrosis, ulceration, and level of injury. It cannot determine extent and severity of injury.**

  E.   **Nursing diagnoses**

    1.   Impaired Gas Exchange

    2.   Ineffective Breathing Patterns

    3.   Ineffective Airway Clearance

    4.   Ineffective Individual/Family Coping

    5.   Fear/Anxiety/Powerlessness

  F.   **Planning and implementation**

ffl   1.   **Monitor hemodynamic status, especially with high levels of PEEP due to effect of decreased venous return on CO.**

    2.   Provide supplemental humidified oxygen CPT and bronchodilators.

    3.   Be aware that intubation and mechanical ventilation with PEEP remains the most effective approach in managing smoke inhalation injury.

    4.   Obtain cultures at regular intervals.

    5.   Monitor ABGs and continuous SpO_2.

    6.   Maintain turning, positioning, and suctioning as needed.

ffl   7.   **Monitor ECG and SaO_2 because of potential for severe hypoxemia.**

    8.   Obtain CXR as ordered.

    9.   Use closed, in-line suctioning systems.

    10.   Use specialty bed as indicated.

G. Evaluation

    1. The patient experiences reduced anxiety/fear as evidenced by calm and trusting appearance and verbalized fears and concerns.

    2. The patient maintains effective airway clearance.

    3. The patient effectively communicates needs and concerns.

    4. The patient verbalizes basic understanding of pathophysiology of disease and treatment modalities.

XVII. Atelectasis

A. Description

    1. Collapse of lung tissue at any of its structural levels (segmental, basilar, lobar, microscopic).

    2. Patchy atelectasis is the term used for collapse throughout the lung.

B. Etiology and incidence

    1. Atelectasis is frequently a complication of impaired diaphragmatic movement following upper abdominal surgery, ascites, obesity, and failure to deep breathe postoperatively.

    2. Also seen with compression of lung tissue (tumors), effusions, pneumothorax, hemothorax, empyema, and chest wall disorders (kyphoscoliosis, flail chest).

    3. Risk factors include conditions that decrease the inspiratory effort of the client such as:

        a. CNS dysfunction: coma, neuromuscular disorders, oversedation

        b. localized airway obstruction: mucous plugging, foreign body aspiration, bronchiectasis

        c. insufficient pulmonary surfactant: ARDS, inhalation anesthesia, oxygen toxicity

        d. pulmonary damage: lung contusion, aspiration of gastric contents, smoke inhalation

        e. increased elastic recoil: interstitial fibrosis (silicosis, radiation pneumonitis)

C. Pathophysiology

    1. Airway obstruction (resorptive atelectasis) results when gas is obstructed from reaching alveoli.

    2. May be caused by mucous plug, foreign body, aspirated material, or tumors.

    3. The gas below the obstruction is absorbed into the circulation because O_2 tension in pulmonary arteries is lower than in the alveoli.

    4. Compression by space-occupying lesions of the chest decreases the number of ventilated alveoli.

    5. Ineffective ventilation is the main postoperative complication that is reversible by lung hyperinflation.

D. Assessment

    1. Usually atelectasis is first detected on CXR which shows patchy atelectasis and diaphragmatic elevation on the affected side.

    2. Symptoms include dyspnea, restlessness, crackles, and diminished or absent sounds.

    3. ABGs will show a decreased PaO_2 and $PaCO_2$.

    4. With persistent atelectasis, signs of pneumonia may be noted.

    5. In severe cases, a tracheal shift toward atelectatic side and decreased chest movement on the involved side will be seen.

E. Nursing diagnoses
1. Impaired Gas Exchange
2. Risk for Fluid Volume Deficit
3. Ineffective Breathing Patterns
4. Pain
5. Ineffective Individual/Family Coping
6. Fear/Anxiety/Powerlessness

F. Planning and implementation

 1. **The best treatment is prevention.**
2. Compression atelectasis is usually relieved once the precipitating cause is removed such as drainage of an effusion or removal of tumor.
3. Lung hyperinflation, with use of incentive spirometry, helps to open alveoli.
4. Coughing, ETT suctioning, vigorous chest PT, or therapeutic bronchoscopy are standards of care.
5. Early ambulation and frequent position changes in the postoperative patient can prevent atelectasis.
6. Humidification and adequate hydration to keep secretions loose and enhance expectoration is often indicated.
7. Assess respiratory status and for evidence of hypoxemia and intervene appropriately.

G. Evaluation
1. The patient is able to maintain effective airway clearance.
2. The patient is able to maintain adequate oxygenation and prevent progression to pneumonia.

XVIII. Near drowning

A. Description: survival for at least 24 hours after suffocation by submersion in a fluid medium.

B. Etiology and incidence
1. Between 4000–5000 persons drown in the U.S. each year, especially during the summer owing to recreational water activities.
2. Wet near-drowning: aspiration of fluid into lungs, which accounts for nearly 90% of cases.

 3. **Dry near-drowning: results from acute laryngospasm, which prevents both air exchange and aspiration of significant amounts of fluid into lungs. These victims have highest successful resuscitation rate.**

 4. **Immersion syndrome: associated with cold-water drowning, with sudden death occurring from vagally induced cardiac arrest or VF from sudden immersion into cold water.**

 5. **Hyperventilation–submersion syndrome: usually occurs after intentional hyperventilation to increase underwater swimming time. Hyperventilation induces hypocapnia, which suppresses the central respiratory drive, causing loss of consciousness before spontaneous central respiratory efforts resume.**
6. Secondary drowning (post-immersion syndrome or delayed drowning): occurs after initial recovery from overwhelming organ dysfunction that body defenses cannot overcome.

C. **Pathophysiology**

    1. In general, hypoxemia with resultant hypoxia affects organs in near drowning.

    2. Hypoxia from near drowning without aspiration results from airway obstruction caused by laryngospasm.

    3. Near drowning with aspiration causes damage which is dependent on the particular fluid aspirated: components, contaminants, and amount.

    4. Must also consider aspirated contaminants such as sand, algae, chlorine, vomit, and bacteria.

    5. In fresh-water drowning, hypotonic liquid is thought to damage the type II alveolar cells, causing decreased ability of pulmonary surfactant to prevent alveolar collapse.

    6. Surfactant inactivation causes alveolar collapse and impaired gas exchange.

    7. Pulmonary edema results, and leads to intrapulmonary shunting of blood, decreased lung compliance with decreased FRC, and increased ventilation–perfusion mismatching.

    8. **The resulting effect is clinically observed hypoxemia, which is compensated for by increased shunting of blood to the lungs, compounding the already-present pulmonary edema.**

    9. In salt-water drowning, hypertonic liquid may directly damage the alveolar capillary membrane.

   10. Salt water also changes osmotic pressure, permitting water and plasma proteins to be drawn into the interstitial spaces and alveoli, which dilute pulmonary surfactant.

   11. Diffuse pulmonary edema results from overwhelming amounts of fluid in alveoli.

D. **Assessment**

    1. **The clinical picture for both fresh and sea water is similar but a number of factors affect prognosis:**
        a. length of time submerged
        b. fluid temperature
        c. amount/type of fluid aspirated
        d. age and physical condition of victim
        e. underlying causes and associated injuries
        f. speed and aggressiveness of resuscitation efforts

    2. Findings may be affected by the precipitating cause of the event such as alcohol, drugs, seizures, myocardial infarction, neurologic injuries, and abuse.

    3. Other factors that alter assessment include the presence of alveolar and interstitial pulmonary edema, alterations in surfactant production, and direct alveolocapillary membrane damage.

    4. **Persistent hypoxia is often the earliest symptom of impending respiratory failure, but this may not develop for up to 24 hours.**

    5. Pulmonary symptoms may include:
        a. Cough with pink, frothy sputum
        b. Dyspnea, tachypnea, shallow, gasping respirations

        c.   Substernal burning or pleuritic chest pain

        d.   Crackles, rhonchi, wheezes

   6.   Initial ABGs usually show a metabolic acidosis

   7.   Other body systems are affected as follows:

        a.   Cerebral edema, manifested by irritability, restlessness, confusion, lethargy progressing to seizures, coma, and loss of reflexes may take 24 hours to develop.

        b.   Myocardial ischemia resulting from hypoxia, acidosis, hypothermia, and electrolyte disturbances are indicated by tachycardia, ventricular dysrhythmias, and chest pain.

        c.   Hypotension due to decreased CO from decreased cardiac contractility may occur.

        d.   Rhabdomyolysis/myoglobinuria secondary to muscle trauma and renal hypoperfusion secondary to decreased CO may contribute to acute tubular necrosis, manifested by oliguria, proteinuria, increased blood urea nitrogen (BUN) and creatinine.

        e.   Vomiting and anorexia related to large volumes of swallowed fluids and decreased perfusion of GI organs may also be noted.

E. **Nursing diagnoses**

   1.   Impaired Gas Exchange

   2.   Risk for Fluid Volume Deficit

   3.   Ineffective Breathing Patterns

   4.   Ineffective Airway Clearance

   5.   Ineffective Individual/Family Coping

   6.   Fear/Anxiety

   7.   Altered Tissue Perfusion: Cardiopulmonary

   8.   Altered Tissue Perfusion: Cerebral

   9.   Hypothermia

F. **Planning and implementation**

   1.   Initial nursing interventions focus on restoring and maintaining pulmonary, cardiac, and neurologic function.

        a.   Maintain patent airway.

        b.   Support adequate ventilation.

        c.   Improve gas exchange.

        d.   **Monitor for the development of MODS hours to days post-submersion.**

        e.   Maintain body alignment with repositioning q2hr.

        f.   Maintain humidification and oxygen therapies.

        g.   **Anticipate and prepare for possible intubation.**

        h.   Assess for changes in neurologic status.

        i.   **Assess for hypoxemia.**

        j.   **Maintain airway while protecting the C-spine until cleared by radiologic reports.**

        k.   **Place in position for maximum lung inflation, which is head and chest down for seawater to drain lungs. This maneuver is of no use in fresh-water drowning, because water is quickly absorbed into circulation and is no longer in the lungs.**

m 2. Anticipate development of ARDS.

m 3. Assess vital signs:
- a. fresh water expands blood volume and increases BP
- b. salt water pulls water from circulation into alveoli, decreasing blood volume and causing hypotension
- c. presence of crackles or pulmonary congestion on x-ray may not indicate fluid overload with salt water aspiration due to additional fluid pulled from interstitium into alveoli

G. Evaluation
1. Patient maintains effective airway clearance.
2. Patient is able to oxygenate adequately and further complications or systemic involvement are avoided.
3. Patient maintains normal volume balance.

H. Home health considerations
1. Poolside safety to prevent drowning includes installing fencing around pool; observing small children; avoiding use of alcohol and other mind-altering substances when in water; not swimming alone.
2. Ocean safety entails heeding lifeguard warnings and not swimming alone.

XIX. Oxygen delivery systems (Display 6-7)
  A. Categories of oxygen delivery
1. Low flow provides partial oxygenation, with patient breathing a combination of supplemental oxygen and room air.

DISPLAY 6-7.
Oxygen Administration and Nursing Implications

Nasal cannula 1–6 LPM (24%–45% FIO_2) prongs into nares low flow; used temporarily during meals for patients wearing face masks; mouth breathing does not affect delivery; delivery rate varies with client f and Vt; can irritate nares and ears

Simple face mask 8–10 LPM (35%–60% FIO_2) vent holes on each side low flow; prehospital and postoperative oxygenation; high-liter flow needed to prevent CO_2 buildup in mask; may cause claustrophobia; oxygen may leak from mask top and cause eye irritation.

Tracheostomy collar 4–6 LPM (35%–45% FIO_2) vent hole at tracheostomy low flow; provides humidification and insertion site oxygen; discomfort due to feeling of air on neck

Face tent 8–10 LPM (24%–45% FIO_2) fits under chin low flow; provides extra humidity; good for those with burns or facial trauma because allows unrestricted facial access

Venturi mask 3–6 LMP (24%–50% FIO_2) mask with bottom O_2 high flow; most precise O_2 administration flow regulator (24%, 28%, 30%, 35%, 40%, and 50%); for those who need exact liter flows due to chronic CO_2 retention (COPD)

Partial rebreather 6–10 LPM (60%–90% FIO_2) has reservoir bag with low flow; bag should only deflate about 1/3; mask holds 500–1000 mL; patient exhales out one-way valve and inhales combination of oxygen and exhaled air

Nonrebreather 10–15 (70%–100% FIO_2) has reservoir bag with high flow; provides greatest O_2 mask; holds 500–1000 mL concentrations without intubation; one-way valves between mask and bag and ot exhalation side vents. Prevents breathing of room air and prevents exhaled air from mixing with reservoir oxygen.

      2.   High flow provides all necessary oxygenation, with patient breathing only oxygen supplied from the mask and exhaling through a one-way vent.

B.   **Planning and implementation**

      1.   Prevent skin breakdown by checking nares, lobes, nose bridge, and applying gauze/cotton PRN.

      2.   Ensure that COPD patients receive low flow oxygen because these persons respond to hypoxia, not increased CO_2 levels, as is normal.

XX.   **Chest physiotherapy**

    A.   **Indications**

      1.   Part of routine treatment for persons with disorders such as COPD, cystic fibrosis, lung abscess, bronchiectasis, and pneumonia.

      2.   **Based on the fact that mucous can be knocked or shaken from airway walls and helped to drain from lungs.**

      3.   Primary techniques may be used alone, but are most effective when used together. Client ability to tolerate these procedures may limit the vigor with which they are applied, so positioning and clapping techniques may need modification.

    B.   **Techniques**

      1.   Percussion: produces energy wave that is transmitted through the chest wall to the bronchi.

          a.   Chest is struck rhythmically with cupped hands over the area where secretions are located.

          b.   Care must be taken to avoid striking over the spine or kidneys, on female breasts, or on incisions or broken ribs. Do not percuss over soft tissue or areas where the technique causes increased pain.

          c.   Cup hands and lightly and rhythmically strike chest wall. A hollow, deep sound indicates correct technique.

          d.   Each area should be percussed for 1–2 minutes.

          e.   Gas-powered or electric percussors are available.

      2.   Vibration: works similarly to percussors.

          a.   Hands placed on client's chest and gently but firmly, rapidly and vigorously vibrate hands against thoracic wall over percussed area during client exhalation.

          b.   May help dislodge secretions and stimulate a cough.

          c.   Should be done at least 5–7 times during patient exhalation.

      3.   Postural drainage: use of gravity to aid in the drainage of secretions.

          a.   Patient is placed in various positions to promote flow of drainage from different lung segments using gravity.

          b.   **Areas with secretions are placed higher than other lung segments to promote drainage.**

          c.   Drainage/mucus enters larger airways and is more easily removed.

          d.   Positions vary depending on the lobe/s to be drained.

          e.   Patient should maintain each position for at least 5 minutes.

          f.   At the end of each positioned period, the client should cough and deep breathe before the next position.

g. Trendelenburg position can increase shortness of breath in the client with COPD because of diaphragmatic pressure from abdominal organs. This position can increase ICP and should be used cautiously for clients with head injuries. It also can be stressful for those with cardiac problems.

 h. Contraindicated in patients with cyanosis/dyspnea resulting from the techniques; increased pain/discomfort with techniques. Suction equipment not available for client with copious sputum, patients with prolonged bleeding/clotting times, extremely obese patients, and those with a history of predisposition to pathologic fractures.

C. Evaluation
  1. Patient assumes specific postural drainage position for 5 minutes.
  2. The area is percussed for 1–2 minutes.
  3. The area is vibrated.
  4. Client is encouraged to cough up and expectorate any sputum.
  5. Different postural drainage position is assumed and the technique repeated.

D. Teaching
  1. Although patients cannot perform techniques completely on themselves, they may perform tapping movements on chest wall by using fingertips of both hands, which may loosen secretions.
  2. Teach family how to perform vibration and percussion.
  3. Perform oral hygiene after procedure.
  4. Perform at least 30 minutes before meals or at least 2 hours after a meal.
  5. Encourage use of tissues during coughing to inspect sputum characteristics.

XXI. **Artificial airways**
  A. Oral airways
  1. These are shorter and often have a larger lumen than nasal airways.
  2. Their use may necessitate the use of "bite block"/oral airway to prevent biting down on the tube and causing airway occlusion.
  3. Patient must be able to orally suction and perform oral hygiene.

  B. Nasal airways
  1. These are usually longer and have smaller lumens, which causes greater airway resistance.
  2. They are less irritating and easier to stabilize than oral airways.

  C. Tracheostomy
  1. Creation of a temporary or permanent surgical opening into the trachea at one of the tracheal rings.
  2. Insertion of a tube to allow ventilation and removal of secretions.
  3. Indications
      a. Indicated for emergency airway access in cases of tracheal edema from trauma/allergic response, airway burns, mechanical airway obstruction, and sleep apnea.

b. Useful in patients who are unable to clear secretions, secondary to upper airway bleed, and laryngeal or tracheal tear.

c. Prevention of aspiration in unconscious client.

d. Need for long-term mechanical ventilation or airway maintenance with upper airway blockage.

4. Planning and implementation

a. Use the shortest tube possible and secure with Velcro or twill tape.

b. Maintain tracheostomy care and ostomy site.

c. Identify complications such as:
   ▶ Right mainstem bronchus intubation
   ▶ Skin breakdown/pressure necrosis
   ▶ Tracheoesophageal fistula
   ▶ Innominate artery erosion
   ▶ Tracheal stenosis/necrosis due to excessive cuff pressure on tracheal walls; use minimal air leak technique to decrease incidence

XXII. Mechanical ventilation

A. Introduction and indications

1. Mechanical ventilation is used to correct hypoxemia and hypoventilation when the client cannot sustain spontaneous and effective respirations.

2. Indicated for various conditions that lead to inadequate ventilation or oxygenation.

B. Types

1. Pressure-cycled
   a. delivers gas until preset pressure is reached
   b. volumes vary based on needed delivery pressure

2. Volume-cycled
   a. delivers gas until preset volume is reached
   b. pressures vary based on needed delivery volumes

3. Time-cycled is the most commonly used method in pediatrics.

4. Settings: various settings are programmed into the ventilator in order to provide optimal oxygenation. Some of these include:
   a. Tidal volume (Vt): amount of air delivered with each breath; set at 10–15 mL/kg body weight
   b. Respiratory rate (Vf): number of breaths per minute
   c. FIO_2: oxygen percentage delivered (21%–100%)
   d. Sigh volume: provides a deeper breath than Vt; promotes alveolar expansion
   e. Peak flow: speed of air flow in liters per minute (LPM)
   f. Sensitivity: the amount of effort needed to initiate a breath
   g. Pressure limit: highest pressure allowed by the machine; mechanical inspiration is stopped when this limit is reached
   h. I:E ratio: inspiration to expiration time; normal is 1:2

C. Modes of mechanical ventilation (Fig. 6-2)

1. Assist-control ventilation (A/C)
   a. Preset to deliver total breathing cycle as needed.

   b. **Client can initiate spontaneous breaths, at which time the machine delivers set volume.**

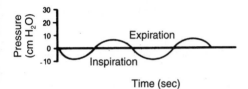

Spontaneous Breathing
Patient has full work of breathing: determining rate, Vt, and rhythm.

Controlled Ventilation
Patient has no work breathing: ventilator will rhythmically deliver Vt at preset rate.

Assist-Control
Patent has minimal work of breathing during initial expansion of chest, then ventilator will deliver preset Vt.

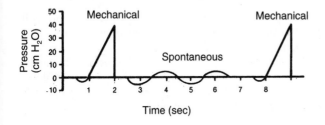

Intermittent Mandatory Ventilation (IMV)
Patient has a variable work of breathing: the mandatory ventilated breaths occur at a preset rate and Vt, but the patient may take spontaneous breaths between the machine-delivered breaths.

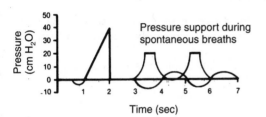

IMV with Pressure Support (12 cm H₂O)
Patent has low-to-moderate work of breathing: the spontaneous breaths are supported with a preset pressure assistance.

FIGURE 6-2.
Modes of mechanical ventilation.

        c.   Provides variable work of breathing, oxygen consumption, and comfort.

        d.   Provides minimal conditioning.

        e.   Resistane factors include tubing (dead space) and small artificial airway size.

    2.   Intermittent mandatory ventilation (IMV)

        a.   **Preset to deliver a specified rate and volume; may result in "stacking" if patient is inhaling when ventilator delivers inhalation.**

        b.   Client initiates spontaneous breathing between ventilator breaths.

        c.   Work of breathing varies with rate.

        d.   Oxygen consumption varies with rate.

        e.   Comfort depends on rate, inspiratory time, and circuit characteristics.

        f.   Provides for strengthening during spontaneous breathing.

        g.   Resistance factors depend on circuit (internal or external) and artificial airway size.

    3.   Synchronized intermittent mandatory ventilation (SIMV): preset as with IMV, but delivers breaths to correspond to client respiratory pattern.

        a.   Ventilator will not initiate breath if patient is inhaling spontaneously.

        b.   **Positive end-expiratory pressure (PEEP) prevents or decreases alveolar collapse at end-expiration, and helps to reinflate collapsed alveoli.**

        c.   Used for clients receiving mechanical ventilation.

    4.   Continuous positive airway pressure (CPAP): same principle as PEEP, but used for non–ventilator-dependent clients.

    5.   Pressure support ventilation

        a.   Assists in overcoming increased airway resistance by providing preset positive pressure assistance when patient inhales.

        b.   Decreases work of breathing, increases comfort, and provides endurance training during weaning.

        c.   **Decreases work resistance related to tube size, mechanical obstacles, and circuit characteristics.**

    6.   "T" piece: humidified oxygen supplied via tube to ETT/tracheostomy so client can spontaneously breathe as a "test" before extubation.

    7.   Jet ventilation: "dog-panting"; rapid rates with small Vt

D.   Troubleshooting alarms

    1.   Low-pressure alarms may be initiated by:

        a.   disconnection

        b.   overbreathing

    2.   High-pressure alarms may be initiated by:

        a.   suctioning

        b.   tubing kinks

        c.   biting on tube

    d.   coughing

    e.   bronchospasm

 3.   If unable to find the problem, disconnect, and ventilate patient manually.

E.   Complications of mechanical ventilation

    1.   intubation/tracheostomy problems

    2.   decreased cardiac output

    3.   pulmonary trauma/pneumothorax

    4.   respiratory muscle dysfunction/failure

    5.   fluid retention

    6.   gastric distention

 7.   oxygen toxicity: excessive amounts of oxygen may cause permanent injury

    8.   infection

    9.   psychological dependence

F.   Assessment (see Display 6-8)

 1.   Evaluate presence of anxiety versus a change in neurologic status.

    2.   Decreased CO is often noted with use of PEEP, therefore monitoring of cardiovascular parameters is important.

    3.   Monitor vital signs and assess respiratory parameters.

    4.   Assess for evidence of stress ulceration.

    5.   Monitor renal status and assess for evidence of decreased urine output, which occurs secondary to increased aldosterone production with PEEP.

    6.   Assess skin temperature, color, and capillary refill.

G.   Nursing diagnoses

    1.   Impaired Verbal Communication

    2.   Ineffective Airway Clearance

    3.   Impaired Gas Exchange

    4.   Ineffective Breathing Pattern

DISPLAY 6-8.
Assessment and Setup of Ventilator Settings

1. Set the machine to deliver tidal volume required (10 to 15 mL/kg).
2. Adjust the machine to deliver the lowest concentration of oxygen to maintain normal PaO_2 (80–100 mm Hg). This setting may be set high and gradually reduced based on arterial blood gas results.
3. Record peak inspiratory pressure.
4. Set mode (assist-control or intermittent mandatory ventilation) and rate according to physician order.
5. If the ventilator is set on assist-control mode, adjust sensitivity so that the patient can trigger the ventilator with a minimal effort (usually 2 mm Hg negative inspiratory force).
6. Record minute volume and measure carbon dioxide partial pressure (PCO_2), pH, and PO_2, after 20 minutes of continuous mechanical ventilation.
7. Adjust setting (FIO_2 and rate) according to results of arterial blood gases to provide normal values or those set by the physician.
8. If patient suddenly becomes confused or agitated or begins bucking the ventilator for some unexplained reason, assess for hypoxemia and manually ventilate on 100% oxygen with a resuscitation bag.

5. Anxiety/fear/powerlessness
6. Risk for alteration in tissue perfusion
7. Dysfunction weaning response
8. Inability to sustain spontaneous ventilation
9. Risk for infection

H.   Planning and implementation

1. **Administer sedatives to keep patient calm. Restrain only if necessary.**
2. Note ETT position at lips/nares and change ETT side-to-side as needed.
3. Auscultate breath sounds and assess for hypoxia and hypercapnia.
4. Monitor ventilator settings including humidifier, temperature, peak airway pressure, Vt, FIO_2, Vf, I:E ratio, and sensitivity.
5. Monitor cuff pressures and maintain at 20 mm Hg or per protocol.
6. Change tubing circuits per policy.
7. Drain condensed water from ventilatory tubing.
8. Perform CPT as indicated.
9. Monitor ABGs.
10. Assess for position changes if certain positions initiate respiratory distress.

11. **Provide alternative communication measures: letter/picture board, paper and pencil, ask closed-ended questions.**

12. **Be aware of potential complications: respiratory insufficiency, atelectasis, oxygen toxicity, decreased cardiac output, GI bleeding.**

I.   Suctioning review: current concepts

1. Suction only when necessary, not routinely.
2. Hyperoxygenate and hyperventilate with 3–5 breaths before and after suctioning.
3. Remember that using a manual resuscitation device makes it nearly impossible to deliver 100% FIO_2; hyperoxygenate through ventilator, if possible.
4. Do not instill normal saline for irrigation; it irritates bronchial mucosa.
5. Use the smallest appropriate suction catheter and know the size of your ETT.
6. Three passes of the catheter is the maximum, with 10 seconds permitted for each catheter pass.
7. Limit suction pressure to not more than 120 mm Hg and less for tracheostomy suctioning.
8. Intermittent and continuous pressure both damage airway tissues, thus either way is acceptable.
9. Assessment should include vital signs and oxygen saturation.

XXIII.   Weaning from mechanical ventilation

A.   Introduction and indications

1. Weaning involves removing the person from mechanical ventilation as the person's spontaneous respiratory efforts improve to the point that assistance is no longer needed.

2. The time needed for this process is individualized, taking longer for clients with long-term diaphragm weakness than for those with brief periods of intubation.

B. Parameters

1. Can attempt weaning when PaO_2 is over 70–80 mm Hg on FIO_2 under 0.5.
2. $PaCO_2$ should be within normal limits for the client.
3. Acceptable general respiratory status based on clinical assessment.
4. Correction of underlying problem which instigated mechanical ventilation.

C. Assessment of respiratory muscle strength

1. Assess respiratory demand and work of breathing.
2. Be able to differentiate between dyspnea of respiratory distress and recovery efforts to spontaneously breathe.
3. Evaluate the following:
   a. oxygen supply vs. demand
   b. tidal volume
   c. cough/deep breathe ability

D. Process

1. There are four essential components to successful weaning:
   a. Establishment of trust: psychological dependency on ventilator develops with long-term patients. The patient must be comfortable with the nurse during weaning.
   b. Nutrition: Adequate nutrition is essential to weaning. It is recommended that the patient be placed on a high-fat, low-carbohydrate diet. Diet should be approximately 45% fat, 25% protein, 30% CHO.

   c. **Tissue oxygenation: supply = demand. Assessment for adequate tissue oxygenation should include evaluation of vital signs, ABGs, and SaO_2 all WNL for the client. The Hgb/Hct should be 10–14 g/dL.**
   d. Lung mechanics includes such factors as airway patency, which is affected by secretions, bronchospasm, and inflammation, resistance, and compliance.
2. Increasing respiratory strength requires frequent physical and occupational therapies.
3. Communication/resocialization/relaxation exercises are useful in assisting the client to control dyspnea and anxiety before successful weaning.
4. Methods: keep airway in place until respiratory parameters indicate the likelihood of successful spontaneous respiratory efforts.
   a. T-Piece/CPAP: allows total spontaneous breathing by client.
   b. SIMV/IMV: allow spontaneous breathing with some ventilator back-up.
   c. PSV: allows spontaneous initiation of respirations by supporting respiratory muscles.

E. Terminal weaning

1. Definition: gradually removing mechanical ventilation from a patient with a terminal illness or a progressively deteriorating condition with a negative prognosis.

2.   Involves a complex needs assessment of pain, anxiety, dyspnea, and fever which can done on the medical-surgical floor or in the home.

3.   Family needs liberal visiting times, the ability to spend time with the patient, and participation in care if they wish.

4.   Process

a.   Teaching: explain the procedure, emphasizing that without adequate spontaneous respiratory effort the patient will experience dyspnea/shortness of breath during the process.

b.   Needs assessment: establish need for nourishment/hydration if the patient cannot take oral nutrients.

c.   Ventilator settings: gradually tapered until machine is turned off.

5.   Other issues: end-of-life decision

XXIV.   Chest tubes

A.   **Description: a chest tube is used to drain fluid and air out of the mediastinum or pleural space and into a collection chamber. By withdrawing air and fluid from the pleural space, chest drainage helps to re-establish normal negative pressure for lung re-expansion.**

B.   Indications

1.   Open heart surgery is a common indication for chest drainage. Chest tubes must be placed in the pericardium postoperatively for drainage of residual blood from mediastinum

2.   **All lung surgery patients except for total pneumonectomy patients because surgical incision causes positive pressure to develop in the pleural space around the affected lung, allowing the lung to collapse.**

C.   Procedure

1.   Chest tube is inserted into the affected chest wall at the level of the second to third intercostal space (ICS) to release trapped air.

2.   **For significant amounts of fluid drainage, a second tube may be placed in the inferior posterior portion of pleural space, as gravity will cause the fluid to flow in that direction.**

3.   A single tube is used to release both air and fluid, and is usually placed in the mid-axillary region at the fourth ICS.

4.   Connecting suction to the other end of the chest tube unit facilitates the flow of drainage. The fluid stays in the collection and the air continues on into an adjacent chamber.

5.   There are two types of systems:

a.   **Wet: usually filled with 20 cm of water. When the negative pressure generated by the suction source exceeds this level, atmospheric air enters chamber through a vent and bubbles up through the water, relieving excess pressure.**

b.   **Dry: contains no water, employs one of two methods of limiting amount of negative pressure. The first is a restrictive orifice mechanism, which is an opening that can be made larger or smaller to increase or decrease the amount of negative pressure. The other is a regulator** that automatically adjusts to changes in negative pressure from the suction source or within the client.

6. The water seal chamber is a calibrated manometer that measures normal pressure changes in the chest associated with breathing.

    a. **Some fluctuations during inspiration in this chamber indicate tube patency. The pattern is reversed in clients on mechanical ventilation because ventilator breaths are provided under positive pressure.**

    b. It contains about 2 cm water.

    c. Incoming air bubbles up through the water, which serves as a one-way valve to prevent air from flowing back into the lung through the system.

    d. Air then exits the water seal and enters the suction control chamber, which regulates the maximum amount of negative pressure that can be applied to the pleural space.

D. **Assessment**

1. **Note the development of pneumothorax or pleural effusion. These are the two most common complications of chest drainage in cardiothoracic surgical patients.**

2. Note color and rate of drainage. Postoperatively there should be gradual reduction in amount and change from bright to dark red color to a pink or straw color.

3. **Assess for gradual reduction in drainage and change in color to pink or straw.**

4. Assess the water seal chamber for air leaks.

5. Note bubbling in the chamber and pattern. In the event of a client lung leak, you will see intermittent pattern corresponding with respiration. If the patient is on PEEP, a leaking lung is most likely to produce continuous bubbling.

6. If continuous bubbling during spontaneous respiration is noted, suspect a drainage system leak.

    a. **Using a toothless tubing clamp, close the chest tube at the point where it exits the chest. Do not apply the clamp for more than a few seconds because of the potential for pneumothorax.**

    b. If bubbling in water seal chamber stops, the leak is in the lung, but if it continues, the leak is between the clamp and the chamber

    c. If bubbling continues, gradually move clamp toward the drainage unit, checking the water seal chamber each time. The clamp is between the leak and the drainage unit if bubbling stops.

    d. Persistent bubbling after this assessment means that the drainage unit itself is leaking in which case you need to replace the entire drainage system

E. **Planning and implementation**

1. **Suction control chamber: maintain between –10 cm H_2O and –20 cm H_2O.**

2. There should be just gentle bubbling in the suction control chamber.

3. **Vigorous bubbling causes faster water evaporation and is unnecessarily noisy.**

4. **If wall suction is not being applied, detach it from the suction tubing so air can leave the system.**

5. Post–chest tube insertion, have client take several deep breaths to help to reinflate collapsed lung and restore negative pressure.

6. Clamp only to assess how the patient will tolerate removal of the chest tube. A trial is usually done 12 hours before tube removal.

7. Be aware of potential complications:
    a. Accidental tube dislodgment/removal
    b. Correct by submerging distal end of tube in container with 2 cm of sterile fluid (saline or distilled water) to form a temporary water seal until the tube is reconnected to the drainage unit.

XXV. Bronchoscopy

A. **Description: the passage of a lighted bronchoscope into the bronchial tree. Performed with rigid steel or flexible fiberoptic instruments for direct visualization of the trachea and tracheobronchial tree.**

B. Indications

1. Diagnostic
    a. Tissue examination
    b. Visual examination, identification, and evaluation of a tumor, obstruction, or foreign body for potential resection
    c. Diagnostic collection of tissue specimens
    d. Evaluation of bleeding sites
    e. Assess for ETT dysfunction

2. Therapeutic
    a. Foreign body removal
    b. Removal of tenacious, copious secretions/mucous plugs
    c. Treat postoperative atelectasis, drain of an abscess, and improve bronchial clearance
    d. Destroy and remove lesions

    e. **Treatment of bronchopulmonary infections if client cannot or will not effectively cough despite suctioning. May be particularly helpful in promoting drainage of purulent material associated with lobar atelectasis, bronchiectasis, or lung abscesses.**

C. Assessment

1. Before the procedure:
    a. Explain procedure to client and family and obtain informed consent.
    b. Maintain NPO 6 hours before procedure.
    c. Before sedation, remove dentures, contact lenses, and other prostheses.
    d. Have patient lay supine with head hyperextended.

2. During the procedure:
   a. Sedate to suppress cough, and relieve anxiety.
   b. Spray topical anesthetic into back of throat.
   c. Observe and assess client.
3. After the procedure:
   a. Throat may be sore, with some initial difficulty swallowing.
   b. Assess vital signs per protocol.

   m
   c. **Observe for respiratory distress: dyspnea, changes in rate, use of accessory muscles, and changes in or absent breath sounds.**
   d. Observe expectorated secretions for hemoptysis.

   m
   e. **Maintain NPO until cough and gag reflexes returned (1–2 hours), then begin with ice chips and small sips of water.**

D. Nursing diagnoses
   1. Impaired Gas Exchange
   2. Ineffective Airway Clearance
   3. Pain
   4. Fear/Anxiety/Powerlessness
E. Planning and implementation
   1. Assess respiratory status
   2. Maintain humidification and oxygen therapies
   3. Assess for hypoxemia
   4. Ensure adequacy of airway
F. Evaluation
   1. Patient is able to maintain effective airway clearance.
   2. Patient experiences reduced anxiety/fear as evidenced by calm and trusting appearance, and verbalized fears and concerns.

Bibliography

Andrews, L. (1994). Medical management of pulmonary emboli. *Med-Surg Nurs* 3(1), 31–35.

Apple, S. (1996). New trends in thrombolytic therapy. *RN* 59(1), 30–35.

Aubier, M., Murciano, D., & Lecoguic, Y. (1985). Effects of hypophosphatemia on diaphragmatic contractility in patients with acute respiratory failure. *N Engl J Med* 313, 420–424.

Aubier, M., Viires, N., & Piquet, J. (1985). Effects of hypocalcemia on diaphragmatic strength generation. *J Appl Physiol* 58, 2054–2061.

Black, J., & Matassarin-Jacobs, E. (Eds.). (1993). *Luckman and Sorenson's medical-surgical nursing: A psychophysiological approach* (4th ed.). Philadelphia: Saunders.

Calianno, C., Clifford, D. W., & Titano, K. (1995). Oxygen therapy: Giving your patient breathing room. *Nursing* 25(12), 33–38.

Carpenito, L. J. (1997). *Handbook of nursing diagnosis* (7th ed.). Philadelphia: Lippincott.

Carroll, P. (1995). A med/surg nurse's guide to mechanical ventilation. *RN* 58(2), 26–35.

Carroll, P. (1994). Safe suctioning PRN. *RN* 57(5), 32–37.

Carroll, P. (1994). Speed: The essential response to anaphylaxis. *RN* 57(6), 26–31.

Glankler, D. M. (1993). Caring for the victim of near drowning. *Crit Care Nurse* 13(4), 25–32.

Glass, C. A., & Grap, M. J. (1995). Ten tips for safer suctioning. *AJN* 95(5), 51–53.

Gold, J. (1994). Ask about latex. *RN* 57(6), 32–34.

Gordon, P. A., Norton, J.M., & Merrell, R. (1995). Refining chest tube management: analysis of the state of practice. *Dimens Crit Care Nurs* 14(1), 6–13.

Gross, S. B. (1993). Current challenges, concepts, and controversies in chest tube management. *AACN Clin Issues Crit Care Nurs* 9(2), 260–275.

Gulanick, M., Klopp, A., Galanes, S., Gradishar, D., & Puzas, M. K. (1994). *Nursing care plans: Nursing diagnosis and intervention* (3rd ed.). St. Louis: Mosby.

Hudak, C. M., & Gallo, B. M. (1994). *Critical care nursing: A holistic approach* (6th ed.). Philadelphia: J. B. Lippincott.

Mays, D. A. (1995). Turn ABGs into child's play. *RN* 58(1), 36–39.

McGaffigan, P. A. (1996). Hazards of hypoxemia: How to protect your patient from low oxygen levels. *Nursing* 26(5), 41–46.

McKinley, M. G. (1989). Near drowning: A nursing challenge. *Crit Care Nurse* 9 (10), 52–60.

Molloy, D. W., Shingra, S., & Solven, F. (1984). Hypomagnesium and respiratory muscle power. *Am Rev Resp Dis* 129, 497–498.

Nelson, N. P., & Beckel, J.(1990). Patient care guidelines: Near drowning. *J Emerg Nurs* 16(2), 119–123.

North American Nursing Diagnosis Association (NANDA). (1996). *Nursing diagnoses: Definitions & classification 1997–1998.* Philadelphia: Author.

Repasky, T. M. (1994). Tension pneumothorax. *AJN* 94(9), 47.

Skipper, A. *Dietician's handbook of enteral and parenteral nutrition.* Rockville, MD: Aspen.

Smeltzer, S. C., & Bare, B. G. (1996). *Brunner & Suddarth's textbook of medical-surgical nursing.* (8th ed.). Philadelphia: Lippincott-Raven.

Zaloga, G. P. (1994). *Nutrition in critical care* (pp. 647–661). St. Louis: Mosby.

STUDY QUESTIONS

1. Which one of the following delivery systems provides the most precise oxygen concentrations?
   a. non-rebreather mask
   b. Venturi mask
   c. partial rebreather mask
   d. simple face mask

2. When a patient questions you about the phrase "dead space," your best answer is to describe it as:
   a. an area in your lung that does not exchange air
   b. a small area of dead tissue that causes infection
   c. the part of the lower airway that brings in fresh air
   d. any part of your lungs that traps mucous

3. Which one of the following principles of tracheostomy suctioning is correct?
   a. To ensure removal of a larger amount of secretions, suction should be on continuously when entering and leaving the respiratory tract.
   b. The maximum amount of time for the procedure is 15 seconds going in and 15 seconds coming out.
   c. To ensure consistent removal of secretions, the catheter should be withdrawn straight out, without twisting.
   d. To minimize hypoxia, the entire suctioning procedure (from start to finish) should not exceed 15 minutes.

4. Which one of the following nursing actions is most helpful in reducing chronically thick respiratory tract secretions?
   a. maintaining continuous oxygen therapy
   b. keeping the patient in semi-Fowler's position as much as possible
   c. maintaining an adequate fluid intake for the patient
   d. instilling 3 mL of NSS intratracheally before suctioning

5. Which one of the following presents the most appropriate reason for suctioning a patient?
   a. Suctioning once per shift is part of the routine nursing assessment.
   b. The patient is unconscious and is unable to cough up secretions.
   c. The patient has a capped tracheostomy.
   d. The physician has ordered suctioning every hour.

6. Mr. Parks has COPD. His nurse has taught him pursed lip breathing, which helps him in which one of the following ways?
   a. increases carbon dioxide concentration, which stimulates breathing in a patient with COPD
   b. teaches him to lengthen inspiration and shorten expiration
   c. enables him to lengthen expiration, which increases CO_2 retention in a patient with COPD
   d. decreases the amount of air that is trapped in the alveoli after expiration

7. Leticia Padilla, a patient with emphysema, is receiving low-dose oxygen at 1.5 L/minute by nasal cannula because:
   a. This is the maximum of oxygen that can be given by nasal cannula.
   b. Her alveoli are unable to absorb higher oxygen concentrations because of her emphysema.
   c. Her alveoli are so damaged that higher oxygen concentrations may cause alveolar rupture.
   d. Her respiratory center needs low oxygen concentrations to stimulate breathing.

8. Which one of the following groups of signs indicates early hypoxia?
   a. bradypnea, dyspnea, cyanosis
   b. bradycardia, lethargy, disorientation
   c. hypotension, dyspnea, pulse deficit
   d. restlessness, tachycardia, diaphoresis

9. Which one of the following is an initial finding at assessment of a patient with atelectasis?
   a. wheezes at lung bases
   b. decreased or absent breath sounds in some areas
   c. stridor on inspiration
   d. crackles and rhonchi at lung bases

10. In which order should the following medications be given to an asthmatic patient?
    a. intranasal steroid, inhalation bronchodilator
    b. inhalation bronchodilator, intranasal steroid
    c. it depends on whether the asthma is new onset or chronic
    d. the steroids should be given according to the client's circadian rhythm; the bronchodilator may be given any time

11. The xanthine bronchodilator Theo-Dur (theophylline) is effective in treating obstructive airway disease because it:
    a. decreases respiratory muscle strength
    b. stimulates ciliary motility of the respiratory tree
    c. decreases cardiac output
    d. has a mild diuretic action

12. Theophylline is being given to your asthmatic patient, who smokes cigarettes. You must tell her that smoking:
    a. decreases the half-life of theophylline, which means that an increased dosage may be needed
    b. decreases the half-life of theophylline, which means that a decreased dosage may be needed
    c. increases the half-life of theophylline, which means that a decreased dosage may be needed
    d. increases the half-life of theophylline, which means that an increased dosage may be needed

13. Which one of the following blood levels is completely within the normal range for theophylline?
    a. 7.2–12.9 mcg/mL
    b. 13.0–17.5 mcg/mL
    c. 17.5–25.0 mcg/mL
    d. The answer will vary, depending on whether the person smokes.

14. Respiratory failure occurs when the respiratory system and heart are unable to
    a. maintain adequate oxygenation
    b. retain adequate CO_2
    c. maintain a PaO_2 of 80 mm Hg
    d. maintain a $PaCO_2$ of less than 45 mm Hg

15. Early respiratory failure initially is demonstrated by:
    a. cyanosis and pallor
    b. restlessness and irritability
    c. hypotension and tachycardia
    d. dyspnea and nasal flaring

16. When assessing a chest tube drainage system, several major items must be checked. From the following, choose the item(s) that is/are to be assessed:
    a. water seal at 2 cm of water
    b. tubing taped to bed
    c. tubing and collection system visible above bed
    d. sign above bed stating "chest tubes present"

17. Intermittent bubbling is noted in the water seal chamber of a left pleural chest tube. Which of the following actions is appropriate?
    a. Clamp the chest tube.
    b. Encourage the client to cough.
    c. Change the drainage unit.
    d. Notify the physician immediately.

ANSWER KEY

1. Correct response: b

The Venturi (Venti) mask can be set to administer a precise amount of oxygen.

a, c, and d. A non-rebreather mask provides close to 100% oxygen but cannot be exactly measured, nor can any other type of mask.

Knowledge/Physiologic/NA

2. Correct response: a

b, c, and d. Dead space does not participate in gas exchange (upper airway, ventilator tubing), and is not greatly responsible for trapping of mucus.

Application/Physiologic/Implementation

3. Correct response: d

a. Suction must be off during catheter insertion, on during removal from the respiratory tract;

b, c, and d. The maximum time for one catheter pass is 10 seconds, with the catheter being withdrawn by using a twisting motion to prevent adherence to mucous membranes and assist with maximum removal of secretions

Application/Safe care/Implementation

4. Correct response: c

Hydration will help to reduce chronically thick secretions

a. Oxygen therapy may provide humidification needed to help with dry cough,

b. Semi-Fowler's position makes it easier for the client to breathe, but these do nothing the reduces the viscosity of secretions.

d. Instillation of intratracheal NSS has been proven to be of no benefit; in fact it can be dangerous to the client.

Comprehension/Physiologic/NA

5. Correct response: b

There is no "routine suctioning" time; the nurse must assess the client to make individualized determinations of need.

Application/Safe care/Assessment

6. Correct response: d

b. Pursed lip breathing encourages the client to inhale through the nose and exhale slowly and forcefully out of the mouth to help him the exhale as much as possible.

a and c. This does not affect CO_2 level

Application/Health promotion/Implementation

7. Correct response: d

a, b, and d. After years of chronically high CO_2 levels, the baroreceptors no longer respond to this normal breathing stimulus and so the body only responds to hypoxia as a stimulus for breathing.

c. This has no relationship to alveolar rupture.

Application/Physiologic/Implementation

8. Correct response: d

Neurologic signs are often the first findings in early hypoxia; tachycardia and hypertension are seen in early compensation, as are dyspnea and diaphoresis.

a. Cyanosis and bradypnea are very late signs.

b. These are later signs of hypoxia.

c. Pulse deficit does not have a classic relationship to hypoxia.

Knowledge/Physiologic/Assessment

9. Correct response: b

Atelectasis, or collapse of alveoli, prevents the normal bronchovesicular sounds.

a, c, and d. Wheezes and stridor are due to constricted airways, whereas crackles and rhonchi are due to fluid accumulation.

Knowledge/Physiologic/Assessment

10. *Correct response: b*

The bronchodilator is administered so that the airways can be widened and can then receive the full benefits of the inhalation steroid.

c and d. This order is followed in both new-onset and chronic asthma, and has nothing to do with the circadian rhythm.

Application/Physiologic/Planning

11. *Correct response: b*

a. As a bronchodilator, it does not directly affect respiratory muscle strength.

c. It is a sympathomimetic agent, which increases cardiac output.

d. Xanthine derivatives such as theophylline do have mild diuretic properties, but these are secondary effects and not primary effects on airway clearance.

Knowledge/Physiologic/Implementation

12. *Correct response: a*

Persons who smoke cigarettes excrete theophylline at twice the normal rate, so they need twice the dose to maintain the same blood levels as those found in a non-smoker.

Application/Physiologic/Implementation

13. *Correct response: b*

Normal level is 10–20 mcg/mL, regardless of other circumstances such as smoking.

Knowledge/Physiologic/Evaluation

14. *Correct response: a*

b. The cardiopulmonary system does not try to retain CO_2 during respiratory crises.

c and d. It is also not realistic to expect that all clients have "normal" blood gases; clients with COPD who are not in respiratory failure often have

$PaCO_2$s greater than 45 mm Hg and PaO_2s of less than 80 mm Hg.

Knowledge/Physiologic/NA

15. *Correct response: b*

Neurologic signs are often the initial presenting problems in impending respiratory failure.

a and d. Cyanosis, pallor, and nasal flaring are ominous late signs.

c. Tachycardia is a compensatory response, as is elevated blood pressure.

Knowledge/Physiologic/Assessment

16. *Correct response: a*

b. Tubing must be intact from the insertion point to the suction system, but should not be taped to limit client movement.

c. The tubing and collection system must be kept below heart/lung level to promote drainage.

d. A sign is not necessary because no special precautions need be taken for clients with functioning chest tubes, the same reason that signs are not placed over the beds of clients with Foley catheters or nasogastric tubes.

Application/Self care/Assessment

17. *Correct response: b*

a. Chest tubes are ONLY to be clamped for several hours before their removal, to assess if the client is able to maintain normal cardiopulmonary function and gas exchange without the tubes.

b, c, and d. Intermittent bubbling is an expected finding, and the client should be encouraged to cough to get rid of the excess air and promote the return of the chest to its normal state of negative pressure.

Application/Self care/Assessment

The Gastrointestinal System

I.   The anatomy and physiology of the GI system

A.   Structures include the mouth, esophagus, stomach, small intestine, large intestine, liver, biliary tract, and pancreas.

    1.   Mouth

        a.   Lips

        b.   Oral cavity

▸ Teeth: mastication

▸ Tongue: mastication and deglutition

▸ Hard palate: separates mouth from nose

▸ Soft palate: separates mouth and pharynx

▸ Salivary glands: Parotid, submaxillary, sublingual

    2.   Pharynx

        a.   Nasopharynx

        b.   Oropharynx

        c.   Laryngeal pharynx

    3.   The esophagus is a 9.2- to 10-inch hollow muscular tube extending from the lower end of the pharynx to the stomach.

        a.   The upper esophageal sphincter is also called the hypopharyngeal sphincter. It contracts to open during swallowing and propels food into the esophagus.

        b.   The lower esophageal sphincter is not an anatomic sphincter, but rather an area of high pressure (also called the cardiac and gastroesophageal sphincter). It opens between the esophagus and stomach during swallowing or vomiting. Otherwise it remains contracted to prevent gastric reflux.

4. Stomach shape and size vary with contents, digestive stage, body structure, sex, and positioning.
   a. Cardia: proximal end
   b. Fundus: left of cardia
   c. Body: central portion
   d. Antrum: greater curvature
   e. Pylorus: distal end
   f. Layers: serous, muscular, submucosal, and mucosal
5. Openings
   a. Lower esophageal sphincter (LES)
   b. Pyloric sphincter is the opening between stomach and duodenum.
6. Small intestine
   a. A coiled tube measuring about 23 feet in length and 1 to 1.1 inches in diameter.
   b. Begins at the pylorus and ends at the ileocecal valve.
   c. There are three villi-lined sections to the small intestine. This is where the digestive enzymes are produced.
   d. The sections are named the duodenum, jejunum, and ileum.
7. Large intestine
   a. A hollow muscular tube about 6 feet long and 2 inches in diameter.
   b. Begins at the ileocecal valve and ends at the anus.
   c. Consists of the ascending colon, transverse colon, descending colon, sigmoid colon, rectum, and anus.

B. Function
1. Motility, the movement of nutrients through the tract. Normally the nutrients move at a rate that allows for digestion and absorption to occur.
2. Digestion and motility begin in the mouth by masticating the food.
3. Lubrication also occurs as the salivary glands provide watery secretions with salivary amylase.
4. Food is swallowed and passes through the esophagus to the stomach. There is no digestion or absorption in the esophagus.
5. In the stomach, digestion continues as pepsinogen is released and is then converted to pepsin.
   a. Pepsin begins protein breakdown.
   b. Gastric secretions increase and mix with the food.
6. Food then passes to the small intestine after several hours in the stomach (time frame is dependent on meal size). Digestion is completed; most of absorption occurs in the small intestine.
7. The large intestine now receives the digested material and absorbs water and electrolytes. Feces are formed until defecation takes place.

II. Overview of GI pathology
A. Assessment
1. Assess mouth, teeth, tongue, pharynx, and neck for deformities or irregularities.
2. Assess abdomen in at least four quadrants.
3. Inspect for pulsations, abnormal masses, or peristaltic movements. Some findings on inspection include:
   a. Hernias

      b.   Splinting

      c.   Ascites

      d.   Spider angiomas

4. Auscultate using the diaphragm of the stethoscope for the following:

      a.   Borborygmi or hyperactive bowel sounds

      b.   Hypoactive bowel sounds

5. Percuss to determine size and position of abdominal organs, masses, or ascites.

6. Palpate and observe the expression of the patient at the same time.

      a.   Light palpation: use to detect areas of tenderness.

      b.   Deep palpation: use to further delineate organs and deeper areas of pain and tenderness.

7. Assess rectal and anal region.

8. Obtain a health history including:

      a.   Present illness or chief complaint

      b.   Past medical history specific to GI concerns

      c.   Pain: document location, character, intensity, and duration; pay attention to timing in relation to food consumption

      d.   Bowel elimination patterns: document color, odor, consistency, and amount

9. Nutritional assessment should use a 24-hour recall chart with attention to:

      a.   height and weight

      b.   food intolerance

      c.   appetite

      d.   nausea and vomiting

      e.   cultural and religious values

      f.   food allergies

      g.   food accessibility

      h.   personal habits

      i.   eating behaviors

      j.   dietary additions and restrictions

      k.   medication usage

B. Laboratory studies

1. Miscellaneous serum tests

      a.   Serum glucose: evaluates hyper- and hypoglycemia and the liver's ability to store glycogen and utilize insulin

      b.   Galactose: evaluates the ability of the liver convert galactose to glycogen

      c.   D-Xylose test: evaluates the absorption of xylose (reduced in cirrhosis, regional ileitis, sprue, diverticula)

      d.   Shilling test: evaluates vitamin B12 absorption

2. Liver function tests

      a.   Serum bilirubin: evaluates the liver's ability to conjugate and excrete bilirubin; measured in total, direct, and indirect values

      b.   Serum liver enzymes: evaluates enzyme stores in the liver (Display 7-1)

3. Serum protein metabolism test: evaluates the liver's ability to synthesize metabolic products

      a.   Serum total protein

      b.   Serum albumin

DISPLAY 7-1.
Liver Enzymes

Aspartate aminotransferase (AST)
Alanine aminotransferase (ALT)
Lactic dehydrogenase (LDH)
Alkaline phosphatase (ALP)
5'Nucleotidase
Leucine aminopeptidase
Gamma-glutamyl transpeptidase (GGTP)
Gamma-glutamyltransferase (GGT)

    c.   Globulins
    d.   Serum ammonia and urea
    e.   Prothrombin time
4.   Serum alpha-fetoprotein (AFP): evaluates hepatocellular dysfunction
5.   Serum hepatitis B surface antigen: evaluates the presence of latent or active hepatitis B virus
6.   Pancreatic function tests
    a.   Serum amylase
    b.   Serum lipase
    c.   Secretin test
7.   Fecal analysis
    a.   Occult blood: evaluates GI bleeding
    b.   Fat (lipids): evaluates presence of liver and biliary tract disease
    c.   Urobilinogen: evaluates the decrease in biliary obstruction

C.   **Diagnostic testing**
   1.   Radiologic studies

    a.   **Upper GI studies (barium swallow): observes the movement of the contrast medium utilizing fluoroscopy; identifies esophageal, stomach, or duodenal disorders**
    b.   Small bowel series: views the terminal ileum 20 minutes after contrast medium is ingested
    c.   Lower GI study: identifies polyps, tumors, or lesions of the colon by administering a barium enema and then observing the contrast using fluoroscopy
    d.   Flat plate of the abdomen: an x-ray examination of the abdominal structures

    e.   **Ultrasound: uses ultrasound waves to detect abdominal masses and gallstones**
   2.   Endoscopic studies
    a.   Esophagoscopy: views mucosal lining of the esophagus, stomach and duodenum
    b.   Gastroduodenoscopy: views stomach and duodenum
    c.   Fiberoptic colonoscopy: visualization of the colon up to the ileocecal valve

        d.   Endoscopic retrograde cholangiopancreatography: visualization of duodenum, common bile duct, and pancreatic ducts; gallstone removal is also possible

   3.   Invasive studies

        a.   Liver biopsy: obtains hepatic tissue; high risk of bleeding with this procedure

        b.   Peritoneal lavage: evaluates the presence of blood in the peritoneal cavity, post-trauma

D. **Nutritional considerations**

   1.   Inflammatory bowel disease (IBD)

        a.   Crohn's disease and ulcerative colitis are the major forms of idiopathic IBD. Crohn's disease can involve any part of the GI tract, whereas ulcerative colitis is usually limited to the large intestine.

        b.   In both cases, treatment may require one or more intestinal resections and multiple medications. Protein–calorie malnutrition is the most common deficiency associated with IBD.

        c.   The cause of the malnutrition may be due to any one, or a combination of the following:

            ▶ Decreased nutrient intake
            ▶ Malabsorption
            ▶ Protein-losing enteropathy
            ▶ Maldigestion of fat
            ▶ Drug-nutrient interaction
            ▶ Increased caloric requirements

        d.   Protein malnutrition associated with IBD leads to immunologic impairment, poor wound healing, infection, weight loss, and growth failure.

        e.   These deficits can be addressed with increased nutrient intake and protein delivery.

        f.   Vitamins and trace elements are lost in diarrheal fluids and fistula output, resulting in deficiencies.

        g.   These losses can impair protein synthesis, and can cause iron deficiency or B12 deficiency.

        h.   Considerations for medical nutrition therapy:

            ▶ The overall goal is to increase the nutrient intake to achieve caloric balance and meet intake needs.
            ▶ A multivitamin containing 1 to 5 times the recommended daily allowance is advised.
            ▶ If being fed by mouth, generally the diet consists of 40–45 kcals/kg and 1.5–2 g/kg of protein.
            ▶ The diet is modified according to complications (Table 7-1).

   2.   Peptic ulcer disease and stress gastritis

        a.   By definition, an ulcer is a break in the mucosa that extends through the muscularis mucosa.

        b.   Nutrition support for the ulcer patient who has had surgery is the same as that for any postoperative patient.

TABLE 7-1.
GI Problems and Dietary Modifications

PROBLEM	MODIFICATION
Steatorrhea	Low-fat diet with medium chain triglycerides (MCT oil)
Calcium oxalate stones	Low-oxalate/low-fat diet
Strictures	Low fiber
Lactose intolerance	Lactose-reduced diet
Severe diarrhea	High-fiber bile-binding resins

   c.   **If the patient is not expected to regain GI function quickly or if the patient was grossly malnourished preoperatively, then parenteral support may be appropriate.**

   d.   Postoperative complications can include dumping syndrome, bile reflux, and gastritis to name a few.

   e.   Early nutrition intervention has been shown to reduce severe bleeding and ulcer perforation.

   f.   Stress gastritis and ulceration are well-recognized in critically ill patients.

   g.   Generally, the more severe the underlying disease, the greater the chance of gastric mucosal damage and subsequent bleeding.

   h.   Frequently H_2 receptor antagonists (cimetidine and ranitidine) and Carafate are used for the management of stress gastritis.

   i.   The patient may also be infused with parenteral nutrition, which is a cost-effective method of preventing complications.

   j.   Enteral nutrition exists as an option for feeding in the treatment of stress-induced gastritis for patients who require surgery.

   k.   Needle jejunostomy may be the best route of administration because the risk of aspiration pneumonia is markedly decreased.

   l.   However, stress ulceration medications are usually required to maintain the gastric pH.

   m.   Considerations for medical nutrition therapy

      ▸ The overall goal is to increase the nutrient intake to achieve caloric balance and meet intake needs.

      ▸ Elevate head of bed to reduce risk of pulmonary aspiration.

      ▸ Advance diet as tolerated, avoiding caffeine, spicy foods, alcohol, and foods not tolerated.

3. Gastrointestinal fistula

   a.   **Most GI fistulas occur after abdominal surgery when there is unrecognized trauma to the bowel or breakdown of an anastomosis.**

b. It is prudent to provide aggressive nutritional support in these cases.

c. **The rate of spontaneous closure has been found to be as much as 70% and the overall mortality as low as 6.5% with the use of hyperalimentation.**

d. Initial nutrients are given intravenously, followed by the enteral route if fistula drainage is not markedly decreased.

e. Enteral nutrition may decrease infection by maintaining the gut integrity and decreasing bacterial translocation.

f. **In proximal fistulas, it may also be possible to place a nasoenteric tube past the fistula or place a feeding jejunostomy.**

g. Considerations for medical nutrition therapy

   ▶ The overall goal is to increase the nutrient intake to achieve caloric balance and meet intake needs.

   ▶ If parenteral nutrition is used, monitor vitamin and mineral deficiencies that may effect wound healing.

   ▶ Enteral nutrition can be initiated if fistula output is low and feeds do not cause output to increase.

4. Short bowel syndrome

   a. Short bowel syndrome (SBS) occurs in patients with less than 150 cm of small intestine.

   b. Nutritional care hinges on providing appropriate fluid and electrolyte management and instituting nutritional repletion.

   c. Parenteral nutrition is often required due to inadequate GI function.

   d. The initiation of some form of enteral feeding is important to maintain the gut integrity if the patient can tolerate it.

   e. Thus, the provision of nutritional support, both enteral and parenteral, stimulates the process of intestinal adaptation.

   f. Considerations for medical nutrition therapy:

   ▶ The overall goal is to increase the nutrient intake to achieve caloric balance and meet intake needs.

   ▶ Early parenteral and/or enteral nutrition intervention is advised if the patient is unable to tolerate oral intake.

E. Psychosocial implications

1. Self-perception and self-concept pattern can be altered with GI disorders, often leading to feelings of depression, rejection and despair, and alterations in body image.

2. Contributing factors include:

   a. Overweight

   b. Underweight

   c. Ostomies

3. Role-relationship pattern

   a. Chronic illness such as cirrhosis, alcoholism, hepatitis, and those requiring ostomies may cause changes in roles and relationships.

      b.   Support groups are helpful in adjusting to changes in body image.

      c.   Sexuality: reproductive pattern changes can arise with GI disorder, such as obesity, anorexia, ascites, ostomies, alcoholism.

F.   **Commonly used medications of the GI system**

     1.   Antacids are used to buffer or neutralize hydrochloric acid and cause an increase in the pH of the stomach. Most antacids are derived from nonsystemic metal ions:

        a.   Aluminum (Amphojel)

        b.   Calcium (Tums)

        c.   Magnesium

        d.   Sodium

     2.   Antiemetics are utilized to reduce and control nausea and vomiting. Commonly used antiemetics are:

        a.   Anticholinergics

        b.   Antihistamines

        c.   Promethazine hydrochloride

        d.   Metoclopramide hydrochloride

        e.   Prochlorperazine

        f.   Corticosteroids

     3.   Emetics are used with poisonings to induce vomiting. Ipecac syrup is an example.

     4.   Antiulcer agents

        a.   Sucralfate: produces a protective acid-resistant barrier over the ulcer along the mucosa.

        b.   Omeprazole: inhibits the gastric acid pump by binding with the hydrogen/potassium ATPase enzyme.

        c. H_2 receptor antagonists: prevent histamine from stimulating the H_2 receptors, resulting in a decrease in the volume of gastric acid being secreted, also affecting the concentration of gastric acid. Examples include cimetidine, ranitidine, famotidine, and nizatidine.

        d.   Laxatives: induce defecation. They are classified according to their source and action (Display 7-2).

III. **Esophageal varices**

    A.   **Description: fragile overdistended veins which develop in the distal esophagus and are very susceptible to rupture.**

    B.   **Etiology and incidence**

DISPLAY 7-2.
Actions of Specific Laxatives

Saline laxatives—retain and increase water in the stool

Stimulant laxatives—increase peristalsis by irritation

Bulk laxatives—absorb water and increase volume, which in turn distends the bowel

Intestinal lubricants—mechanical lubrication

Hyperosmotic agents—draw water into the bowel and therefore increase volume

Softening agents—mix water and fatty substances in the feces, which eases the passage of stool.

     1.   Fibrotic liver changes with advanced disease, resulting in hepatic vein obstruction and portal hypertension.

     2.   Mortality rate increases with hemorrhage of varices.

C. **Pathophysiology (see Chapter 8)**

     1.   With advancing cirrhosis, there is an eventual development of collateral circulation in bordering organs, the distal esophagus, stomach, and mesentery.

     2.   The portal blood flow system uses these collateral vessels as a conduit to the systemic circulation. With increasing demands on the collateral circulation, the pressure within the portal vein rises, causing increased distention in the fragile varix, resulting in rupture.

D. **Assessment**

     1.   Health history of the patient should include evaluation of:
- a. Chief complaint
- b. Past history, including chronic alcohol abuse and cirrhosis

     2.   Clinical manifestations
- a. Bright red blood flowing from the mouth
- b. Changes in level of consciousness
- c. **Signs and symptoms of hypovolemic shock (see Chapter 13)**
- d. Decreased blood pressure, increased heart rate, and increased respiratory rate
- e. Decreased urinary output

     3.   Laboratory and diagnostic tests
- a. Diagnostic endoscopy
- b. CBC with differential
- c. Serum chemistries
- d. PT/PTT
- e. Urinalysis
- f. Type and screen
- g. Chest x-ray

E. **Nursing diagnoses**

     1.   Decreased Cardiac Output

     2.   Ineffective Airway Clearance

     3.   Altered Nutrition: Less than Body Requirements

     4.   Pain

     5.   Anxiety

     6.   Knowledge Deficit

F. **Planning and implementation**

     1.   Maintain airway.

     2.   **Monitor vital signs and hemodynamics every 15 minutes until stable. This should include the following parameters:**
- a. **Continuous ECG monitoring**
- b. **Swan-Ganz catheter: PCWP <8 mm Hg**
- c. **CVP: <10 cm H_2O**
- d. **Arterial line**

     3.   Assess pulse oximetry every 1–2 hours and PRN.

     4.   Maintain accurate I and O every 1–2 hours and PRN by:
- a. Foley to gravity

      b.   NPO status

      c.   Nasogastric tube (NGT)—Sengstaken-Blakemore tube

5. Maintain gastric lavage, if ordered.

6. Provide safe environment for the patient.

7. Provide mouth care, as needed.

8. Explain all procedures simply and briefly.

9. Assess anxiety level and allow for verbalization of fears.

10. Promote adequate pain relief:

      a.   Assess and document level of pain on a 1 to 10 scale (include location, character, intensity, and duration).

      b.   Administer pain medications IM or IV and record response.

      c.   Teach relaxation techniques in addition to pain medications.

      d.   Decrease external stimuli.

      e.   Provide emotional support.

11. Maintain adequate nutritional status.

      a.   Obtain baseline nutritional assessment.

      b.   Maintain NPO status until stable. Ensure that NGT patency is maintained.

      c.   Initiate small amounts of liquids when stable.

      d.   Omit consumption of gastric irritants: coffee and other caffeinated beverages and high roughage foods, all of which are irritating to varices.

12. Administer medications, as prescribed:

      a.   Administer analgesics, as prescribed.

𝓶   b.   **Maintain IV therapy at the prescribed rate (note that too-rapid infusion will increase portal pressure).**

      c.   Administer vitamin K, as ordered.

      d.   Administer IV H_2 antagonists.

      e.   Maintain neomycin schedule to prevent hepatic encephalopathy.

      f.   Maintain antacid regimen (if ordered).

      g.   Administer propranolol, as ordered. This medication may be used to decrease heart rate, decrease cardiac output, or decrease hepatic venous pressure.

𝓶 **13.**   **Administer vasopressin with titration to bleeding. This drug is used when sclerotherapy is contraindicated.**

      a.   20 units/100 mL D5W over 20 minutes with maintenance infusion of 0.1–0.5 units/min.

𝓶   b.   **Wean slowly over 24 hours when medication is to be discontinued.**

𝓶   c.   **Phentolamine mesylate is a subcutaneous antidote.**

      d.   Administer through central line only.

      e.   Use with caution in patients with coronary artery disease or prepare to run NTG simultaneous drip.

14. Maintain proper use of Sengstaken-Blakemore tube (Fig. 7-1):

      a.   Explain procedure to patient.

      b.   Check balloons for patency.

      c.   Lavage stomach prior to insertion PRN.

      d.   Monitor patient during insertion of tube by physician.

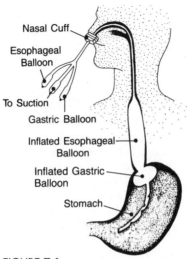

FIGURE 7-1.
Sengstaken-Blakemore tube.

 e. Monitor inflated pressures after insertion.
 f. Connect gastric port to low intermittent suction.
 g. Obtain x-ray to confirm placement.
 h. Maintain traction to tube if ordered.
 i. Label lumens of tube.
 j. Have available at bedside a second NGT, Yankauer suction, and scissors.
 k. Assess for potential complications, including rupture or deflation of balloon(s), pulmonary aspiration, esophageal rupture.

 15. Be familiar with sclerotherapy: injection of a coagulating agent into the varices to stop the bleed.
 a. Paravariceal injection: into the surrounding tissue
 b. Intravariceal injection: into the lumen of the varix

16. Be familiar with endoscopic band ligation (EBL), which involves banding of the varice with no risk of ulcer, strictures, or perforation.

 17. Be aware of the potential need for a transjugular intrahepatic portasystemic shunt (an invasive angiographic procedure done under fluoroscopy to decrease portal hypertension).

18. Surgery may also be indicated:
 a. Nonselective surgical shunt: to decompress the portal system
 b. Selective surgical shunts: to decompress the circulation to esophageal varices

19. Administer preprocedural care that includes patient/family education and baseline assessment.

20. Administer postprocedural patient care.

 n a. **Assess frequently for bleeding: H and H, PT, PTT, decreased blood pressure, tachycardia, and increased abdominal pain.**

      b.   Assess frequently for fluid volume deficit.

      c.   Assess for infection.

  21. Be aware of potential complications including:

      a.   **Bleeding from intrahepatic vessels and/or puncture site**

      b.   Thrombosis

      c.   Development of intrahepatic arteriovenous or arterioportal fistulas

      d.   Stent migration

      e.   Allergic reaction to contrast medium/medications

      f.   Infection

G. **Evaluation**

  1. The patient maintains stable vital signs.

  2. The patient reports absence of pain.

  3. The patient demonstrates independent self-care.

  4. The patient tolerates ordered diet.

  5. The patient demonstrates the ability to cope with ongoing stressors.

H. **Home health considerations**

  1. The client will verbalize understanding of diet:

      a.   Avoid spicy and gas-forming, low-roughage foods.

      b.   Consume frequent, small meals.

  2. The patient will verbalize signs and symptoms to report to physician:

      a.   Increased abdominal girth

      b.   Changes in level of consciousness

      c.   Increased pain

      d.   Changes in vital signs

      e.   Bleeding

  3. The client will maintain medication regimen and will have knowledge of:

      a.   Dose, route, frequency

      b.   Side effects

      c.   Food interactions

  4. The patient will verbalize stress-reducing strategies.

  5. The patient will maintain appropriate physician visitation.

IV. Ulcers

A. **Description: erosion of the GI mucosa into the submucosa and/or deeper. Ulceration can occur anywhere along the tract when the affected area is exposed to pepsin and hydrochloric acid. Sites include:**

  1. Esophagus

  2. Stomach

  3. Duodenum

  4. Margin of gastrojejunal anastomosis. This ulceration occurs post-surgery.

B. **Etiology and incidence**

  1. Men are affected four times more frequently than women.

  2. Ulcer disease may be chronic, with exacerbation associated with infection or stress.

  3. *Helicobacter pylori* **may be a major cause of ulcer development.**

  4. Duodenal ulcers occur more frequently than gastric ulcers, with seasonal occurrence.

  5. There are familial tendencies to have ulcers.

6. **Occurs more commonly in those with type O blood.**
7. Increased incidence in postmenopausal women.
8. Associated with stress, smoking, and drug (NSAIDs) and/or alcohol usage.
9. Stress ulcers: develop secondary to physiologic stress.

C. Pathophysiology
1. The gastric mucosa is protected by columnar epithelial cells that secrete bicarbonate, a mucous gel that is stimulated by prostaglandins and a rich blood supply.
2. Ulcer formation occurs owing to an imbalance in the protective barrier's ability to resist the damage from hydrochloric acid and pepsin. An increase in acid production causes:
   a. Increased acid and/or pepsin-producing cells in the stomach
   b. Increased parietal cell sensitivity to food, alcohol, and caffeine
   c. Excess vagal stimulation
   d. Decreased production of gastric secretions as food passes out of the stomach and into the intestines
3. *H. pylori*: a gram-negative rod bacterium which penetrates the mucosal gel layer and produces large amounts of urease (which splits urea into ammonia, CO_2, and bicarbonate), which leads to ulceration.

D. Assessment
1. Health history should include information regarding:
   a. Positive family history
   b. Alcohol abuse
   c. Cigarette smoking
   d. Chronic renal failure
   e. COPD
   f. Chronic pancreatitis
2. Medication history should include:
   a. Aspirin usage
   b. NSAID usage
   c. Corticosteroid usage
3. Clinical manifestations include pain, anxiety, irritability, anemia, and guaiac-positive stools.
4. Symptoms specifically related to a gastric ulcer include pain, and burning pressure in the high left epigastrium radiating to the back and upper abdomen.
   a. Pain is aggravated 1–2 hours after food consumption
   b. Nausea and vomiting occasionally occur.
   c. Weight loss occurs.
5. Symptoms specifically related to a duodenal ulcer include burning pain and cramping across the epigastrium:
   a. Pain occurs 2–4 hours after meals, in mid-afternoon, in the middle of the night, and is intermittent.
   b. Pain is relieved by foods and antacids.
   c. Nausea and vomiting occur occasionally.
6. Laboratory and diagnostic studies may include:
   a. Upper GI series
   b. Upper GI endoscopy
   c. Gastric acid analysis

> d. Serum gastric level test
> e. CBC, PT, PTT
> f. Serum electrolytes
> g. Liver enzymes
> h. Urinalysis
> i. Guaiac stool

E. Nursing diagnoses
1. Knowledge Deficit
2. Pain
3. Ineffective Individual Coping
4. Altered Nutrition: Less than Body Requirements
5. Risk for Injury
6. Impaired Adjustment

F. Planning and implementation
1. Promote pain relief.
   a. Promote physical and emotional rest with a quiet, calm environment.
   b. Identify stressful situations and assist patient with relaxation techniques and other methods to cope with stress.
   c. Encourage smoking cessation.
   d. Increase water consumption according to physical status.
   e. Administer medications as ordered.
2. Maintain adequate nutritional status.

   𝖓 a. **Eliminate foods and beverages that promote production of HCL and pepsin secretion.**
   b. Encourage regularly scheduled meals in a relaxed environment.
3. Administer medications as ordered:
   a. Proton pump inhibitor: omeprazole inhibits acid secretion regardless of the source of stimulation. It is given orally after bleeding is controlled.

   𝖓 b. **Anticholinergics: inhibit cholinergic stimulation of gastric secretion.**
   c. **Antisecretory: H_2 receptor antagonists.**
   d. **Cytoprotective: produces an acid resistant barrier.**
   e. **Antacids: decrease gastric acidity and the acid content of chyme that enters to duodenum.**
   f. Antibiotics: treat *H. pylori*.
4. Prepare the patient for surgical intervention if necessary. Types of surgeries include:
   a. Gastrectomy
   b. Vagotomy
   c. Pyloroplasty
5. Maintain optimal postoperative care:
   a. Monitor fluid balance.
   b. Observe for signs of hemorrhage.
   c. Observe for signs of infection.

   𝖓 d. **Splint abdominal suture line to prevent rupture.**
   e. Observe for signs and symptoms of dumping syndrome.

6.   Be aware of potential complications:

  a.   Hemorrhage: most common complication with peptic ulcer disease, with the most commonly occurring site being the distal portion of the duodenum.

  b.   **Perforation: life-threatening without immediate treatment. Perforated duodenal ulcers are located on the posterior mucosal wall. Perforated gastric ulcers are commonly found on the lesser curvature of the stomach. Peritonitis is a complication of perforation.**

  c.   Gastric outlet obstruction: occurs when scar tissue forms from healing and then breaks down. This commonly occurs in the antrum, pre-pyloric, and pyloric areas.

G.   Evaluation

  1.   The patient reports less pain.
  2.   The patient will maintain adequate nutritional status.
  3.   The patient will maintain medication regimen.
  4.   The patient demonstrates and complies with life-style modifications.

H.   Home health considerations

  1.   Teach client life-style changes.
  2.   Encourage client to stop smoking.
  3.   Instruct patient on medication regimen.
  4.   Encourage rest and stress reduction.
  5.   Maintain adequate diet.
  6.   Teach the client signs and symptoms of potential complications.

V.   Gastrointestinal hemorrhage

A.   Description: any degree of injury to the epithelium along the GI tract, resulting in bleeding characterized by hematemesis, melena, or hematochezia.

  1.   Upper GI bleed: site of bleeding above the ligament of Treitz at the duodenojejunal junction
  2.   Lower GI bleed: site of bleeding below the ligament of Treitz

B.   Etiology and incidence

  1.   Bleeding from the GI tract may range from chronic, intermittent, to massively severe. Upper GI bleed affects 50 to 150 people per 100,000 population.
  2.   Causes of upper GI bleeding include peptic ulceration, Mallory-Weiss tears, esophagogastric varices, and reflux esophagitis.
  3.   Causes of lower GI bleeding include carcinoma of the left colon, diverticular disease, polyps, and inflammatory bowel disease.

C.   Pathophysiology

  1.   **Upper GI bleeding: there is generally a loss of 25% of intravascular blood volume. It is usually a slower flow from venous or capillary vessels and presents with vomiting of blood or black, tarry stools or both.**
  2.   Lower GI bleeding presents with passage of bright red blood from the rectum.
  3.   The severity of the bleeding depends on the origin:

    a.   Venous

    b.   Capillary

    c.   Arterial

D. **Assessment**

    1.   Health history should include:

        a.   Past health history of peptic ulcer disease, previous bleeding episodes and treatment used, smoking, and/or use of alcohol.

        b.   **Medication history indicating usage of aspirin, NSAIDs, corticosteroids and anticoagulants.**

    2.   Clinical manifestations include:

        a.   **Changes in level of consciousness or restlessness**

        b.   **Vital sign changes such as tachycardia and hypotension**

        c.   Appearance of neck veins

        d.   Skin color and temperature: pale, cool, clammy, jaundice

        e.   Decreased capillary refill

        f.   Abdomen may be distended with guarding and decreased peristalsis

    3.   Laboratory and diagnostic tests

        a.   H and H, CBC, PT/PTT

        b.   Clotting times

        c.   Type and crossmatch

        d.   Serum electrolytes

        e.   BUN and creatinine

        f.   Serum glucose

        g.   Urinalysis

        h.   Guaiac stools

        i.   Chest x-ray and abdominal films

        j.   Liver function enzymes

        k.   Upper GI studies or endoscopy

        l.   ECG

E. **Nursing diagnoses**

    1.   Fluid Volume Deficit

    2.   Altered Tissue Perfusion: Peripheral

    3.   Altered Tissue Perfusion: Renal, Cerebral

    4.   Anxiety

    5.   Ineffective Individual Coping

    6.   Altered Nutrition: Less than Body Requirements

    7.   Impaired Adjustment

F. **Planning and implementation**

    1.   Promote pain relief.

        a.   **Assess and record description, location, duration, and character of pain q2hr–q4hr and PRN.**

        b.   Instruct patient to use relaxation and distraction techniques.

        c.   Administer pain medications as ordered and document outcome.

        d.   Provide back rubs.

    2.   Ensure adequate nutrition:

        a.   Obtain baseline nutritional assessment.

        b.   Maintain patient NPO.

      c.   Maintain NGT until stable.

      d.   Maintain accurate I and O.

3.   Administer medications as ordered and appropriate.

      a.   Administer IM/IV analgesics, as ordered.

      b.   **IV replacement with Ringer's lactate and normal saline to replace vascular volume at the rate it was lost. Observe for fluid overload.**

      c.   Administer blood products (if ordered).

      d.   Administer IV histamine receptor antagonists: inhibits the action of histamine on the H_2 receptors, therefore decreasing gastric acid output and concentration.

      e.   Antacids, as ordered.

      f.   Vasopressin infusion, as ordered.

4.   Be aware of technical interventions:

      a.   Endoscopic electrocoagulation: sealing the vessel thermally

      b.   Transcatheter embolization: injection of a selected embolic material through the catheter into the bleeding artery

      c.   Photocoagulation: coagulation achieved through lasers

5.   Be aware of surgical interventions:

      a.   Upper GI bleed: refers to ulcer disease

      b.   Lower GI bleed: colectomy, segmental resection, colon resection

6.   Be aware of potential complications:

      a.   Gastrointestinal perforation

      b.   Peritonitis

      c.   Sepsis

      d.   Hypovolemic shock

      e.   Death

G.   **Evaluation**

1.   The patient will maintain adequate fluid balance.

2.   The patient will maintain stable vital signs.

3.   The patient will demonstrate the ability to cope with ongoing stressors.

4.   The patient will tolerate diet as prescribed.

H.   **Home health considerations**

1.   Activity level recommendations include:

      a.   Gradual return to full activity, alternating periods of rest with activity

      b.   **Avoidance of heavy activity and straining**

2.   Dietary recommendations include:

      a.   Follow prescribed diet, avoiding irritating foods.

      b.   Eat frequent small meals.

      c.   Avoid stress during and after meals.

      d.   Provide rest periods after meals.

3.   Medication recommendations include:

      a.   Maintain compliance with medication therapy.

      b.   Avoid acetylsalicylic acid (ASA) or medications containing ASA.

      c.   **Avoid NSAIDs and over-the-counter medications.**

4. Reportable signs and symptoms the client needs to understand include: presence of pain, abdominal distention, nausea, vomiting, or diarrhea or blood in stool.

VI. Bowel obstruction

A. Description: the lack of movement of intestinal contents through the GI tract. Classified by the area of the bowel affected and also classified as mechanical or functional obstructions.

1. Small bowel: small intestine affected most frequently, with the ileum most commonly affected.
2. Large bowel: accounts for only 15% of all obstructions, with the sigmoid colon most commonly affected.

B. Etiology and incidence

1. Bowel obstruction can occur anywhere throughout the GI tract. Sixty percent of all small bowel obstructions are related to adhesions.
2. Functional causes of obstruction include:
   a. Sepsis
   b. Intestinal ischemia
   c. Hypokalemia
   d. Peritonitis
   e. Narcotic usage
   f. Prolonged intestinal distension
2. Mechanical causes of obstruction include those:
   a. Contained within the lumen: neoplasms, meconium, intussusception, large gallstones
   b. Extending into bowel wall: radiation, neoplasms, diverticulitis, congenital stenosis, congenital atresia
   c. Outside the bowel: adhesions, hernias, abscesses, neoplasms, volvulus, and stomal stenosis

C. Pathophysiology

1. Intestinal contents, fluid, and gas collect proximal to the obstruction, causing distension.

2. **With distension, there is an increase in fluid and pressure within the lumen of the bowel.**
3. **Increased pressure leads to increased capillary permeability and movement of fluid and electrolytes into the peritoneal cavity, which may cause the bowel to rupture.**
4. Extravasation of fluids into the peritoneal cavity decreases the circulating blood volume, resulting in hypovolemic shock.
5. A closed-loop obstruction is one in which the intestinal lumen is blocked in two different areas.
6. A volvulus is a strangulating obstruction that is life-threatening.

D. Assessment

1. A complete health history, particularly including past surgical information, is helpful.
2. Clinical manifestations vary depending on location:
   a. Abdominal distension
   b. Obstipation
   c. Constipation
   d. Cramping abdominal pain

       e.   High-pitched bowel sound above the area of obstruction

       f.   Emesis

       g.   Hypokalemia and dehydration with prolonged obstruction

  3.   Laboratory and diagnostic tests

       a.   CXR

       b.   Abdominal x-rays (upright and lateral)

       c.   Barium enema: helpful in diagnosis of large bowel obstruction: however, is not used when a perforation is suspected

       d.   Sigmoidoscopy

       e.   Colonoscopy

       f.   CBC

       g.   Serum electrolytes, amylase, BUN

E. **Nursing diagnoses**

  1.   Acute Pain

  2.   Ineffective Breathing Pattern

  3.   Fluid Volume Deficit

  4.   Potential for Impaired Skin Integrity

  5.   Potential for Aspiration

  6.   Anxiety

  7.   Ineffective Individual Coping

  8.   Altered Nutrition: Less than Body Requirements

F. **Planning and implementation**

  1.   Pain relief will be achieved.

       a.   Administer analgesics and record outcome.

       b.   Assess vital signs q2hr and PRN.

       c.   Teach and encourage relaxation techniques.

       d.   **Assess and document description, location, and duration of pain q2hr–q4hr and PRN.**

       e.   Promote a relaxing, restful environment.

  2.   Maintain adequate nutritional status:

       a.   **Nasogastric and intestinal tubes are initially used for decompression.**

       b.   Explain all procedures to the patient.

  3.   Position patient appropriately:

       a.   Semi- to high-Fowler's for NGT

       b.   Right side with intestinal tube

  4.   Assess tube for patency q4hr and PRN.

  5.   Provide mouth care PRN.

  6.   Maintain accurate I and O.

  7.   Administer medications as prescribed.

  8.   Maintain IV therapy.

  9.   Prepare for surgical intervention if necessary.

  10.   Teach patient turning, coughing, and deep breathing and demonstrate use of incentive spirometry.

  11.   Postoperative wound care:

       a.   **Observe for signs and symptoms of hemorrhage and infection at site.**

       b.   Splint abdominal incision when moving patient PRN.

12. Be aware of potential complications:
    a. Bowel necrosis: impaired circulation with volvulus and closed-loop obstruction
    b. Perforation: results from overdistension with sepsis; results in a very high mortality rate

G. Evaluation
1. The patient has relief from intestinal obstruction.
2. The patient exhibits return of normal bowel function.
3. The patient verbalizes minimal to no pain.
4. The patient demonstrates appropriate nutritional status with return of fluid and electrolyte values to normal.
5. The patient demonstrates appropriate coping mechanisms.

H. Home health considerations
1. Inform the client to avoid heavy lifting at home and to slowly return to previous level of activity.
2. Follow prescribed diet and avoid stress during and after meals.
3. Assess wound for signs and symptoms of infection and cleanse and dress wound as ordered.

VII. Gastrointestinal cancer

A. Description: malignant neoplastic disease that can occur throughout the GI tract (Display 7-3).
1. Esophageal: squamous cell carcinoma is the most common form, with the incidence increasing with age.
2. Gastric: an adenocarcinoma that may be caused by such factors as carcinogenic chemical and oncogenic viruses.
3. Small intestine: cancer of the small intestine is extremely rare; adenocarcinoma is the most common type and occurs most frequently in the duodenum and/or the upper part of the jejunum.
4. Large bowel/rectum: this type of cancer is the second most common cause of death in the United States; it is a malignant tumor that develops from the epithelial lining of the bowel and/or rectum, usually an adenocarcinoma.

B. Nursing diagnoses
1. Colonic Constipation or Diarrhea
2. Abdominal pain
3. Anxiety
4. Body Image Disturbance
5. Altered Nutrition: Less than Body Requirements
6. Knowledge Deficit

C. Planning and implementation
1. Promote pain relief.
    a. Teach patient techniques to decrease the pain.
    b. **Assess and document location, duration, and character of pain q2hr–q4hr and PRN using the 1 to 10 scale.**
    c. Reposition q2hr and PRN.
    d. Instruct patient in relaxation and diversionary activities.
    e. Administer pain medications, as ordered.
    f. Splint incision during turning, coughing, and deep breathing immediately postoperatively.
    g. Assess incision for tenderness and abdominal distention.

DISPLAY 7-3.
Etiology, Pathophysiology, Manifestations, and Diagnostic Studies Related to GI Cancer

ESOPHAGEAL

Etiology: Unknown, predisposing risk factors include: cigarette smoking, excessive alcohol intake, poor oral hygiene, spicy foods, and chronic trauma.

Pathophysiology: Malignant tumors form along middle to end of the esophagus. May penetrate through the muscular layer and protrude outside the esophageal wall.

Manifestations: Progressive dysphagia and belching. Substernal epigastric pain develops later. May penetrate into the back and radiate to the neck. Pain increases with swallowing. Weight loss is common and there may be regurgitation of blood-streaked esophageal contents with esophageal stenosis.

Diagnostic studies: Barium swallow esophagoscopy with biopsy, endoscopic ultrasonography, bronchoscopy, CBCPT/PTT

GASTRIC

Etiology: Unknown. Ingestion of nitrates can form nitrosoamines and nitrosomides through digestion. Refrigeration of foods and vitamin C intake inhibit nitrosocarcinogen. Increased incidence with blood type A. 75% of carcinomas found in the distal third of the stomach.

Pathophysiology: Protruding mass which invades both the lumen and wall of the stomach. Found most often in the antrum. May occur as a superficial tumor involving only the gastric mucosa (rare).

Manifestations: When advanced: anorexia, weight loss, abdominal pain. With an obstructive mass: dysphagia, substernal pain, weight loss, some regurgitation of food several hours after a meal. With an ulcerated mass: pain after food consumption not relieved by food or antacids.

Diagnostic studies: Esophagoscopy with biopsy, endoscopy, cytology, gastric secretory studies, serum CEA, FSA

SMALL BOWEL

Etiology: Unknown.

Pathophysiology: Lymphomas found along the distal portion impair motility as nerve endings are affected.

Manifestations: Depending on location: abdominal pain, mass in right abdomen, vomiting, weight loss, diarrhea, intermittent bowel obstruction, GI bleeding possible.

Diagnostic studies: Barium x-ray, abdominal ultrasound, esophagoscopy

LARGE BOWEL/RECTUM (COLORECTAL)

Etiology: Unknown. High-calorie, high-fat diet of the western world plays a part. Increased incidence with age and family history of cancer. History of ulcerative colitis and with familial polyps. The incidence of tumors of the right side of the colon is slowly increasing; however the majority still originate in the sigmoid and rectum.

Pathophysiology: Adenocarcinoma is the most common. The cancer seems to develop from adenomatous polyps. The growth rate of the tumors are slow. By the time symptoms do appear, it may have spread into the layers of the colon.

Manifestations: Present according to size, location, and extent of the tumor. Right-sided—melena, dull abdominal pain, weight loss, anorexia, lethargy, and complaints of indigestion. Left-sided—changes in bowel habits, abdominal distention, rectal bleeding, constipation and diarrhea, ribbon-like stools, and feeling of incomplete emptying.

2. Promote adequate nutrition during medical or surgical treatment.
    a. Maintain TPN or enteral feedings, as ordered.
    b. Maintain accurate I and O.
    c. Weigh patient daily.

 d. **Instruct patient at discharge the importance of a high-fiber, low-fat diet, as tolerated.**
    e. Provide a calm, stress-free environment during meals.
    f. Avoid gas-forming foods if ileostomy/colostomy is in place.
3. Maintain medication regimen:
    a. Evaluate IV therapy, as ordered.
    b. Administer chemotherapy (if ordered).
    c. Maintain radiation schedule (if ordered).
4. Prepare patient for surgical intervention, if necessary:
    a. Teach pre-operative breathing and positioning.
    b. Demonstrate use of incentive spirometry.
    c. Explain or clarify procedure with patient and family, as needed.
    d. Arrange for consultation with enterostomal therapist, as needed.
5. Maintain wound/stoma care.
    a. Assess wound for signs and symptoms of infection at least q4hr.
    b. Assess stoma for integrity every shift.
    c. Maintain adequate skin integrity on an ongoing basis.

d. **Assess abdomen for distention and tenderness.**
    e. Teach proper use of sitz baths for perineal area as needed.
6. Be aware of potential complications:
    a. Intestinal obstruction
    b. Intra-abdominal bleeding
    c. Peritonitis
    d. Paralytic ileus
    e. Metastatic disease

D. Evaluation
1. The patient verbalizes decreased pain.
2. The patient demonstrates adequate nutritional intake.
3. The patient exhibits adequate coping strategies.
4. The patient demonstrates appropriate colostomy care.
5. The patient maintains normal bowel function.

E. Home health considerations: implement teaching strategies as in bowel obstruction

VIII. Ischemic bowel

A. Description: insufficient arterial mesenteric vascular supply of the celiac axis, the superior mesenteric artery, and the inferior mesenteric artery.

B. Etiology and incidence
1. Occurs in patients over 50 years old with a history of diabetes mellitus, arteriosclerosis, and impaired cardiac output.
2. Thrombosis or embolus is in the splanchnic bed.

    3. Drug-overdose patients may incur ischemic bowel after treatment for hypovolemia.

    4. Post–angioplastic surgery for ruptured aortic aneurysm.

    5. Prolonged hypotensive states.

    6. Sepsis.

C. Pathophysiology

    1. A transient or prolonged interruption to the oxygenated vascular supply to the splanchnic vessels can cause necrosis.

    2. Intestinal hypoxia causes edema and mucosal lesions, which can lead to hemorrhage.

    3. Lesions may become infected with pathogenic organism specific to the colon.

D. Assessment

    1. Health history will reveal a positive history of diabetes mellitus, atherosclerosis, cardiac failure.

    2. The patient may report a weight loss.

    3. Clinical manifestations include:

        a. Insidious onset of symptoms

        b. Complaints of obscure diffuse abdominal pain especially after eating

        c. Possible bloody diarrhea

        d. Abdominal distention and tenderness

        e. Nausea and vomiting

        f. Fever and leukocytosis

        g. Fluid and electrolyte imbalances

    4. Laboratory and diagnostic tests

        a. CBC

        b. ABG

        c. Serum electrolytes, amylase, and alkaline phosphatase

        d. Abdominal x-rays

        e. Barium enema (only if vascular disease is ruled out)

        f. Mesenteric arteriography

E. Nursing diagnoses

    1. Pain

    2. Anxiety

    3. Altered Nutrition: Less than Body Requirements

    4. Altered Tissue Perfusion: Intestinal

    5. Fluid Volume Deficit

F. Planning and implementation

    1. Manage pain adequately:

        a. Assess and document pain on a scale of 1 to 10 noting onset, location, duration.

        b. Administer IV or IM analgesics as ordered.

        c. Teach relaxation techniques.

        d. Provide a calm, relaxing environment.

    2. Promote adequate nutrition:

        a. Insert NGT and maintain NPO status to rest compromised bowel.

        b. Maintain IV therapy pre- and postoperatively.

        c. Postoperatively, advance diet as patient tolerates.

       d.   Maintain accurate I and O.

       e.   Weigh patient daily.

  3. Administer medications, as ordered:

       a.   Initially, IV therapy consists of crystalloid solutions to treat hypotension and shock.

       b.   Administer blood if bleeding is present.

       c.   Administer IV vasodilator, as ordered.

       d.   Initiate and maintain IV antibiotics, as ordered.

  4. Prepare patient for surgical intervention:

       a.   Explain operative procedure as needed.

       b.   Teach postoperative turning, coughing, and deep breathing.

       c.   Insert nasogastric tube if not already done.

  5. Maintain wound/stoma:

       a.   Assess for signs and symptoms of hemorrhage.

       b.   Assess for signs and symptoms of infection.

       c.   Splint incision during turning, coughing, and deep breathing.

       d.   Reinforce stoma teaching from enterostomal therapist.

  6. Be aware of potential complications such as intestinal infarction and gangrenous necrosis.

G. **Evaluation**

  1. The patient will express relief of pain.

  2. The patient will demonstrate adequate nutritional status.

  3. The patient will maintain adequate fluid and electrolyte balance.

  4. The patient will maintain adequate intestinal perfusion.

H. **Home health considerations**

  1. Visitation of home health nurse on a regular weekly basis.

  2. Establishment of wound/stoma care regimen.

  3. Compliance with follow-up physician visitation.

IX. **Abdominal trauma (see Chapter 13)**

X. **Gastrointestinal fistula**

A. **Description: an abnormal tunnel or tract between two or more structures.**

B. **Etiology and incidence**

  1. Predisposing contributors include irradiation, cancer, ulcerative colitis, Crohn's disease, trauma, diverticulitis, and small bowel obstruction.

  2. Failure of abdominal incision to close is the most common cause.

C. **Pathophysiology**

  1. Categorized specifically to location in the body.

  2. The fistulas can also be categorized according to volume of output.

       a.   **High output: greater than 500 mL/24 hours.**

       b.   **Low output: less than 500 mL/24 hours.**

  3. There is usually an infected mucosal abrasion.

D. **Assessment**

  1. Clinical manifestations include:

       a.   Drainage of fluid or feces through an opening in the skin with external fistulas

       b.   Passage of feces, gas through the urethra or vagina with an internal fistula

       c.   Fever

2.   Laboratory and diagnostic tests:
 a.   Fistulogram
 b.   Gastrografin enema
 c.   Tampon placement into the vagina with methylene blue instillation
 d.   CBC, serum electrolytes
 e.   Effluent analysis for volume and composition

E.   Nursing diagnoses
1.   Pain
2.   Altered Nutrition: Less than Body Requirements
3.   Impaired Skin Integrity
4.   Fluid Volume Deficit

F.   Planning and implementation
1.   Maintain medication regimen:
 a.   Administer pain medication and analgesics, as ordered.
 b.   Promote a relaxing environment and utilize relaxation techniques.
 c.   Record pain on a scale of 1 to 10 noting onset, intensity, location, and duration.
2.   Maintain adequate nutritional status:
 a.   Maintain accurate I and O every shift.
 b.   Obtain daily weights.
 c.   Administer parenteral and enteral solutions as ordered.
 d.   Document daily caloric intake with calorie counts.
 e.   Monitor serum electrolytes, protein and albumin levels.
3.   Maintain skin integrity and wound care:
 a.   Reposition q2hr.
 b.   Prevent shearing or friction.
 c.   Apply moisture barriers to affected areas as ordered.
 d.   Teach patient to us a pouch as needed on stoma.
4.   Be aware of potential complications such as bowel necrosis and GI abscess.

G.   Evaluation
1.   The patient reports decreased pain.
2.   The patient demonstrates adequate nutritional intake.
3.   The patient demonstrates appropriate skin care measures.
4.   The patient is free from fever.

H.   Home health considerations
1.   Visitation of a home health nurse to ensure proper skin care should be arranged.
2.   Stress importance of adequate caloric intake for tissue repair.
3.   Ensure adherence to medication regimen.

XI.   Peritonitis

A.   Description: an acute or chronic inflammatory process of the peritoneum resulting from trauma or rupture of an abdominal organ into the peritoneal space.

B.   Etiology and incidence
1.   Chemical irritants such as blood, bile, and pancreatic enzymes can lead to peritonitis.

2. Bacterial invasion status after ruptured appendix, perforated bowel, and ruptured intestines contributes to peritonitis. The most common organism found is *Escherichia coli* or *Streptococcus*.
3. Can also present following abdominal surgery.

M. **Pathophysiology**

1. **Immune and inflammatory responses are activated when bacteria come in contact with the peritoneal space.**
2. Continued peritoneal exposure causes mast cells to release histamine and vasoactive substances, increasing capillary permeability.
3. Fibrinous exudates form, in an attempt to contain the offending agent.
4. Third spacing and hypovolemia can occur, secondary to action of vasoactive substances.

D. **Assessment**

1. **Clinical manifestations include boardlike abdominal rigidity, abdominal pain, rebound tenderness, abdominal distension, diminished or absent bowel sounds, nausea, vomiting, fever, tachypnea, tachycardia, restlessness, acidosis, oliguria, confusion, and/or disorientation.**
2. Laboratory and diagnostic tests:
   a. CBC, serum electrolyte
   b. Liver and renal function studies
   c. Blood cultures
   d. ABGs
   e. Abdominal x-rays
   f. Ultrasound and CT scans
   g. Paracentesis to examine for bacteria, blood, bile, amylase, and pus

E. **Nursing diagnoses**

1. Abdominal Pain
2. Fluid Volume Deficit
3. Altered Nutrition: Less than Body Requirements
4. Anxiety
5. Ineffective Breathing Pattern

F. **Planning and implementation**

1. Pain management will be implemented:
   a. Monitor for pain q2hr and PRN.
   b. Administer analgesics as ordered and document response.
   c. Reposition for comfort.
2. Maintain adequate nutrition:
   a. Weigh daily.
   b. Maintain TPN as ordered.
   c. Accurately monitor I and O.
   d. Monitor serum electrolyte levels.
    e. **Administer antiemetics as ordered to decrease nausea and vomiting.**
    f. **Maintain NPO status and NGT maintenance.**

 3. **Adhere to medication regimen after offending organism has been identified including antibiotics and sedatives or narcotics.**

4. Prepare patient for laparotomy or peritoneal lavage, if indicated:
    a. Monitor respiratory status carefully.
    b. Position in semi-Fowler's position.
    c. Monitor vital signs as ordered and PRN.
5. Ensure adequate wound care is maintained:

   a. **Assess wound for signs and symptoms of inflammation.**
   b. Maintain patency of Jackson-Pratt drain and/or Penrose drain.
   c. Protect skin around drains and incision.

6. **Be aware of potential complications:**
    a. **Hypovolemic shock**
    b. **Septicemia**
    c. **Intra-abdominal abscess**
    d. **Paralytic ileus**
    e. **Organ failure (liver and kidney)**

G. Evaluation
1. The patient will verbalize adequate abdominal pain relief.
2. The patient will maintain sufficient nutritional intake.
3. The patient will have resolution of inflammation.

XII. Necrotic bowel (see Ischemic bowel)
XIII. Perforated bowel

A. Description: a hole in the bowel that causes the contents to flow into the peritoneal cavity.

B. Etiology and incidence
1. Results from ruptures of the appendix and diverticulum.
2. Secondary to surgical procedures of the bowel or adjacent organs.
3. Secondary to diagnostic tests such as an endoscopy.
4. Status after ingestion of foreign bodies.
5. Secondary to trauma.
6. Chronic constipation.

C. Pathophysiology (see Peritonitis). The most commonly found organisms are *E. Coli, Staphylococcus, Pneumococcus, Streptococcus, Pseudomonas aeruginosa* and *Clostridium perfringens*.

D. Assessment
1. Health history may include diverticulitis.

2. **Clinical manifestations include abdominal pain with boardlike rigidity, hypoactive bowel sounds, and leukocytosis. With progressive peritonitis, fever, dehydration, oliguria, shock, and death may occur.**
3. Laboratory and diagnostic tests
    a. Abdominal x-rays
    b. Upper GI x-ray with water-soluble contrast media
    c. CBC, serum electrolytes
    d. Blood and urine culture and sensitivity

E. Nursing diagnoses
1. Acute Pain
2. Ineffective Breathing Pattern
3. Decreased Cardiac Output
4. Anxiety

       5.   Potential for Aspiration

       6.   Potential for Infection

       7.   Ineffectual Individual Coping

  F.   **Planning and implementation**

       1.   Assess for presence of abdominal pain and treat appropriately.

       2.   Maintain adequate nutritional status by monitoring patient for changes in weight, I and O, and lab work.

       3.   Assess and maintain IV therapy with TPN implementation, as ordered.

       4.   Maintain medication regimen and ensure administration of oxygen therapy to decrease intestinal hypoxia.

       5.   Prepare patient for surgery by providing education and consultation with enterostomal therapist.

       6.   Manage postoperative wound care:

          a.   Assess for signs and symptoms of infection.

          b.   Maintain skin integrity around incision and any drains.

          c.   Change dressing as needed, noting color, odor, consistency, and amount of any drainage.

       7.   Be aware of potential complications such as shock, abscess, and death.

  G.   **Evaluation**

       1.   The patient will verbalize the absence of abdominal pain.

       2.   The patient will demonstrate adequate nutritional status.

       3.   The patient will demonstrate proper technique when performing wound care.

XIV. **Hypovolemic shock (see Chapter 13)**

XV. **Interventions in GI pathology: Whipple procedure—indicated with pancreatic carcinoma**

  A.   **Involves proximal pancreatectomy, duodenectomy, and partial gastrectomy**

  B.   **Palliative treatment may also include cholecystojejunostomy**

Bibliography

Beare, P. G., Myers, J. L. (1994). *Principles of adult health nursing* (2nd ed.). St. Louis: Mosby–Year Book.

Beyea, S. C. (1996). *Critical pathways for collaborative nursing care.* Menlo Park: Addison-Wesley Nursing.

Bouley, G., Grimshaw, K., Lendewall-Motto, D., & Kiernan, L. (1996). Transjugular intrahepatic portosystemic shunt: An alternative. *Crit Care Nurse* 16(1), 23–29.

Bowers, A. C., Thompson, J. M. *(1992). Clinical manual of health assessment.* St. Louis: Mosby–Year Book.

Clochesy, J. M., Brew, C., Cardis, S., Whittaker, A. A., & Rudy, E. B. (1996). *Critical care nursing* (2nd ed.). Philadelphia: W.B. Saunders.

Digestive tract cancers. Knowledge for practice: Part 1. (1995, December 6–12). *Nursing Times,* 91(49).

Digestive tract cancers. The art of nursing the patient with gastrointestinal cancer, and the use of self in counseling can help patients to understand their condition. (1995, December 13–19). *Nursing Times,* 91(50).

Fitzgerald, M., Berg-Gulcher, L. (1995). Pharmacological highlights: Diagnosis and treatment of *Helicobacter pylori* infection in peptic ulcer disease. *J Am Acad Nurse Pract* 7(5), 233–235.

LeMone, P., Burke, K. *(1996). Medical surgical nursing: Critical thinking in client care.* Menlo Park: Addison-Wesley Nursing.

Lewis, S. M., Collier, I. C., & Heitkemper, M. M. (1996). *Medical surgical nursing: Assessment and management of clinical problems* (4th ed.). St. Louis: Mosby–Year Book.

Marotta, R. B., Floch, M. H. (1991). Diet and nutrition in ulcer disease. *Med Clin North Am* 75, 967–979.

McKenry, L. M., Salerno, E. (1995). *Pharmacology in nursing.* St. Louis: Mosby–Year Book.

Moynihan, B. G. A. (1905). On duodenal ulcers: With notes of 52 Operations. *Lancet* i, 340–346.

North American Nursing Diagnosis Association (NANDA). (1996). *Nursing diagnoses: Definitions & classification 1997–1998.* Philadelphia: Author.

Pagano, K. D., Pagano, T. J. (1994). *Diagnostic testing and nursing implications: A care study* (4th ed.). St. Louis: Mosby–Year Book.

Perkal, M. F., Seashore, J. H. (1989). Nutrition and inflammatory bowel disease. *Gastroenterol Clin North Am* 18, 129–155.

Ruppert, S. D., Kernicki, J. G., & Dolan, J. T. (1996). *Dolan's critical care nursing: Clinical management through the nursing process* (2nd ed.). Philadelphia: F.A. Davis.

Saunders, C. E., Ho, M. T. (1992). *Current emergency diagnosis & treatment* (4th ed.). Norwalk, CT: Appleton & Lange.

Thelan, L. A., Davie, J. K., & Urden, L. D. (1990). *Textbook of critical care nursing: Diagnosis & management.* St. Louis: C.V. Mosby.

Zaloga, G. P. (1994). *Nutrition in critical care.* St. Louis: Mosby.

Zuckerman, G. R., Shuman, R. (1987). Therapeutic goals and treatment options for prevention of stress ulcer syndrome. *Am J Med* 83(Suppl. 6A), 29–35.

STUDY QUESTIONS

1. Assessment findings for a patient with esophageal varices would include:
   a. increased blood pressure
   b. increased heart rate
   c. decreased respiratory rate
   d. increased urinary output

2. The nurse would anticipate using which medication if sclerotherapy has not been used?
   a. neomycin
   b. propranolol
   c. vasopressin
   d. cimetidine

3. The nurse must be alert for complications with Sengstaken-Blakemore intubation including:
   a. pulmonary obstruction
   b. pericardiectomy syndrome
   c. pulmonary embolization
   d. cor pulmonale

4. Peptic ulcer disease may be caused by:
   a. *Helicobacter pylori*
   b. *Clostridium difficile*
   c. *Candida albicans*
   d. *Staphylococcus aureus*

5. Pain control with peptic ulcer disease includes all of the following except:
   a. promoting physical and emotional rest
   b. identifying stressful situations
   c. eating meals when desired
   d. administering medications that decrease gastric acidity

6. Peritonitis can occur as a complication of:
   a. septicemia
   b. multiple organ failure
   c. hypovolemic shock
   d. peptic ulcer disease

7. Nitrosocarcinogen production can be inhibited with intake of:
   a. vitamin C
   b. vitamin E
   c. carbohydrates
   d. fiber

8. A patient has become very depressed postoperatively after receiving a colostomy for GI cancer. He does not participate in his colostomy care or look at the stoma. An appropriate nursing diagnosis would be:
   a. Ineffective Individual Coping
   b. Knowledge Deficit
   c. Impaired Adjustment
   d. Anxiety

9. Abdominal assessment includes:
   a. inspect, percuss, palpate, auscultate.
   b. inspect, auscultate, palpate, percuss.
   c. inspect, auscultate, percuss, palpate.
   d. inspect, palpate, percuss, auscultate.

10. The nurse can expect a 60-year-old patient with ischemic bowel to report a history of:
   a. diabetes mellitus
   b. asthma
   c. Addison's disease
   d. cancer of the bowel

11. During initial assessment of a patient post-endoscopy, the nurse notes absent bowel sounds, tachycardia, and abdominal distention. The nurse would anticipate:
   a. ischemic bowel
   b. peritonitis
   c. hypovolemic shock
   d. perforated bowel.

12. Medication administered while caring for the patient described in question 11 above would include:
   a. cephalosporin, metronidazole, aminoglycosides
   b. metronidazole, cimetidine, famotidine
   c. famotidine, aminoglycosides, vitamin K
   d. aminoglycosides, vitamin K, clindamycin

ANSWER KEY

1. **Correct response: b**
   Tachycardia is an early sign of compensation.
   a, c, d. The opposite occurs in each response in response to hypovolemia.
   Analysis/Physiology/Assessment

2. **Correct response: c**
   Vasopressin is the drug of choice when sclerotherapy is contraindicated.
   a. Is used to prevent encephalopathy when blood is broken down.
   b. May or may not be used to decrease cardiac output and hepatic venous pressure.
   d. H_2 antagonists are commonly used.
   Application/Physiologic/Planning

3. **Correct response: a**
   Rupture or deflation of the balloon can result in upper airway obstruction.
   b, c, and d are not related to the Sengstaken-Blakemore tube.
   Analysis/Safe care/Assessment

4. **Correct response: a**
   H. pylori may be a major cause of ulcer development.
   b, c, and d are unrelated.
   Knowledge/Physiologic/NA

5. **Correct response: c**
   Meals should be regularly spaced in a relaxed environment.
   a, b, and d all are important interventions in providing pain control.
   Analysis/Health promotion/ Implementation

6. **Correct response: d**
   Perforation is a life-threatening complication of peptic ulcer disease and can result in peritonitis.
   a, b, and c apply directly to complications of peritonitis.
   Analysis/Physiologic/Assessment

7. **Correct response: a**
   Vitamin C and refrigeration of foods inhibit nitrosocarcinogen.

b, c, and d are not related to nitrosocarcinogen.
Knowledge/Health promotion/Planning

8. **Correct response: a**
   The patient is dealing with a disturbance in self-concept and difficulty coping with the newly established stoma.
   b, c, d. Initially the postoperative patient is just beginning the education process.
   Analysis/Psychosocial/Analysis

9. **Correct response: c**
   Auscultation is done before palpation because the nurse does not want to stimulate peristaltic movement, distorting auscultory sounds.
   a, b, and d are out of abdominal assessment sequence.
   Knowledge/Physiologic/Assessment

10. **Correct response: a**
    Ischemic bowel occurs in patients over 50 with a history of diabetes mellitus.
    b, c, and d are unrelated to ischemic bowel.
    Knowledge/Health promotion/ Evaluation

11. **Correct response: d**
    Invasive diagnostic testing can cause perforated bowel.
    a is not usually related; **b** can be a complication after initial perforation; **c** can occur if peritonitis is allowed to continue.
    Analysis/Safe care/Assessment

12. **Correct response: a**
    All and/or a combination of these medications can be administered.
    b, c, d. Although some of these are used for peritonitis, none are used consistently.
    Knowledge/Safe care/Analysis

The Biliary System

8

I. Anatomy and physiology
A. Structures
1. Liver
a. The liver is the largest organ in the body, weighing 3 pounds. It is encased in a fibrous capsule and lies in the upper right quadrant of the abdomen.

b. The liver is composed of four lobes containing lobules that are the functioning units of the liver. The four lobes are: the right, left, caudate, and quadrate.

c. Each lobule is composed of hepatocytes (liver cells) and its own blood supply called sinusoids. The phagocytic Kupffer cells are located within the sinusoids.

d. The main blood supply to the liver is transported via the hepatic artery and the portal vein emptying into the inferior vena cava via the hepatic veins.

e. The hepatic artery receives blood directly from the aorta and the portal vein drains the blood from the spleen and intestines.

f. Fibers from the vagus (parasympathetic) and celiac plexus (sympathetic) comprise the liver's nerve supply.

2. Biliary system
a. Hepatic lobules are the functional unit of the liver. The lobules consist of a network of small ducts called canaliculi.

b. The hepatic duct receives bile via the canaliculi that join to create larger bile ducts.

c. The common bile duct is formed by the joining of the hepatic and cystic ducts located in the liver and gallbladder respectively. The liquid contents of these ducts drain into the duodenum via the sphincter of Oddi.

d. Relaxing of the sphincter of Oddi permits the passage of bile into the duodenum.

e. The gallbladder is a pear-shaped hollow organ, 3 to 4 inches long, located on the undersurface of the right lobe of the liver.

f. Normal bile capacity is approximately 50 to 75 mL.

3. Pancreas
a. The pancreas is a long, slender organ, approximately 6 to 9 inches in length, which is situated behind the stomach and consists of three segments: head, body, and tail.

b. The organ is composed of lobules that form lobes.

c. The lobules have enzyme-producing acini that release their secretions into the duct of Wirsung or pancreatic duct.

d. The pancreas produces exocrine and endocrine secretion. The exocrine secretions are via the acini cells for digestive purposes. The endocrine secretions are associated with the islets of Langerhans whose cells are involved in the regulation of carbohydrate metabolism.

B. Functions
1. Liver

a. **The liver is the first organ to receive blood carrying the final products of digestion and decomposition products.**

      b.   From this blood the liver begins its enormous role in maintaining normal body functions.

  2. Major liver functions

      a.   Maintains normal serum glucose levels by means of glycogenesis, glycogenolysis, and gluconeogenesis.

      b.   Deaminizes amino acids, forming ammonia that is then converted into urea. Synthesizes nonessential amino acids, plasma proteins (albumin), vitamin A, and coagulation factors (fibrinogen, prothrombin), and is the source of heparin, an anticoagulant.

      c.   Breaks down triglycerides and fatty acids and stores and synthesizes excess fats. Also synthesizes cholesterol, lipoprotein, phospholipid, and excess fat.

      d.   Serves as a storage place for the fat-soluble vitamins A, D, E, K and B12, iron, and trace elements.

      e.   Detoxifies potentially harmful substances, eg, alcohol, poisons, and various toxic substances produced by the body. Metabolizes drugs and excretes their breakdown products.

      f.   Continuously secretes and excretes bile.

  3. Bile components:

      a.   Bile is composed of bilirubin, cholesterol, mucin, electrolytes, bile salts, fatty acids, lecithin, water, and various inorganic and organic substances.

      b.   Biliverdin: oxidation of bilirubin forming the greenish color in the bile.

      c.   Bilirubin: pigment from phagocytosed hemoglobin removed from the blood and chemically modified by conjugation to glucuronic acid and formed by the hepatocytes into bile.

      d.   Bile salts: synthesized from cholesterol, conjugated with amino acids for fat emulsification; recycling is achieved by reabsorption through the ileal mucosa and into the portal circulation for transport to the liver.

  4. Biliary system

      a.   Bile from the hepatocytes is transported to the gallbladder via an intricate drainage system.

      b.   Cholecystokinin, a duodenal hormone, stimulates the gallbladder to contract, thereby relaxing the sphincter of Oddi and releasing bile for digestion.

  5. The pancreas is composed of two basic cell types, endocrine and exocrine. Endocrine cells are discussed in Chapter 11. Functions of the pancreatic exocrine cells (acini) include:

      a.   production of a watery pancreatic juice rich in enzymes for digestion and bicarbonate to neutralize the acidic chyme

      b.   production of enzymes for digestion, consisting of amylase (hydrolyzes starch), trypsin (proteolytic enzyme that catalyzes the hydrolysis of peptide bonds), and lipase (breaks triglycerides into fatty acids and glycerol)

II. Overview of biliary pathology

  A. **Assessment**

    1. Determine the liver size by percussing along the right midclavicular line.

       a.   Percuss upward from tympany to dullness to assess the lower border.

       b.   Percuss downward from lung resonance until the tone changes to dullness for upper boarder assessment.

  2.   To estimate the liver span, mark each tone change and measure and record the distance between the marks.

  3.   Palpate the liver by utilizing two methods:

       a.   At the right midclavicular line along the costal margin gently place the fingertips deeply in and up and ask the patient to take a deep breath.

       b.   With fingers hooked over the right costal margin, press in and up and have the patient take a deep breath.

       c.   If the liver is palpable, assess for firmness, size, shape, pain, tenderness, and nodules; document all findings.

B. **Laboratory studies**

  1.   Liver function tests:

       a.   Direct, indirect, and total serum bilirubin

       b.   Urinary bilirubin

       c.   Urinary and fecal urobilinogen

       d.   Serum enzymes: alkaline phosphatase (ALP), serum glutamic-oxaloacetic transaminase (SGOT) or aspartate aminotransferase (AST), serum glutamic pyruvic transaminase (SGPT) or alanine aminotransferase (ALT), and gamma-glutamyl transferase (GGT)

       e.   Serum isoenzymes LDH

       f.   Serum total protein

       g.   Alpha-fetoprotein (AFP) serum markers for liver cancer

       h.   Serum ammonia levels

       i.   Coagulation studies

       j.   Serum cholesterol and glucose

       k.   Complete blood count (CBC) and platelets

       l.   Serum antigen and antibody for hepatitis

       m.   Serum electrolytes

       n.   Albumin/globulin (A/G) ratio

  2.   Indocyanine green (ICG) dye excretion test

       a.   Evaluates the liver's ability to take up and excrete dye.

       b.   Dye amount is based on the patient's weight, is injected, and blood samples are drawn q5min for 30 minutes

  3.   Aminoprine breath test

       a.   Assesses the liver's ability to metabolize compounds; determines prognosis, residual function, and response to therapy.

       b.   Dye, based on the patient's weight, is administered intravenously and breath samples are taken over a 2-hour period or longer, at specific intervals.

  4.   Pancreatic laboratory studies:

       a.   Serum amylase

       b.   Serum lipase

       c.   Urinary amylase

       d.   Renal amylase-creatinine clearance ratio

       e.   Fecal fat determination

   f. SGOT

   g. Serum glucose, calcium and triglycerides

   h. Carcinoembryonic antigen (CEA) levels

 5. Diagnostic testing: invasive and noninvasive diagnostic studies of the liver, biliary system, and pancreas

   a. Liver biopsy: A core of hepatic tissue is obtained via a needle insertion and analyzed for diagnoses of local or diffuse liver disease.

   b. Hepatobiliary ultrasound is used to identify tumors, cysts, abscesses, and visualize hepatic ducts.

   c. Liver scan is used to determine hepatomegaly, hepatic malignancy, cysts, or abscesses, and hepatocellular disease.

   d. Nuclear imaging scans will show shape, size, and position of an organ, along with any structural defects and functional disorders.

   e. Computed tomography (CT) scan can be done with or without contrast medium. This study can detect tumors, cysts, pseudocysts, abscesses, hematomas, and obstructions of the liver, biliary tract, and pancreas.

   f. **Ultrasonography aids in distinguishing between an obstruction and a nonobstruction, jaundice, and is helpful in the diagnosis of cholecystitis, gallstones, hematomas, pancreatitis, and metastatic disease. It also identifies edema, inflammation, fatty or fibrotic infiltrates, or calcifications.**

   g. Oral cholecystography visualizes and determines the patency of the gallbladder and biliary duct system.

   h. Cholescintigraphy is helpful in the diagnosis of early biliary duct obstruction and acute cholecystitis.

   i. Biliary drainage test or duodenal drainage test analyzes the color, volume, and contents of bile, which aids in detecting structural and functional hepatobiliary changes.

   j. Gallbladder ultrasound reveals gallstones and can be used for patients who are allergic to contrast media.

   k. Percutaneous transhepatic cholangiogram (PTC) reveals strictures or obstruction from tumors and/or stones and distinguishes between hepatic and extrahepatic jaundice.

   l. Splenoportogram evaluates the quality of portal blood flow.

   m. Magnetic resonance imaging (MRI) detects hepatic neoplasms, cysts, abscesses, and hematomas.

   n. Endoscopic retrograde cholangiopancreatography (ERCP) permits direct visualization of pancreatic and common bile ducts. It also can be used to take biopsy specimens from tumors for analysis, dilate strictures, retrieve a gallstone from the distal common bile duct (CBD), and aid in the diagnosis of pancreatitis and pancreatic cancer.

C. **Nutritional considerations**

 1. Acute pancreatitis

   a. Some controversy exists over the provision of parenteral nutrition with acute pancreatitis.

      b.   Although it has no immediate effect on the course of pancreatic inflammation, recent studies indicate potential complications of catheter infection, higher insulin requirements, and hyperglycemia. However, these risks are minimal in most cases.

      c.   Parenteral nutrition has been shown to significantly reduce morbidity and mortality rates if started within 72 hours of admission, particularly among malnourished patients.

      d.   Jejunal feeding has also been looked at as a potential route of nutrition support. New research has shown that intrajejunal feeds may not stimulate the pancreas. Besides maintaining gut integrity, this method avoids the inherent risks of parenteral nutrition.

      e.   Considerations for medical nutrition therapy

          ▶ The overall goal is to increase the nutrient intake to achieve caloric balance and meet intake needs.

          ▶ Monitor electrolytes and replace as required.

          ▶ Advance as tolerated to a high-carbohydrate, high-protein, low-fat diet.

  2. Chronic pancreatitis

      a.   Malabsorption tends to be the most significant of the dietary concerns, particularly of fat.

      b.   A high-fat diet may exacerbate the patient's symptoms.

      c.   Peripheral edema, hypoalbuminemia, hypovitaminosis, and essential fatty acid deficiency may also be evident.

      d.   Glucose intolerance is another major problem found in 40%–90% of patients. The onset of diabetes is usually 7 or more years after the diagnosis of chronic pancreatitis.

      e.   Considerations for medical nutrition therapy

          ▶ The overall goal is to increase the nutrient intake to achieve caloric balance and meet intake needs.

          ▶ A low-fat diet and/or diabetic diet as tolerated.

          ▶ Attention to fat-soluble vitamins must be considered.

  3. Liver disease

      a.   Nutritional deficiencies are common in liver disease.

      b.   Related factors that cause the deficits are decreased dietary intake, decreased absorption and hepatic storage, altered metabolism, and alcoholism.

      c.   Once failure is established, a mass of secondary complications can arise, such as malabsorption of fat.

      d.   Errors in metabolism of protein, carbohydrate, and vitamins occur as well.

      e.   There may also be marked depletion of muscle mass and lack of adequate glucose stores.

      f.   There is an alteration in the plasma amino acid pattern, with a rise in the aromatic amino acids (AAA) and a fall in the branch chain amino acids (BCAA).

      g.   Some speculate that the BCAAs, taken up by the extrahepatic tissue, provide a better source of protein.

h. Liver disease can pose a difficulty in evaluating nutritional status.

i. **The four major plasma proteins (albumin, prealbumin, retinol-binding protein, and transferrin) are synthesized by the liver and cannot be relied on as a marker for malnutrition.**

j. Midarm muscle circumference for somatic measures, and triceps skinfold for fat stores, may be skewed due to subclinical edema.

k. The use of blood urea nitrogen levels to interpret nitrogen balance may be affected by alterations in nitrogen metabolism.

l. Hypercatabolism often accompanies liver failure.

m. Increased glucagon, cortisol, and epinephrine levels stimulate the basal metabolic rate and the resting energy expenditure is altered.

n. Fat is used as a primary fuel source due to poor glucose and protein metabolism.

o. Considerations for medical nutrition therapy

  ▶ The overall goal is to increase the nutrient intake to achieve caloric balance and meet intake needs.

  ▶ Protein administration of 0.6–1.2 g/kg of body weight and 25–35 kcal/kg of body weight. If there is evidence of protein intolerance as evidenced by mental status changes, then the lower range should be administered. If there is no need for restrictions, then the upper range may be given.

  ▶ Use of enteral and parenteral formulas containing BCAAs are preferred in the treatment of hepatic encephalopathy.

  ▶ The carbohydrate source should provide approximately 40%–50% of the total calories. The addition of insulin may be necessary to control glucose intolerance.

  ▶ Medium chain diglyceride oil is beneficial as a fat source in short-term use. It requires less involvement from the liver than other fats.

D. **Psychosocial implications**

  1. Patients with disorders of the liver, biliary, or pancreatic system may encounter coping/stress tolerance difficulties associated with:

  a. Progression of the disease process

  b. Acute and/or chronic essence of the disease process

  c. Remorse related to the circumstances surrounding the disease process

  d. Functional restraints

  e. Pain

  2. Self-perception/self-concept difficulties may be influenced by:

  a. Performance of expected role/relationship in the family, social and work structure

  b. Changes in sexual function

  c. Dissatisfaction with personal sexuality

  d. Attitude involving body image and general self worth

  e. Potential self-care deficit

  f. Interruption of normal life-style may potentiate a mental health disorder.

E.   Commonly used medications

1.   Dramamine and Tigan are antiemetics used as supportive drug therapy in hepatitis.

m 2.   **Immune globulin (IG) is administered prophylactically as soon as possible after exposure to hepatitis A.**

3.   **Hepatitis B immune globulin (HBIG) provides temporary passive immunity after exposure to blood positive for hepatitis B surface antigen.**

4.   **Heptavax-B and Recombivax HB, administered in a series of three injections, is the most effective prevention method against HBV infection.**

5.   Spironolactone (Aldactone), amiloride (Midamor), or triamterene (Dyrenium) are potassium-sparing diuretics used for management of ascites in cirrhosis of the liver.

6.   Furosemide (Lasix), a loop diuretic, may be used in combination with a potassium-sparing diuretic.

m 7.   **Vasopressin (Pitressin), a vasoconstrictor, is administered intravenously to stop bleeding from esophageal varices. Vasopressin can cause tissue necrosis if infiltration occurs. Because of its vasoconstricting effects, a patient with cardiovascular disease should not receive this drug.**

8.   Nitroglycerin, a vasodilator, is administered in combination with vasopressin to prevent or reduce angina from constriction of the coronary arteries.

9.   Propranolol (Inderal), a beta-blocking agent, may be administered to prevent bleeding from esophageal varices by decreasing portal venous pressure. This drug is usually used with sclerotherapy treatment or balloon tamponade.

m 10.   **Neomycin sulfate, an aminoglycoside antibiotic, may be administered orally to prevent hepatic encephalopathy from the release of ammonia in the intestinal bacteria flora and from the breakdown of red blood cells. This drug is a derivative of gentamicin with side effects of nephrotoxicity and ototoxicity.**

m 11.   **Lactulose (Cephulac), a hyperosmotic laxative, may also be used to treat hepatic encephalopathy by converting ammonia to a nonabsorbable form and excreting the ammonia in feces by its laxative effect.**

12.   Vitamin K (AquaMEPHYTON), may be required to promote clotting.

13.   Normal saline solution (NSS) or other crystalloids are given to maintain adequate intravascular volume.

14.   Packed red blood cells (RBCs), fresh frozen plasma (FFP), platelets, and albumin are used to maintain vascular volume and promote clotting.

15.   Cimetidine (Tagamet), famotidine (Pepcid), ranitidine (Zantac), and histamine (H_2) blockers, are used to decrease gastric acidity. Gastritis is not uncommon in cirrhosis.

16.   Magnesium sulfate, a magnesium replacement, may be administered as a result of hypomagnesemia that occurs with liver function.

17. Thiamine is a water-soluble vitamin of the B-complex group. It is an essential coenzyme in carbohydrate metabolism, used in liver disease and when a patient is suspected of alcohol abuse.

18. Folic acid is a member of the vitamin B complex. It stimulates RBC and WBC production. It is used in patients with primary liver disease and suspected alcohol abuse.

19. Dopamine produces direct action on alpha- and beta-adrenergic receptors and specific dopaminergic receptors in mesenteric and renal vascular beds. It is used to correct hemodynamic imbalance.

20. Meperidine HCl (Demerol), a narcotic agonist analgesic, relieves moderate-to-severe pain. Should be given IV rather than IM to prevent bleeding at the site.

21. Dicyclomine HCl (Bentyl) is an anticholinergic antispasmodic that relieves muscle spasms in the GI and biliary systems.

22. Pancrelipase (Viokase, Cotazym, Cotazym-B) is an enzyme digestant that aids in the digestion and absorption of fats and proteins.

23. Somatostatin is indicated in the treatment in acute pancreatitis. It inhibits release of pancreatic enzymes.

24. Fluorouracil (5-fluorouracil, 5-FU), methotrexate sodium, and doxorubicin HCl (Adriomycin), are antineoplastic, antimetabolite, immunosuppressant drugs that may be used as a direct infusion through the hepatic artery via an implantable pump to prolong survival and improve the quality of life in liver failure. May also be used as adjunctant therapy after surgery.

25. Medications used to prevent liver transplant rejection:
    a. Cyclosporine (Sandimmune): acts specifically on T-helper cells and prevents secretion of interleukin-2 (IL-2) and IL-1 from macrophages. Its nephrotoxic and hepatotoxic adverse effects seem to be dose related and respond to dose reduction.
    b. Azathioprine (Imuran): an antimetabolite that interrupts DNA synthesis and inhibits cellular division and the activation of B lymphocytes and cytotoxic T cells. Because of its bone marrow suppression effects and cumulative effects with decreased renal function, low doses are prescribed in the treatment of rejection.
    c. OKT3 (Orthoclone OKT3): a monoclonal antibody directed against the T lymphocyte. It is prophylactically used for rejection via IV bolus and is used as rescue therapy in acute rejection episodes when other rejection efforts have failed. The greatest reaction occurs with the first dose (30–60 minutes)
    d. F-K 506 is the newest immunosuppressant drug that decreases production of IL-2 and other lymphokines that help in the proliferation of T cells. The best method of administration has not yet been identified. It is used in combination with other immunosuppressants and steroids. Method of action is similar to cyclosporine.
    e. Methylprednisolone (Solu-Medrol), prednisone: these steroids are given parenterally and orally, respectively, and are anti-inflammatory agents that decrease the production of activated T-helper cells and cytotoxic cells, decreasing the antigenic activity of the graft. IV boluses of Solu-Medrol (40–100 mg) must be given over 20–30 minutes.

III.　Acute pancreatitis

A.　Description: Pancreatic enzymes activated prematurely initiate an acute or chronic inflammatory process, varying from mild edema to severe hemorrhage and necrosis.

B.　Etiology and incidence

　　1.　The most common causes are alcohol abuse and cholecystitis.

　　2.　Other associated factors include surgery or abdominal trauma, pancreatic tumors, common bile duct obstruction, infectious process, third trimester or ectopic pregnancy, ERCP, total parenteral nutrition (TPN), hypercalcemia, and hypertriglyceridemia.

　　3.　Drug reactions or toxic doses of medications, such as corticosteroids, furosemide, thiazide diuretics, estrogens, NSAIDs, tetracycline, procainamide, and sulfonamides, have also been known to cause pancreatitis.

　　4.　Alcoholism and trauma account for the higher incidence in men, whereas acute pancreatitis in women is predominately associated with cholecystitis.

C.　Pathophysiology

　　1.　Pancreatic enzymes are secreted by the acini cells in an inactive form and are activated in the intestine by enterokinase.

　　2.　When enzymes are activated prematurely a cyclic destruction of the pancreatic parenchyma occurs with autodigestion of the pancreas as the net result.

　　3.　The proteolytic and lipolytic enzymes cause pathologic changes ranging from a mildly inflamed and edematous interstitium to a severe inflammatory, hemorrhagic, and necrotic degradation of the pancreatic cells.

　　4.　Trypsin, thought to be the activating source of the proteolytic enzymes, causes a chain of events that result in increased capillary permeability, leading to third-space fluid in the retroperitoneal space and the peritoneal cavity, and thrombosis, hemorrhage, and necrosis of the acinar cells.

　　5.　Management goals for patients with acute pancreatitis are aimed at fluid and electrolyte replacement, resting the pancreas, pain management, nutritional support, and prevention or treatment of complications.

　　6.　Surgical intervention is usually reserved for pseudocysts and acute necrotizing pancreatitis. A cholecystectomy, ERCP, or endoscopic sphincterotomy may be performed if gallstones are the cause of the disease process.

D.　Assessment

　　1.　Clinical manifestations include:

　　　　a.　Abdominal pain usually in the left upper quadrant (LUQ) or maybe in the midepigastric region.

　　　　b.　Abdominal tenderness with guarding.

　　　　c.　Decreased or absent bowel sounds are indicative of a paralytic ileus.

　　　　d.　**Grey Turner's sign (ecchymosis of flank).**

　　　　e.　**Cullen's sign (periumbilical ecchymosis)**

　　　　f.　Fever

    g. Hypotension, tachycardia, adventitious breath sounds, hypoxemia

    h. Jaundice

    i. Nausea, vomiting, and steatorrhea

  2. Laboratory findings include:

    a. Elevated serum and urine amylase

    b. Elevated serum lipase

    c. Elevated WBCs

    d. Hyperlipidemia and hyperglycemia

    e. Hypocalcemia and hypomagnesium

    f. Elevated bilirubin, SGOT, LDH, and alkaline phosphatase with liver and/or biliary involvement

    g. Amylase-creatinine clearance test >6%

  3. Diagnostic studies include:

    a. Chest x-ray (CXR) that may show a pleural effusion

    b. ERCP

    c. Ultrasound and abdominal x-ray

    d. CT scan or MRI

E. Nursing diagnoses

  1. Pain

  2. Fluid Volume Deficit

  3. Ineffective Breathing Pattern

  4. Altered Nutrition: Less than Body Requirements

  5. Anxiety

  6. Altered Protection

  7. Decreased Cardiac Output

F. Planning and implementation

  1. Assess degree and nature of pain and administer an antispasmodic, dicyclomine (Bentyl) and meperidine (Demerol), an analgesic, as prescribed.

  2. Reassess for pain relief approximately 30 minutes after administration of pain medication.

  3. Promote bed rest with minimal activities, and frequent position changes for comfort.

  4. Observe nasogastric tube (NGT) drainage, and monitor for patency. Removal of gastric secretions prevents stimulating the pancreas to produce more enzymes.

  5. Possible administration of antacids, cimetidine (Tagamet), ranitidine (Zantac), or famotidine (Pepcid), via NGT to repress gastric acid.

  6. Maintain semi-Fowler's or Fowler's position as tolerated to maintain optimal lung expansion.

  7. Fluid resuscitation with colloids, crystalloids, albumin, and blood or blood products and monitor response.

  8. Monitor hemodynamic status: PCWP, PAP, CVP, CO, and CI. Monitor cardiac and respiratory assessments, vital signs, intake and output q1hr or PRN.

  9. Administration of dopamine, a vasoconstrictor, may be instituted if response to fluid therapy fails.

  10. Monitor laboratory results: BUN, creatinine, blood sugar, liver function studies (LFS), CBC, ABGs, and electrolytes, especially calcium, magnesium, and potassium.

11.   Monitor electrolyte replacement therapy for signs of calcium and potassium toxicity.

 12.   **Observe cardiac monitor for dysrhythmias.**

13.   Administer supplemental oxygen via nasal cannula and monitor pulse oximetry.

14.   Observe strict NPO initially, then small frequent feedings with high carbohydrates, protein, low fat, no stimulants (caffeine or alcohol), supplemental fat-soluble vitamins, and commercial liquid or TPN for vitamin deficiencies.

15.   Be aware of potential complications:
a.   Pancreatic abscess and pseudocysts: collection of purulent fluid and products of necrosis situated within the pancreas. This complication can be fatal if not treated.
b.   Diabetes mellitus (see Chapter 11)
c.   Hypovolemic shock (see Chapter 13)
d.   Disseminated intravascular coagulopathy (DIC) (see Chapter 13)
e.   Adult respiratory distress syndrome (ARDS) (see Chapter 13)
f.   Acute renal failure (see Chapter 10)
g.   Gastrointestinal hemorrhage (see Chapter 7)

G.   Evaluation
1.   The patient experiences relief of pain.
2.   The patient exhibits improved fluid and nutritional balance.
3.   The patient experiences improved respiratory function.

IV.   Pancreatic cancer

A.   Description: malignant tumors arising in the head, body, or tail of the pancreas.

B.   Etiology and incidence
1.   The cause of pancreatic cancer is unknown.
2.   Major risk factors are:
a.   Cigarette smoking >2 packs/day
b.   Ingestion of a diet high in fat
c.   Diabetes mellitus
d.   Chronic pancreatitis or history of pancreatitis
e.   Exposure to environmental toxins or industrial chemicals
3.   In the United States it is the fourth leading cause of death from cancer. It more prevalent in men than women and in African Americans than Caucasians. Increase in incidence peaks between the fifth and seventh decades.

C.   Pathophysiology and management
1.   Although pancreatic cancer most often occurs in the head of the pancreas, other sites within the gland may be the primary source.
2.   In addition to the common manifestations, each site has distinctive characteristics specific to its origin.

3.   **The poor prognosis is related to the nonspecific symptoms and the advancement of the disease before a diagnosis is made. After the initial diagnosis, death usually occurs within 12 months.**
4.   Therapeutic management may include:
a.   Surgery, curative or palliative.

      b.   Radiation therapy, most effective for pain relief.

      c.   Chemotherapy with limited success.

D. **Assessment**
1. The most common manifestations are anorexia, nausea, weight loss, and dull abdominal pain initially.
2. Abdominal pain increases in severity with disease progression.
3. More specific manifestations depend on the location such as jaundice, clay-colored stools, dark- or mahogany-colored urine, and pruritis commonly seen in cancer of the pancreatic head. Cancer of the pancreatic body causes abdominal pain radiating to the midback and is more prominent when lying supine and eating. Cancer of the pancreatic tail often has no overt symptoms until metastases.
4. Laboratory and diagnostic studies include:
   a. Elevated serum amylase.
   b. Elevated carcinoembryo antigen (CEA).
   c. Elevated CA19-9 radioimmunoassay (RIA), which is a specific tumor marker associated with pancreatic cancer.
   d. Ultrasound and CT scan identify a tumor mass.
   e. ERCP through direct visualization of the pancreatic ductal system identifies a mass.
   f. Cancer cells are identified in the pancreatic secretion test.
   g. Positive tissue biopsy.

E. **Nursing diagnoses**
1. Pain
2. Altered Nutrition: Less than Body Requirements
3. Ineffective Denial
4. Risk for Impaired Skin Integrity

F. **Planning and implementation**
1. Assess pain parameters and administer pain medication as ordered. Demerol or morphine sulfate is given via PCA to control severe pain.
2. Monitor weight and report changes.
3. Administer supplemental feedings or TPN as prescribed.
4. Monitor laboratory values such as serum glucose, coagulation studies, and LFTs.
5. **Administer pancreatic enzymes as prescribed.**
6. **Administer before or with meals and snacks. Antacids may decrease their effectiveness. Do not crush or chew because the enteric coating will be destroyed.**
7. Prepare the patient and family members for a pancreatoduodenectomy (Whipple's procedure), which is a resection of the pancreas and surrounding organs for palliative or possible curative management.
8. Encourage communication between nurse, patient, and family members to support successful resolution of grief and the completion of the grieving process.
9. Maintain parenteral fluids and monitor the amount of fluids, flow rate, and the site for infection
10. Assess heart rate and rhythm and lung fields for adventitious breath sounds.

11. Monitor vital signs q4hr or PRN.
12. Administer supplemental oxygen and pulse oximetry.
13. Be aware of potential complications:
   a. Bleeding: this can occur from decreased vitamin K levels and abnormal coagulation factors or as a complication of surgery.
   b. Ascites: accumulation of fluid in the abdominal cavity
   c. Metastasis: the spread of cancer to adjacent abdominal organs or via the lymph system to other bodily organs.
   d. Hyperinsulinism: a complication from a tumor (benign or malignant) of islet cells (islets of Langerhans), resulting in hypersecretion of insulin and an excessive rate of glucose metabolism.

G. Evaluation
1. The patient displays adequate fluid and nutritional status.
2. The patient verbalizes only minimal discomfort.
3. The patient demonstrates no respiratory compromise.
4. The patient exhibits gradual progression through the stages of the grieving process.

V. Cirrhosis of the liver

A. Description: a focal or diffuse degeneration and destruction of hepatocytes with occurring necrosis and irreversible fibrotic regeneration resulting in chronic liver dysfunction with eventual failure.

B. Etiology and incidence
1. The four major causes of cirrhosis are listed in order of incidence.
   a. Alcohol abuse and/or nutritional deficiencies causing changes in lipid metabolism leading to fatty infiltrates with eventual atrophy and hardening of the liver (Laennec's cirrhosis).
   b. Complication of hepatitis (B and C), intoxication with industrial chemicals, infection, and metabolic disorders resulting in a small, nodular liver (post-necrotic after cirrhosis).
   c. Chronic bile flow obstruction, stasis of bile in the hepatic ducts, and infection lead to inflammation, necrotic process, and hepatic scar tissue (biliary cirrhosis).
   d. Severe right-sided heart failure, decompensated cor pulmonale, prolonged constrictive pericarditis, or atrioventricular valve disease can eventually cause hepatomegaly, hepatocellular death from anoxia, and fibrotic scarring (cardiac cirrhosis).
2. Incidence is higher in men than women and can occur at any age with peak incidence after age 40.

C. Pathophysiology and management
1. Initially in cirrhosis, lipid metabolism is impaired, leading to fatty infiltrates within the parenchymal cells, with eventual degeneration and destruction of the cells.
2. The liver exerts its ability to regenerate liver tissue. Normal liver tissue and regenerated fibrotic and scarred tissue become nodular in appearance.
3. **The normal flow of blood and bile is compromised by enlarged liver cells and the fibrotic changes. Sequelae of these irreversible changes include jaundice, portal hypertension, esophageal varices, hepatic encephalopathy, and eventual liver failure.**

    4. Liver dysfunction results in impaired metabolism, bile production and secretion, detoxification, filtration, absorption, and coagulation.

D. Assessment

    1. Early manifestations include:

        a. Dyspepsia

        b. Nausea and vomiting

        c. Diarrhea or constipation

        d. Right upper quadrant or epigastric pain

        e. Fever

        f. Slight weight loss

        g. Enlarged, firm, nodular liver

    2. Late manifestations include:

        a. Jaundice

        b. Ascites

        c. Peripheral edema

        d. Splenomegaly

        e. Dilated superficial arterioles on the face and truck

        f. Hematologic disorders

        g. Peripheral neuropathies

        h. Nonpalpable liver

        i. Bruising and bleeding

    3. Diagnostic studies include:

        a. Elevated AST, ALT, GGT, LDH, and alkaline phosphatase

        b. Decreased total protein, albumin, and cholesterol

        c. Prolonged prothrombin time

        d. Elevated serum and urine bilirubin

        e. Retention of indiocyanine green (ICG) dye

        f. Liver biopsy reveals destruction and fibroses of tissue

E. Nursing diagnoses

    1. Altered Nutrition: Less than Body Requirements

    2. Activity Intolerance

    3. Impaired Skin Integrity

    4. Fluid Volume Excess

    5. Altered Thought Processes

    6. Pain

    7. Altered Protection

F. Planning and implementation

    1. Ensure low-protein, high-caloric intake. Provide low or restricted sodium if ascites or edema is present.

    2. Provide small, frequent feedings.

    3. Administer antiemetics, Tigan, PRN or as prescribed.

    4. Provide activity and scheduled periods of rest.

    5. Protect skin from injury by applying emollients to skin, mittens to hands, and reposition q2hr.

    6. Monitor for bleeding gums, epistaxis, ecchymosis, petechiae, melena, hematuria, and hematemesis.

    7. Monitor vital signs q4hr or PRN.

    8. Administer vitamin K as prescribed with a small-gauge needle or slowly IV over 1 hour.

9. Administer diuretics, (Aldactone, Lasix), albumin, and protein supplements as prescribed.
10. Monitor accurate intake and output.
11. Measure and record abdominal girth daily.

12. **Avoid narcotics and barbiturates if possible or cautiously administer sedatives if prescribed. Metabolism of medications is altered due to liver damage.**
13. Assess and record changes in orientation and mental status and level of consciousness.
14. Reduce dietary protein and increase carbohydrate intake.
15. Provide a warm and draft-free environment to decrease risk of infections.
16. Administer medications and enemas (lactulose and neomycin sulfate) as ordered.

17. **Cautiously administer antispasmodics if prescribed.**
18. Monitor hemodynamic stability, PCWP, CVP, and urine output.
19. Monitor laboratory values including coagulation studies, platelets, hemoglobin and hematocrit, and electrolytes.
20. Maintain and monitor infusion rate of intravenous fluids. Do not administer Ringer's lactate or D5LR because they will contribute to acidosis.
21. Observe cardiac monitor for dysrhythmias.
22. Administer thiamine and folic acid as prescribed.
23. Assist with invasive treatments and/or procedures such as insertion of a Sengstaken-Blakemore tube for esophageal varices, paracentesis for ascites, or liver biopsy study.
24. Be aware of potential complications:
    a. Portal hypertension: increased blood pressure within the portal circulation resulting from destruction and compression of the portal and hepatic veins and sinusoids. The development of collateral circulation coupled with increased hydrostatic pressure within the vessels are contributing factors in the development of esophageal varices and ascites.
    b. Ascites: accumulation of serous fluid in the abdominal cavity. The mechanisms involved are hypoalbuminemia, hyperaldosteronism, and leakage of proteins from the portal circulation into the lymphatic system, with the eventual movement of proteins and water into the peritoneal cavity.
    c. Esophageal varices: distended, tortuous, fragile veins located in the lower esophagus and upper gastric region that are formed from collateral circulation. The fragility of these veins brings about rupture with moderate provocation.
    d. Hepatic encephalopathy: disturbances in the central nervous system (CNS) caused by the inability of the liver to metabolize proteins and convert ammonia to urea for excretion. This dysfunction causes motor and cognitive changes in the brain.
    e. Hepatorenal syndrome: a functional renal failure with no structural abnormality. Redistribution in renal blood flow or hypovolemia secondary to ascites are thought to be the causative factors.

G. Evaluation
1. The patient demonstrates increased tolerance for activities.
2. The patient exhibits increased nutritional intake.
3. The patient experiences no incidence of bleeding.
4. The patient demonstrates an increased level of consciousness.
5. The patient exhibits improved skin integrity.
6. The patient verbalizes decreased episodes of pain.

VI. Cancer of the liver

A. Description: primary liver tumors can be benign or malignant. Primary carcinoma of the liver is rare, with metastatic tumors being more common.

B. Etiology and incidence
1. Benign adenomas are associated with oral contraceptives or androgens.
2. Primary malignant hepatoma occurs primarily in men.
3. Exposure to hepatotoxic chemicals, androgen therapy, anabolic steroid use, cigarette smoking combined with alcohol use, history of cirrhosis, and hepatitis are factors associated with primary tumors.
4. Metastatic liver tumors are approximately 20 times more frequent than primary tumors.

C. Pathophysiology and management
1. The majority of primary liver tumors originate in the parenchymal cells. The remaining tumors are cholangiomas (bile duct carcinomas).

2. **The liver's abundant blood flow and extensive capillary network makes it an ideal site for metastasis from other parts of the body.**
3. The most common routes of metastasis include direct extension from surrounding organs, transportation through the portal circulation or lymphatic channels, and seeding from diagnostic and/or surgical procedures.
4. The disease is usually not diagnosed until the advanced stage, resulting in a poor prognosis. If the patient is unresponsive to therapy, a 4–7 month survival time is predicted.
5. Because of their vascularity, a benign adenoma can rupture, causing hemorrhage and possible death.
6. Treatment may be palliative (surgery and/or chemotherapy) or involve transplantation.

D. Assessment
1. The most common clinical manifestations include:
   a. Dull pain in the epigastric or right upper quadrant regions
   b. Weight loss and extreme weakness
   c. Anorexia, nausea, and vomiting
   d. Hepatomegaly, ascites, jaundice, and peripheral edema
   e. Bruit or friction rub may be auscultated over the liver
   f. Liver mass on palpation
2. Relevant laboratory studies include:
   a. Elevated alkaline phosphatase and reversal of albumin-globulin (A/G) ratio
   b. Hypoproteinemia

      c.   Increased bilirubin, SGOT, and LDH
      d.   Elevated alpha-fetoprotein
   3.   Pertinent diagnostic studies include:
      a.   Positive liver biopsy: this is usually the definitive diagnostic test, although there is a high risk of bleeding after the procedure.
      b.   Liver scan
      c.   ERCP
      d.   CT scan, MRI, and ultrasonography are helpful in locating liver tumors.

E.   **Nursing diagnoses**
   1.   Anxiety
   2.   Pain
   3.   Anticipatory Grieving
   4.   Risk for Infection
   5.   Altered Nutrition: Less than Body Requirements
   6.   Additional diagnoses are related to the degree of liver function.

F.   **Planning and implementation**
   1.   Administer analgesics for pain as prescribed. Assess pain relief and consult physician to change medication if pain is not relieved.

   2.   **Prescribed pain medication should be administered with caution because of decreased metabolic and detoxification functions of the diseased liver.**
   3.   Monitor and report signs of infection
   4.   Observe the surgical incisions, dressings or any drainage apparatus for drainage and patency, and the incisional site for signs of infection.
   5.   Maintain aseptic techniques when performing wound care or when assisting with invasive procedures (eg, paracentesis, peritoneovenous shunt).
   6.   Provide increased calories, fats, and carbohydrates; limit protein intake.
   7.   Monitor laboratory values for liver function tests, especially BUN, nitrogen balance, and albumin.
   8.   Perform a frequent neurologic assessment and monitor serum ammonia levels.
   9.   Initiate home health care follow-up.
   10.   Encourage the patient and family members to verbalize their feelings and provide emotional support.
   11.   Assist the patient and family members to identify coping strategies or develop new strategies to cope with the diagnosis and prognosis of cancer, and support the identified behavior.
   12.   Explain to the patient and family members all prescribed treatments and procedures (chemotherapy, radiation therapy, surgical resection, and liver transplantation) and the rationale for each.
   13.   Assess for signs of grieving, explain its stages, and support behaviors evoking successful resolution of grief.

G.   **Evaluation**
   1.   The patient reports adequate relief of pain.
   2.   The patient is free of infection.

3. The patient and family members demonstrate a beginning progression through the grieving process.
4. The patient and family members verbalize their fears and anxieties.
5. The patient and family members effectively use available support systems.
6. The patient verbalizes an understanding of the plan for follow-up home health or hospice care.

VII. Hepatitis

A. Description: an acute, occasionally chronic, inflammatory process of the liver, stemming from viruses and toxic or drug-induced agents. The process involves the parenchyma, Kupffer cells, bile ducts, and blood vessels.

B. Etiology and incidence: although hepatitis can be idiosyncratic or a direct result of specific chemicals, infections from hepatitis A, hepatitis B, hepatitis C (non-A non-B), delta hepatitis, and hepatitis E are the most prevalent types of virus (Display 8-1).

C. Pathophysiology and management

1. Inflammation of liver tissue, deterioration and necrosis of the hepatocytes, and enlargement of the Kupffer cells occurs as a result of the body's immune response to the virus.
2. Interruption of bile flow from inflammation impedes excretion of conjugated bilirubin. Serum bilirubin is elevated with eventual diffusion into the tissues and accumulation of bile salts in the skin.
3. Resultant effects of the liver changes are hepatomegaly and splenomegaly.

4. The average incubation period varies according to the type:
   a. hepatitis A: 28–30 days
   b. hepatitis B: 60–90 days

DISPLAY 8-1.
Specific Types of Hepatitis

Hepatitis A: An RNA virus transmitted by the fecal-oral route (infectious contaminated liquids and food, especially shell fish, hepatitis) and by infected food handlers. The greatest risk occurs at 15 years or younger and is most severe in the fourth decade of life and beyond.

Hepatitis B: A DNA virus disseminated via blood or blood products (serum body secretions, punctures from contaminated needles) and maternal perinatal exposure. Those with an increased incidence are health care workers, dialysis patients, recipients of multiple transfusions (blood and blood products), those with many sexual contacts, IV drug abusers, and those with poor hygiene habits.

Hepatitis C: Similar in transmission and risk factors to those (non-A, non-B) of hepatitis B. Additional spread may be by an asymptomatic carrier and possibly by the fecal-oral route.

Delta hepatitis: A defective RNA virus, which can only be replicated in the presence of hepatitis B. Transmission is the same as with hepatitis B. High-risk populations are IV drug abusers and transfusion recipients.

Hepatitis E: An RNA virus, is spread via fecal-oral route, food or water contamination, and poor sanitation. It is predominately seen in developing countries and is rare in the United States.

Toxic Hepatitis: Occurs from an idiosyncratic effect or from dose-related medications or chemicals (eg, isoniazid, phenytoin, quinidine, halothane, acetaminophen, aspirin, benzene, carbon tetrachloride, and tetracyclines, industrial toxins, paint removal products, and chemicals necessary for developing chemicals).

      c.   **hepatitis C: 56 days**

      d.   **hepatitis D: varies because hepatitis B virus must precede its development**

      e.   **hepatitis E: 26–42 days**

  5. If the course of the disorder is uncomplicated, regeneration of the liver cells with returning normal function usually begins within 2 weeks of onset of jaundice.

  6. Prevention and immunization are the first defenses against hepatitis.

D. **Assessment**

  1. The patient can be asymptomatic. This is particularly true in young patients. Symptoms usually occur in three phases (Display 8-2).

  2. Diagnostic findings include:

      a.   Elevated SGOT, SGPT, LDH.

      b.   Increased GGT.

      c.   Decreased albumin.

      d.   Elevated urinary bilirubin and urobilinogen.

      e.   Prolonged prothrombin time.

      f.   Elevated alkaline phosphatase.

      g.   IgM-positive indicates current infection for hepatitis A.

      h.   IgG-positive indicates past infection for hepatitis A.

      i.   HBsAg-positive indicates active infection, carrier state (after 6 months), or chronic hepatitis B virus.

      j.   HBeAg-positive measures infectivity.

      k.   Anti–hepatitis D virus in the presence of HBsAg indicates present infection of hepatitis D (delta).

      l.   Liver biopsy is performed if mixed etiology is present or a more severe form is suspected.

E. **Nursing diagnoses**

  1. Altered Nutrition: Less than Body Requirements

  2. Activity Intolerance

  3. Knowledge Deficit: Hepatitis

F. **Planning and implementation**

  1. Provide small frequent meals high in carbohydrate, protein, and calories.

  2. Administer antiemetics (eg, Tigan) 30 minutes before meals.

  3. Record accurate intake and output and weight every shift.

  4. Maintain parenteral fluids if indicated.

DISPLAY 8-2.
Assessing Signs and Symptoms of Hepatitis

Phases and manifestations

Pre-icteric: anorexia, nausea, vomiting, diarrhea or constipation, right upper quadrant discomfort, malaise, headache, fever, weight loss, arthralgias, urticaria, hepatomegaly, lymphadenopathy and splenomegaly; infective phase.

Icteric: pruritus, dark urine, bilirubinuria, clay-colored stools, fatigue, weight loss, hepatomegaly, right upper quadrant tenderness, jaundice (most common symptom).

Post-icteric: malaise, early fatiguability, symptoms subsiding when jaundice abates.

5. Gradually increase activity, with planned rest periods, especially after meals.

 6. **Administer mild analgesic as prescribed. To decrease further liver damage, medications not metabolized by the liver are preferred.**

7. Assess patient's feeling about disease process and appearance.

8. Teach the patient about the infectious process, modes of transmission, diet, activities allowed, necessity of follow-up care, and the avoidance of alcohol.

9. Instruct the patient in ways to prevent spread of the infection related to the specific type of hepatitis (Display 8-3).

10. Instruct the patient not to donate blood.

11. Be aware of potential complications:

  a. Chronic persistent hepatitis is a benign sequelae from either hepatitis B or hepatitis C viral infections. The patient's major complaints are fatigue and hepatomegaly. Although liver function tests are abnormal for a period of time, follow-up visits every 6–12 months are the only treatment.

 b. **Chronic active hepatitis most often progresses to cirrhosis. There is higher incidence in cases of hepatitis B, hepatitis C, and hepatitis D. Signs and symptoms vary but are usually similar to hepatitis, with fatigue as the most common manifestation. When signs and symptoms together with persistent abnormal liver function tests last longer than 6 months, chronic active hepatitis is suspected and a differential diagnosis is made by a liver biopsy study. The approved treatment, alpha interferon, has proven to be beneficial for some patients.**

  c. Fulminant hepatitis is a serious complication with a high rate of mortality. Massive widespread necrosis of the parenchyma with rapid clinical deterioration takes place. Liver transplantation is the treatment of choice.

G. Evaluation

1. The patient demonstrates progressive increase in activity.
2. The patient maintains adequate caloric and fluid intake.
3. The patient exhibits a positive adaptation to body image.
4. The patient verbalizes an understanding of the infectious process, follow-up care, and preventive measures.

DISPLAY 8-3.
Hygiene Measures and Hepatitis

Hepatitis A: good personal hygiene practices, passive immunization with immune globulin.

Hepatitis B: good personal hygienic practices; personal items such as razors, toothbrush, washcloths, cigarettes, etc., should not be shared; use of condoms with sexual contact; administration of specific hepatitis B immunoglobulin.

Hepatitis C: same as hepatitis B

Hepatitis D: same as hepatitis B

VIII. **Lacerated liver**

    A. Description: a severe abdominal injury occurring from blunt or penetrating trauma.

    B. Etiology and incidence

        1. Penetrating injuries of the abdomen usually result from gunshot wounds, stab wounds, or impalement. The spleen and liver are the most commonly involved organs.

        2. Depending on the velocity of a gunshot or missile (bullet), surgery is almost always required to determine tissue damage. The depth and location of stab wounds determine whether surgical or conservative treatment is indicated.

        3. Blunt trauma may consist of direct blows, falls, or crushing injuries. This type of injury is a potential time bomb because of possible hidden injuries.

        4. Lacerated liver or degree of liver injury depends on the speed and/or force associated with the injury.

        5. The majority of injuries involving the liver are a result of motor vehicle accidents.

    C. Pathophysiology and management

        1. Because of its vascularity and ductal system, the primary insult to the liver determines the extent of damage.

        2. Injuries from a high velocity missile (bullet) penetration can cause extensive tissue, blood vessel, or bile duct damage, with resultant hemorrhage.

        3. Liver injuries resulting from blunt trauma can range from hematomas to hemorrhage. Rib fractures from blunt trauma can cause lacerations of the liver tissue. The degree of injury is paramount to the liver's ability to produce sufficient amounts of clotting factors.

        4. Blunt injuries to the liver may have little external evidence and a delay in detection and treatment may result.

        5. Management depends on the severity of insult to the liver. The liver may be packed to control hemorrhage, with surgical repair within a few days after removal. Whether segmental resection or debridement is indicated depends on the size of the laceration. Nonoperative management is reserved for a small percentage of injuries.

    D. Assessment

        1. Clinical manifestations include:

            a. Decreased blood pressure

            b. Increased heart and respiratory rate

            c. Abdominal pain, distention, and rigidity

            d. Decreased or absent bowel sounds

            e. Contusions, abrasions over abdomen

            f. Cullen's sign: ecchymosis around the umbilicus

            g. Hematuria

            h. Visible, external abdominal wound

        2. Laboratory findings include:

            a. Decreased hemoglobin and hematocrit

            b. Increased bilirubin

            c. Abnormal urinalysis

        d.   Increased WBC

   3.   Diagnostic studies include:

        a.   Chest x-ray and abdominal x-ray

        b.   CT scan to determine extent of injury

        c.   Diagnostic peritoneal lavage

E. **Nursing diagnoses**

   1.   Decreased Cardiac Output

   2.   Ineffective Breathing Pattern

   3.   Fluid Volume Deficit

   4.   Altered Tissue Perfusion: Cardiopulmonary, Renal

   5.   Risk for Infection

F. **Planning and implementation**

   1.   **Monitor nasogastric drainage for color, odor, consistency, and amount.**

   2.   Administer crystalloids, lactated Ringer's (LR) or normal saline solution (NSS) as prescribed.

   3.   Infuse packed RBCs as prescribed and observe for transfusion reaction.

   4.   Monitor laboratory values including electrolytes, CBC, coagulation factors, BUN, creatinine, and LFTs.

   5.   Monitor for respiratory distress and prepare for possible intubation.

   6.   Administer oxygen via a non-rebreather and monitor ABGs.

   7.   Monitor vital signs, blood pressure, level of consciousness, and oxygen saturation.

   8.   Maintain accurate intake and output (report urine output <30 mL/hr).

   9.   Monitor hemodynamic parameters: PAP, CVP, CO.

  10.   Monitor heart and lung sounds.

  11.   Assess for jaundice.

  12.   Observe wounds, IV, and drain sites for infection.

  13.   Obtain cultures as needed and administer antibiotics as prescribed.

  14.   Maintain sterile technique with all dressing changes.

  15.   Maintain optimal nutrition: TPN, tube feedings, or oral feedings as ordered.

  16.   Observe cardiac monitor for dysrhythmias and treat per hospital protocol.

  17.   **Be aware that administration of pain medications may mask symptoms.**

  18.   Be aware of potential complications:

        a.   Hypovolemic shock: a decrease in circulating blood volume from trauma, surgery or rupture of a major artery (see Chapter 13).

        b.   Sepsis: an ischemic episode leading to necrosis and infarction. Gram-negative bacteria from an abdominal organ leaks into the bloodstream causing septicemia. Septic shock can develop.

        c.   Hepatic abscess: develops as a result of the destruction of liver cells by bacterial toxins. The necrotic cells stimulate phagocytosis. A liquid containing liquefied liver cells, dead leukocytes, and bacteria is the aftermath of this destruction. Bacterial cholangitis and portal vein bacteremia are predisposing factors.

      d.   Adult respiratory distress syndrome (ARDS): a sudden progressive disorder involving pathophysiologic lung changes (see Chapter 13).

      e.   Disseminated intravascular coagulopathy (DIC): a serious coagulation disorder occurring secondary to another disease process. Several disease processes, tissue damage, and shock states may trigger the clotting mechanism, exhausting the normal clotting factory and thereby effecting the blood's ability to clot, which predisposed a patient to hemorrhage (see Chapter 13).

G. **Evaluation**

  1.   The patient shows no evidence of bleeding, as evidenced by stable H/H and hemodynamic parameters.

  2.   The patient maintains optimal fluid and electrolyte balance and nutrition intake.

  3.   The patient exhibits no tissue breakdown or signs of infection.

  4.   The patient maintains adequate oxygenation.

  5.   The patient and family verbalize fears and concerns and are receiving emotional support.

IX. **Hepatic encephalopathy**

A. **Description: a progressive depression of the central nervous system as a consequence of severe liver disease, injury, or failure.**

B. **Etiology and incidence**

  1.   Proposed precipitating factors include:

      a.   Hepatic parenchyma destruction and necrosis.

      b.   Marked liver failure

      c.   Absorption of toxic agents from the GI tract.

      d.   Bypassing the portal circulation (portal shunting) causing direct blood flow into the septemic circulation.

  2.   Research proposes that false neurotransmitters can be produced by faulty protein metabolism, thus precipitating the encephalopathic condition.

  3.   The encephalopathic process depends on the severity of the liver disorder.

C. **Pathophysiology and management**

  1.   When blood proteins, bacteria, and enzymatic digestion of dietary protein are increased in the gastrointestinal tract increased serum ammonia levels ensue.

  2.   The destruction or necrotic process of the hepatic parenchyma renders the organ or liver incapable of detoxifying and converting ammonia to urea.

  3.   **The abnormal concentration of ammonia in the septemic circulation cross the blood–brain barrier causing toxic effects on the neurologic system.**

D. **Assessment**

  1.   Signs and symptoms are described in stages (Display 8-4).

  2.   Laboratory studies include:

      a.   Decreased serum albumin

      b.   Decreased clotting factors

      c.   Increased ammonia levels

DISPLAY 8-4.
Stages and Clinical Manifestations of Hepatic Encephalopathy

Stage I: Restlessness, irritability, decreased concentration, day–night pattern reversed, personality and mental changes, mild asterixis.

Stage II: Increased drowsiness, disorientation, lethargy, agitation, asterixis, behavioral changes, fetor hepaticus.

Stage III: Hyperactive deep-tendon reflexes, asterixis, diminished verbal stimuli responses, aroused with difficulty, stuporous, incoherent, rigid extremities.

Stage IV: Absence of asterixis and reflexes with positive Babinski's reflex, flaccid extremities, decorticate and decerebrate posturing, no response to painful stimuli, comatose.

d. Increased serum bilirubin
e. Increased hepatic enzymes (SGOT, SGPT)
f. Abnormal ABGs
g. Decreased electrolytes
h. Abnormal EEG

E. Nursing diagnoses
1. Altered Thought Processes
2. Altered Nutrition: Less than Body Requirements
3. Sleep Pattern Disturbance
4. Impaired Social Interaction
5. Risk for Infection
6. Risk for Impaired Skin Integrity
7. Risk for Ineffective Breathing Pattern
8. Risk for Fluid Volume Deficit

F. Planning and implementation

1. **Administer oral lactulose to reduce ammonia absorption via its cathartic effect. If stool consists of watery diarrhea, suspect overdose.**
2. Administer neomycin to decrease ammonia production.
3. Maintain restricted or low-protein, high-calorie diet
4. Monitor for GI bleeding; this will increase ammonia levels secondary to breakdown of RBCs in the gut.

5. **Monitor neurologic function and level of consciousness and immediately report abnormalities.**
6. Observe concentration level, attention span, problem-solving abilities, and any memory deficits.
7. Observe for behavior and psychological changes.

8. **Observe and immediately report seizure activity.**
9. Administer thiamine to patients on TPN or with a history of alcohol abuse.
10. Elevate head of bed 45 degrees to prevent aspiration.
11. Maintain parenteral fluid and electrolyte replacement.
12. Record intake and output and daily weights.
13. Monitor laboratory values.

m   14.   Avoid administration of benzodiazepines to patients with liver dysfunction.

m   15.   Avoid use of opiates and use caution with administration of narcotics, sedatives, and tranquilizers. Frequent monitoring is necessary.

16.   Assess for asterixis (liver flaps).

17.   Monitor vital signs and blood pressure q4hr or PRN.

18.   Provide supplemental oxygen or prepare for intubation and mechanical ventilation as indicated and maintain patent airway.

19.   Teach patient and family members about disease process, dietary and medication restriction, administration and side effects of prescribed medications, the importance of follow-up appointments, and any changes in mental functions.

   F.   Evaluation

     1.   The patient displays no evidence of motor or cognitive impairment.

     2.   The patient exhibits no tissue breakdown or signs of infection.

     3.   The patient maintains optimal fluid balance and nutritional intake.

     4.   The patient maintains normal laboratory values.

     5.   The patient verbalizes an understanding of the necessity of follow-up care and abstinence of alcohol.

X.   **Liver transplant**

   A.   Description: transplantation of a liver with tissue antigens that closely resemble the recipient's, to improve the beneficiary's quality of life.

   B.   Indications

     1.   Cholestatic diseases (primary biliary cirrhosis, sclerosis cholangitis, biliary atresia)

     2.   Hepatocellular diseases (viral hepatitis, drug and alcohol-induced liver disease, Wilson's disease)

     3.   Vascular diseases (Budd-Chiari syndrome)

     4.   Fulminant hepatic failure

     5.   Irreversible advanced chronic liver disease

     6.   Metabolic liver disease

     7.   Confined hepatic malignancy

   C.   Assessment

     1.   ABO typing

     2.   Tissue typing

     3.   HIV screening

     4.   Platelet and leukocyte counts

     5.   Dental examination to detect any infections

     6.   Gynecologic examination for women

     7.   Urine analysis and urine culture & sensitivity

     8.   CXR

     9.   Psychological evaluation and social history

     10.   Purified protein derivative for tuberculosis

     11.   Possible GI, gallbladder, kidney studies

   D.   Nursing diagnoses

     1.   Decreased Cardiac Output

     2.   Fluid Volume Excess

     3.   Altered Tissue Perfusion: Cardiopulmonary

  4. Pain
  5. Impaired Gas Exchange
  6. Altered Protection
  7. Risk for Infection
  8. Risk for Altered Urinary Elimination
  9. Risk for Impaired Skin Integrity
  10. Risk for Anxiety
  11. Risk for Loneliness

E. Planning and implementation
  1. Assess hemodynamic parameters: apical rate and rhythm, PCWP, CVP, PAP, CO.
  2. Observe cardiac monitor for dysrhythmias.

 3. **Assess for signs and symptoms of rejection and infection.**
  4. Perform vital signs and intake and output q1hr or PRN.
  5. Monitor wound, IV, and drain sites for signs of infection. Maintain sterile technique with all dressing changes.
  6. Monitor drainage vehicle (Foley, Jackson-Pratt, Hemovac, NGT, chest tube, etc.) for color, consistency, and amount of drainage.
  7. Monitor neurologic and respiratory status.
  8. Administer platelets, fresh frozen plasma, and other blood products as prescribed and observe for transfusion reactions.
  9. Monitor endotracheal tube and ventilator for adequate oxygenation and patency and perform sterile suctioning.
  10. Cautiously administer pain medication as prescribed.
  11. Administer immunosuppressant agents:
     a. Imuran (may cause liver damage, jaundice, and increased susceptibility to infection)
     b. Monoclonal antibody-CD3 (orthoclone OKT3)
     c. Cyclosporine (only administer in a glass container)
     d. FK 506 (an investigative drug)
     e. Steroids (eg, Solu-Medrol) (may mask signs and symptoms of infection)
  12. Prepare the patient for liver biopsy surgery and ultrasound if rejection if suspected.
  13. Teach the patient and the family the importance of adherence to therapeutic regimen, signs and symptoms of rejection, and importance of follow-up care.
  14. Encourage open communication between the patient and nurse and family and nurse.
  15. Be aware of potential complications:
     a. Infection: increased susceptibility for infection is caused by the administration of immunosuppressant agents needed to prevent rejection. This complication is the leading cause of death after transplantation.

 b. **Rejection: the recipient's immune system recognizes the transplanted organ as a foreign antigen. Symptoms of acute rejection are fever, tachycardia, right upper quadrant or flank pain and increased jaundice. Between the fourth to tenth postoperative days is the most common period for rejection.**

    c.   Hemorrhage: blood loss due to the liver's inability to synthe-size coagulation factors (see Chapter 4).

    d.   Acute renal failure: decreased renal blood flow as a result of insufficient circulating blood volume, hepatic failure, acute re-jection, and administration of nephrotoxic antibiotics and im-munosuppressant agents (see Chapter 10).

    e.   Biliary complications: infection or biliary anastomosis leakage or obstruction can lead to abscess formation, peritonitis, bac-teremia, or cirrhosis.

G. Evaluation

1. The patient displays an effective cardiac rate and rhythm.
2. The patient maintains cardiac parameters within normal limits.
3. The patient maintains optimal fluid balance and nutritional intake.
4. The patient exhibits no evidence of infection, rejection, or skin breakdown.
5. The patient maintains adequate oxygenation as evidenced by ABGs within normal limits.
6. The patient and family verbalize an understanding of the informa-tion imparted at teaching sessions.
7. The patient verbalizes fears and is receiving emotional support.

Bibliography

Ambrose, M. A. & Dreher, H. M. (1996). Pancreatitis: Managing a flare up. *Nursing 96* 26(4), 33–39.

Black, J. M. & Matassarin-Jacobs, E. (1993). *Luckman and Sorenson's medical-surgical nurs-ing: A psychophysiologic approach* (4th ed.). Philadelphia: W. B. Saunders.

Carpenito, L. J. (1995). *Nursing care plans and documentation* (2nd ed.). Philadelphia: J. B. Lippincott

Corley, M. C. & Sneed, G. (1994). Criteria in the selection of organ transplant recipients. *Heart Lung* 23(6), 446–455.

Cox, H. C. (1993). *Clinical applications of nursing diagnosis: Adult, child, women's psychi-atric, gerontic and home health considerations* (2nd ed.). Philadelphia: F. A. Davis.

Fischer, J. E. (1989). Hepatobiliary dysfunction associated with total perenteral nutrition. *Gastroenterol Clin North Am* 18, 645–666.

Hudak, C. M. & Gallo, B. M. (1994). *Critical care nursing: A holistic approach* (6th ed.). Philadelphia: J. B. Lippincott.

Lewis, S. M., Collier, I. C., & Heitkemper, M. M. (1996). *Medical-surgical nursing: Assessment and management of clinical problems* (4th ed.). St. Louis: Mosby–Year Book.

Mark, J. F. (1993). Viral hepatitis: Unscrambling the alphabet. *Nursing 93* 23(1), 34–41.

McCullough, A.J., Mullen, K.D., & Smanik, E.J. (1989). Nutritional therapy and liver dis-ease. *Gastroenterol Clin North Am* 18, 619–643.

North American Nursing Diagnosis Association (NANDA). (1996). *Nursing diagnoses: Definitions & classification 1997–1998*. Philadelphia: Author.

Phipps, W. J. & Cassmeyer, V. L. (1995). *Medical-surgical nursing: Concepts and clinical practice* (5th ed.). St. Louis: Mosby–Year Book.

Robin, A. P., Campbell, R., & Palani, C.K. (1990). Total parenteral nutrition during acute pancreatitis: Clinical experience with 156 patients. *World J Surg* 14, 572–579.

Shannon, M. T., Wilson, B. A., & Stank, C. L. (1992). *Govoni and Hayes' drugs and nursing implications* (7th ed.). Norwalk, CT: Appleton and Lange.

Shronts, E. P. (1988). Nutritional assessments of adults with end stage hepatic failure. *Nutr Clin Pract* 3, 113–119.

Siconolfi, L. A. (1995). Clarifying the complexity of liver function tests. *Nursing 95* 25(5), 39–44.

Springhouse Corporation. (1996). *Handbook of critical care nursing.* Springhouse, PA: Springhouse.

Thelan, L. A. (1994). *Critical care nursing* (2nd ed.). St. Louis: Mosby–Year Book.

Zaloga, G. P. (1994). *Nutrition in critical care* (pp. 617–646). St. Louis: Mosby.

STUDY QUESTIONS

1. You are caring for a patient in a hepatic coma. Which evaluation criteria would be the most appropriate?
   a. The patient demonstrates an increase in level of consciousness.
   b. The patient exhibits improved skin integrity.
   c. The patient experiences no evidence of bleeding.
   d. The patient verbalizes decreased episodes of pain.

2. To inhibit pancreatic secretions, which pharmacologic agent would you anticipate administering to a patient with acute pancreatitis?
   a. nitroglycerin
   b. somatostatin
   c. pancrelipase
   d. Pepcid

3. Which of the following tests can be useful as a diagnostic and therapeutic tool in the biliary system?
   a. ultrasonagraphy
   b. magnetic resonance imaging (MRI)
   c. endoscopic retrograde cholangiopancreatography (ERCP)
   d. computed tomography (CT) scan

4. Which of the following laboratory values would be the most important to monitor for a patient with pancreatic cancer?
   a. serum glucose
   b. radioimmunoassay (RIA)
   c. creatine phosphokinase (CPK)
   d. carcinoembryo antigen (CEA)

5. Which statement by a patient with cirrhosis of the liver would require additional teaching by the nurse:
   a. "I guess I'll have to read the food labels when I'm grocery shopping."
   b. "I'll have a glass of wine with my meals instead of a bottle of beer."
   c. "Watching my diet is going to be difficult, but I will try my best."
   d. "I love meat but I guess I'll have to change my eating habits."

6. You observe changes in mentation, irritability, restlessness, and decreased concentration in a patient with cancer of the liver. Hepatic encephalopathy is suspected and the patient is ordered neomycin enemas. Which information in the patient's history would be a contraindication of this order?
   a. left nephrectomy
   b. glaucoma in both eyes
   c. myocardial infarction
   d. peripheral neuropathy

7. What is the primary nursing diagnosis for a 4th to 10th day postoperative liver transplant patient?
   a. Fluid Volume Excess
   b. Risk for Rejection
   c. Impaired Skin Integrity
   d. Decreased Cardiac Output

8. A nursing intervention for a patient with hepatitis B would include which of the following types of isolation?
   a. universal precautions
   b. blood transfusion precautions
   c. enteric isolation
   d. strict isolation

9. A patient is admitted with a lacerated liver as a result of blunt abdominal trauma. Which of the following nursing interventions would NOT be appropriate for this patient?
   a. Monitor for respiratory distress.
   b. Monitor coagulation studies.
   c. Administer pain medication as ordered.
   d. Administer normal saline, crystalloids as ordered.

ANSWER KEY

1. **Correct response: a**
   Increased level of consciousness indicates resolving of a comatose state.
   b, c, d. These are important evaluations but do not evaluate a patient in a hepatic coma who is responding to external stimuli.
   Application/Physiologic/Evaluation

2. **Correct response: b**
   Somatostatin, a treatment for acute pancreatitis, inhibits the release of pancreatic enzymes.
   a. Nitroglycerin is a vasodilator and does not affect pancreatic secretions.
   c. Pancrelipase is an enzyme that aids in the digestion and absorption of fats and proteins.
   d. Pepcid is a histamine (H_2) blocker and is used to decrease gastric motility.
   Comprehension/Physiologic/Planning

3. **Correct response: c**
   An ERCP permits direct visualization of the pancreatic and common bile duct. Its therapeutic value is in retrieving gallstones from the distal common bile duct and dilating strictures.
   a. Ultrasonography aids in the diagnosis of cholecystitis, gallstones, pancreatitis, and metastatic disease. Also identifies edema, inflammation, and fatty or fibrotic infiltrates or calcifications.
   b. MRI detects hepatic neoplasms, cysts, abscesses, and hematomas.
   d. CT scan can be done with or without contrast dye. It can detect tumors, cysts, pseudocysts, abscesses, hematomas, and obstructions of the liver, biliary tract, and pancreas.
   Knowledge/Safe care/Assessment

4. **Correct response: a**
   In pancreatitis, hypersecretion of insulin from a tumor may affect the islets of Langerhans, resulting in hyperinsulinemia, a complication of pancreatic cancer.

   b, d. These tests should also be monitored to measure the effects of therapy, but hypoglycemia may be life-threatening.
   c. Creatine phosphokinase (enzyme) reflects normal tissue catabolism; elevated serum levels indicate trauma to cells with high CPK content. CPK and CPK-isoenzymes are used to detect a myocardial infarction.
   Comprehension/Safe care/Assessment

5. **Correct response: b**
   Cirrhotic patients must abstain from drinking alcoholic beverages.
   a, c, d. These comments by the patient indicate an understanding of dietary intake.
   Application/Health promotion/Evaluation

6. **Correct response: a**
   Neomycin prevents the release of ammonia from the intestinal bacteria flora and from the breakdown of red blood cells. Common side effects of this drug are nephrotoxicity and ototoxicity. Patients with renal disease or renal impairment should not take this drug.
   b, c. These diseases are not affected by neomycin.
   d. Peripheral neuropathy is a chronic complication of diabetes mellitus.
   Analysis/Physiologic/Implementation

7. **Correct response: b**
   Risk for rejection is always a possibility, especially during the 4th to 10th day postoperatively.
   a, c, d. These nursing diagnoses are always possibilities for every postoperative patient.
   Knowledge/Physiologic/Planning

8. **Correct response: a**
   Universal precautions are indicated for the patient with hepatitis B. Hepatitis B is contracted via blood and blood products, body secretions, and punctures from contaminated needles.

b. This type of precaution is not sufficient with hepatitis B because of the additional types of transmission.

c. This type of isolation is indicated with the fecal-oral transmission route.

d. This type of isolation is indicated with direct contact and respiratory involvement.

Application/Safe care/Implementation

9. *Correct response: c*

Pain medication may mask signs and symptoms of hemorrhage, further de-

crease blood pressure, and interfere with assessment of neurologic status and additional abdominal injury.

a, b, d. These interventions would be appropriate for this patient.

Application/Physiologic/Implementation

Hematology
and Immunology

I. **The immune system**
   A. Granulocytes
   B. Monocytes
   C. Complement, which system
   D. Lymphocytes

II. **Lymphoid system**
   A. Bone marrow
   B. Thymus
   C. Secondary lymphoid organs
   D. Spleen
   E. Lymphatics
   F. Immunoglobulins
   G. Actions of antibodies
   H. Primary and secondary immune response

III. **Structures and functions of the hematopoietic system**
   A. Blood characteristics
   B. Plasma
   C. Plasma proteins
   D. Erythrocytes
   E. Erythropoiesis
   F. Hemoglobin (Hgb)
   G. Factors needed for erythropoiesis
   H. Control of RBC production
   I. Platelets
   J. Normal hemostasis
   K. Hemostatic mechanism
   L. Blood coagulation
   M. Laboratory studies
   N. Diagnostic testing
   O. Nutritional considerations
   P. Nutritional considerations: cancer

   Q. Nutritional considerations: acquired immunodeficiency syndrome (AIDS)
   R. Psychosocial implications
   S. Commonly used medications

IV. **Anemia**
   A. Description
   B. Etiology and incidence
   C. Pathophysiology
   D. Assessment
   E. Nursing diagnoses
   F. Planning and implementation
   G. Evaluation
   H. Home health considerations

V. **Aplastic Anemia**
   A. Description
   B. Etiology and incidence
   C. Pathophysiology
   D. Assessment
   E. Nursing diagnoses
   F. Planning and interventions
   G. Evaluation

VI. **Hemolytic Anemia**
   A. Description
   B. Etiology and incidence
   C. Pathophysiology
   D. Assessment
   E. Nursing diagnoses
   F. Planning and implementation
   G. Evaluation

VII. Sickle cell anemia/sickle cell crisis
  A. Description
  B. Etiology and incidence
  C. Pathophysiology
  D. Assessment
  E. Nursing diagnoses
  F. Planning and implementation
  G. Evaluation
VIII. Hemophilia
  A. Description
  B. Etiology and incidence
  C. Pathophysiology
  D. Assessment
  E. Nursing diagnoses
  F. Planning and implementation
  G. Evaluation
  H. Home health considerations
IX. Leukemias
  A. Description
  B. Acute lymphocytic leukemia (ALL)
  C. Acute myelocytic leukemia (AML)
  D. Chronic lymphocytic leukemia (CLL)
  E. Chronic myelocytic leukemia (CML)
  F. Nursing diagnoses
  G. Planning and implementation
  H. Evaluation
  I. Home health considerations
X. Multiple myeloma
  A. Description
  B. Etiology and incidence
  C. Pathophysiology
  D. Assessment
  E. Nursing diagnoses
  F. Planning and implementation
  G. Evaluation
  H. Home health considerations
XI. Malignant lymphoma
  A. Description
  B. Etiology and incidence
  C. Pathophysiology

XII. Hodgkin's disease
  A. Description
  B. Etiology and incidence
  C. Assessment
  D. Planning and implementation
  E. Evaluation
  F. Home health considerations
XIII. Non-Hodgkin's lymphoma (NHL)
  A. Description
  B. Etiology
  C. Pathophysiology
  D. Assessment
  E. Nursing diagnoses
  F. Planning and implementation
  G. Evaluation
  H. Home health considerations
XIV. Oncologic emergencies
  A. Description
  B. Sepsis and infection
  C. Hemorrhage
  D. Thrombocytopenia
  E. Hypercoagulability
  F. Hyperleukotic syndrome
XV. Metabolic emergencies
  A. Hypercalcemia of malignancy
  B. Tumor lysis syndrome
  C. SIADH
  D. Hypoglycemia
XVI. Cardiopulmonary emergencies
  A. Malignant pericardial tamponade
  B. Superior vena cava (SVC) syndrome
XVII. Neurologic emergencies
  A. Parenchymal brain metastasis
  B. Malignant spinal cord compression
  C. Disseminated intravascular coagulation (DIC)
XVIII. Bone marrow transplant
  A. Description
  B. Preparation
  C. Surgery
  D. Nursing diagnoses

I. The Immune system

A. Granulocytes: these cells are the first line of defense against microbial invasion. They are a category of white blood cells (WBCs) composed of neutrophils, eosinophils, and basophils (Display 9-1).

1. **Neutrophils are phagocytic cells that recognize, ingest, and kill microorganisms.**

   a. Neutrophils attach to blood vessel endothelium to move through the capillary wall. This is a process known as diapedesis, in which foreign particles are engulfed and trapped within the phagocytic cell.

   b. During infection, bone marrow produces and releases more neutrophils in various developmental stages. These may include:

   ▶ bands or immature neutrophils that possess less phagocytic activity

   ▶ segmented or mature neutrophils that possess greater phagocytic activity

   c. A larger percentage of immature cells increases the chance for infection, due to less phagocytic activity.

DISPLAY 9-1.
Type and Function of WBCs

Type	% of Total WBC	Function
Neutrophils Bands (immature) Segmented (mature)	40–75	Phagocytosis
Eosinophils	2–5	Phagocytosis allergy: suppresses inflammation; granulocyte migration
Basophils	0.2–0.5	Inflammatory mediator release
Monocytes (macrophages)	2–6	Phagocytosis; monokine production
Lymphocytes	20–35	Adaptive immunity: cell-mediated; humoral

    d.   Presence of excess numbers of immature neutrophils is called a shift to the left on complete blood count. A right shift is characterized by an increased percentage of mature neutrophils.

2.   Eosinophils are a type of WBC that deactivates histamine and the slow reactive substance of anaphylaxis (SRS-A) to decrease severity of allergic/inflammatory reactions.

3.   Basophils are cells that contain heparin, SRS-A, and eosinophil chemotactic factor of anaphylaxis. They are released as needed, such as in allergen stimulation.

    4.   In order for phagocytes to accomplish their defensive purpose, they must:

        a.   accumulate in sufficient numbers at the right place
        b.   attach to the foreign material or agent
        c.   envelop or engulf the agent
        d.   dispose of the debris

B.   **Monocytes: macrophages are a large category of WBC that consists of both circulating and stationary cells.**

    1.   They are responsible for removal of antigens, damaged or old cells, and cellular debris by phagocytosis.

    2.   They secrete substances that help with inflammatory regulation and fever. Other substances are involved in the tissue repair processes necessary for wound healing.

    3.   Monocytes also secrete natural killer cells that have direct tumoricidal and microbicidal activity. In the lung these cells are called alveolar macrophages. In the liver they are referred to as Kupffer's cells. The spleen and bone marrow also have cells that can assist with RBC synthesis via returning iron to transferrin for transport

C. **Complement system: a group of proteins that circulate in the blood in an inactive form, but when activated provide a mechanism for beginning and enhancing the inflammatory process.**

    1.   When stimulated, each activated complement component sequentially acts on the next. This is called the complement cascade.

    2.   This cascade results in:

        a.   opsonization of microorganisms and immune complexes, which promotes their phagocytosis

        b.   chemotaxis and phagocyte activation, including macrophages and neutrophils

        c.   target cell lysis triggered by antigen-antibody complexes, which activates either the classical or the alternate pathway

        d.   Various fragments are activated during progression of the cascade, some of which have specific effects including vasoconstriction, changes in vascular permeability, and halting of anaphylaxis.

        e.   The final phase of the complement cascade produces a protein called the membrane attack complex (MAC).

D. **Lymphocytes are nonphagocytic cells that function to protect the body against specific antigens. They originate from stem cells in bone marrow and differentiate into either B or T cells.**

    1.   When stimulated by an antigen, B cells differentiate into cells that secrete antibodies into body fluids, which mediates humoral immunity. They originate from common stem cells in bone marrow.

    2.   The surface of B cells is coated with immunoglobulin or antibody that enables the B cell to proliferate and differentiate.

    3.   Once activated, B cells develop into either plasma (short-lived) or memory (long-lived) cells. This activation of B cells and the production of antibodies by plasma cells is called humoral immunity.

    4.   The memory cells circulate between the blood, lymphoid system, and tissues for about a year, and are responsible for the enhanced and faster immune response that occurs with repeated exposure to the same antigen.

    5.   Both T and B lymphocytes are constantly recirculating among blood, lymph, and lymph nodes.

    6.   T cells are responsible for cell-mediated immunity (CMI) and interact directly with foreign invaders. Cells mature in the thymus and are functionally divided into four cell types:

        a.   Cytotoxic cells kill foreign/infected cells, virus-infected cancer cells, and transplanted cells.

        b.   Helper cells recognize foreign cells/antigens and help to activate B cells and cytotoxic T cells.

        c.   Inducer T cells induce development of the different types of T cells.

        d.   Suppressor T cells suppress responses of the other cells and provide for feedback regulation.

    7.   T cells are distinguished by means of specific markers called cluster designations (CD) located on their cell surfaces:

        a.   All mature T cells carry markers known as T2 (CD2), T3 (CD3), T5(CD5), T7(CD7).

        b.   Helper T cells carry a T4 (CD4) marker.

    c.   Cytotoxic T cells carry a T8 (CD8) marker.

    d.   Unlike B cells, which recognize free antigen, T cells can only recognize antigen in close association with their cell surface markers.

    e.   CMI includes any immune response in which antibodies play a lesser role, such as that seen with viruses, slow-growing bacteria, and fungal infections.

    f.   A component of the immune response that is largely responsible for the rejection of transplanted tissue is the delayed hypersensitivity reaction.

    g.   The main function of T cells is to recognize and eliminate infected cells

    h.   Stimulation of a T-cell response results in formation of T memory cells, which have a longer life-span, lasting months to years.

    8.   Lymphocytic disorders include viral disorders such as HIV, mumps, rubella, rubeola, hepatitis, and varicella, pertussis, and chronic lymphocytic leukemia.

II.   Lymphoid system

    A.   **Bone marrow**

        1.   Found inside the long bones

        2.   Major site for stem cells to replicate and mature into specific immune cells.

    B.   **Thymus**

        1.   Large in newborns and children and gradually becomes smaller with age.

        2.   Within the thymus, T lymphocytes multiply and become capable of immune response.

    C.   **Secondary lymphoid organs (Fig. 9-1)**

        1.   Include lymph nodes, spleen, tonsils, and adenoids

        2.   Other areas of lymphoid tissue are mucosal areas of the GI (Peyer's patches) and respiratory and genitourinary tracts

    D.   **Spleen**

        1.   Contains both phagocytic and lymphoid tissues

        2.   Role is to prevent organisms from entering the body via mucosa-lined structures that are open to the external environment

        3.   Enlargement of the spleen is called splenomegaly.

    E.   **Lymphatics**

        1.   Lymphocytes eventually return to circulation through the thoracic duct or right lymphatic duct.

        2.   Lymph nodes are dispersed along lymphatic vessels, grouping into clusters in the neck, axillae, abdomen, and groin.

        3.   Interstitial fluid is drained by the lymphatic vessels. This fluid then filters through the lymph nodes, where antigens are trapped and presented to lymphocytes.

        4.   Lymphocytes then multiply, which manifests as an enlarged, palpable lymph node.

    F.   **Immunoglobulins: antibodies produced by plasma cells. There are five types: IgG, IgA, IgM, IgD, IgE.**

        1.   IgG

            a.   Role is to seek out infectious organisms.

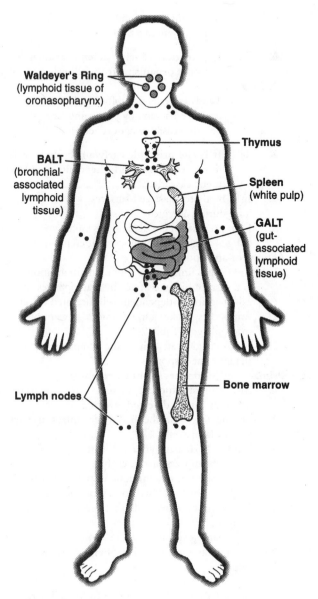

Waldeyer's Ring
(lymphoid tissue of
oronasopharynx)

Thymus

BALT
(bronchial-
associated
lymphoid
tissue)

Spleen
(white pulp)

GALT
(gut-
associated
lymphoid
tissue)

Bone marrow

Lymph nodes

FIGURE 9-1.
Normal immune system.

b.   By opsonizing or coating microorganisms, it speeds their up-
     take by phagocytic cells and can activate the complement cas-
     cade that subsequently increases the immune response.

 c.   **It is the only immunoglobulin that can cross the placenta
     and offer passive immunity to the newborn.**

2.   IgA

a.   It is present in seromucous secretions such as saliva, tears, colostrum, breast milk, and secretions of the respiratory, GI, and reproductive tracts.

 b. It provides primary defense against local infections and prevents organisms from adhering to mucosal surfaces.

3. IgM
    a. Tends to remain in blood, where it is effective against gram-negative bacteria by producing large antigen clumps that can be more easily phagocytized.

 b. It is the principle early antibody seen in the primary immune response and the main activator of the complement cascade.

4. IgE: binds to mast cell surfaces, where it stimulates histamine release during allergic response.
5. IgD: present on circulating B lymphocytes and may be involved in antigen-triggered lymphocyte differentiation.

G. Actions of antibodies
1. Antibodies function in antigen neutralization or by increasing antigen susceptibility to attack by macrophages and neutrophils. This is called antibody-dependent cell-mediated cytotoxicity.
2. Antibodies make antigen more susceptible to phagocytosis by macrophages (Table 9-1).
3. IgG and IgM can activate the complement cascade to help enhance the immune response

H. Primary and secondary immune response
1. After antigen exposure, there is a latent period in which little or no antibody can be detected in serum.
2. During this time the B cell recognizes antigen and differentiates into a plasma cell.
3. Within 4–10 days after the first exposure, serum antibody levels rise. IgM appears first, then IgG.
4. This is the primary immune response that is characterized by peak antibody levels followed by a rapid decrease.
5. However, memory cells that are produced are able to recall this antigen.
6. With later exposure to the same antigen, antibody is produced faster, lasts longer, and is often much higher than in the primary response.
7. Cytokine
    a. This is is the general term for cell-derived factors that mediate intercellular interactions.
    b. Some of these factors are called interleukins, which provide regulatory signals between various leukocytes.
8. Interferons
    a. These are a group of proteins secreted by various leukocytes and by infected body cells.
    b. They protect noninfected cells from viral invasion.
    c. When activated by either lymphocytes, tumor cells, or bacterial endotoxin, monocytes and macrophages synthesize and secrete regulatory mediators called monokines. Two of these are interleukin 1 and interleukin 2 (Display 9-2).

TABLE 9-1.
Allowable Transfusion Blood Types

TYPE	ANTIBODIES	CAN DONATE TO	CAN RECEIVE FROM
A	B	A	A, O
B	A	B	B, O
O	A, B	Universal	O
AB	None	AB	Universal
RH+		RH+	RH+/−
RH−		RH+/−	RH−

9. Tumor necrosis factor (TNF) provides protection via tumoricidal action.
   a. Produces tumor necrosis by occluding the blood supply
   b. Also protects against various organisms by activating eosinophils, neutrophils, macrophages, and cytotoxic cells
   c. TNF also has harmful effects. In response to sepsis, it initiates a series of reactions involving activation of endothelial cells, macrophages, and neutrophils.
   d. Several mediators are released, resulting in platelet aggregation and fibrin deposition, which eventually cause intravascular coagulation and tissue damage.

III. Structures and functions of the hematopoietic system
   A. Blood characteristics
      1. Circulating blood volume is approximately 70–75 mL/kg body weight.

      2. **Adult men have a blood volume of 5–6 L and women 3.5–4.5 L.**
      3. Plasma, the fluid part of the blood, comprises 55% of blood volume, with the rest being composed of various cells and other suspended solid particles.
      4. The proportion of RBCs to plasma is known as the hematocrit.

DISPLAY 9-2.
Major Interleukins and Their Principal Effects

Interleukin-1: Lymphocyte activation, macrophage and neutrophil stimulation, stimulation of acute-phase proteins, fever and sleep, pituitary hormone regulation

IL-2: Enhances T-cell growth and function

IL-3: Stimulates differentiation of hematopoietic cells (colony-stimulating factor)

IL-4: B-cell growth factor

IL-5: B-cell growth and differentiation

IL-6: B-bell growth and differentiation; stimulates acute phase response

        5.   Arterial blood has a higher oxygen concentration than venous blood and is bright red, versus the darker red of venous blood.

B. **Plasma**

    1.   The volume of plasma in adults ranges from 2.5–3.5 L.

    2.   **Plasma maintains circulatory volume and transports proteins, electrolytes, and small molecules throughout the body.**

    3.   It is composed of over 90% water, with the rest made up of protein, electrolytes, glucose, urea, and lipids.

C. **Plasma proteins: There are over 100 different proteins with various functions**

    1.   Albumin makes up most of the plasma protein concentration.

        a.   It is involved in maintenance of plasma colloidal osmotic pressure.

        b.   It acts as a carrier by transporting free fatty acids and bilirubin to the liver for catabolism and excretion.

        c.   It also acts as a carrier for the hormones thyroxine and cortisol.

    2.   Globulins are classified by structure that are glycoproteins and lipoproteins, or by size.

    3.   Fibrinogen: one of the largest plasma proteins.

    4.   Most plasma proteins are synthesized in the liver except:

        a.   immunoglobulins (B cells)

        b.   parts of complement system (macrophages)

        c.   some apolipoproteins (intestinal cells)

        d.   Von Willebrand factor (endothelial cells)

    5.   **Larger proteins cannot cross the capillary membrane and remain in the blood vessels, whereas smaller ones (albumin) can leak extravascularly to be returned to circulation by lymph system.**

D. **Erythrocytes (RBCs): perfectly shaped for transporting oxygen from the lungs to body cells.**

    1.   Biconcave disc shape makes them flexible and provides a large surface area for gas diffusion. This allows cell volumes to increase and decrease without causing cell rupture.

    2.   Conditions that change the shape of RBCs and reduce surface area available for gas exchange may occlude passage through blood vessels

E. **Erythropoiesis**

    1.   **The average life-span of an RBC is 120 days.**

    2.   Adult RBC production occurs in bone marrow of vertebrae, sternum, ribs, iliac crest, and the proximal ends of the femur and humerus.

    3.   RBCs arise from a common, undifferentiated stem cell that differentiates into the mature RBC.

F. **Hemoglobin (Hgb): the main component of the erythrocyte. It is made up of a protein (globin) and pigment (heme) that give it its color.**

    1.   Each of the 4 Hgb subunits can bind with one iron atom.

    2.   Iron is bound to Hgb. Each iron atom in its reduced (ferrous)

state, binds with one oxygen atom. Each molecule of Hgb thus can bind with 4 oxygen atoms when completely saturated.

3. Hgb is a transport molecule, picking up and binding oxygen in lungs to form oxyhemoglobin (see oxyhemoglobin dissociation curve, Chapter 6).

4. The RBC changes shape depending on whether it needs to pick up or release carbon dioxide.

G. Factors needed for erythropoiesis

1. Iron
   a. The majority of body iron supply is used to maintain Hgb content of RBC, with the rest attached to muscle cells, used by bone marrow for additional RBC production, or stored in spleen and liver.
   b. Dietary sources include red meats (especially liver), some fruits and vegetables (beans, spinach, kale, greens), and egg yolks.
   c. Ingested iron is actively transported into the cells of the small intestine, where iron binds to a protein to form ferritin for storage.

2. Vitamin B12 and intrinsic factor
   a. These are needed for RBC maturation.
   b. The body needs intrinsic factor, which is produced by the parietal cells of gastric mucosa, to act as a carrier before it can be absorbed from the ileum.
   c. It is stored in the liver until needed by the bone marrow for RBC production.

3. Folic acid
   a. Folic acid (folate) is a B vitamin.
   b. Dietary sources include green vegetables, beans, nuts, liver, and fruits.

4. Copper (abundantly supplied in regular diets)

H. Control of RBC production

1. RBC production is under the control of erythropoietin, which is manufactured and secreted by the kidneys in response to tissue hypoxia.

2. Stimulation of erythropoietin results in increased RBC production and release from bone marrow.

3. Regulation is best maintained with adequate iron stores for erythropoiesis.

4. RBC destruction occurs when old and damaged cells are removed from circulation and phagocytized by macrophages in the spleen, liver, and bone marrow.

I. Platelets (also called thrombocytes): they arise from bone marrow and contain granules that release clotting factors and substances to promote wound healing.

1. Average life span of a thrombocyte is 7.5 days

2. Two thirds of platelets are in circulating blood and one third are located in the spleen.

J. Normal hemostasis

1. Initially there is rapid contraction of blood vessels at the site of injury and surrounding area.

  2.   Platelet plug formation occurs and substances are released that promote vasoconstriction and coagulation.
  3.   Blood coagulation is via both intrinsic and extrinsic systems.
K.   Hemostatic mechanism
  1.   Rapid vasoconstriction is an immediate response after blood vessel injury; this may be related to the release of serotonin and other platelet substances.
  2.   Approximately 80% of platelets are circulating in blood and the rest are in the spleen.
    a.   Initially platelets help to stop bleeding by platelet plug formation and later they help with plug stabilization.
    b.   Formation of the plug begins seconds after vessel injury, by platelet adhesion to exposed blood vessel wall tissue.
    c.   Initial adhesion of platelets to connective tissue is followed by platelet aggregation, where platelets adhere to each other to further seal the injured area.
    d.   Other substances such as collagen, thrombin, vasopressin, and epinephrine also stimulate aggregation, but only in the presence of extracellular calcium.
    e.   Platelets in contact with collagen fibers are stimulated to produce prostaglandins and thrombi A2, which is a platelet aggregating and vasoconstricting substance.
    f.   All aspects of platelet function work together to form the temporary platelet plug that eventually will be converted into the stable fibrin clot.
L.   Blood coagulation
  1.   The goal of all the interactions of the coagulation factors is the formation of thrombin, which stabilizes the platelet plug and results in the change of fibrinogen to fibrin. This forms a coagulated mass that is called a clot.
  2.   Clotting of blood can be initiated in two ways:
    a.   Extrinsic pathway, which is initiated by factors not normally found in blood. In this pathway, factor III is released at the injury site, and reacts with factor VII and calcium to convert factor X to its active form.
    b.   Intrinsic pathway, which is initiated by factors contained within the plasma. It is stimulated when factor XII contacts a foreign surface such as collagen or skin. It proceeds as a sequence of enzymatic reactions, with the active form of each factor activating the next.
  3.   Both of these systems culminate in the common pathway.
    a.   Activated factor X initiates the conversion of prothrombin to thrombin, with involvement of factor V, platelet factor 3, and calcium.
    b.   Thrombin then divides the fibrinogen molecule to form a loose fibrin mesh.
    c.   Through interaction of factor XIII and calcium, a tough, insoluble fibrin clot is formed.
    d.   This clot holds the aggregated platelets onto the injured blood vessel surface, thus preventing or minimizing blood loss.

      e.   Platelet contraction then results in clot retraction away from blood flow within vessel

M. **Laboratory studies**
1. CBC with differential count
2. Hgb and Hct
3. Platelet levels, bleeding times, clotting times
4. ABGs
5. Erythrocyte sedimentation rate, reticulocyte count
6. Serum immunoglobulin testing

N. **Diagnostic testing**
1. Bone marrow studies
2. X-rays
3. CT scan/MRI

O. **Nutritional considerations**
1. Studies have shown that immunocompromised patients who are malnourished tend to have worse outcomes than those who are well-nourished.
2. Although malnutrition is not usually the principal cause of immunosuppression, it does exacerbate conditions such as infection, injury, and cancer.
3. The initiation of nutrition support, especially maintaining the integrity of the gut, can positively affect patient outcome.
4. The gut is an active metabolic and immune organ, participating in substantial interorgan nitrogen transfer and immune output following injury and infection.
5. The gut's epithelial cells turn over every 2 to 3 days and have specific requirements during the catabolic response to stress.
6. If metabolic and immune breakdown occurs in the gastrointestinal tract during critical illness because of a failure to provide appropriate nutrition, loss of mucosal integrity and function may occur.
7. Loss of GI barrier function can lead to a state of gut-derived sepsis, organ dysfunction, and death.

P. **Nutritional considerations: cancer**
1. Protein calorie malnutrition is a common problem in the cancer patient. The disease itself and the treatments contribute to the malnourished state of cancer patients.
2. Metabolic abnormalities include derangements in protein, carbohydrate, lipid, and energy metabolism.
3. Malnutrition in the cancer patient is associated with increased morbidity and mortality from surgery, chemotherapy, and radiation therapy.
4. Once established, tumor growth and metastases may significantly alter nutrient intake.
5. Although nutritional intake is required, controversy exists regarding the phenomenon of nutrient-induced accelerated tumor growth.
6. Questions remain as to the effectiveness of nutrition support and the clinical outcome in cancer patients undergoing antineoplastic therapy.
7. It is generally accepted that preoperative conventional nutritional support results in a significant reduction in postoperative morbidity only in severely malnourished patients.

8. Considerations for medical nutritional therapy
   a. The overall goal is to increase the nutrient intake to achieve caloric balance and meet intake needs.
   b. Vitamin and mineral supplementation is recommended.
   c. Closely monitor levels of potassium, magnesium, and phosphorus.
   d. Problems with oral intake (Table 9-2)

Q. Nutritional considerations: acquired immunodeficiency syndrome (AIDS)

   1. Clinical manifestations of AIDS include many symptoms that affect nutritional status and intake.
   2. Oral and esophageal lesions cause pain during eating, fever increases energy requirements and adversely alters food intake, nausea and vomiting decreases nutritional intake, and opportunistic intestinal infections and lesions lead to malabsorption and diarrhea.
   3. Food and drug interactions often interfere with nutrient metabolism and tolerance of food.
   4. Considerations for medical nutrition therapy
   a. The overall goal is to increase the nutrient intake to achieve caloric balance and meet intake needs.
   b. Maintain body weight and normal nitrogen balance.
   c. Monitor total protein, albumin, pre-albumin, and transferrin for visceral protein status.
   d. Intake needs can range from 30–35 kcals/kg/day and from 1.0–2.5 g protein/kg/day.
   e. If there is normal gut function, a high-calorie, high- protein, low-fat diet is the initial recommendation.

TABLE 9-2.
Problems and Interventions with Oral Intake

PROBLEM	MODIFICATION
Anorexia/early satiety	Small, frequent meals high-calorie foods
Dysgeusia (impaired taste)	Offer foods at room temperature or cold
Mouth dryness	Add sauces, gravies, and fats to food Suggest liquid foods Offer extra liquid and flavored ice
Esophagitis/stomatitis	Avoid spicy and acidic foods Offer soft or pureed, foods Offer hard candy and popsicles
Nausea/vomiting	Avoid excessively sweet or strong-flavored foods Use carbonated beverages or salty foods to relieve nausea Avoid odorous foods

      f.   Medical nutritional supplements with multivitamin and multimineral supplements should be used if oral intake is reduced.

      g.   Give special attention to B12, B6, and folate levels; these may be deficient in this population.

R.   **Psychosocial implications**

    1.   Living with a chronic disease with a progressive and sometimes irreversible or fatal symptomatology is a psychosocial challenge to patients.

    2.   Patients may experience difficulty with employment due to length of time needed for treatments.

    3.   Chronic disease also entails financial constraints.

    4.   Adjustments in time management must be made.

    5.   There are possible altered role performance, self-concept, and body image changes.

    6.   Many patients also will face possible altered self-care abilities.

    7.   Changes in energy levels related to blood/immune system alterations may also occur.

S.   **Commonly used medications: see Table 9-4**

IV. Anemia

A.   **Description: condition resulting from hematopoietic disease, characterized by decreased number or function of circulating RBCs/hemoglobin.**

B.   **Etiology and incidence**

    1.   High risk in clients with dietary iron deficiency or those who cannot metabolize iron adequately.

    2.   Some forms of anemia are hereditary.

    3.   Commonly seen in conditions in which there is chronic/gradual blood loss without replacement.

    4.   Associated with chronic renal failure.

    5.   Also associated with instances of massive blood loss or hemolysis.

C.   **Pathophysiology**

    1.   General effects of anemia are due to decreased oxygen-carrying cell capacity, but clinical manifestations are related to underlying pathophysiology.

    2.   **Tissue hypoxia occurs when oxygen is unavailable or insufficient at the cellular level for vital metabolic processes.**

    3.   Compensatory mechanisms include:

        a.   Increased synthesis of 2, 3-DPG at the cellular level, which shifts oxyhemoglobin dissociation curve so that more oxygen is released to tissues at higher oxygen tension.

        b.   Entails the use of all available blood vessels to increase tissue perfusion to vital areas, which leads to decreased blood flow to skin and kidneys.

        c.   Vasoconstriction and deoxygenated Hgb contribute to pallor in anemic clients.

        d.   Increased erythrocyte production occurs due to erythropoietin stimulation, except in patients with chronic renal failure.

        e.   Increased bone marrow production of RBCs may cause generalized pain in active areas.

       4. Failure of compensatory mechanisms may result in angina pectoris, intermittent claudication, and night cramps due to lactic acidosis accumulation.

       5. In cases of chronic anemia the blood volume remains normal because of compensatory increased plasma volume.

       6. In instances of acute anemia both volume and blood components are lost.

D. Assessment
    1. Systemic manifestations include:
       a. fatigue, weakness, dyspnea
       b. tachycardia with activity
       c. orthostatic hypotension and chest pain with exertion
    2. Neurologic manifestations include:
       a. headache, lightheadedness, "roaring in the ears"
       b. faintness, irritability, restlessness, or depression

E. Nursing diagnoses
    1. Decreased Cardiac Output
    2. Risk for Injury
    3. Activity Intolerance

F. Planning and implementation
    1. Monitor Hgb and Hct.
    2. Prioritize care to reduce fatigue and conserve oxygen.
    3. Anticipate need for PRBC transfusion.
    4. Administer erythropoietin alfa to stimulate erythropoiesis.
    5. Educate patient and family about foods high in iron.

G. Evaluation
    1. The patient is able to achieve adequate activity tolerance and is able to perform activities of daily living (ADLs).
    2. Hematologic parameters will return to pre-illness levels.

H. Home health considerations
    1. Clients will generally require long-term iron supplements.
    2. Home health nurses will need to assess the home for safety issues secondary to the hypotension and fatigue experienced by the client.

V. Aplastic anemia

A. Description: deficiency disorder brought about by stem cell failure, resulting in decreased leukocyte production and decreased platelets, causing pancytopenia.

B. Etiology and incidence: one half of cases are idiopathic and half develop after exposure to certain drugs, chemicals, viruses, or other environment agents (Display 9-3).

C. Pathophysiology: stem cell changes may result from:
    1. suppression of blood cell production processes by the immune system or suppression by drug/chemotherapy
    2. metabolic dysfunctions during cellular differentiation
    3. genetic abnormalities

D. Assessment
    1. Patients may experience increasing malaise, fatigue, and dyspnea due to poor tissue oxygenation.
    2. There is an increased susceptibility to infection.

DISPLAY 9-3.
Suspected Causes of Aplastic Anemia

Drugs: chloramphenicol, phenylbutazone, diphenylhydantoin, mephenytoin, tolbutamide, sulfonamides, chlorpromazine, alkylating agents, antimetabolites

Toxic chemicals: benzene insecticides (Ddt): organic solvents (glue fumes)

Infections: tuberculosis, hepatitis, viruses

Immune dysfunction: humoral, cellular

Environmental: radiation

Genetic

3. Bruising and epistaxis from thrombocytopenia may be seen.
4. Pallor, petechiae, or purpura may be present.
5. Laboratory studies include:
    a. thrombocytopenia (decreased platelet count); bleeding time, capillary fragility, and clot retraction indicate thrombocytopenia
    b. diagnosis confirmed by bone marrow biopsy

E. **Nursing diagnoses**
1. Risk for Infection
2. Risk for Injury
3. Knowledge Deficit: Anemia
4. Activity Intolerance

F. **Planning and interventions**
1. Interventions are directed at discontinuation of possible toxic medications and removal from exposure to toxic environmental agents.
2. Transfuse blood components as ordered and appropriate.
3. Administer corticosteroids and androgens to help stimulate remaining bone marrow function
4. Administer antithymocytic globulin as indicated.
5. Prevent or treat infection with reverse isolation.
6. Prepare for splenectomy when indicated.
7. Prepare for bone marrow transplantation when indicated.
8. Explain functions of blood elements.
9. Explain need for possible bone marrow biopsy for diagnosis and possible transplantation (HLA typing).
10. Monitor for signs of systemic infection and protect wounds to prevent contamination.
11. Monitor lab studies, including platelets.
12. Assess skin for bruising/petechia and check for epistaxis, urinary, gum, or GI tract bleeding (blood in stools or urine).
13. **Institute bleeding precautions, which are necessary when platelet count falls under 50,000/mm^3.**
14. **Avoid rectal procedures that can stimulate bleeding.**
15. Plan ADLs with patient to reduce fatigue.

G. **Evaluation**
1. The patient will show reduced risk of infection as evidenced by normal WBCs and absence of fever.

2. The patient will describe known facts about disease and treatment plan.
3. The patient will have a reduced bleeding risk.
4. The patient will be able to participate in self care at adequate activity levels.
5. The patient will verbalize feelings about self and condition.

VI. Hemolytic anemia

A. **Description: increased rate of destruction of erythrocytes (RBCs), resulting in a shortened life span to under 120 days.**

B. **Etiology and incidence**
1. May be caused by drugs such as penicillin, levodopa, phenacetin, methyldopa, quinidine, aspirin, nitrites, sulfonamides, vitamin K, dapsone, thiazide diuretics, and chloramphenicol.
2. May be immune-mediated as in ABO incompatibility and systemic lupus erythematosus.
3. Inherited anemias include sickle cell disease, G6PD deficiency, and the thalassemias.
4. RBC trauma–related causation includes burns, cardiopulmonary bypass, and prosthetic valves.
5. Other causes include infectious agents, surgery, pregnancy, psychological stress, snake/spider venoms, near-drowning, hepatic disease, and lead exposure.

C. **Pathophysiology**
1. Defective or old RBCs are taken out of circulation and destroyed in the liver or spleen. This is the most common form of hemolysis.
2. When RBCs are lysed, free Hgb is released into the circulation.
3. The released Hgb is removed by the reticuloendothelial system (RES). When degradation capacity is exceeded, breakdown products enter glomerular filtrate causing hemoglobinuria.
4. Jaundice and pigmented gallstones may result from severe hemolysis.
5. RBC membrane particles circulating in plasma can trigger DIC.

D. **Assessment**
1. Symptoms range from those associated with mild anemia to a severe hemolytic process.
2. Hepatomegaly and splenomegaly may be present.
3. Lab findings depend on etiology. Generally the Hct and Hgb are decreased, with an elevated reticulocyte count during bone marrow regeneration. Red cell survival studies may be ordered.

E. **Nursing diagnoses**
1. Fatigue
2. Risk for Infection
3. Impaired Gas Exchange

F. **Planning and implementation**
1. Identify the underlying cause and prepare for treatment.
2. Improve tissue oxygenation and support cardiovascular function.
3. Administer blood transfusions as needed, recognizing that crossmatching is difficult to accomplish with severely impaired oxygen-carrying capacity.
4. Administer steroids and other immunosuppressive drugs in immune-mediated hemolytic processes as ordered.

       5.   Prepare patient for splenectomy when extravascular hemolysis in spleen is major problem.

       6.   Provide skin care for jaundiced clients with pruritus. Use soothing, emollient lotions, not soap.

  G. **Evaluation**

       1.   The patient will verbalize appropriate infection precautions.

       2.   The patient will demonstrate adequate tissue perfusion and gas exchange.

       3.   The patient will demonstrate decreased fatigue.

VII. **Sickle cell anemia/sickle cell crisis**

  A. **Description: a form of hereditary hemolytic anemia, with the gene being autosomally dominant in transmission.**

  B. **Etiology and incidence**

       1.   Occurs in about 10% of the African American population.

       2.   Sickle cell trait is an asymptomatic homozygous condition.

       3.   Sickle cell disease causes chronic hemolysis and acute, episodic vaso-occlusive crises that can lead to organ failure.

  C. **Pathophysiology**

       1.   Erythrocytes carrying the hemoglobin S of sickle cell anemia become deformed and sickle-shaped when there are decreased oxygen concentrations, pH decreases, or increases in the concentration of 2,3-diphosphoglycerate (DPG).

       2.   Sickling increases blood viscosity and impairs smooth flow. Occlusions of small vessels in different organs may occur when large numbers of sickled cells are in circulation.

       3.   Sickling is usually reversible if oxygenation is restored.

       4.   Sickle cell crisis is a potentially fatal complication caused by painful blood vessel blockages in various organ systems (kidney, liver, spleen, musculoskeletal, lungs, brain, eyes, corpus cavernosum of penis, uterus).

       5.   It may also cause temporary but total halt of erythropoiesis, resulting in rapid decreases in levels of hemoglobin and hematocrit.

  D. **Assessment**

       1.   Similar to that found with that other forms of anemia.

       2.   Assess for pain, dysrhythmias and fever.

       3.   Jaundice is possible due to extensive hemolysis.

       4.   Patients often have physical and sexual developmental retardation and cholelithiasis.

       5.   Patients will show an increased susceptibility to infection due to splenic dysfunction and complement system dysfunction.

       6.   Chronic leg ulcers can occur.

       7.   There is a high risk of stroke during acute sickling episode.

  E. **Nursing diagnoses**

       1.   Decreased Cardiac Output

       2.   Risk for Injury

       3.   Risk for Infection

       4.   Pain

       5.   Fluid Volume Deficit

       6.   Activity Intolerance

F. **Planning and implementation**

1. **Interventions are directed at maintaining hemostasis to prevent and manage sickling and aplastic crisis.**
2. Administer blood transfusions as ordered and as appropriate.
3. Provide supplemental oxygen
4. **Avoid dehydration and acid–base alterations. Provide for increased fluid intake to maintain adequate hydration status.**
5. Prevent infection; implement aggressive management of infection if it occurs.
6. Use care with venipunctures.
7. **Provide pain relief with narcotic analgesics. Assess level of pain and implement aggressive management due to disseminated vascular occlusions.**
8. Be aware that hydroxyurea decreases incidence of sickling crises.
9. Monitor vital signs and peripheral pulses, hemodynamic parameters, and ECG.
10. Assess skin for color, warmth, turgor, and edema.
11. Assess for jugular venous distention.
12. Assess heart and breath sounds and report shortness of breath, cough, or production of frothy sputum.
13. Monitor weight, intake and output.
14. Maintain neurologic checks.
15. Elevate head of bed.
16. Promote restful environment.
17. Provide skin care and ensure frequent position changes.

G. **Evaluation**

1. Early assessment and intervention for bleeding will be provided and the patient will suffer no injury.
2. The patient will verbalize relief of pain.
3. The patient will verbalize understanding of disease, treatment, and home care.
4. Infection will not develop.
5. Optimal physical mobility will be maintained.

VIII. **Hemophilia**

A. **Description: an inherited inability to maintain hemostasis due to defect in clotting mechanisms.**

B. **Etiology and incidence**

1. Hemophilia A is a genetic disease characterized by deficiency of factor VIII; considered to be a sex-linked recessive trait.
2. Von Willebrand's disease: autosomal dominant trait, affecting both sexes equally.

C. **Pathophysiology**

1. Hemophilia is characterized by a defect in cells lining the blood vessel walls, which either cannot produce or properly use factor VIII precursors.
2. This leads to decreased amounts of factor VIII, which is vital for normal function of the intrinsic pathway.
3. The normal platelet adhesion role is impaired during primary hemostasis.

      4. Continued impaired interaction between platelets and blood vessel lining occurs during the clotting process.

      5. Bleeding onset is usually delayed for hours or days after injury, but once started may continue for weeks.

      6. Spontaneous bleeding is rare in mild cases. Exsanguination may occur if severe cases are untreated.

D. **Assessment**

      1. Symptom severity is directly proportional to blood levels of clotting factors.

      2. Frequently there is a family history of excessive bleeding after trauma, surgery, or childbirth.

      3. Localized/systemic bleeding problems are manifested by bruising, ecchymoses, hematomas without development of petechiae or purpura, and spontaneous hematuria.

      4. Joint hemorrhages can occur, therefore pain assessment and management are indicated.

      5. Laboratory studies include a prolonged bleeding time, normal platelet count, decreased platelet adhesiveness, and reduced factor VIII precursors.

E. **Nursing diagnoses**

      1. Risk for Injury

      2. Decreased Cardiac Output

      3. Altered Tissue Perfusion: (Cerebral, Cardiopulmonary, Renal, GI, and Peripheral)

      4. Pain

      5. Anxiety

      6. Ineffective Individual Coping

F. **Planning and implementation**

      1. Apply pressure and cold during bleeding episodes.

      2. **Anticipate the need for blood replacement: O-negative blood should be immediately available.**

      3. **Be aware that during emergency situations, antihemophilic factor concentrate is given every 10–12 hours due to short duration of action and the need to attain nearly normal levels.**

      4. **Be aware that factor VIII activity rapidly decreases after transfusion (half-life of 12 hours), so transfusions are needed until bleeding stops. Cryoprecipitate may also be used.**

      5. Prompt administration of analgesics at regular intervals via PTCA if available. Avoid products containing aspirin.

      6. Assess sites likely to bleed for bruising/bleeding.

      7. Measure abdominal girth.

      8. Monitor laboratory studies: Hgb and Hct, platelets.

G. **Evaluation**

      1. Early assessment and intervention for bleeding will occur and the patient will suffer no injury

      2. The patient will verbalize pain relief.

      3. The patient/family will verbalize understanding of diseases, treatment, and home care.

      4. Patient will be free of infection.

     5. Optimal physical mobility will be maintained.

  H. **Home health considerations**
1. Explain recessive sex-linked genetic inheritance.
2. Teach client:
   a. about disease severity, treatment plans, and measures to prevent injury
   b. to avoid aspirin products
   c. to notify all health care providers and dentist about the disease; in many instances prophylaxis with coagulation factors before surgery or dental manipulation is indicated
   d. to avoid contact sports
   e. to use caution with tools/devices that can cut
   f. not to go barefoot
   g. that bleeding into joints may cause serious chronic disability and vocational retraining may be necessary

IX. Leukemia

  A. **Description**
1. Leukemia is a disease characterized by overproduction of malignant WBC precursors (leukemic cells) in bone marrow, resulting in anemia, granulocytopenia, and thrombocytopenia.
2. Characterized by replacement of bone marrow with developing leukemia cells, which spread to the blood and invade the liver, spleen, lymph nodes, bone marrow, and other sites (Table 9-3).

TABLE 9-3.
Stages of Leukemia

STAGE I	STAGE II	STAGE III
Chronic phase: median duration of 3–6 years.	Accelerated stage: patients have been under chronic treatment and have shown disease progression but do not yet meet blastic disease criteria.	Blastic phase: aggressive, rapidly terminal phase into which all patients enter; refractory to treatment.
Leukostasis may lead to thromboembolic episodes and bleeding of major blood vessels, especially in the pulmonary or central nervous systems. Excessively high WBC is a medical emergency: WBC count must be quickly lowered with hydroxyurea and/or leukopheresis.	Time of progression to accelerated phase greatly affects survival. First evidence of accelerated stage may be failure to respond to drugs that were previously effective during the chronic stage. Rapidly increasing leukocyte formation (time needed to double shortens to 20 days or less). Signs and symptoms include fatigue, anemia, recurrence of splenomegaly, thrombocytopenia, hypermetabolic signs (night sweats, decreased appetite, weight loss). Periosteal infiltrates may cause bone pain and sternal pain.	Tremendous increase in blasts in bloodstream; bone marrow treatment: bone marrow transplant the only curative treatment. Assessment: fatigue, pallor, dyspnea, anemia, anorexia, weight loss, sternal tenderness, splenomegaly. Laboratory studies; Philadelphia chromosome (Ph1) present.

3. Anemia, bleeding, coagulation disorders, and loss of normal WBC are usual causes of death.
4. Disease either acute or chronic.
5. Classification of leukemias is according to WBC origin:
   a. Lymphocytic leukemia shows malignant cells of lymphocytic origin.
   b. Granulocytic or myelocytic leukemia shows malignant cells of granulocytic origin.
6. Additional classification is based on cell maturity:
   a. Immature (blastic) cells are categorized as acute.
   b. Mature or stable cells are categorized as chronic.
   c. Acute leukemia is known to be severe and aggressive.

B. Acute lymphocytic leukemia (ALL)
   1. Description: absence of mature white cells and overabundance of immature lymphocytes.

   a. **Normally when stem cells divide, one of the daughter cells matures and is functionally committed while the other remains as an uncommitted stem cell retaining the properties necessary for normal blood cell functions.**
   b. This ratio is altered in ALL because leukemia results in an interruption of the cell differentiation process, causing the proportion of stem cells to increase.
   2. Etiology and incidence
      a. Specific risk factors include genetic disorders and exposure to ionizing radiation from nuclear reactions. ALL is usually seen in young children.
      b. May have a viral etiology.

C. Acute myelocytic leukemia (AML)
   1. Description: absence of mature white cells and overabundance of immature granulocytes
      a. In AML there is in an interruption of the cell differentiation process.
      b. This causes the proportion of stem cells to increase, which interrupts normal blood cell functioning.
   2. Etiology and incidence
      a. Multinodal therapy increases survival. Median age at diagnosis is about 50 years.
      b. Specific risk factors include genetic disorders, exposure to benzene (in unleaded gasoline, rubber cement, and cleaning solvents), exposure to ionizing radiation from nuclear reactions and from occupational and therapeutic radiation. AML is usually seen in young adults.
      c. May also have a viral etiology.
   3. Assessment

      a. **Presence of Auer bodies on blood smear.**
      b. Platelet count is generally less than $20,000/mm^3$.
      c. The patient suffers from recurrent infections unresponsive to standard oral antibiotics.
      d. Easy bruising, epistaxis, or gingival bleeding reflect thrombocytopenia.

e.   Increased number of immature blast cells are associated with anemia and thrombocytopenia.

f.   Marrow aspirate shows myeloblasts comprising the majority of the nucleated cells.

D.   Chronic lymphocytic leukemia (CLL)

1.   Description: CLL is a disease of immunoglobulin-secreting cells characterized by continuous replication of nonfunctional stem cells that survive for longer than normal periods and accumulate. Most often these are B cells.

2.   Etiology and incidence

a.   CLL is more a result of genetic predisposition than environmental influences.

    b.   **There is a strong correlation between CLL and autoimmune disorders.**

3.   Assessment

a.   Assess for skin and respiratory infections

b.   Nearly one-half of the bone marrow is infiltrated before laboratory blood count is altered.

c.   Lymphocytosis: peripheral WBC count may exceed 50,000/mm^3, with more than 90% immature lymphocytes.

d.   Rai clinical staging system is based on lymphocytes, lymphadenopathy, and splenomegaly. Staging progresses from stage 0 to stage IV, with each stage indicating decreased length of survival.

e.   Malaise, anorexia, fatigue, and lymphadenopathy develop in later stages of the disease.

f.   GI and GU complaints are related to abdominal lymphadenopathy.

g.   Abdominal discomfort or a sense of fullness is related to splenomegaly, hepatomegaly, and anemia.

E.   Chronic myelocytic leukemia (CML)

1.   Description: disorder characterized by proliferation of the granulocytes, with the malignant WBC appearing as mature and well-developed, though functioning abnormally.

2.   Etiology and incidence

a.   Most commonly occurs between 20–60 years of age

b.   Associated with radiation or benzene exposure

c.   Not clearly associated with alkylating agents or hereditary factors

F.   Nursing diagnoses

1.   Risk for Injury

2.   Altered Nutrition: Less than Body Requirements

3.   Body Image Disturbance

4.   Ineffective Individual/Family Coping

5.   Risk for Infection

6.   Anticipatory Grieving

G.   Planning and implementation

1.   Treatment goal is cure, with treatment divided into two phases: induction and post-remission therapy.

2. Be aware of treatment modalities:
   a. Bone marrow transplant: bone marrow is harvested from the client (autologous transplant) or from a histocompatible donor (allogeneic transplant).
   b. Best results are obtained when performed early in the chronic phase.
   c. Recurrent disease therapy is aimed toward achieving remission. It is difficult to attain remission after relapse and these remissions rarely last more than 1 year.
   d. Radiation therapy.
3. Assess support systems.
4. Offer support through the grieving process.
5. Discuss community resources such as the Leukemia Society of America and American Cancer Society.
6. Administer medications on time to maintain therapeutic blood levels. Types of antineoplastic medications include:
   a. Induction chemotherapy: cytarabine with anthracycline
   b. Single-agent: chlorambucil (alkylating agent), cyclophosphamide, prednisone, fludarabine
   c. Busulfan (oral alkylating agent)
   d. Hydroxyurea: ribonucleotide reductase inhibitor of DNA synthesis
   e. Interferon
   f. Combination chemotherapy
7. Prepare for splenectomy:
   a. This procedure does not influence survival but may be indicated for hematologic disorders refractory to systemic therapy.
   b. Indicated in a patient with persistent symptomatic splenomegaly who is responding to chemotherapy.
8. Be aware of future treatments:
   a. Biologic therapies such as with monoclonal antibodies and gamma interferon.
   b. Biologic response modifiers and growth factors such as interleukins, TNF, and colony-stimulating factors. These are under investigation.
9. Provide protective isolation for neutropenia. Screen visitors and encourage handwashing.
10. Be aware of potential complications of radiation treatments:
   a. scar tissue development under skin, resulting in taut, shiny skin
   b. telangiectasis (spider veins) due to small surface blood vessel damage
   c. skin ulcers or failure of wounds to heal due to blood vessel and circulatory changes
   d. dry skin that persists after treatment due to permanent damage to sweat and oil glands

H. **Evaluation**
1. The patient will progress through the grieving stages toward acceptance of this potentially fatal disease.
2. The patient will verbalize basic understanding of pathophysiology

of disease, necessary life-style adjustments, methods to maintain optimal wellness, and correct use of medications.

3. The patient will experience reduced anxiety and fear as evidenced by effective communication of needs and concerns.

I. **Home health considerations**

1. Teach etiology, pathophysiology, and signs/symptoms of the disease process.
2. Clarify the difference between acute and chronic disease.
3. Explain diagnostic process, treatments, complications, and prognosis.
4. Avoid use of soaps, lotions, powders, and cosmetics.
5. Avoid sun exposure. Do not use tanning salons.
6. Wear loose clothing made of cotton.
7. In instances of radiation to the neck and face, do not shave or use electric razor.
8. Dry skin well after hygiene.
9. Swim only in fresh water; chlorine and salt can irritate skin.
10. Avoid extreme heat and cold exposure of skin. Monitor weather changes, showers, heating pads, and cold packs.
11. Encourage adequate nutrition.
12. Teach client to watch out for signs and symptoms of infection and prevent infection.
13. Take care to prevent bruising of the skin.

X. **Multiple myeloma**

A. **Description: cancerous production of plasma cells involving bone marrow and resulting in bone destruction and systemic effects**

B. **Etiology and incidence**

1. Higher incidence in the late middle-aged to the elderly.
2. Etiology is unknown, but there are possible genetic and environmental links.
3. May have a prodromal period of up to 20 years

C. **Pathophysiology**

1. **There normally is a certain combination of different types of plasma cells, but with multiple myeloma, only one type of cell replicates (clones), resulting in an excess of one type of immunoglobulin.**
2. The abnormal immunoglobulin, known as the M protein, is ineffective in antibody production. One of the immunoglobulins—usually IgG—produces excessive "clones" of itself. IgG is the most commonly affected immunoglobulin.
3. Excess numbers of abnormal plasma cells infiltrate the marrow. Tumors develop and destroy the bone, and invade soft tissues such as the lymph nodes, liver, spleen, and kidneys.
4. The malignant cell is called a plasma cell, which proliferates in bone marrow.
5. Neoplastic cells cause excessive calcium resorption from the bone into the serum.

D. **Assessment**

1. The major symptom is severe bone pain.

2. Weakening of the bones leads to spontaneous and compression fractures of thoracic and lumbar vertebrae, pelvis, ribs, and proximal long bones.

3. Laboratory studies may show:
   a. Pancytopenia; proteinuria; increased BUN, uric acid, and creatinine levels.
   b. Hypercalcemia, which is manifested by anorexia nervosa, constipation, lethargy, muscle weakness, and confusion.

 c. **Presence of Bence Jones protein that the kidneys cannot clear. It precipitates in renal tubules resulting in impaired renal function.**

 d. **Hyperviscosity syndrome is characterized by circulatory impairment and blockage of small vessels, producing intermittent claudication, visual and neurologic changes, and hypervolemia.**

4. X-ray findings include:
   a. Fragile, abnormal porous areas of bone called osteolytic lesions.
   b. These are usually seen in the spine but also in the skull, sternum, pelvis, and ribs.
   c. Pathologic fractures.

E. **Nursing diagnoses**
1. Pain
2. Fluid Volume Deficit
3. Risk for Injury

F. **Planning and implementation**

 1. **Assess and treat pain. Administer analgesics early before pain becomes severe. Be aware that back pain is a common complaint.**

2. Provide fluid management and force fluids (2–3 L/day).
3. Maintain meticulous I and O.
4. If NPO, administer IV fluids to prevent hypercalcemia and renal damage.
5. Administer medications as ordered by physician:
   a. VBMCP: vincristine, carmustine (BCNU), melphalan, cyclophosphamide, prednisone: repeat cycle every 35 days for at least 1 year.
   b. MP regimen: melphalan & prednisone, repeat cycle every 28 days for at least 1 year. This regimen is used in patients over age 70 and/or with decreased mobility.
6. Monitor chemotherapy treatments for development of adverse reactions.
7. Maintain ADLs as possible. Mobility decreases calcium loss from bones, decreases constipation from narcotics and inactivity, and increases muscle strength.
8. Monitor lab tests such as Hgb, Hct, and platelets.

9.   Avoid unnecessary trauma:

a.   Draw all bloods with one venipuncture.
b.   Avoid rectal temperatures.
c.   Prevent constipation.

10.   Instruct patient to use soft toothbrushes and to use an electric razor only.
11.   Observe for bruising, melena, and hematuria.
12.   Instruct patient to avoid aspirin-containing medications, which affect platelet functioning.
13.   Place sign at the bedside about bleeding precautions.
14.   Refer to other support systems such as social services or chaplaincy, as needed.
15.   Be aware of complications of radiation (see Leukemia).

G.   Evaluation

1.   The calcium level will be maintained as close to normal range as possible.
2.   Patient maintains renal function at pre-illness level.
3.   Pain will be alleviated.
4.   Risk of fractures will be minimized.
5.   Patient will progress through grieving stages towards acceptance of fatal disease.
6.   Patient will verbalize basic understanding of pathophysiology of disease, necessary life-style adjustments, methods to maintain optimal wellness, and correct use of medications.
7.   Patient will experience reduced anxiety and fear as evidenced by effective verbalization of fears and concerns.

H.   Home health considerations (see Leukemia)

XI.   Malignant lymphoma

A.   Description: presence of malignant, enlarged, painless lymph nodes that spread from site of origin to other parts of the lymphatic system, eventually involving the spleen, liver, and bone marrow, blood, and thymus.

B.   Etiology and incidence: disease process is considered lethal without aggressive, effective treatment

C.   Pathophysiology

1.   Lymphocytes originate in bone marrow.
2.   They develop into several different types of mature cells.
3.   At any stage of development, the normal cell may become malignant, specific to the stage in which the cell became transformed.

XII.   Hodgkin's disease

A.   Description

1.   A disorder that spreads in a predictable manner from one lymph node to the adjacent nodal groups without becoming blood-borne.
2.   Presents with positive serum tests for Reed-Sternberg cells, which are giant multinucleated transformed lymphocytes.
3.   Complete remission and long-term survival probable by using a combination chemotherapy of nitrogen mustard, Oncovin (vincristine), procarbazine, and prednisone (MOPP).

B. **Etiology and incidence**
   1. Most common cancer of young adults, peaking in 20s–30s and declining until age 45, when it increases to a second peak in the 60s–70s.
   2. There is no strong evidence that specific etiologic factors exist, although a viral etiology or immune system disturbance has been implicated.
   3. Genetic and occupational predispositions may also exist.
C. **Assessment**
   1. Lymphadenopathy, pruritus, fever, weight loss, night sweats, and alcohol-induced pain may be noted.
   2. Diagnosis involves a biopsy of the enlarged node. Ann Arbor Staging Classification divides this into four stages (Display 9-4).
D. **Planning and implementation**
   1. Treatment includes radiation therapy to nodal areas: MOPP and ABVD (adriamycin, bleomycin, vinblastine, dacarbazine): either is given in 28-day cycles for minimum of six cycles (see Table 9-4).
   2. Be aware of long-term effects of treatment. Gonadal dysfunction and sterility have resulted following treatment.
   3. Assess support systems and support through the grieving process.
   4. Discuss community resources such as the American Cancer Society.
   5. Administer medications on time to maintain therapeutic blood levels.
   6. Assess anxiety level (mild, moderate, severe) and intervene appropriately.
   7. Administer analgesics/antianxiety agents as necessary.
   8. Be aware of potential complications:
      a. secondary disease development; lung and colon cancers occur with greatest frequency
      b. treatment-related
      c. chemotherapy-induced secondary malignancies such as acute nonlymphocytic leukemia and epithelial tumors
      d. gonadal dysfunction resulting in sterility and infertility
      e. radiation therapy resulting in gonadal dysfunction, sterility, infertility, and pneumonitis

DISPLAY 9-4.
Ann Arbor Staging Classification of Lymphomas

Stage I: Involvement of single lymph node region or of single extralymphatic organ or site

Stage II: Involvement of two or more lymph node regions on the same side of the diaphragm

Stage III: Involvement of lymph node regions on both sides of the diaphragm

Stage IV: Disseminated involvement of one or more extralymphatic organs or tissues

A–No systemic symptoms

B–Systemic symptoms present

text continued on page 356

TABLE 9-4.
Medications Used in the Treatment of Cancer

MEDICATION	SIDE EFFECTS (**NOTE: Many clients with alopecia have alterations in body image, which must be addressed)	ADVERSE REACTIONS	NURSING CONSIDERATIONS
Antimetabolites			
Fluorouracil (5-FU)	Alopecia, anorexia, nausea, vomiting, erythema, pruritus, lethargy, dark discoloration of soles, palms, and nailbeds in people of color	Hyperthermia, chills, severe diarrhea, stomatitis, dark stools, increased bleeding tendency, heartburn, esophagitis	Assess for anemia, dyspnea, signs of infection, bleeding; meticulous oral hygiene; assess for chest pain, diarrhea, tarry stools, hematemesis; give bland foods and avoid high-acid foods; meds PRN
Methotrexate (Mexate)	Anorexia, nausea, vomiting, erythema, stomatitis	Black diarrhea stools, hematemesis, hyperthermia, chills, stomatitis, increased bleeding tendency (intrathecal: seizures, disorientation, vertigo, vision changes), esophagitis, rash, conjunctivitis	Meds PRN; monitor for allergic reaction, bleeding, dyspnea, infection; assess for tarry stools, hematemesis, monitor renal studies for impairment; assess for allergic reaction right after administration
Alkylating Agents			
Cyclophosphamide (Cytoxan)	Alopecia, anorexia, nausea, vomiting dark discoloration of fingernails and skin	Hyperthermia, chills, irregular menses, increased bleeding tendency, leg edema, dysarthria, dyspnea	Meds PRN; assess menstrual patterns; elevate legs; measures to relieve respiratory distress, measures to treat hyperthermia
Mechlorethamine (Mustargen)	Anorexia, nausea, vomiting, metallic taste in mouth	Hyperthermia, chills, increased bleeding tendency, painful rash, joint pain, leg edema, amenorrhea, tinnitus	Meds PRN; assess menstrual patterns; elevate legs; measures to relieve respiratory distress, measures to treat hyperthermia

Cisplatin (Platinol)	nausea, vomiting, anorexia	Tinnitus/hearing loss, hyperthermia, chills, increased bleeding tendency, anemia, GI upset, joint pain, leg edema, impaired taste and vision, peripheral neuropathy	Meds PRN; assess for hearing/vision loss; treat hyperthermia; assess for bleeding; monitor for Hgb and Hct, elevate legs, promote foods less likely to affect taste
Antibiotics			
Doxorubicin (Adriamycin)	Alopecia, anorexia, nausea, vomiting, red-colored urine	Hyperthermia, chills, increased bleeding tendency, stomatitis, esophagitis, erythematous rash, joint pain, leg edema, dyspnea, GI upset, cardiotoxicity	Meds PRN; assess for dyspnea, tachycardia, crackles, CHF development; teach that urine discoloration is expected and temporary; monitor ECGs
Vinca Alkaloids			
Vinblastine (Velban)	Alopecia, anorexia, nausea, vomiting, muscle aches and pains, constipation	Somewhat less toxic than others: hyperthermia, chills, increased bleeding tendency, leg edema, peripheral neuropathy, paralytic ileus	Meds PRN; monitor for paresthesias, jaw pain decreased DTRs in legs; encourage high-fiber diet with activity and stool softeners
Vincristine (Oncovin)	Alopecia, anorexia, nausea, vomiting, rash, flatulence, constipation, insomnia	Neurotoxicity: diplopia/blurred vision, paresthesias, ataxia, decreased DTRs, peripheral neuropathy; ptosis, jaw pain, headache, GI upset, leg edema, disorientation, depression, seizures; pulmonary problems when given with mitomycin	Meds PRN; monitor for paresthesias, jaw pain, decreased DTRs in legs; encourage high-fiber diet with activity and stool softeners, monitor respiratory status during administration, assess for chest pain

        f.   cranial radiation that causes confusion, headache, motor function disabilities, seizures, nausea, vomiting, slurred speech, and vision changes

        g.   potential complications of radiation treatments (see Leukemia)

E. Evaluation

1. Compliance with treatment regimen will be maintained to increase chances for long-term remission/cure.
2. Patient will progress through grieving stages toward acceptance of fatal disease.
3. Patient will verbalize basic understanding of pathophysiology of disease, necessary life-style adjustments, methods to maintain optimal wellness, and correct use of medications.
4. Patient will experience reduced anxiety and fear as evidenced by verbalization of fears and effective communication of concerns.

F. Home health considerations

1. Teach:
   a. signs and symptoms of infection including fever, chills, pain, erythema, swelling, pus formation
   b. monitoring of fluid intake and output
   c. self-care measures, potential for injury from walking, changes in sensation, muscle strength
   d. chronic nature of the disease etiology, hematopoietic changes, pathophysiology signs and symptoms, diagnostic process, treatments, complications, prognosis
2. Avoid use of soaps, lotions, powders, and cosmetics.
3. Avoid sun exposure and do not use tanning salons.
4. Wear loose clothing made of cotton.
5. In instances of radiation to neck and face do not shave or use electric razor.
6. Dry skin well after hygiene.
7. Swim only in fresh water; chlorine and salt can irritate skin.
8. Avoid extreme heat/cold exposure of skin including weather, showers, heating pads, and cold packs.

XIII. Non-Hodgkin's lymphoma (NHL)

    A. Description: diffuse lymphomas that invade the entire lymph node in an erratic and unpredictable pattern, destroying the normal node structure and function

1. B cell lymphomas include:
   a. Small lymphocytic diffuse type, well-differentiated lymphocytic lymphoma, Burkitt's lymphoma
   b. Immunoblastic sarcoma of B cells
   c. Plasmacytoid lymphocytic lymphoma (with secretion of antibody) ·
2. T cell lymphomas include:
   a. Small lymphocytic T cell lymphoma
   b. Convoluted T-cell lymphoma
   c. Cutaneous T-cell lymphoma and Sézary's syndrome
   d. Immunoblastic sarcoma of T cells

    B. Etiology

1. It is thought to possibly be an immune abnormality.

2. Greatest incidence in persons with:
   a. congenital immunodeficiencies, organ transplants
   b. autoimmune disease, immunosuppression, infections

C. Pathophysiology

1. It is presumed to develop with chronic deficiency in immunocompetence, which promotes lymphocyte development and proliferation.

 2. Most lymphomas arise from B cells, which could occur with abnormal CD8 suppressor cells or when CD4 helper cells are promoting B-cell growth.

 3. In Burkitt's lymphoma, Epstein-Barr virus acts to cause B-cell proliferation.

 4. T cells then regulate this proliferation, resulting in either no disease or infectious mononucleosis.

5. Staging (see Table 9-5)
   a. Indolent (low grade): survival measured in years
   b. Aggressive (intermediate grade): survival measured in months
   c. Highly aggressive (high grade): survival measured in weeks

TABLE 9-5.
TNM Classification System

T* subclasses

Tx—tumor cannot be adequately assessed
T0—no evidence of primary tumor
TIS—carcinoma *in situ*
T1, T2, T3, T4—progressive increase in tumor size and involvement

N† subclasses

Nx—regional lymph nodes cannot be assessed clinically
N0—regional lymph nodes demonstrably normal
N1, N2, N3, N4—increasing degrees of demonstrable abnormalities of regional lymph nodes

M‡ subclasses

Mx—not assessed
M0—no (known) distant metastasis
M1—distant metastasis present, specify site(s)

Histopathology

G1—well-differentiated grade
G2—moderately well-differentiated grade
G3,G4—poorly to very poorly differentiated grade

*T = Primary tumor
†N = Regional lymph nodes.
‡M = Distant metastasis.
(American Joint Committee on Cancer. Manual for Staging of Cancer. Chicago, American Joint Committee.)

D.   Assessment
1.   The primary symptom is painless lymphadenopathy in the neck.
2.   Lymphadenopathy is more generalized than that of Hodgkin's disease and often involves abdominal nodes and extranodal sites including the bone marrow, liver, and GI tract.
3.   Symptoms of vague abdominal discomfort, back pain, and ascites may occur.
4.   There are no specific lab studies. CBC is usually normal, as with Hodgkin's disease.

E.   Nursing diagnoses
1.   Risk for Injury
2.   Alteration in Nutrition: Less than Body Requirements
3.   Body Image Disturbance
4.   Ineffective Individual/Family Coping
5.   Risk for Infection
6.   Anticipatory Grieving

F.   Planning and implementation
1.   Assess support systems and support through the grieving process.
2.   Discuss community resources such as the American Cancer Society.
3.   Provide protective isolation for neutropenia such as screening visitors and promoting good handwashing.
4.   Administer medications on time to maintain therapeutic blood levels.
5.   Assess anxiety level and intervene appropriately.
6.   Administer analgesics/antianxiety agents as necessary.
7.   Be aware of potential complications:
    a.   Disease-related: superior vena cava syndrome, CNS and/or spinal cord involvement
    b.   Treatment-related (see Hodgkin's disease)
    c.   Potential complications of radiation treatments (see Leukemia)

G.   Evaluation
1.   The patient will progress through the grieving stages toward acceptance of fatal disease.
2.   The patient will verbalize basic understanding of pathophysiology of disease, necessary life-style adjustments, methods to maintain optimal wellness, and correct use of medications.
3.   The patient will experience reduced anxiety/fear as evidenced by verbalization of fears and effective communication of concerns.

H.   Home health considerations (see Leukemia)

XIV.   Oncologic emergencies
A.   Description
1.   Acute complications in cancer increases as treatment becomes more effective.
2.   Cancer-associated emergencies are usually systemic and usually fall into one of four categories:
    a.   Hematologic-septic: DIC
    b.   Metabolic: hypercalcemia
    c.   Cardiovascular: SVC
    d.   Neurologic: increased intracranial pressure

B.   Sepsis and infection
1.   This is the most common cause of death in cancer patients.
2.   Assessment
    a.   Assess for evidence of fever and neutropenia.

      b.   Fever with neutropenia is often the first sign that bacteremia is present in a cancer patient.

      c.   A neutrophil count below about 500/mm^3 indicates infection.

      d.   Neutropenic clients may look fine early on, but their condition often quickly declines.

      e.   Assess possible sites for infection sources (ie, catheter sites, skin, ears, sinuses, oropharynx, abdomen, and perineum).

   3.   Planning and implementation

      a.   Administer broad-spectrum antibiotics to cover both gram-negative and gram-positive organisms as ordered and appropriate.

      b.   **If possible, administer the IV antibiotics at home or clinic to decrease chance of nosocomial exposure.**

      c.   Expect to administer biologic response modifiers (granulocyte and monocyte colony stimulating factors) to decrease incidence and extent of infection limit when given before development of neutropenia.

      d.   Educate patients regarding prevention and recognition of infection.

C. **Hemorrhage: often occurs due to thrombocytopenia or decreased clotting factors, but may also be due to hypercoagulability or DIC**

D. **Thrombocytopenia**

   1.   This is the most frequent predisposing factor for bleeding.

   2.   It usually results from chemotherapy and from decreased platelet production, but also may be due to radiation or cancer infiltration into bone marrow.

   3.   Because ASA and other NSAIDs inhibit platelet action, instruct clients to avoid these agents.

E. **Hypercoagulability**

   1.   Leg swelling or shortness of breath may be the first signs.

   2.   Anticoagulants are rarely helpful with cancer-associated hemorrhage, owing to clotting factor dysfunctions.

   3.   Treatment involves insertion of an inferior vena cava filter to decrease mortality from pulmonary embolus.

F. **Hyperleukotic syndrome**

   1.   This results from blast crisis in chronic myelocytic leukemia or acute myelocytic leukemia.

   2.   **When the WBC rises above 100,000/mm^3, the preponderance of poorly developed cells drastically increases blood viscosity.**

   3.   Hyperviscous blood damages blood vessels, especially in the pulmonary and central nervous systems.

   4.   This extra resistance also may cause cardiac failure.

   5.   **Excess WBCs also deplete glucose and release potassium as they lyse, causing pseudohypoglycemia, pseudohypoxia, and pseudohyperkalemia.**

   6.   Assessment involves recognition of marked dyspnea and hypoxia, along with CNS changes such as headache, confusion, and neurologic deficits.

   7.   Treatment is use of leukapheresis or chemotherapy to lyse white cells.

XV. Metabolic emergencies
A. Hypercalcemia of malignancy
  1. This is the most common metabolic cancer, usually occurring in conjunction with multiple myeloma and breast cancer.
  2. Causes include:
    a. Increased bone resorption or inability to excrete calcium via renal system.
    b. Parathyroid hormone stimulates osteoclast activity and bone destruction
    c. Metastasis to bone also causes bone destruction.
  3. Assessment
    a. **Dehydration with a normal blood pressure is a major indicator of hypercalcemia, and is due to smooth-muscle contraction resulting from excessive calcium.**
    b. Chronic hypercalcemia produces nephrogenic diabetes insipidus, resulting in dehydration, polydipsia, and polyuria.
    c. Other symptoms include fatigue, constipation, nausea, vomiting, and subtle mental status changes.
  4. Treatment
    a. Rehydration with saline and/or lactated Ringer's solution
    b. Administration of loop diuretics to increase calcium excretion
    c. Avoid use of thiazide diuretics, which decrease calcium excretion
    d. Steroids may be indicated
  5. Long-term treatment
    a. Encourage early physical mobilization.
    b. Administer plicamycin (mithramycin) to inhibit RNA synthesis and interfere with parathormone and vitamin D production.
    c. Hemodialysis may be indicated.
B. Tumor lysis syndrome
  1. Description
    a. Characterized by rapid breakdown of cells and consequent release of intracellular contents into bloodstream, which overwhelms the excretion system, leading to the syndrome.
    b. This occurs between 6–72 hours after chemotherapy.
    c. It is usually associated with leukemias, lymphoma, and solid tumors.
  2. Assessment
    a. Most common symptoms are weakness and malaise due to severe hyperkalemia.
    b. Hypertension, hyperuricemia, and severe renal insufficiency may occur.
    c. Hypophosphatemia with secondary hypocalcemia is noted.
  3. Treatment involves administration of allopurinol and aggressive hydration.
C. **SIADH: usually associated with small-cell lung cancer, as well as antineoplastic agents (vincristine, cyclophosphamide) (see Chapter 11)**
D. Hypoglycemia
  1. Manifested by seizures and focal neurologic abnormalities, which often are due to secreting islet-cell tumor.

      2. Treatment involves resection, radiation, and dietary modification.

XVI. Cardiopulmonary emergencies

    A. Malignant pericardial tamponade (fairly common)

    B. Superior vena cava (SVC) syndrome

      1. Definition: increased venous pressure in head, neck, and upper extremities caused by compressive pressure to or elevated obstructive pressure within the SVC.

      2. Causes are usually due to malignant disease, mostly lung cancer.

      3. Signs and symptoms include swelling of the head, neck, and upper extremities without other edema, dyspnea, feeling of head fullness, cough, and chest pain.

      4. Diagnosis is made through:

        a.   Sputum cytology

        b.   Thoracentesis

        c.   Thoracotomy: last choice for detection but extremely accurate

      5. Treatment

        a.   Elevate head of bed to decrease or prevent facial and brain edema.

        b.   Provide supplemental oxygen.

        c.   Be aware of inconclusive effect concerning use of corticosteroids and diuretics.

        d.   Mediastinal radiation may be used to shrink obstruction.

        e.   May prevent this syndrome by percutaneous placement of intravascular stent to keep vein open.

XVII. Neurologic emergencies

    A. Parenchymal brain metastasis stems from lung, breast, GI, and GU cancers, and melanomas.

      1. Pathophysiology: Edema occurs around the tumor and causes many of the obvious signs and symptoms.

      2. Symptoms:

        a.   Headache, nausea, vomiting, dysphasia, ataxia, and personality changes are symptoms.

        b.   Symptoms are the most severe on waking due to hypoventilation during sleep, which increases CO_2 retention, with resulting cerebral vessel dilation and increased edema.

      3. Diagnosis is made by use of CT and MRI. Skull films are of no value.

      4. Treatment: must be treated aggressively to prevent death.

        a.   intubation and hyperventilation with target CO_2 of 25–30 mm Hg

        b.   seizure treatment

        c.   **Steroids, especially dexamethasone, are beneficial because of potency with minimal mineralocorticoid effect.**

        d.   Radiation therapy

    B. Malignant spinal cord compression: usually results from an extradural source

      1. Sites of compression are the thoracic spine, lumbar, then cervical vertebrae.

      2. The major symptom is pain.

3.   Treatment involves administration of corticosteroids, chemotherapy, radiotherapy, and surgery.

C.   **Disseminated intravascular coagulation (DIC) (see Chapter 13)**

XVIII.   Bone marrow transplant

   A.   **Description**

   1.   Bone marrow transplant is the standard curative method to restore immunologic and hematologic function in persons with immunologic deficiencies, leukemias, or several other disorders.

   2.   It is also used to eliminate bone marrow toxicities resulting from chemotherapy and/or radiation therapies.

   3.   Three major types (autologous, allogeneic, and syngeneic) are named to indicate source of donor marrow. The recipient must be matched with a compatible donor, based on human leukocyte antigen (HLA) typing and mixed lymphocyte culture (MLC) results.

      a.   Syngeneic: donor and recipient are identical twins and successful transplantation is assured.

      b.   HLA-matched allogeneic transplants: occurs between compatible sibling or nonsibling donor and recipient.

      c.   HLA-mismatched donor and recipient transplant: due to development of technique to remove harmful mature T cells from donor marrow, HLA–half-matched parents can be donors.

      d.   Autologous: patient's own marrow is frozen and stored for reinfusion after chemotherapy and radiation to destroy the underlying malignant growth.

   B.   **Preparation:**

   1.   Recipient must be immunosuppressed before procedure.

   2.   Set up laminar airflow room. Clean all articles in room with germicidal agent. Have client bathe BID with agents such as chlorhexidine (Hibiclens). Ensure sterile clothing and sheets.

   3.   The GI tract is sterilized with nonabsorbable IV antibiotics.

   4.   Women receive antibacterial and antifungal agents intravaginally.

   5.   **Following the procedure to eliminate normal flora, the patient undergoes immunosuppression, which reduces incidence of graft rejection, removes malignant cells, and prepares bone marrow spaces for engraftment.**

   6.   The typical regimen includes total body irradiation (TBI) for 4 days followed by IV chemotherapy for 2 days.

   7.   Chemotherapeutic agents commonly used are cyclophosphamide (Cytoxan), procarbazine (Matulane), and human antilymphocyte globulin.

   C.   **Surgery**

   1.   Transplant marrow is obtained by multiple aspirations from donor's posterior and anterior iliac crests.

   2.   After the marrow has been prepared, it is transfused into the recipient over several hours via a specialized catheter in a peripheral vein. The transplant itself closely resembles a blood transfusion.

   D.   **Nursing diagnoses**

   1.   Risk for Infection

   2.   Risk for Injury

   3.   Altered Nutrition: Less than Body Requirements

4. Anxiety/fear/powerlessness
5. Pain

E. Planning and implementation
1. Explain procedure and complications to patient.
2. Assess for bleeding as evidenced by epistaxis, bleeding gums, melena, hematemesis, hemoptysis, hematuria, and vaginal bleeding.
3. Assess for signs of liver dysfunction. Symptoms usually take 1–3 weeks to develop:
   a. Sudden weight gain, hepatomegaly, right upper quadrant pain
   b. Jaundice, tea-colored urine, ascites
   c. Dyspnea, confusion, lethargy/fatigue
4. Encourage mobility as possible.
5. Discuss transfusion of blood components.
6. Explain actions, purposes, side effects of medications.
7. Discuss neutropenic precautions (private room, laminar air flow, etc.).
8. Monitor labs: CBC/differential, serum iron, TIBC, total protein, albumin.

F. Potential complications
1. The critical period is 2–4 weeks after transplantation.
2. The person is most susceptible to infection and bleeding during this time.
3. Graft-versus-host disease (GVHD): newly grafted immunocompetent cells recognize antigens of recipient as foreign.
   a. Primarily affects the skin, GI tract, liver.
   b. May present in acute or chronic form.
   c. Onset is marked by development of red maculopapular rash 7–14 days after transplant.
   d. Rash usually begins on the face, palms of hands, and soles of feet, then progresses to trunk and extremities.
   e. Skin may become dry and peel or may develop blisters.
   f. May first be treated with high-dose steroids. If there is no improvement, antithymocyte globulin may be administered.
   g. Nonsystemic treatments are provided to decrease the severity and discomfort of the numerous disease manifestations.

G. Evaluation
1. Successful engraftment as evidenced by improvement in laboratory studies within 10–30 days after transplantation.
2. Successful engraftment as evidenced by development of RBC, WBC, and platelets in bone marrow.
3. WBC differential should show increased PMNs if bone marrow is functioning normally.

H. Home health considerations
1. Encourage handwashing, neutropenic precautions, and low-bacterial diet (well-cooked meats, fruits washed well).
2. Promote hygiene by use of a separate towel or cloth for each infected area, to prevent cross-contamination. Use careful oral hygiene (Display 9-5).

XIX. Human immunodeficiency virus (HIV)
A. Description:
1. A virus is believed to be responsible for the disease known as acquired immunodeficiency syndrome (AIDS).

DISPLAY 9-5.
Household Tips After Bone Marrow Transplant

> Frequent handwashing
> Meticulous oral and body hygiene
> Avoid crowds
> Avoid cleaning cat litter boxes, fish tanks, and bird cages
> Do not handle dog or human feces; avoid contact with barn-yard animals
> Avoid swimming in public pools

    2.   The disease is characterized by a low number of T-helper lymphocytes or a lower ratio of helper cells to T-suppressor cells, which leads to decreased immunity, increasing the risk of opportunistic infections, any of which may be life threatening.

B.   **Etiology and incidence**

    1.   Development may depend on dose/virulence of pathogen and host resistance.

    2.   Those at greatest risk are:

        a.   Men who have unprotected sex with men

        b.   Persons with multiple sex partners

        c.   Persons who are intravenous drug abusers (IVDA) or those who have sexual contact with an IVDA without barrier protection

        d.   Infants of HIV+ mothers

        e.   Minority populations in urban settings

        f.   Adolescent heterosexuals who do not use safer sex practices

        g.   Heterosexuals with high-risk sexual practices

C.   **Pathophysiology**

    1.   A retrovirus is a piece of genetic information, either RNA or DNA, protected by a protein coat.

    2.   Normally, genetic information goes from DNA to RNA protein.

    3.   A retrovirus reverses the process and makes itself into DNA.

    4.   Steps in virus replication include:

        a.   HIV recognizes T4 (helper) cells, which normally coordinate immune system responses.

        b.   HIV's newly made DNA copies itself into the genetic material of the helper cell.

        c.   With foreign antigen stimulation, the T4 cell reproduces the HIV virus instead of itself.

        d.   The new virus infects other T4 cells.

    5.   In an intact immune system, there are twice as many T4 helper cells as T8 cells; however, with increasing numbers of HIV cells, the number of T4 cells decreases, leading to immunosuppression.

D.   **Progression**

    1.   Virus is replicating but does not yet produce antibodies. This is a "window period" with appropriate immune system response.

    2.   CD4 activates, thus activating HIV.

    3.   HIV is released and reproduced.

4. The immune response decreases and CD4 count lowers as more of them become infected with HIV.

 5. **HIV should be conceptualized as a continuum of infection from asymptomatic to seriously ill with life-threatening opportunistic infections and malignancies.**

E. Transmission

1. Transmission is person-to-person via body fluids.

 2. **The HIV must enter via damaged skin and mucous membranes, due to the fact that it has no DNA of its own. It needs a T cell to attach to so it can penetrate.**

3. Sexual contact: Individuals do not need to be symptomatic to spread the disease. The longer time one is infected with HIV, the greater the chance of spreading the disease with a single sexual encounter.

4. Blood-to-blood—IVDA: The risk of transmission is small, especially when compared with the risk of acquiring hepatitis.

5. Prenatal: May be transmitted before birth or by contamination with instruments and blood during delivery.

6. The risk of a child developing HIV has been dramatically decreased by giving AZT to the mother during pregnancy, IV during labor, then syrup to the baby for 6 weeks.

7. Artificial insemination

8. Breastfeeding

9. Vaginal secretions

10. Saliva: Centers for Disease Control and Prevention recommends no deep kissing

F. No documented transmission

1. Casual contact, including living in the same house

2. Tears, urine, stool

G. Uncertain transmission

1. Amniotic fluid

2. Pericardial fluid

3. Synovial fluid

4. Spinal fluid

5. Pleural fluid

H. Testing

1. The median period between HIV conversion and AIDS diagnosis is 9–11+ years.

2. Antibodies are not formed until 3 weeks to 6 months, or longer, after exposure.

3. ELISA (enzyme-linked immunosorbent assay) detects antibodies in serum.

4. Western blot is used to confirm all positive ELISA tests.

5. The P24 antigen test evaluates antibodies that bind to the main protein of HIV. It is used to measure viral activity to evaluate replication and medication effectiveness.

 6. **Polymerase chain reaction (PCR) detects HIV's DNA and can detect an extremely small viral load.**

7. The presence of HIV in blood does not mean the person has AIDS.

8. A positive ELISA and western blot provide "reasonable proof" of HIV.

9. The presence of antibody confirms seropositive HIV, positive P24 antigen test or PCR indicates seropositivity.
10. Testing after exposure is recommended if the test is negative; retest at 6 weeks, 3 months, and 6 months.

I. Assessment

1. **A diagnosis of AIDS is given to someone with a positive HIV test and a CD4 count of 200 or less per mm^3.**
2. Evaluate for diagnosed opportunistic disease.
3. Assess for decreased CD4 count.
4. Lymphadenopathy (lymph node enlargement) is a common finding.
5. Constitutional symptoms include weight loss, anorexia, persistent diarrhea, fatigue, headache, and dizziness.
6. Monitor for unexplained bleeding from mucous membranes/body orifices.
7. Pulmonary symptoms include shortness of breath and a persistent cough.
8. Neurologic symptoms include memory loss, loss of coordination, and paralysis.

J. Nursing diagnoses

1. Impaired Gas Exchange
2. Pain
3. Altered Protection
4. Activity Intolerance
5. Risk for Impaired Skin Integrity
6. Altered Sexual Patterns
7. Self-Esteem Disturbance
8. Powerlessness
9. Ineffective Individual Coping

K. Planning and implementation

1. Administer medications as ordered by physician:
    a. Zidovudine (Retrovir), formerly azidothymidine (AZT): as with all nucleoside analogs, AZT inhibits HIV replication by mimicking HIV particles. HIV then incorporates the drug into its own genetic makeup and thus cannot completely develop. AZT does not remove HIV from already-infected cells.
    b. Other medications used to treat HIV/AIDS include didanosine or dideoxyinosine (ddI, Videx), zalcitabine, dideoxycytidine/zalcitabine (Hivid, ddC); protease inhibitors: indinavir (Crixivan), saquinavir mesylate (Invirase), ritonavir (Norvir) (Table 9-6).
2. Assess anxiety level (mild, moderate, severe) and intervene appropriately.
3. Encourage expression of feelings.
4. Administer analgesics and anti-anxiety agents as necessary.
5. Refer to other support systems: social services, spiritual.
6. Be aware of potential complications:

    a. **Opportunistic infections occur as CD4 cells become more depleted; organisms with normal virulence cause dangerous infection (Table 9-7).**

text continued on page 370

TABLE 9-6.
Primary Medications Used to Treat HIV/AIDS

MEDICATION	MAIN USES/ACTIONS	SIDE EFFECTS/ADVERSE REACTIONS	MISCELLANEOUS
Zidovudine (Retrovir)	Blocks action of reverse transcriptase (key enzyme is HIV replication); HIV with CD4 under 500/mm³;	Bone marrow suppression (neutropenia, anemia, leukopenia), nausea, vomiting, headache, decreased efficacy over time	Decreases risk of fetal transmission if taken during pregnancy, labor, and given to infant post-delivery
Didanosine (ddl, Videx)	Blocks action of reverse transcriptase (key enzyme is HIV replication); HIV with CD4 under 500/mm³; treatment of adults who are intolerant of Retrovir	Bone marrow suppression, anemia; do not give to those with pancreatitis; may elevate liver enzymes	Take on empty stomach (do not mix with milk or acidic juices)
Zalcitabine (ddC, HIVID)	Blocks action of reverse transcriptase (key enzyme is HIV replication); HIV with CD4 under 300/mm³; used in combination with Retrovir or alone for those intolerant to Retrovir	Peripheral neuropathy, pancreatitis; esophageal ulceration; CHF; ana-phylaxis, hepatic failure, stomatitis, insomnia	Stop use with pancreatitis develop-ment
Didehydrothymidine (d4T, Zerit)	Blocks action of reverse transcriptase (key enzyme is HIV replication); HIV with CD4 under 300/mm³; treatment of those who are intolerant to or unable to benefit from other approved treatments	Peripheral neuropathy; hepatotoxicity, anemia with less bone marrow suppression than Retrovir	Possible alternate to ddl/Retrovir in monotherapy
Lamivudine (3TC, Epivir)	Combination therapy with Retrovir	Headache, insomnia, fatigue, peripheral neuropathy	
Saquinavir (Invirase) Ritonavir (Norvir) Indinavir (Crixivan)	Protease inhibitors for monotherapy or in combination with Retrovir or similar drug	Usually well tolerated; nausea, vomiting, diarrhea, circumoral numbness, hyper-bilirubinemia, nephrolithiasis	

TABLE 9-7.
Opportunistic Infections Found in AIDS

OPPORTUNISTIC INFECTION	SITE AFFECTED	PATHOPHYSIOLOGY	MANIFESTATIONS	DIAGNOSIS	TREATMENT
Protozoal:					
Pneumocystis carinii pneumonia (PCP)	Lungs	Forms spores that attach to alveolar wall and multiply to form cysts in alveolar spaces; results in decreased surfactant, thus causing respiratory distress	Fever, dry cough, pleuritic chest pain, DOE, sputum hypoxemia, clear sputum	CXR, bronchoscopy, sputum specimen	TMP/SMX, pentamidine, dapsone
Cryptosporidium enteritis	Intestine	Shrinks digestive surface area by fusing villi, thus decreasing enzyme production and fermenting malabsorbed nutrients	Profuse diarrhea (fermentation leads to gas, which increases GI osmotic load so fluid pulled into bowel)	Stool sample	Rest bowel, TPN if needed for symptomatic diarrhea
Toxoplasma gondii	Focal	Organism contracted by eating undercooked meat or exposure to contaminated cat feces	Extremity weakness, ataxia, altered mental status, headache	Test for organism	Pyrimethamine (Daraprim) and leucovorin (Wellcovorin)
Fungal:					
Candida albicans	Mouth, esophagus, vagina	Organism thrives on immuno-suppression; initial presenting symptom for many HIV+ women	Based on location: dysphagia, substernal pain, burning, pruritus	Inspection, culture, esophagoscopy	Mycostatin/nystatin to affected area

Cryptococcal meningitis	Central nervous system	Most concentrated in pigeon feces and nesting areas (window ledges); inhaled after drying and becoming airborne	Fever, malaise, nausea, vomiting, headache, nuchal rigidity	Lumbar puncture with CSF culture, test for cryptococcal antigen	Amphotericin B, fluconazole, itraconazole
Viral:					
Cytomegalovirus (CMV)	Retina, colon, lungs, esophagus	Humans the only reservoir	Based on location: retinitis, abdominal pain, diarrhea, cough, dyspnea, dysphagia, burning, pain	Examination, culture, antigen testing	Gancyclovir (Foscarnet) is palliative
Herpes simplex virus (HSV)	Genitals, mouth, eyes	Not known	Single/multiple painful vesicles	Examination, culture	Acyclovir
Bacterial:					
Mycobacterium avium-intracellulare complex (MAC)	Disseminated	Scrofulaceum, ubiquitous environmental organisms	Fever, weight loss, diarrhea, night sweats, cough	Culture	Rifabutin, clarithromycin, amikacin, clofazimine, ethambutol, rifampin, azithromycin
Mycobacterium tuberculosis	See Chapter 6				

369

      b.   Cancer and malignancies: as persons with AIDS live longer, neoplasms have more time to develop during times of low CD4 levels.

      c.   Kaposi's sarcoma (KS): systemic development of tumors in blood vessel walls, causing painless purple macular and/or papular areas on the skin of the arms, chest, legs, and face. These may enlarge to occlude circulation. Treatment is palliative.

      d.   Lymphoma: primary (brain), non-Hodgkin's

      e.   Cervical cancer

      f.   Anal cancer

L.   **Evaluation**

    1.   The patient will have minimized incidence of contracting opportunistic infections.

    2.   The patient will be able to verbalize basic understanding of pathophysiology of disease, necessary life-style adjustments, methods to maintain optimal wellness, and correct use of medications.

    3.   The patient will be able to select the treatment plan that is best, based on individual needs and concerns.

    4.   The patient will be able to progress through grieving stages toward acceptance of fatal disease.

    5.   The patient will experience reduced anxiety and fear as evidenced by verbalization of fears and effective communication of needs and concerns (Displays 9-6 and 9-7).

M.   **Home health considerations**

    1.   Encourage client to return to optimal ADLs in the home environment.

    2.   Stress that even if both partners are HIV+, use of safer sexual practices could decrease the incidence of contracting new HIV strains.

    3.   Teach IVDA prevention measures:

      a.   Before preparing injection, clean "works" with solution of one-half water and one-half bleach.

      b.   Soak for at least 30 seconds before rinsing.

    4.   Teach safer sex methods.

    5.   Be aware that use of some substances impairs judgment and increases chance of high-risk behaviors.

    6.   Household teaching:

      a.   Do not share toothbrushes or razors.

      b.   No need to separate dishes; the virus is killed by soap and water.

    7.   Ensure that client is aware that:

      a.   Donor blood has been screened since 1985. Although you cannot guarantee donor blood is HIV negative, there is a minimal chance that a unit is HIV+.

      b.   HIV cannot be acquired by donating blood.

XX. **Anaphylactic shock**

    A.   **Description: an often rapidly developing, severe hypersensitivity reaction to an antigen to which an individual was previously sensitized. It is characterized by severe respiratory tract mucosal edema and cardiovascular collapse secondary to extreme systemic vasodilation.**

DISPLAY 9-6.
HIV Community Phone Numbers

AIDS Clinical Trials Information Service (800) TRIALS-A

AIDS Data Treatment Network (212) 268–4196

National AIDS and HIV Hot Line: English, (800) 342–2437

Spanish, (800) 344–7432

AIDS LINE—Prepared by National Library of Medicine; extracted from MEDLINE

AIDS Coalition to Unleash Power (ACT UP) (212) 564–2437

AIDS National Interfaith Network (202) 842–0010

Represents multiple organized AIDS ministries in the United States. Publishes a quarterly newsletter and has published two books (*AIDS and Your Religious Community: A Hands-On guide for Local Programs* and the HIV/AIDS Housing Handbook)

HIV/AIDS Treatment Information Service (800) 448–0440

Hearing impaired (800) 243–7012

Run by CDC and staffed by information specialists who draw on National Library of Medicine database; offers information for clients, families, and health providers on treatment guidelines. Spanish-speaking operators available.

National Hemophilia Foundation
(212) 219–8180

National HIV/AIDS Education & Training Centers Program (301) 443–6364

Network of regional centers with multiple local sites that provide multidisciplinary HIV education and training programs for health care providers.

Gay Men's Health Crisis AIDS Hot Line
(212) 807–6664

Jewish Family and Children Services–AIDS Support Services: (609) 424–1333

Names Project (Quilt)—"Threads of Love"; (415) 882–5500

DISPLAY 9-7.
HIV Community Access

Computer Sites: AIDS Treatment Data Network (800) 734–7104
611 Broadway, Suite 613, New York, NY, 10012
htp://health.nyam.org.8000public_html/network/-index.html
e-mail: AIDSTreatD@AOL.COM

A home page on the Internet for those with AIDS and their caregivers that provides information on approved and experimental treatments for AIDS-related conditions. It also publishes a quarterly directory of clinical trials on HIV and AIDS (English/Spanish).

AMA HIV/AIDS Information Center
World Wide Web site (http://www.ama-assn.org)

Offers clinical updates, news, and information on social and policy questions. Cosponsored by Glaxo Wellcome, Inc.

Gay Men's Health Crisis (GMHC)
Site on the World Wide Web (http://www/gmhc.org)

Provides on-line forums hosted by GMHC representatives.

DISPLAY 9-8.
Common Causes of Anaphylaxis

Foods: fish, shellfish, strawberries, nuts, milk products, eggs, chocolates

Medications: antibiotics (PCN most common), sulfonamides, sulfa diuretics, dilantin, aspirin, anesthetics

Volume substitutes: transfused blood/blood products or substitutes

Insect stings/bites: bees, yellow jackets, hornets, wasps, fire ants

Other causes: exercise induced, radiologic contrast media, vaccines, latex, chemotherapeutic agents, allergenic extract

B. **Etiology and incidence (Display 9-8)**
C. **Pathophysiology**
1. First exposure to substance rarely causes symptoms. Reactions are allergic and develop from the production of allergen-specific immunoglobulin E (IgE) antibody, which causes release of histamine, SRS-A, and other vasoactive substances.
2. It is only after the antigen has been introduced into the body that the immune system identifies it as foreign and builds up antibodies against it.
3. This results in:
   a. Increased capillary permeability, producing edema
   b. Smooth muscle constriction, causing bronchospasm
   c. Vasodilation, which can lead to decreased PVR, compensatory tachycardia, decreased venous pressure, and hypotension, followed by shock.
4. **Note that parenteral medication administration allows antigen to access the bloodstream more quickly, resulting in a more serious reaction.**
D. **Assessment**
1. Main assessment findings are related to cardiovascular, respiratory, and integumentary systems.
2. Patients may experience fear, panic, and a feeling of impending doom.
3. Lightheadedness, syncope, weakness, hypotension, and tachycardia may occur.
4. Angioedema (swelling) of the mouth, tongue, extremities (especially hands), and around eyes is common.
5. Laryngeal edema is manifested by labored breathing, difficulty talking, hoarseness, tightness in the throat, prolonged exhalation, stridor, and coughing.
6. Other pulmonary symptoms include wheezing, tightness in the chest, prolonged exhalation, tachypnea, increasing $PaCO_2$ with decreasing pH, the use of accessory ventilatory muscles, cyanosis, and bronchospasm.

7. Urticaria is characterized by flushing, hives, tingling, and warm, dry, pruritic skin.
8. Hemodynamic parameters indicative of shock include:
   a. SVR under 800 dynes/sec/cm^{-5}
   b. CI under 2.5 L/min/m^2; CO under 4 L/min
   c. PCWP under 8 mm Hg
   d. Urine output under 30 mL/hr

E. Nursing diagnoses
   1. Ineffective Breathing Pattern
   2. Decreased Cardiac Output
   3. Impaired Gas Exchange
   4. Fear/Anxiety/Powerlessness
   5. Possible Knowledge Deficit: Anaphylaxis

F. Planning and implementation
   1. Initial treatment is to administer drug therapy to decrease mediator formation, decrease mediator release, or alter mediator effects.
   2. Medications include:
      a. Epinephrine: to reverse laryngeal edema and hypotension IV, SQ, IM, depending on severity of reaction. Massage site to speed absorption. Inhalation epinephrine is indicated if stridor is present.
      b. Antihistamines: compete for receptor sites. If the situation is critical, give epinephrine followed by antihistamines. Otherwise first administer antihistamine (diphenhydramine PO, IV, IM)
      c. Hydroxyzine for urticaria symptoms.
      d. Corticosteroids: to decrease pulmonary inflammation; IV or via inhalation
      e. Aminophylline IV drip

   3. Assume most comfortable respiratory position, assess for bronchospasm and laryngeal edema, and provide nonrebreather mask as necessary.
   4. Monitor BP and attach cardiac monitor/pulse oximetry, and hemodynamic parameters.
   5. Assist with rapid intubation tracheostomy, or cricothyrotomy. Oral airways/manual respiratory bagging are ineffective with laryngeal edema.
   6. Start an IV of normal saline solution (NSS)/lactated Ringer's as ordered by physician.
   7. Identify source of reaction. If it is an IV source, stop the infusion immediately and keep vein open with NSS.
   8. If food is the cause, assist with lavage.
   9. If bites/injected agents are the cause, apply tourniquet above site but ensure perfusion to distal area by briefly loosening it q10min.
   10. If you see an embedded insect stinger, do not forcefully remove it: this could cause remaining venom to be injected. Try to flick with a fingernail or plastic card.
   11. Observe for and treat allergic reactions of skin such as flushing, rashes, and edema.

12. Decrease anxiety/fear/powerlessness as possible.
13. Be aware of potential complications such as recurrence. Many persons experience recurrence within 24 hours, and the second reaction may be just as serious as the first.
14. **Be sure someone can stay with client at home for the first day after discharge.**

G. Evaluation
1. The patient will maintain a patent airway and effective gas exchange.
2. The patient will attain and maintain adequate hemodynamic parameters.
3. The patient will maintain adequate fluid volume.
4. The patient will show decreased urticaria and concomitant discomfort.
5. The patient will experience decreased anxiety and fear by verbalizing understanding of allergic reaction, prevention, and treatment.

H. Home health considerations
1. The client is likely to have another reaction if exposed to the substance. If antigen has not been identified, go for follow-up and possible skin testing.
2. Notify all health team members, including client's dentist and pharmacist, of allergy. If caused by an OTC medication, be sure that it can be identified by both generic and brand name.
3. For food reactions:
    a. Know how meals are prepared and what ingredients are used at restaurants.
    b. Avoid dishes with unknown hidden components (casseroles).
    c. Read food labels carefully.
4. For insect reactions:
    a. Avoid bright colors outside. Dark colors or white are least likely to attract insects.
    b. Avoid perfumes and scented hair sprays, deodorants, and sunscreens.
    c. If insect approaches, do not swat at it. Remain still until it goes away.
    d. Do not walk barefoot outdoors (for reactions to fire ants).
5. Obtain a MedAlert necklace/bracelet at pharmacy or through MedicAlert Foundation, PO Box 1009, Turlock, CA 95381-1009; (800) ID-ALERT.
6. At discharge, prepare for use of self-treatment device.
7. To avoid reactions while in the hospital, nurses should ask about:
    a. previous blood transfusions/reactions
    b. type of reaction to contrast media and whether pretreatment is indicated
    c. medication allergies
    d. Due to risk of recurrence, patient should remain in clinic, office, or emergency department for at least 30 minutes after receiving medications.
    e. **Be careful giving cephalosporins to patients with PCN allergy: up to 10% are allergic to this also.**

XXI. **Latex allergy**

   A. Description: a delayed hypersensitivity reaction caused by continued exposure to latex-containing (rubber) products (Display 9-9)

   B. Etiology and incidence

   1. Increasingly common among health care team members, who use latex-containing supplies during routine daily activities.

   2. Develops in those who have sustained latex exposure due to chronic health problems that necessitate frequent, long-term bowel and bladder control using latex tip enemas and latex Foley catheters.

   C. Pathophysiology

   1. This is an allergic response to rubber gloves.

   2. It is usually characterized by localized reactions. The most frequent symptom is urticaria.

   3. Also may have flushing, cough, rhinitis, wheezing, and conjunctivitis.

   4. The reaction usually resolves spontaneously or responds to topical hydrocortisone and PO antihistamines.

    5. **Latex-induced systemic anaphylaxis is a life-threatening event occurring when latex comes into contact with internal mucous membranes such as the intestines, respiratory tract, peritoneum, and vagina.**

   6. Latex may also directly enter the circulatory system via injection or parenteral line.

   D. Assessment and nursing diagnoses (see Anaphylactic shock)

   E. Planning and implementation

   1. Prepare to assist with administration of skin prick test.

      a. Drop of liquid latex is diluted in saline and placed on skin.

      b. Area is pricked with needle and observed for 10 minutes.

      c. A wheal and flare reaction indicates allergy.

DISPLAY 9-9.
Latex-containing Products

Household products

Balloons, dental dams, and condoms
Dishwashing gloves, diaphragms
Infant feeding nipples
Rubber balls, rubber bands
Telephone cords

Hospital products

Adhesive bandages anesthesia masks and BP cuffs/tubing
Urinary and IV catheters, endotracheal tubes
Injection posts on IV, gloves, hot water bottles
Manual resuscitation bags
Oral and nasal airways, nasogastric and nasointestinal tubes
Rubber vial stoppers, tourniquets

2. If nonallergic, use powderless latex surgical gloves to prevent airborne spread of antigen.
3. Stock all hospital carts with both vinyl and plastic supplies: gloves, oral and nasal airways, oxygen delivery devices, urethral catheters, and tourniquets.
4. Use IV bags and tubing with nonlatex injection ports, if possible. Otherwise, use stopcocks on IV tubing and cover latex ports with tape to prevent withdrawal or injection of fluid.
5. **Use medications that come in glass ampules rather than vials with latex stoppers. Otherwise remove rubber stopper before fluid withdrawal. This prevents latex protein transmission during parenteral use.**
6. Notify operating room/short procedure unit of allergy preoperatively.
7. Assess history of swelling after dental work, blowing up balloons, or using condoms or diaphragms.

F. **Potential complications and home health considerations (see Display 9-9)**

Bibliography

Baum, M. K., Mantero, A., Tienza, E., & Shor-Posner, G. (1991). Association of vitamin B6 status with parameters of immune function in early HIV-1 infection. *J Acquir Immune Defic Syndr* 4, 1122–1132.

Black, J. M. & Matassarin-Jacobs, E. (1994). *Luckman and Sorenson's medical-surgical nursing: A psychophysiologic approach* (4th ed). Philadelphia: Saunders.

Campbell, M. K. & Pruitt, J. J. (1996). Radiation therapy: Protecting your patient's skin. *RN* 59(1), 46–47.

Carroll, P. (1994). Speed: The essential response to anaphylaxis. *RN* 57(6), 26–31.

Donaldson, S. S. (1984). Nutritional support as an adjunct to radiation therapy. *JPEN* 8, 302–309.

Gold, J. (1994). Ask about latex. *RN* 57(6), 32–34.

Greifzu, S. (1996). Chemo quick guide: Antimetabolites. *RN* 59(3), 32–33.

Greifzu, S. (1996). Chemo quick guide: Antitumor antibiotics. *RN* 59(4), 35–36.

Greifzu, S. (1996). Chemo quick guide: Hormonal agents. *RN* 59(5), 41–42.

Greifzu, S. (1996). Chemo quick guide: Plant alkaloids. *RN* 59(6), 36–37.

Harriman, G.R., Smith, P.D., Hone, M.K., (1989). Vitamin B12 malabsorption in patients with AIDS. *Arch Intern Med* 149, 2039–2041.

Kaiser, H. B., Kaliner, M. A., & Scott, J. L. (1991). Anaphylaxis: When routine turns nightmare. *Patient Care* 25(9), 16.

Kee, J. L. (1995). *Laboratory & diagnostic tests with implications* (4th ed). Norwalk, CT: Appleton & Lange.

North American Nursing Diagnosis Association (NANDA). (1996). *Nursing diagnoses: Definitions & classification 1997–1998*. Philadelphia: Author.

Newman, C. F. (1991). Practical dietary recommendations in HIV infection. In D. P. Kotler (Ed.), *Gastrointestinal manifestations of AIDS*. New York: Raven Press.

O'Brien, J. F. (1996). The oncologic crisis. Part 1: Septic, hematologic, and metabolic emergencies. *Emerg Med* June, 24–38.

O'Brien, J. F. (1996). The oncologic crisis. Part 2: Cardiorespiratory and neurologic emergencies. *Emerg Med* July, 21–44.

Otto, S. E. (1994). *Oncology nursing* (2nd ed.). St. Louis: Mosby–Year Book.

Raiten, D. J. (1991). Nutrition in HIV infection. *Nutr Clin Pract* 6(Suppl.), 1–94.

Schweid, L., Etheredge, C., & Werner-McCullough, M. (1994). Will you recognize these oncological crises? *RN* 57(9), 22–29.

Waite, L. G. & Krumberger, J. M. (1994). *Noncardiac critical care nursing*. Albany, NY: Delmar.

Zaloga, G. P. (1994). *Nutrition in critical care*. St. Louis: Mosby.

STUDY QUESTIONS

1. Which one of the following immunoglobulins is the principal early antibody seen in the primary immune response?
   a. IgM
   b. IgA
   c. IgG
   d. IgD

2. Your client has blood type B–. Which one of the following types of blood can she receive?
   a. B+
   b. O–
   c. A+
   d. AB–

3. Your client has blood type O+. Which one of the following types of blood can she receive?
   a. B+
   b. O–
   c. A+
   d. AB–

4. Which of the following symptoms are commonly found in the client with anemia?
   a. fatigue, orthopnea, chest pain
   b. fatigue, dyspnea, tachycardia
   c. tachycardia, chest pain, fatigue
   d. orthopnea, inspiratory pain, pallor

5. Which of the following are included when a client needs bleeding precautions?
   a. avoidance of rectal temperatures
   b. assessment of skin for bruising or petechiae, assessment for occult blood
   c. avoidance of unnecessary venipunctures
   d. all of the above

6. Which one of the following describes the rationale for pain during a sickle cell crisis?
   a. occlusion of blood vessels and tissue hypoxia
   b. occlusion of blood vessels and increased bone marrow activity
   c. tissue hypoxia and decreased bone marrow activity

   d. increased bone marrow activity and metabolic acidosis

7. Which one of the following activities should the client with hemophilia avoid?
   a. swimming
   b. golf
   c. football
   d. tennis

8. Which one of the following is found in the blood of a client with acute myelocytic leukemia?
   a. Reed-Sternberg cells
   b. Bence Jones proteins
   c. Epstein-Barr bodies
   d. Auer bodies

9. Which of the following describes the progressive stages of chronic myelocytic leukemia?
   a. chronic, accelerated, blastic
   b. chronic, blastic, accelerated
   c. blastic, accelerated, chronic
   d. accelerated, blastic, chronic

10. Which one of the following is contraindicated in the client with multiple myeloma?
   a. 3 servings of grapes per day
   b. 3 servings of skim milk per day
   c. 3 servings of orange juice per day
   d. 3 servings of asparagus per day

11. Which one of the following is found in the blood of a client with multiple myeloma?
   a. Reed-Sternberg cells
   b. Bence Jones proteins
   c. Epstein-Barr bodies
   d. Auer bodies

12. Which of the following are included when teaching the client with multiple myeloma?
   a. Drink plenty of fluids, take special care when brushing teeth.
   b. Avoid taking nonsteroidal anti-inflammatory drugs (NSAIDs).
   c. Notify the physician if stools become tar-colored.
   d. All of the above

13. Which one of the following is found in the blood of a client with Hodgkin's disease?
   a. Reed-Sternberg cells
   b. Bence Jones proteins
   c. Epstein-Barr bodies
   d. Auer bodies

14. Which of the following contributes to the hypercalcemia of malignancy?
   a. increased bone resorption
   b. inability to excrete calcium via renal system
   c. stimulation of parathormone
   d. all of the above

ANSWER KEY

1. *Correct Response: a*
IgM is the major early antibody seen, followed by IgG; the others arrive, peak, and recede during different phases of the immune response.
Knowledge/Physiologic/NA

2. *Correct Response: b*
A person with type B blood can safely receive only type B or type O (universal donor). However, a person without the Rh factor (Rh–) must receive Rh– blood to avoid a reaction, thus making answers a, c, and d incorrect.
Application/Physiologic/Implementation

3. *Correct Response: b*
A person with type O blood can safely receive only type O (universal donor). In addition, the presence of the Rh factor allows this person to receive either Rh+ or Rh– blood. Therefore answers a, c, and d are incorrect.
Application/Physiologic/Implementation

4. *Correct Response: b*
Fatigue, dyspnea, and tachycardia result from insufficient tissue oxygenation.
a. Orthopnea occurs in such disorders as emphysema, not with anemia.
c. Chest pain may occur, although it is an uncommon finding.
d. Inspiratory pain indicates possible pulmonary or rib injury.
Knowledge/Physiologic/Assessment

5. *Correct Response: d*
Any intervention that will decrease the incidence of bleeding is included with bleeding precautions. Rectal temperatures can damage rectal mucosa; bruising or petechia signals subcutaneous bleeding; occult bleeding may occur from multiple sites; and all types of skin punctures and incisions should be avoided as much as possible to reduce the risk of bleeding.
Application/Safe care/Planning

6. *Correct Response: a*
Occlusion of blood vessels results in tissue hypoxia, which causes ischemic pain.
b. There is minimal to no bone marrow activity during acute sickle cell crisis; lack of bone marrow activity is not related to pain.
c, d. Metabolic alterations vary depending on concomitant disorders, but are not part of the sickle cell process.
Comprehension/Physiologic/NA

7. *Correct Response: c*
Clients with hemophilia must avoid contact sports such as football, basketball, hockey, etc.
a, b, d. Swimming, golf, and tennis are safe sports as long as there is no threat of bodily injury.
Application/Health promotion/Planning

8. *Correct Response: d*
Reed-Sternberg cells are found with Hodgkin's Disease; Bence Jones proteins with multiple myeloma; Epstein-Barr bodies with mononucleosis and other disorders.
Knowledge/Physiologic/Assessment

9. *Correct Response: a*
The chronic stage occurs first, and may last for a relatively long period of time. The accelerated phase occurs as the disease progresses, ending with the blastic phase, which is rapidly terminal.
Knowledge/Physiologic/NA

10. *Correct Response: b*
Milk and high-calcium products must be avoided in clients with multiple myeloma.
a, c, d. Grapes, orange juice, and asparagus are low-calcium foods that are permitted on such a diet.
Application/Health promotion/Implementation

11. *Correct Response: b*

Bence Jones proteins are found in patients with multiple myeloma.

   a. Reed-Sternberg cells are found with Hodgkin's Disease.

   c. Epstein-Barr bodies are found in mononucleosis and other disorders.

   d. Auer bodies are found with AML.

Knowledge/Physiologic/Assessment

12. *Correct Response: d*

It is essential that the client with multiple myeloma drink plenty of fluids to maintain hydration and decrease the chances of the development of hypercalcemia; bleeding precautions must be followed, thus the client needs to be careful during mouth care and avoid the use of NSAIDs; because of the risk of occult bleeding, the physician must be notified of tarry stools.

Knowledge/Health promotion/
Implementation

13. *Correct Response: a*

Reed-Sternberg cells are found with Hodgkin's Disease.

   b. Bence Jones proteins are found with multiple myeloma.

   c. Epstein-Barr bodies are found in mononucleosis and other disorders.

   d. Auer bodies are found with AML.

Knowledge/Physiologic/Assessment

14. *Correct Response: d*

Hypercalcemia is further increased due to breakdown of bone and resulting calcium release into the bloodstream; renal injury prevents normal calcium excretion; abnormal production of parathormone stimulates calcium production; and tumor metastasis can exacerbate all of the above mentioned conditions.

Comprehension/Physiologic/NA

The Renal System

I. Anatomy and physiology
A. Structure
1. The kidney is located retroperitoneally at the level of L-3 and T-12.
2. The right kidney is lower than the left due to liver position.
3. The kidney is composed of an outer cortex (85% of tissue) and an inner medulla (15% of tissue).
4. It is composed of multiple triangular areas called pyramids.
5. The blood supply is from the renal arteries, which branch off at the aorta.
6. The circulatory system for the kidneys is composed of:
    a. Peritubular capillaries, which supply nutrients to the renal tissue;
    b. Vasa recta, which help with renal metabolic functions.
B. Function (Fig. 10-1)
1. The nephron is the functional unit of the kidney. There are approximately 1 million per kidney.
2. Renal function is maintained with 33% functional nephrons.
3. The glomerulus is located inside Bowman's capsule, a cluster of tightly coiled capillaries that produces an ultrafiltrate, a portion of which eventually becomes urine.

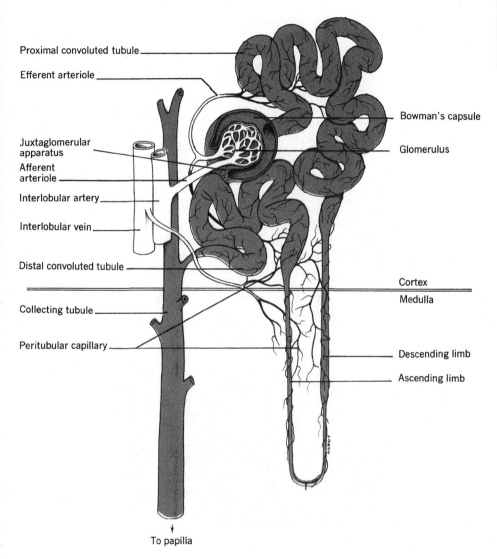

Proximal convoluted tubule

Efferent arteriole

Bowman's capsule

Juxtaglomerular apparatus

Glomerulus

Afferent arteriole

Interlobular artery

Interlobular vein

Distal convoluted tubule

Cortex

Medulla

Collecting tubule

Peritubular capillary

Descending limb

Ascending limb

To papilla

FIGURE 10-1.
The nephron, the functional unit of the kidney.

4. The tubules play a role in filtration. Filtrate enters the:
    a. Proximal convoluted tubule—80% reabsorption occurs here
    b. Then it enters the loop of Henle
    c. The countercurrent mechanism impacts on filtration
    d. Filtrate then enters the distal convoluted tubule for final concentration
    e. From the collecting duct, the filtrate that is now urine enters the renal pelvis, and continues through the ureters and bladder for excretion via the urethra.

5.   Renal blood flow (RBF)
   a.   Blood enters the nephron via the afferent arteriole, then flows into the glomerulus for filtration.
   b.   It is composed mainly of plasma, as red blood cells (RBCs) and other proteins do not normally cross the glomerular membrane.
6.   Autoregulation allows for the constriction/dilation of afferent arterioles to alter RBF.
7.   The basic functions of the kidneys:
   a.   Excretion of protein metabolism wastes
   b.   Regulation of water and electrolytes
   c.   Regulation of blood pressure
   d.   Secretion of erythropoietin
   e.   Regulation of extracellular volume
   f.   Regulation of extracellular osmolarity
   g.   Regulation of pH (acid–base balance)
   h.   Stimulation of RBC production
   i.   Hormone production
   j.   Vitamin D metabolism
   k.   Drug excretion, but not detoxification
8.   Sodium feedback mechanism
   a.   Aldosterone is sensitive to the concentration of sodium in the blood.
   b.   Renin also plays a role in the development of renal hypertension.
   c.   Active reabsorption of sodium results in passive transport of chloride and bicarbonate. This helps to maintain acid–base balance.
   d.   It also affects potassium. As reabsorption of sodium is increased by aldosterone, reabsorption of potassium is decreased. The increased concentration of potassium stimulates aldosterone production.

II.   Overview of renal pathology
A.   Laboratory studies (Table 10-1)
   1.   Blood urea nitrogen (BUN)
   2.   Creatinine
   3.   Filtration tests
   4.   Creatinine clearance—measures glomerular filtration rate (GFR). It depends on muscle mass and is collected as a 24-hour specimen.
   5.   Tubular function tests
      a.   Fishberg concentration test—measures ability to concentrate urine when deprived of water from dinner to 12:00 the next day. This test measures urine osmolality.
      b.   Specific gravity
      c.   Urine/plasma osmolality
      d.   Normal urine osmolality = 500–800 mOsm/L
      e.   Normal plasma osmolality = 280–295 mOsm/L
      f.   Urinalysis—measures specific gravity, electrolytes, cells, metabolic wastes, urea, creatinine, ammonia, and volume (Table 10-2)

TABLE 10-1.
Serum Indicators of Renal Function

TEST	NORMAL	RENAL
BUN	10–20 mg/dL	Increased
Creatinine	0.5–1.5 mg/dL	Increased
BUN:creatinine ratio	20:1	Increased
pH	7.35–7.45	Decreased
Sodium	135–145 mEq/L	Decreased
Magnesium	1.5–2.5 mEq/L	Increased
Calcium	8.5–10.5 mg/dL	Decreased
Phosphorus	2.5–4.5 mg/dL	Increased
Carbon dioxide	24–30 mEq/L	Decreased

B. Nutritional considerations

1. Critical care nutrition for patients with renal failure focuses on the management of acute renal insufficiency. It is important to note that the nutritional management differs from that of chronic renal failure.
2. The goals of nutritional therapy for acute renal failure are to maintain good nutritional status, promote recovery of renal function, prevent further renal damage, and prevent or minimize toxicity and metabolic derangements.
3. Patients with acute renal failure are frequently catabolic and may succumb to rapid nutritional deterioration.
4. This catabolic state is characterized by protein breakdown, lipolysis, water retention, and disorders of electrolyte and acid–base balance.
5. Malnutrition in acute renal failure can result in serious complications. These include compromised immune status, increased susceptibility to infections, impaired healing, and increased morbidity and mortality.

TABLE 10-2.
Normal Urinalysis Findings

PARAMETER	ASSESSMENT FINDINGS
Color	Pale yellow to dark amber depending on the concentration of solutes
Specific gravity	1.005–1.025
Osmolality	300–900 mOsm/kg
pH	4–8
Presence of foreign material	None to trace: RBC, WBC. None: ketones, bacteria, casts/sediment, glucose, protein

6.   These complications may result in further worsening of nutritional status.
7.   Attention to metabolic and nutritional details can help avoid complications while awaiting the return of renal function.
8.   Over the past few years, there has been a move away from parenteral toward enteral nutrition, and a move away from protein restriction and the use of essential amino acid formulas.
9.   Considerations for medical nutrition therapy:
    a.   The overall goal is to increase the nutrient intake to achieve caloric balance and meet intake needs.
    b.   Protein should be 70% High Biological Value (HBV)—protein that contains a full complement of essential amino acids. HBV protein facilitates reduction of serum urea levels.
    c.   Closely monitor fluid status. Fluid requirements depend on residual excretory capacity, gastrointestinal fluid losses, and insensible water losses (eg, fever and sweating). Many patients require 1500–2000 mL of water per day to replace losses.
    d.   Serum levels of sodium, potassium, phosphorus, and magnesium should be monitored daily. Patient requirements for these elements change according to metabolic status.

C.   Psychosocial implications
1.   It is a challenge to live with a chronic disease that has a progressive and sometimes irreversible symptomatology
2.   There are difficulties with employment because of the length of time needed for treatments; there are also financial constraints.
3.   Adjustments in time management need to be made.
4.   The patient may experience possible altered role performance and self-concept, body image changes, and altered self-care abilities.
5.   Patients will also need to adjust to fluid and food restrictions.

D.   Commonly used medications
1.   Electrolyte inhibitors or replacements
2.   Diuretics and antihypertensives to regulate fluid balance and blood pressure
3.   Vitamin and mineral supplements
4.   Ammonia-lowering agents

III.   Acute renal failure (ARF)

A.   Description: sudden loss of renal function due to decreased renal blood flow, glomerular damage, or tubular changes. The syndrome is associated with acute suppression of renal function, which usually develops rapidly.

B.   Etiology and incidence
1.   Renal blood flow can be reduced by hypotension, hypovolemia, or shock. Obstructed renal blood flow and tubular dysfunction also can be caused by calculi or tumors.
2.   Glomerular filtration rate (GFR) or tubular damage can result from toxic precipitates. For example, proteins and hemoglobin (Hgb) released from muscles (injured by burns or infections) that become concentrated in tubules may cause tubular damage.
3.   Some medications impair renal blood flow, especially in the elderly—including NSAIDs, certain antibiotics (streptomycin), and heavy metals (mercury).

C. **Pathophysiology: ARF is usually reversible if identified and treated before the onset of permanent renal damage. Irreversible failure leads to uremia and chronic renal failure.**

    1. Stages of ARF:

        a. Oliguric: urine output is under 400 mL per day. This stage is characterized by hypertension and acidosis, and usually lasts up to 2 weeks.

        b. Diuretic: increasing urine output, sometimes more than 3 L per day.

        c. Recovery

    2. Prerenal renal failure

        a. **Results from decreased renal perfusion**

        b. Can be caused by arterial or venous problems such as acute renal arthritis; aortic dissection; renal artery stenosis, thrombosis, or occlusion; and renal vein thrombosis.

        c. Commonly seen following episodes of decreased volume, as in hemorrhage, third spacing, diarrhea, burns, vomiting, and diabetes insipidus (DI).

        d. Vasodilation can also contribute to this as in sepsis, anesthesia, anaphylaxis, and ganglionic blockade.

        e. Pump failure, as in myocardial infarction (MI), congestive heart failure (CHF), and pulmonary embolism (PE), will result in prerenal failure

        f. Episodes of increased renal vascular resistance, as in anesthesia, hepatorenal syndrome, and surgery, can also play a role.

    3. Intrarenal renal failure

        a. **This is due to the inflammatory/immunologic process affecting glomeruli. Acute tubular necrosis (ATN) is the most common cause.**

        b. Occurs with ischemic injury, which is any condition that decreases renal blood flow for more than 40 minutes.

        c. Hypovolemia/hypotension, cardiac ischemia, renal vasoconstriction, burns, sepsis, peritonitis, and CHF are known causes.

        d. Nephrotoxins: see Display 10-1.

DISPLAY 10-1.
Common Nephrotoxic Substances

> Heavy metals: mercury, gold, lead, arsenic
> Antibiotics: sulfonamides, aminoglycosides, amphotericin, cephalosporins
> Contrast media: radiologic dyes
> Myoglobinuria: strenuous exercise, seizures, crush injuries, CO poisoning, ABO incompatibility
> NSAIDS: aspirin, ibuprofen
> Organic solvents: ethylene glycol, carbon tetrachloride
> Diuretics: furosemide, thiazides
> Other medications: cimetidine, captopril, allopurinol, phenytoin, cyclosporine

e.   Glomerulonephritis, pyelonephritis, diabetic sclerosis, vasculitis, emboli, hemolytic and uremic syndrome have also been identified as causes.

f.   Infections, drug-induced allergies, and hypercalcemia also lead to intrinsic renal failure.

4.   **Post–renal failure is caused by obstruction of the urinary system anywhere from the calyces to the urethral meatus.**

a.   Must rule out this type before assuming another type of failure

b.   Ureteral causes include stones, tumors, fibrosis, and thrombus.

c.   Lower genitourinary (GU) tract causes include bladder stone, tumor, and benign prostatic hypertrophy (BPH).

d.   Obstruction causes increased hydrostatic pressure within the renal system, which decreases renal filtering ability.

D.   Assessment should include evaluation of the following:

1.   Urine volume, quality, sodium, protein, specific gravity

2.   Serum chemistries

3.   Vital signs

4.   Symptoms of fatigue, dyspnea, weakness, and lethargy from anemia

5.   Increased susceptibility to bleeding, as manifested by easy bruising, epitaxis, and GI bleeding

6.   Anorexia, nausea, vomiting, and stomatitis, due in part to acidosis or fluid/electrolyte imbalances

7.   Negative nitrogen balance, which is characterized by decreased serum cholesterol, decreased calorie intake, and decreased protein intake

8.   Delayed or impaired wound healing

9.   Symptoms related to fluid/electrolyte disorders such as oliguria, anuria, and, rarely, polyuria

10.   Pericarditis

11.   Encephalopathy due to ammonia intoxication

12.   Pleural effusion, as noted by dyspnea, pleuritic pain, decreased breath sounds over site, and decreased chest wall movement on affected side

E.   Nursing diagnoses

1.   Altered Tissue Perfusion: Renal

2.   Risk for Infection

3.   Altered Nutrition: Less than Body Requirements

4.   Risk for Injury

5.   Altered Urinary Elimination

6.   Fluid Volume Excess

7.   Altered Protection

F.   Planning and implementation

1.   Monitor for signs of fluid overload such as weight gain, dependent edema, increased blood pressure (BP), tachycardia, jugular venous distention (JVD), crackles, or rhonchi.

2.   Monitor VS, hemodynamic parameters, and laboratory data including Na, K, Hgb, Hct, WBC, and coagulation studies.

3.   Assess skin turgor and mucous membranes.

4.   Observe for symptoms of anemia such as fatigue, pallor, and dyspnea.

5. Monitor for changes in level of consciousness.
6. Palpate bladder for retention, and implement measures to prevent calculi.
7. Ensure frequent position changes and provide skin care.
8. Administer urine-acidifying juices.
9. Assess for hematuria and stones.
10. Weigh daily and maintain strict I and O.
11. Understand that fluid loss includes urine and drainage output, plus about 400 mL/day to account for insensible losses.
12. Distribute fluids evenly throughout the 24-hour day.
13. Give oral medications with meals or with smallest possible amount of fluid.
14. Dilute all IVs in smallest amount of fluid.
15. Limit fat and protein intake.
16. Administer medications such as diuretics, antihypertensives, electrolyte inhibitors or replacements, vitamin and mineral supplements, and ammonia-lowering agents.
17. Administer erythropoietin alfa (synthetic erythropoietin).
    a. Administered 3 times per week to increase Hct and blood viscosity
    b. Can increase BP and thrombus formation in vascular access sites.
    c. Contraindicated with hypertension
    d. Need sufficient ferritin, folic acid, and B12 levels to be effective
18. Ensure that patient has a thorough understanding of the medical diagnosis, prognosis, and treatment plan

G. Evaluation
1. The patient will maintain fluid balance.
2. The patient's laboratory studies will remain within acceptable physiologic parameters.
3. The patient will have clear lung sounds and will demonstrate sufficient gas exchange.
4. The patient will show evidence of decreased catabolism.
5. The patient will be able to verbalize understanding of medical condition and treatment regimen.

IV. **Chronic renal failure/uremic syndrome**
   A. Description: end-stage renal disease (ESRD) is a progressive, irreversible loss of nephron function that occurs with failure of the body to regulate metabolic, fluid, and electrolyte balance, resulting in uremia.
   B. Etiology and incidence: a type of renal dysfunction found with chronic glomerulonephritis, pyelonephritis, polycystic kidney disease, diabetes mellitus, HTN, or systemic lupus erythematosus (SLE).
   C. Pathophysiology
   1. CRF is an irreversible process.
   2. It is characterized by three stages:
      a. Decreased renal reserve
      b. Renal insufficiency
      c. ESRD

3. Decreased kidney function causes:
   a. Sodium and water retention in edema, congestive heart failure, hypertension
   b. Excessive sodium and water excretion, resulting in hypovolemia, hypotension, and worsening of the uremic state
   c. Accumulation of waste products, electrolyte disturbances, sustained effects of drugs, and severe hypertension, resulting in neurologic dysfunction ranging from personality changes to coma
   d. Retention of hydrogen ions and a decreased ability to conserve bicarbonate, resulting in metabolic acidosis
   e. Inability to sufficiently excrete magnesium and potassium, resulting in neurologic and cardiac dysfunction
   f. Impaired phosphorus excretion with reciprocal hypocalcemia and secretion of parathyroid hormone, resulting in bone disease
   g. Decreased production of erythropoietin and the shortened life span of RBCs, secondary to the mechanical effects of hemodialysis, resulting in anemia
   h. Decreased libido, impotence, and amenorrhea, resulting in emotional turmoil

D. Assessment
1. Patients should be assessed for hypertension.
2. Uremia is a syndrome associated with ESRD. Symptoms include halitosis that is similar to the odor of urine. Occurs because of increased nitrogenous wastes and salivary urea.
3. Anemia is associated with ESRD, and is manifested by fatigue, dyspnea, weakness, and lethargy.
4. Patients have an increased susceptibility to bleeding, associated with easy bruising, epistaxis, and gastrointestinal bleeding.
5. Gastrointestinal disorders associated with anorexia, nausea, and vomiting may be noted.
6. Stomatitis is due in part to acidosis or fluid and electrolyte imbalances.
7. Symptoms related to fluid and electrolyte disorders include:
   a. Oliguria, anuria, and (rarely) polyuria
   b. Pericarditis with pericardial friction rub
   c. Encephalopathy due to ammonia intoxication
8. Monitor for development of pleural effusion as noted by the presence of
   a. Dyspnea, and pleuritic pain
   b. Decreased chest wall movement on affected side
   c. Decreased breath sounds over effusion site
9. Assess skin for color, bruising, and hair loss.
10. Neurologic assessment should include evaluation of weakness and confusion.
11. Musculoskeletal symptoms including pathologic fractures and cramping may be seen.

12. Lab results may include:
    a. Hypoalbuminemia, proteinuria, edema, hypovolemia, and increased H and H
    b. Negative nitrogen balance
    c. Decreased serum cholesterol, decreased calorie intake

E. **Nursing diagnoses**
1. Ineffective Management of Therapeutic Regimen
2. Risk for Infection
3. Altered Nutrition: Less than Body Requirements
4. Altered Protection
5. Fluid Volume Excess
6. Activity Intolerance

F. **Planning and implementation**
1. Monitor for signs of fluid overload
    a. Weight gain, dependent edema
    b. Increased BP, tachycardia, JVD, crackles, or rhonchi
2. Monitor VS; hemodynamic parameters; laboratory studies such as Na, K, Hgb, Hct, WBC; and coagulation studies
3. Assess skin turgor and mucous membranes.
4. Observe for symptoms of anemia:
    a. Fatigue, pallor, and dyspnea
    b. Changes in level of consciousness
5. Palpate bladder for retention, and ensure measures to prevent calculi.
6. Assess for hematuria and stones.
7. Weigh daily and maintain strict I and O.
8. Administer oral medications with meals or with smallest possible amount of fluid.
9. Dilute all IVs in smallest amount of fluid.
10. Limit fat and protein intake.
11. Be aware of potential complications:
    a. Anemia, fluid or electrolyte imbalance, GI bleeding
    b. Hyperparathyroidism, pathologic fractures, polyneuropathy
    c. Hypoalbuminemia, CHF, metabolic acidosis
    d. Pleural effusion, pericarditis, cardiac tamponade
12. Administer medications as appropriate and ordered by physician.
13. Administer erythropoietin alfa (synthetic erythropoietin; see ARF).
14. Apply lotion to dry, flaky skin areas.
15. Ensure adequate education so that patient and family can make informed decisions.

G. **Evaluation**
1. The patient will maintain adequate fluid balance.
2. Laboratory studies will be within acceptable physiologic parameters.
3. The patient will have clear breath sounds and will demonstrate sufficient gas exchange.
4. The patient will show decreased catabolism.
5. Vital signs will be within the acceptable range.

H. **Home health considerations: The client will verbalize importance of compliance with medication, fluid restriction, and dialysis regimen.**

V.   Rhabdomyolysis

   A.   Description: disorder stemming from an activity or event that causes muscle damage, resulting in protein breakdown that occludes the renal system.

   B.   Etiology and incidence

   1.   Frequently seen in trauma patients.

   2.   **Associated with any activity or event that causes muscle damage. Such activities include seizures, strenuous exercise, shaking chills accompanying amphetamine or heroin overdoses, and muscular hyperactivity with PCP abuse.**

   3.   Occurs in injured persons who are unable to move, and who lie in one position for a long period of time, such as stroke patients.

   4.   Noted in patients in drug-induced slumber in which the person does not move at all for hours or days.

   C.   Pathophysiology

   1.   Myoglobin is an iron-containing pigment found in skeletal muscle, particularly in muscle that functions in sustained contraction situations.

   2.   The protein from the destroyed tissue turns the urine red or cola colored.

   3.   The muscle cell breakdown releases myoglobin into the bloodstream, which is rapidly filtered by the kidneys, producing the dark red or brown urine.

   4.   The myoglobin can occlude the kidneys, and renal failure may result.

   D.   Assessment

   1.   Assess for recent history of traumatic injury or event producing muscle damage

   2.   Urinalysis reveals hematuria, protein, and is reddish-colored.

   E.   Nursing diagnoses

   1.   Pain

   2.   Altered Tissue Perfusion: Renal

   3.   Altered Urinary Elimination

   4.   Urinary Retention

   F.   Planning and implementation

   1.   Administer volume replacement as necessary to flush kidneys. The goal is to decrease the incidence of protein obstruction of tubular system.

   2.   Administer diuretics such as furosemide or mannitol with volume replacement as ordered and appropriate.

   3.   Be aware of potential complications:

      a.   Resulting renal dysfunction and hemolysis may lead to hyperkalemia.

      b.   Massive necrosis of skeletal muscle may lead to severe hypovolemia and the development of subsequent shock.

   G.   Evaluation

   1.   Urine output will return to pre-injury condition.

   2.   Urinalysis results will return to normal levels.

   3.   Renal function tests will be within normal limits.

VI. **Glomerulonephritis: term that encompasses various diseases, most of which are caused by an immunologic reaction. This reaction, in turn, results in proliferative and inflammatory changes within the glomerular structure.**

VII. **Acute glomerulonephritis**

    A. Description: post–infectious glomerulonephritis and infectious glomerulonephritis.

    B. Etiology aand incidence

        1. Classically, the causative factor of infectious glomerulonephritis is beta-hemolytic streptococcal, viral, or parasitic infection elsewhere in the body.

        2. Other organisms may also be responsible.

        3. It usually occurs during or within a few days of the original infectious process, whereas post–infectious glomerulonephritis occurs about 21 days after respiratory or skin infection.

    C. Pathophysiology

        1. Primary function of the glomerulus is to filter blood. Most cases of glomerulonephritis result from trapping of circulating antigen–antibody complexes within the glomerulus.

        2. The resulting inflammatory damage impedes glomerular function, reducing the glomerular membrane's capacity for selective permeability.

        3. The source of the antigens may be exogenous (post–strep infection) or endogenous (SLE).

        4. Some antigen–antibody complexes may form in situ within the kidney

        5. It can become a fulminating process, but most patients start to recover within 14 days.

        6. Most clinical signs return to normal within several weeks, although the hematuria and proteinuria may be present for longer periods.

    D. Assessment

        1. Classic symptoms are of sudden onset and include hematuria with red cell casts and proteinuria.

        2. Assess for fever, chills, weakness, pallor, anorexia, nausea, and vomiting

        3. Generalized edema, especially facial and periorbital swelling, may be noted.

        4. Assess for presence of ascites, pleural effusion, and CHF.

        5. Headache and moderate-to-severe hypertension are common.

        6. Visual acuity may be decreased due to retinal edema.

        7. Abdominal or flank pain, probably due to kidney edema, may occur.

        8. **Distention of the renal capsule, oliguria, and anuria may be present for several days. The longer this persists, the more irreversible the renal damage.**

        9. In contrast, symptoms may be so mild that the patient reports only vague weakness, anorexia, and lethargy.

       10. Scanty, dark, smokey, cola-colored, or red/brown urine may occur.

       11. Laboratory results may include:

           a. Proteinuria producing persistent and excessive foam

           b. Low urinary pH and specific gravity in mid-to-high-normal range due to decreased renal concentration ability

      c.   Elevated serum urea nitrogen and creatinine levels, C-reactive proteins, and antistreptolysin O titer

      d.   Decreased creatinine clearance, serum complement level, Hct, and Hgb

  12.   Diagnosis is based on the presence of an underlying infection and an elevated antistreptolysin O titer.

E. **Nursing diagnoses**

  1.   Altered Nutrition: Less than Body Requirements

  2.   Fluid Volume Excess

  3.   Activity Intolerance

  4.   Risk for Infection

F. **Planning and implementation**

  1.   Goal is prevention of further renal damage and improvement of renal function.

  2.   Plasmapheresis may be used in conjunction with immunosuppressive therapy.

  3.   **Remove specific circulating antibody or mediator of the inflammatory response.**

  4.   Large volumes of client plasma are cyclically removed and replaced with fresh frozen plasma (FFP) by use of continuous-flow blood cell separator.

  5.   Administer medications as appropriate and ordered by physician.

  6.   Antibiotics, diuretics, antihypertensives, and restriction of dietary sodium and water, are implemented to treat volume overload and hypertension.

  7.   Administer corticosteroids and immunosuppressive agents (azathioprine and cyclophosphamide).

  8.   Be aware of potential complications:

      a.   CHF with pulmonary edema

      b.   Increased intracranial pressure (ICP)

      c.   Renal failure

G. **Evaluation**

  1.   The patient will experience resolution of the inflammatory process.

  2.   Laboratory results will return to pre-illness urine values.

H. **Home health considerations**

  1.   Instruct client regarding methods to avoid infections and stressors on kidneys.

  2.   Level of home health care follow-up depends on the degree of renal damage.

VIII. **Acute tubular nephrosis (ATN)**

A. **Description: the most common cause of intrarenal azotemia and acute renal failure, usually resulting from injury to parenchymal tissue. Commonly associated with intrarenal ischemia, toxins, or both.**

B. **Etiology and incidence**

  1.   **Blood circulates through the kidney approximately 14 times a minute, giving the kidney repeated exposure to all components in the blood.**

  2.   If liver disease is present, the kidney can be overloaded with underdetoxified substances. As these substances await transport, they are held within the renal cells where they may disrupt function.

3. The renal countercurrent mechanism concentrates bodily substances, and, with an increased concentration, these substances can be toxic to the kidney.

4. Nephrotoxic agents include:
   a. Body substances: the renal countercurrent mechanism concentrates bodily substances; with an increased concentration, these substances can be toxic to the kidney.
   b. X-ray contrast media
   c. Drugs: antibiotics, antineoplastics, and anti-inflammatory agents
   d. Biologic substances: toxins, tumor products, and pigments from hemoglobin or myoglobin
   e. Plant and animal substances: poisonous mushrooms and snake venoms
   f. Heavy metals: lead, gold, and mercury
   g. Environmental agents: pesticides and organic solvents

5. Immune processes such as hypersensitivity, autoimmunity, and tissue/organ transplant rejection can lead to ATN.

6. Obstruction of the kidney by tumor, stones, and scar tissue can cause ATN.

7. Trauma or radiation to the kidney can contribute to ATN.

8. Intravascular hemolysis related to a transfusion reaction and disseminated intravascular hemolysis can obstruct renal tubules.

9. Systemic and vascular disorders such as:
   a. Nephrotic syndrome, diabetes mellitus, malignant hypertension, and SLE
   b. Wilson's disease, malaria, renal vein thrombosis, multiple myeloma, and sickle cell disease

10. Pregnancy-related disorders such as septic abortion, preeclampsia, abruptio placentae, intrauterine fetal demise, and idiopathic postpartum renal failure contribute to ATN.

C. Pathophysiology
   1. Ischemic acute tubular necrosis:

   a. Prolonged hypoperfusion to the kidneys with a sustained MAP of <75 mm Hg causes the kidney's autoregulation system to fail. In response, the sympathetic nervous system (SNS) and renin-angiotensin system cause afferent arteriole constriction, which causes decreased glomerular blood flow, decreased glomerular hydrostatic pressure, and decreased glomerular filtration rate (GFR).
   b. The kidneys are unable to synthesize prostoglandins for vasodilation, exacerbating the ischemic injury.
   c. SNS stimulation and angiotensin II redistribute the blood flow from the renal cortex to the renal medulla, worsening tubular ischemia, and further decreasing glomerular capillary blood flow.
   d. The nutrients and oxygen for basic cellular metabolism and tubular transport systems are diminished.
   e. Ischemia causes a decrease in renal cellular potassium, magnesium, and inorganic phosphates, and an increase in intra-

cellular sodium, chloride, and calcium. The increases in calcium and sodium increase cell injury.

    f.   After prolonged tubular ischemia, tubular cells swell and become necrotic, altering the function of the basement membrane.

    g.   Necrotic cells and cast formation causes tubular obstruction, which causes increased tubular and Bowman's capsule hydrostatic pressure, opposing the glomerular hydrostatic pressure, and lowering the GFR.

    h.   Tubular permeability increases, and tubular infiltrate is allowed to leak back into the interstitium and peritubular capillaries.

    i.   The degree of renal cellular damage depends on the length of time of the ischemic episode:

        ▶ Less than 25 minutes causes reversible, mild injury

        ▶ 40–60 minutes causes more severe damage with some recovery after 2–3 weeks

        ▶ 60–90 minutes causes irreversible, severe damage

2. Toxic acute tubular necrosis

    a.   Occurs secondary to renal exposure to nephrotoxic agents and/or toxic products of organisms.

    b.   Injury to tubular cells causes subsequent pathophysiology similar to ischemic ATN, eg, tubular cell necrosis, cast formation, tubular obstruction, and altered GFR.

    c.   The basement membrane is usually intact and the injured areas are more localized than with ischemic ATN.

    d.   Non-oliguric ATN occurs more frequently with toxic ATN.

    e.   Toxic ATN injury is less severe than with ischemic ATN, therefore recovery occurs more quickly.

D. Nursing diagnoses

  1. Altered Tissue Perfusion

  2. Risk for Infection

  3. Altered Nutrition: Less than Body Requirements

  4. Risk for Injury

  5. Altered Urinary Elimination

  6. Fluid Volume Excess

  7. Altered Protection

E. Planning and implementation

  1. Monitor for signs of fluid overload:

    a.   Weight gain, dependent edema

    b.   Increased BP, tachycardia, JVD, crackles, or rhonchi

  2. Monitor VS and hemodynamic parameters, and assess for evidence of hydration status:

  3. Assess skin turgor and mucous membranes.

  4. Observe for symptoms of anemia:

    a.   Fatigue, pallor, dyspnea

    b.   Changes in level of consciousness, apathy

  5. Weigh daily and maintain strict I and O.

  6. Concentrate fluids to provide prescribed medications in as little volume as possible.

7. Limit fat and protein intake.
8. Administer medications as ordered, including erythropoietin alfa.

F. Evaluation

1. The patient will maintain fluid balance.
2. Laboratory studies will be within acceptable physiologic parameters.
3. Lungs will be clear and will demonstrate sufficient gas exchange
4. Catabolism will be decreased.

IX. Sodium regulation and abnormalities

A. Description: normal level is 135–145 mEq/L.

1. **Plays a major role in nerve impulse transmission, muscle contraction, and movement of glucose, insulin, and amino acids.**
2. Na is the major extracellular fluid (ECF) cation.
3. It is the main element in determining plasma osmolality, which is a measure of how concentrated serum is.
4. Along with chloride, it is involved with water and electrolyte movement between body fluid compartments.
5. Most adults need to ingest only 2–4 grams per day.
6. Renal system helps maintain sodium and chloride balance.
7. About 80% of sodium is reabsorbed by kidneys as NaCl, with the rest reabsorbed in exchange for potassium or hydrogen.

8. **If chloride is unavailable for reabsorption, as with acidosis or hypochloremia, then bicarbonate takes its place.**

B. Hyponatremia

1. Description: less than 135 mEq/L
   a. Ratio of sodium to water decreases because body has lost sodium or gained excess water.
   b. Develops when the kidneys cannot hold onto sodium or rid excess fluid by producing dilute urine.
2. Etiology and incidence
   a. Although both sodium and H_2O are lost in sweat, sodium loss is greater.
   b. Sodium is lost through vomiting or diaphoresis.
   c. Hypothyroidism or adrenal insufficiency, and overzealous use of thiazide diuretics, can lead to decreased sodium reabsorption by the kidneys.
   d. Low sodium levels occur in CHF. If fluid overload develops, sodium can drop as the blood becomes more dilute. In patients receiving diuretics for CHF, it occurs as both water and sodium are lost.
   e. SIADH occurs with multiple neurologic disorders. The body secretes excessive amounts of ADH, causing kidneys to hold onto water and excrete sodium.
   f. Drug causes of SIADH include carbamazepine, tolbutamide, cyclophosphamide, and tricyclic antidepressants (TCAs).

   g. **PEEP increases intrathoracic pressure, which decreases the amount of blood returning to the heart or preload. The body perceives this decreased preload as fluid loss and responds by increasing ADH secretion, which in turn causes the kidneys to conserve water.**

      h.   Also occurs in instances of excess intake of plain water and renal failure.

3.   Assessment for the following signs and symptoms should be performed:

      a.   Anorexia, nausea, vomiting, abdominal cramping, headache, and fatigue

      b.   Neurologic changes due to fluid movement into interstitial spaces and brain cells, causing headache, lethargy, restlessness, irritability, disorientation, confusion, seizures, stroke, coma, or death

      c.   low specific gravity of urine (1.001–1.003), which reflects conservation of sodium

4.   Nursing diagnoses

      a.   Altered Nutrition: Less than Body Requirements

      b.   Fluid Volume Excess/Deficit

      c.   Risk for Injury

      d.   Decreased Cardiac Output

5.   Planning and implementation

      a.   Identify and correct underlying cause.

      b.   Replace sodium or restrict free water to restore balance.

      c.   Begin with oral replacement such as salt tablets, salty broths, and electrolyte-rich beverages (Gatorade). For levels under 110 mEq/L, administer hypertonic solution (3% or 5% NaCl). These IV fluids may be started before hyponatremia is severe.

      d.   In severe cases, administer demeclocycline (Declomycin), which blocks ADH and increases renal water excretion.

      e.   Monitor for fluid overload and cerebral edema, both of which can occur due to fluid shifts from cells into interstitial and extracellular spaces to decrease hypertonicity of fluid. If this happens, give a diuretic such as furosemide.

      f.   Monitor to keep sodium increase to no greater than 2 mEq/L/h.

6.   Evaluation: sodium returns to normal levels, with absence of signs and symptoms of electrolyte imbalance.

C. **Hypernatremia**

  1.   Description: over 145 mEq/L

      a.   Excess of sodium in relation to water, which is usually associated with fluid loss.

      b.   Also occurs if sodium intake increases and water intake does not.

  2.   Etiology and incidence

      a.   The elderly are at risk due to the fact that they can be easily dehydrated. As the body ages, the percentage of total body water decreases, making dehydration more likely. They also may be unable to respond to thirst response.

      b.   Severe burns and fever cause increased insensible fluid loss, as can high-protein enteral feeding formulas. The protein draws fluid into the GI tract, causing diarrhea.

      c.   Over-administration of IV hypertonic saline is an iatrogenic cause of hypernatremia.

      d.   In Cushing's syndrome, excess aldosterone prompts the kidneys to conserve more sodium than water.

      e.   A deficiency of ADH prevents the kidneys from reabsorbing water, thus leaving serum concentrated with sodium. Brain masses, head trauma, CNS infection, and granulomatous diseases put patients at risk for this.

      f.   Suspect if urine output exceed 200 mL/hour (5 L/day) and low urine specific gravity is present.

3. Assessment should include evaluation of:
- a. Fatigue, muscle weakness, and thirst
- b. Tachycardia, dyspnea, and crackles
- c. Restlessness, flushing, and low-grade fever
- d. Increased circulating blood volume leading to increased blood pressure and weight gain
- e. Edema, usually beginning peripherally and progressing to anasarca
- f. Hydration status by assessment of mucous membranes

4. Nursing diagnoses
- a. Altered Nutrition: Less than Body Requirements
- b. Fluid Volume Excess/Deficit
- c. Risk for Injury
- d. Decreased Cardiac Output

5. Planning/implementation
- a. Maintain sodium restriction/decrease sodium intake.

   b. **If dehydrated, increase intake of free water IV 0.45% NaCl or D5W. These are hypotonic solutions that are given slowly to prevent rapid shifts in brain fluid composition.**

   c.   Administer vasopressin if condition is secondary to diabetes insipidus.

6. Evaluation: sodium returns to normal levels, with absence of signs and symptoms of electrolyte imbalance.

X. **Chloride regulation and abnormalities.**

  A. **Description: normal chloride level 95–110 mEq/L**
- 1. Chloride is the main ECF anion.
- 2. It is secreted as hydrochloric acid (HCl) by the stomach mucosa, which aids in digestion.
- 3. It helps maintain acid–base balance
- 4. It takes part in oxygen and CO_2 exchange from Hgb in RBCs.

  B. **Hypochloremia**
- 1. Description: less than 95 mEq/L
- 2. Etiology and incidence

   a. **Often accompanies hyponatremia**

   b.   Seen in instances of low-salt diet, chronic respiratory acidosis, severe diaphoresis, prolonged diarrhea, vomiting, and gastric suctioning.

   c.   Also noted with long-term use of some thiazide diuretics

   d.   Can also occur with hypokalemia because K is lost as KCl.

3. Assessment
   a. Muscle weakness, twitching, tetany, agitation

b. Progresses to slowed, shallow respirations and hypoventilation, possibly resulting in respiratory arrest

4. Nursing diagnoses
   a. Altered Nutrition: Less than Body Requirements
   b. Fluid Volume Excess/Deficit
   c. Risk for Injury
   d. Decreased Cardiac Output

5. Planning and implementation:
   a. If deficient only in chloride, use solutions containing KCl or ammonium rather than NaCl
   b. Need to replace chloride without subsequent development of hypernatremia

C. Hyperchloremia

1. Description: chloride level >110 mEq/L
2. Etiology and incidence
   a. Often occurs with hypernatremia and ammonium chloride ingestion
   b. Occurs with hemoconcentration due to dehydration
   c. Occurs in cases of hyperchloremic metabolic acidosis, in which bicarbonate is lost and replaced by chloride in ECF
   d. Necessitates $NaHCO_3$ replacement
   e. Increased bicarbonate levels result in increased chloride excretion

3. Assessment: signs and symptoms similar to hypernatremia, but more severe
   a. Fatigue, muscle weakness, thirst
   b. Tachycardia, dyspnea, crackles
   c. Restlessness, flushing, low-grade fever
   d. Increased circulating blood volume leads to increased blood pressure and weight gain
   e. Edema; usually begins peripherally and progresses to anasarca

4. Nursing diagnoses
   a. Altered Nutrition: Less than Body Requirements
   b. Fluid Volume Excess/Deficit
   c. Risk for Injury
   d. Decreased Cardiac Output

5. Planning and implementation
   a. Treatment is similar to that for hypernatremia.
   b. When giving bicarbonate, note signs of hypokalemia such as ECG changes, confusion, and nausea, because sodium bicarbonate causes potassium to shift intracellularly, preventing it from depolarizing.
   c. Maintain safety measures (eg, quiet environment, seizure precautions, have suction equipment available).
   d. Assess fluid status and check for acid–base and electrolyte changes.
   e. Teach to prevent recurrences. If exercising or working outside during hot weather, replenish fluids with fruit juices, electrolyte-rich beverages, salty drinks.

f. Report prolonged diarrhea or vomiting, especially for the elderly.

6. Evaluation:

a. Sodium returns to normal levels

b. Absence of signs and symptoms of electrolyte imbalance

XI. Calcium regulation and abnormalities

A. **Description: normal total level is 8.5–10 mEq/L; ionized level is 4.50–5.5 mEq/L.**

1. Best known for its role in tooth and bone formation.

2. **Necessary for muscle contractions (including heart muscle), coagulation, transmission of nervous system impulses, and maintaining integrity of cell membrane. Bones contain more than 99% of total body calcium. The rest is in serum and exists in two forms:**

a. Ionized (free) calcium: the only type the body can use

b. Calcium bound to albumin: accounts for about half of the serum calcium

B. **Hypocalcemia**

1. Description: total level less than 8.5 mEq/L or ionized level under 4.5 mEq/L.

2. Etiology and incidence

a. Usually associated with insufficient dietary intake of calcium or vitamin D.

b. Also caused by disorders affecting calcium absorption, such as pancreatitis.

c. Seen in respiratory alkalosis related to hyperventilation. In alkalosis, calcium binds with bicarbonate, resulting in less available calcium.

d. Associated with renal failure, severe burns, and use of loop diuretics (due to excess renal calcium loss).

e. Banked blood has decreased calcium levels, predisposing those who need multiple transfusions to hypocalcemia.

f. Hypoparathyroidism: lack of parathormone decreases calcium, as can low magnesium, which inhibits parathyroid function.

g. Hyperphosphatemia: phosphorus levels are inversely related to calcium levels.

3. Assessment

a. Clinical assessment should observe for the following:

▸ Tetany, carpopedal spasms (Chvostek's and Trousseau's signs)

▸ Seizures, confusion, numbness, tingling of fingertips and toes, pathologic fractures

b. **ECG changes are associated with hypocalcemia and are manifested by a prolonged Q-T interval, dysrhythmias, and AV conduction defects.**

4. Nursing diagnoses

a. Altered Nutrition: Less than Body Requirements

b. Fluid Volume Excess/Deficit

    c. Risk for Injury

    d. Decreased Cardiac Output

  5. Planning and implementation

    a. **Adjust total serum calcium level according to albumin level. Calcium level rises 0.8 mg/dL for every 1.0 mg/dL increase in albumin, and decreases 0.8 mg/dL for every 1 mg/dL decrease in albumin.**

    b. Administer high-calcium, low-phosphorus diet (Display 10-2).

    c. IV calcium gluconate may be given in severe cases, at no more than 1 gram per hour.

    d. May give CaCl2 instead because it is more quickly available for use in muscle contractions.

    e. Implement cardiac monitoring.

    f. Ensure early ambulation and regular deep-breathing exercises.

    g. Treat underlying risk factors.

    h. Keep calcium intake at recommended levels: 1500 mg/day for those over 65 and 1000 mg/day for premenopausal women and men.

  6. Evaluation: Calcium returns to normal levels, with absence of signs and symptoms of electrolyte imbalance.

C. **Hypercalcemia**

  1. Description: total serum calcium above 10 mg/dL or free calcium level above 5.5 mEq/L.

  2. Etiology and incidence

    a. Usually related to malignant tumors that result in decreased bone calcium or release a parathyroid-like substance to increase bone resorption.

    b. **Also related to prolonged immobility, which increases resorption rate. Bones begin to lose calcium from atrophy, and calcium enters the bloodstream.**

    c. Associated with adrenal insufficiency, hyperparathyroidism, hypophosphatemia, hyperthyroidism, renal dysfunction, and thiazide diuretic use.

    d. Has also been noted secondary to vitamin D intoxication and in instances of tuberculosis.

DISPLAY 10-2.
Methods to Increase Blood Calcium Levels

> Calcium-rich foods: milk, cheese, yogurt, and other dairy products
> Vegetables: carrots, green beans, raw broccoli, spinach
> Phosphate binders: Basaljel/Amphojel, take $1\frac{1}{2}$ hrs pc for best absorption
> Dietary supplements: MVI plus calcium

   e. Fresh post–renal transplant patients are at risk because hypercalcemia may develop before the new kidney can excrete calcium.

   f. Excessive calcium intake in diet or in over-the-counter medications can contribute to hypercalcemia.

  3. Assessment:

   a. Assess for lethargy and weakness.

   b. Personality changes may also occur.

  4. Nursing diagnoses

   a. Altered Nutrition: Less than Body Requirements

   b. Fluid Volume Excess/Deficit

   c. Risk for Injury

   d. Decreased Cardiac Output

  5. Planning and implementation

   a. Hydration with IV normal saline solution (NSS) to dilute serum calcium and increase renal excretion of calcium.

   b. Administer loop diuretics to further increase excretion.

   c. Administer steroids to inhibit calcium absorption and decrease tumor size.

   d. Administer oral fluids, if possible.

   e. Administer mithramycin and calcitonin to reduce serum calcium.

   f. IV potassium and sodium phosphates are used only in severe instances.

   g. Dialysis may be needed.

  6. Evaluation: Calcium returns to normal levels, with absence of signs and symptoms of electrolyte imbalance.

XII. **Phosphorus regulation and abnormalities**

 A. **Description: normal level is 2.5–4.5 mEq/L.**

  1. Primary anion in intracellular fluid (ICF).

  2. Functions in the formation of stored energy in cells (ATP).

  3. Aids in bone and tooth formation.

  4. Interacts with Hgb to increase oxygen release to tissues.

  5. Contributes to WBC phagocytic actions.

  6. Helps metabolize proteins, carbohydrates, and fats.

  7. **Essential for normal platelet structure and function.**

  8. Has an inverse relationship with calcium.

  9. Sufficient calcium intake usually indicates adequate phosphorus intake.

 B. **Hypophosphatemia**

  1. Description: serum phosphate level <2.5 mEq/L.

  2. Etiology and incidence

   a. Usually due to disorders that increase renal excretion of phosphorus such as hyperparathyroidism, aldosteronism, hypokalema, and recovery from diabetic ketoacidosis (DKA) due to treatment with insulin, which causes phosphorus to move intracellularly.

   b. TPN preparations often contain insufficient phosphorus.

    c.   Overuse of antacids containing aluminum, magnesium, or calcium decrease GI absorption of phosphorus by binding with it in intestines. This also occurs in cases of chronic alcohol abuse and associated vomiting, diarrhea, and malnutrition.

3.   Assessment: Patients often experience restlessness and irritability.

4.   Nursing diagnoses
    a.   Altered Nutrition: Less than Body Requirements
    b.   Fluid Volume Excess/Deficit
    c.   Risk for Injury
    d.   Decreased Cardiac Output

5.   Planning and implementation
    a.   Ensure diet of foods high in phosphorus such as meat, fish, nuts, dried fruits, and vegetables. Decrease intake of high-calcium foods.
    b.   **IV phosphorus must be given slowly, at no more than 20 mmol over 8 hours, to avoid development of hypocalcemia.**

6.   Evaluation: Phosphorus returns to normal levels, with absence of signs and symptoms of electrolyte imbalance.

C.   Hyperphosphatemia

1.   Description: serum phosphate level >4.5 mEq/L.

2.   Etiology and incidence
    a.   Renal dysfunction is the usual cause.
    b.   Overuse of phosphorus-containing laxatives and excess dietary intake may also cause hyperphosphatemia.
    c.   Increased GI absorption is due to excess vitamin D intake.
    d.   Hypo- and hyperparathyroidism can also lead to phosphate retention.
    e.   Also associated with metabolic acidosis and rhabdomyolysis.
    f.   Can occur with use of chemotherapy and cytotoxic agents.

3.   Assessment
    a.   Symptoms include tetany and numbness or tingling in the fingers and toes.
    b.   Soft tissue calcification can occur.

4.   Nursing diagnoses
    a.   Altered Nutrition: Less than Body Requirements
    b.   Fluid Volume Excess/Deficit
    c.   Risk for Injury
    d.   Decreased Cardiac Output

5.   Planning and implementation
    a.   Administer antacids that lower GI absorption of phosphorus.
    b.   Dialysis clients need to avoid magnesium-containing antacids. Clients with hyperphosphatemia need high-calcium diets to counteract hypocalcemia.
    c.   **Administer IV calcium (usually CaC_{12} or Ca gluconate) for treatment of dangerously high levels, if there is adequate renal function.**

6.   Evaluation: Phosphorus returns to normal levels, with absence of signs and symptoms of electrolyte imbalance.

XIII. **Regulation of potassium and abnormalities**

    A. Description: normal levels 3.5–5.0 mEq/L

        1. Major intracellular fluid cation

        2. Plays a major role in nerve impulse transmission, muscle contraction, and movement of glucose, insulin, and amino acids.

        3. Essential for neuromuscular function, especially cardiac and skeletal activity

        4. Assists with the transmission of electrical impulses and muscular contractions

        5. Continuously moves in and out of cells via the sodium-potassium pump

        6. Most potassium is excreted in the urine. The kidneys do not conserve potassium, so adequate daily intake is necessary.

        7. Plays a role in cell metabolism and growth

        8. Helps maintain osmotic pressure

        9. Helps regulate acid–base balance

    B. **Hypokalemia**

        1. Description: serum potassium level <3.5 mEq/L.

        2. Etiology and incidence

            a. Seen in malnourished states, such as in alcoholics and anorexics.

            b. Observed in use of loop or thiazide diuretics.

            c. Occurs with diarrhea, as in irritable bowel syndrome, food poisoning, and ileostomy patients.

            d. Associated with excessive vomiting and in patients with nasogastric tubes to continuous suction.

            e. Occurs in instances of volume depletion/polyuria. Aldosterone production is stimulated, and retention of sodium with consequent potassium excretion takes place.

            f. Patients with continuous insulin infusions and patients on TPN may show hypokalemia due to hyperinsulinemia.

            g. In DKA, potassium moves out of the cells and into the blood in exchange for hydrogen. Potassium is then osmotically diuresed out of the body.

            h. Once acidosis is corrected, potassium returns intracellularly, leaving serum levels even lower.

            i. Associated with hyperaldosteronism, Cushing's disease, and long-term steroid use.

            j. Potassium moves into the cell during new tissue formation, and leaves the cell during tissue breakdown (catabolism).

            k. Without sufficient oxygen, glucose, or insulin, there is effective K excretion, but little conservation of K.

        3. Assessment

            a. Musculoskeletal symptoms include muscle flaccidity and weakness, generalized body cramps, decreased deep tendon reflexes (DTRs), and lethargy.

            b. Gastrointestinal symptoms include anorexia, nausea, vomiting, and the development of a paralytic ileus.

            c. May progress to hypoventilation, respiratory muscle weakness, and arrest.

  d. Hypokalemia may be shown on the ECG by a prolonged PR interval, U-wave, flat T-wave, S-T segment depression, dysrhythmias, and prolonged Q-T interval.

  e. Hypokalemia increases the risk of digitalis toxicity.

  f. Decreased renal tubular ability to concentrate waste results in increased water loss.

  g. Laboratory assessment includes electrolytes and magnesium levels.

 4. Nursing diagnoses

  a. Altered Nutrition: Less than Body Requirements

  b. Fluid Volume Excess/Deficit

  c. Risk for Injury

  d. Decreased Cardiac Output

 5. Planning and implementation

  a. Promote diet rich in potassium (Display 10-3).

  b. Administer potassium supplements, orally if possible, with food, and increase magnesium intake.

  c. **Never administer potassium by IV push. It can cause rapid dysrhythmias and asystole.**

  d. Monitor IV drip rates, even if using an infusion control device.

  e. Monitor serum electrolytes.

  f. Monitor I and O.

 6. Evaluation: Potassium returns to normal levels, with absence of signs and symptoms of electrolyte imbalance.

C. **Hyperkalemia**

 1. Description: potassium level >5.0 mEq/L.

 2. Etiology and incidence

  a. Often accompanies renal failure, when the kidneys lose their ability to adequately excrete potassium.

  b. **Severe tissue damage from trauma, burns, and large or multiple hematomas results in damaged cells leaking potassium into the bloodstream.**

DISPLAY 10-3.
Food Sources of Potassium

Leafy green vegetables	Bananas
Chocolate	Nuts
Baked potatoes	Red meat
Salt substitutes	Citrus fruits
K+ supplements	Fish
Cola	Cheese
Instant coffee	Peanut butter
Dried fruits	

    c.   In acidosis, hydrogen ions move from the bloodstream into cells in exchange for potassium to raise serum pH.

    d.   **In blood administration, one unit of blood, 1 day old, has about 7 mEq/L of potassium while a 21-day-old unit contains about 23 mEq/L.**

    e.   High blood glucose concentration pulls water and potassium from cells into extracellular compartment.

    f.   Patients with hyponatremia develop hyperkalemia due to the action of the sodium-potassium pump.

    g.   Too much potassium supplementation or replacement can contribute to hyperkalemia.

    h.   Dehydration and use of potassium-sparing diuretics, and ACE inhibitors such as captopril can also raise potassium levels.

    i.   **Pseudohyperkalemia is a condition in which blood cells in a specimen container hemolyze, which releases potassium into serum.**

    j.   Obtain and handle blood specimens carefully to prevent pseudohyperkalemia from hemolysis; this is caused by a tourniquet applied too tightly, a tightly clenched fist throughout the blood draw, or vigorous shaking of the tube after specimen collection.

3.   Assessment

    a.   Clinical assessment includes the following symptoms:

        ▶ Vague muscle weakness, confusion, and decreased DTRs

        ▶ Irritability, slurred speech, restlessness

        ▶ Nausea, cramping, diarrhea

        ▶ **Increasing levels may lead to paresthesia and ascending paralysis, progressing to respiratory arrest.**

4.   **ECG changes include: dysrhythmias, bradycardia, low-amplitude or missing P-waves; shortened and then prolonged P-R interval; first-degree heart block, bradycardia, shortened Q-T interval; and S-T segment elevation or depression. A widening QRS complex and the presence of tall, tented, narrow T waves may signify hyperkalemia.**

5.   Nursing diagnoses

    a.   Altered Nutrition: Less than Body Requirements

    b.   Fluid Volume Excess/Deficit

    c.   Risk for Injury

    d.   Decreased Cardiac Output

6.   Planning and implementation

    a.   Restrict potassium-rich foods.

    b.   Avoid salt substitutes containing potassium.

    c.   **Administer IV calcium to counteract the effects of excess potassium on the heart by raising the threshold, making dysrhythmias less likely to occur.**

   d.   Sodium bicarbonate and insulin are each used to shift K back
        into the cells temporarily. Then you must correct the under-
        lying disturbance.
   e.   Cation exchange resin entails the use of sodium polystyrene
        sulfonate (Kayexalate, SPS Suspension) in sorbitol orally or
        by enema. The resin absorbs potassium in exchange for
        sodium, mainly in the large intestine.
   f.   Sorbitol stimulates diarrhea and subsequently causes potas-
        sium loss.
   g.   Use of loop and thiazide diuretics also help to decrease
        potassium levels.
   h.   The patient may require hemodialysis.
7.   Evaluation: Potassium returns to normal levels, with absence of
     signs and symptoms of electrolyte imbalance.

XIV.   Regulation of magnesium and abnormalities

A.   Description: normal range 1.5–2.5 mEq/L.

   1.   Magnesium is the second most abundant ICF cation.
   2.   Most of body magnesium is in the bones.
   3.   Lesser amounts are in the muscles and soft tissues.
   4.   Minimal amounts are in the RBCs and serum.

B.   Functions

   1.   Magnesium is involved in enzyme reactions that result in ATP pro-
        duction for energy.
   2.   It is responsible for maintaining the correct level of electrical ex-
        citability in nerves and muscle cells, including those of the heart
        and cardiac conduction system.
   3.   Magnesium helps to maintain the structural integrity of heart.
   4.   Most dietary magnesium is absorbed in the small intestine, with
        kidneys excreting the excess and conserving existing supplies in in-
        stances of dietary insufficiency.

C.   Hypomagnesemia

   1.   Description: levels <1.5 mEq/L
        a.   Magnesium is one of the most common electrolyte imbal-
             ances.
        b.   It is often overlooked because lab tests measure only serum
             levels, which account for minimal amounts of total body
             magnesium.
   2.   Etiology and incidence
        a.   Commonly seen in cases of increased renal excretion related
             to loop diuretic or aminoglycoside use, which inhibits mag-
             nesium reabsorption in the loop of Henle.
        b.   Anorexia nervosa and alcohol abuse can cause magnesium
             loss. It is even more problematic when accompanied by liver
             dysfunction, diarrhea, and vomiting
        c.   Diarrhea can be a major problem, because the normally mag-
             nesium-rich lower GI tract does not absorb sufficient quanti-
             ties.
        d.   Lower GI tract dysfunction of the small bowel, pancreatitis,
             and diseases of intestinal mucosa such as ulcerative colitis and
             status post–small bowel resection, can contribute to hypo-
             magnesemia.

e. In DKA, the insulin deficiency forces magnesium out of the cells and into the serum, where it is excreted by the kidneys. Insulin treatment pushes magnesium back into the cells, which further decreases serum levels.

f. A diet low in magnesium occurs with long-term liquid protein diets, prolonged IV therapy, or TPN without magnesium replacement.

3. Assessment

a. **The predominant symptom includes evidence of myocardial irritability, with ventricular dysrhythmias.**

b. **There is an increased risk of digitalis toxicity secondary to intensified cardiac response to the drug.**

c. Neurologic symptoms include ataxia, vertigo, and nystagmus.

d. Muscle spasms, Chvostek's and Trousseau's signs, seizures, and coma can result.

e. Concurrent signs and symptoms of hypocalcemia and hypokalemia also may be seen.

4. Nursing diagnoses

a. Altered Nutrition

b. Fluid Volume Excess/Deficit

c. Risk for Injury

d. Decreased Cardiac Output

5. Planning and implementation

a. Increase dietary intake. The best foods include fruits, vegetables, seafood, cereals, and milk.

b. **Administer IV magnesium slowly over 4 hours for maximum serum retention. You may have to give 1–2 grams $MgSO_4$ over 30 minutes in emergencies, slowing rate if hypotension develops, as ordered and appropriate.**

6. Evaluation: Magnesium returns to normal levels, with absence of signs and symptoms of electrolyte imbalance.

D. Hypermagnesemia

1. Description: levels >2.5 mEq/L

2. Etiology and incidence

a. **A rare occurrence because kidneys can usually excrete excesses, therefore excess is almost always linked to renal failure.**

b. Overuse of magnesium-containing antacids, cathartics, milk of magnesia, and magnesium citrate are common causes.

c. There is an increased incidence in the elderly, who are most likely to use these products.

3. Assessment

a. CNS and cardiovascular depression are the most important symptoms.

b. Hypotension and weakness may be noted.

c. Hot, flushed skin may be associated with dehydration.

d. Nausea and vomiting also may be seen.

e.   Drowsiness and decreased DTRs progress to hypoventilation, respiratory arrest, and complete heart block if untreated.

4.   Nursing diagnoses
    a.   Altered Nutrition: Less than Body Requirements
    b.   Fluid Volume Excess/Deficit
    c.   Risk for Injury
    d.   Decreased Cardiac Output

5.   Planning and implementation
    a.   Hydrate with IV fluids, adding calcium for severe cases. This counteracts the effects of high magnesium. It is given with symptoms of respiratory depression, hypotension, and bradycardia.
    b.   Be prepared to administer loop diuretics.
    c.   Assess for fluid overload.
    d.   Withhold magnesium products.
    e.   If renal failure develops, may need to administer hemodialysis.

6.   Evaluation: Magnesium returns to normal levels, with absence of signs and symptoms of electrolyte imbalance.

XV.   Regulation of water balance and abnormalities

A.   Introduction: disorders of balance refer to disorders in which both sodium and water are lost or gained in relatively equal amounts.

B.   Water
    1.   Accounts for about one-half of adult body weight.
    2.   The highest percentage of water is within cells, but water will shift based on osmotic concentration differences between ICF and ECF.
    3.   Water balance is directly controlled by ADH and indirectly by sodium balance.

C.   Aldosterone
    1.   Aldosterone is sensitive to the concentration of sodium in blood.
    2.   Renin is secreted by the kidneys in response to sensed renal hypoperfusion (Fig. 10-2).
    3.   Sodium reabsorption is vital. It affects the regulation of other electrolytes.
    4.   Active reabsorption of sodium results in passive transport of chloride and bicarbonate, which helps to maintain acid–base balance.
    5.   It also affects potassium. As reabsorption of sodium is increased by aldosterone, reabsorption of potassium is decreased. The increased concentration of potassium stimulates aldosterone production, as does a low sodium concentration.
    6.   When sodium is lost, water follows, and when sodium is retained, water also is retained.

D.   Hypervolemia
    1.   Description: hypervolemia is a primary water excess. Abnormal retention of both water and electrolytes in about the same proportion as normal is characteristic of hypervolemia.
    2.   Etiology and incidence
        a.   It results from renal inability to rid the body of unneeded water and electrolytes.

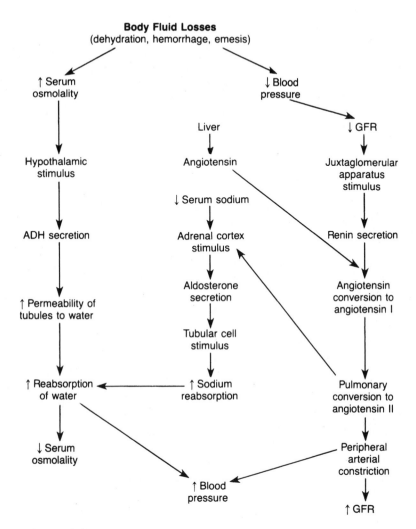

FIGURE 10-2.
Relationship of ADH, renin, and aldosterone to fluid regulation by the kidneys.

    b.   Severe water excess can lead to CHF, especially in patients with underlying cardiovascular dysfunction.

    c.   Cardiac insufficiency, cirrhosis, and ascites are examples of conditions that predispose to hypervolemia.

    d.   Malnutrition, stress/steroid therapy, and renal disease are also causative agents.

    e.   Rapid administration of IV NSS, or more hypertonic solutions, is an iatrogenic cause.

    f.   Mental health disturbances such as psychogenic polydipsia can lead to hypervolemia.

3. Assessment
   a. Clinical findings include:

   ▸ CVP >10, distended neck veins, PCWP >12
   ▸ Hypertension, bounding pulses, tachycardia
   ▸ Increased weight, increased temperature
   ▸ Increased respiratory rate, dyspnea, fine crackles
   ▸ Peripheral edema, taut, shiny skin, puffy eyelids

   b. Diagnostic findings are non-specific. Labs are usually normal because water and electrolytes are gained in the same proportion as normally.

4. Nursing diagnoses
   a. Fluid Volume Excess
   b. Decreased Cardiac Output
   c. Risk for Injury
   d. Impaired Gas Exchange

5. Planning and implementation
   a. Monitor I and O, urine output, specific gravity, and daily weights.
   b. Note presence of edema and rate using 0 to 4 scale.
   c. Limit fluids as prescribed, offering ice chips to minimize thirst.
   d. Frequent oral hygiene to maintain status of mucous membranes.
   e. Limit sodium intake and consider the use of salt substitutes.
   f. Monitor responses to diuretics.
   g. Monitor vital signs and hemodynamic parameters for signs of volume depletion.
   h. **Be aware of potential complications such as overcompensation and hypovolemia, and electrolyte imbalance.**

6. Evaluation: Water balance returns to normal levels, with absence of signs and symptoms of electrolyte imbalance.

E. **Hypovolemia**
   1. Description: primary water deficit is abnormal loss of water and electrolytes in about the same proportions as normal. Hypovolemia can lead to hypovolemic shock, and if prolonged, acute renal failure.
   2. Etiology and incidence
      a. Occurs as a result of increased fluid loss or decreased fluid intake.
      b. Vomiting, fistulas, tap water enemas, diarrhea, and NG suction can contribute to hypovolemia.
      c. Trapped fluids or third spacing occurs secondary to bowel obstruction, peritonitis, burns, and crush injuries.
      d. Other causes include severe diaphoresis, overuse of diuretics, and Addison's disease.
   3. Assessment
      a. Clinical assessment should include evaluation of:

      ▸ Flat neck veins; weak, thready pulses
      ▸ Hypothermia, hypotension, tachycardia
      ▸ Tachypnea, dyspnea

          ▶ Decreased weight

          ▶ Dry mucous membranes, decreased skin turgor

          ▶ Dizziness, syncope

  b. Diagnostic parameters include:

          ▶ Urine output <30 mL/hr

          ▶ CVP <2; PCWP <8

4. Nursing diagnoses

  a. Fluid Volume Deficit

  b. Altered Nutrition: Less than Body Requirements

  c. Fluid Volume Excess/Deficit

  d. Risk for Injury

  e. Decreased Cardiac Output

5. Planning and implementation

  a. Monitor I and O, and urine output, specific gravity, and daily weights.

  b. Maintain intake that initially exceeds output.

  c. Administer PO and IV fluids as ordered, documenting response.

  d. Encourage liberal sodium use if there are no concomitant disorders.

  e. Assess for hidden fluid loss such as insensible losses, abdominal fluid loss, and bleeding.

  f. **Notify physician for decreasing Hgb and Hct that may indicate bleeding. However, remember that decreases in Hgb and Hct are expected with rehydration, and may be accompanied by decreases in serum sodium and BUN levels.**

  g. Increase venous return by placing symptomatic patient supine with legs elevated at 45 degrees.

  h. Maintain security of all tubing connections that may cause fluid loss if disconnected.

  i. Monitor vital signs and hemodynamic parameters for signs of volume overload.

  j. Be aware of potential complications such as overhydration resulting in hypervolemia, especially dangerous when patients have preexisting cardiopulmonary or renal dysfunction.

6. Evaluation: Water balance returns to normal levels, with absence of signs and symptoms of electrolyte imbalance.

XVI. **Acid–base balance disturbances (see Chapter 6)**

XVII. **Hemodialysis (HD)**

  A. **Description**

    1. Removal of toxins and excess fluids via diffusion through a semipermeable membrane outside of the body.

    2. Hemodialysis is performed by specially trained hemodialysis nurses.

  B. **Nursing care: Same as for any renal patient, with special attention given to the arm with the AV graft.**

  C. **Care of the graft**

    1. Priority is given to maintaining the patency of the graft.

    2. No blood pressure cuffs or tourniquets should be applied to that arm, and the patient should be instructed to wear loose clothing and to avoid restricting blood flow to that arm.

3. The graft site should be evaluated for a bruit and a thrill as part of each physical assessment. The doctor should be notified immediately if there are any changes in the quality of the bruit or thrill.

XVIII. Peritoneal dialysis (PD)

   A. Description: use of a peritoneal membrane as dialyzing area to remove nitrogenous wastes and to stabilize body electrolytes and fluids

   B. Etiology and incidence: PD is indicated for clients who need dialysis but cannot tolerate the hemodynamic changes associated with hemodialysis, or clients for whom hemodialysis is inappropriate (Table 10-3).

   C. Physiology

   1. The peritoneal cavity is a semipermeable membrane with a large surface area (Fig. 10-3).
   2. It is permeable to low–molecular weight substances (eg, urea, electrolytes).
   3. It is impermeable to high–molecular weight substances (large proteins).
   4. Fluid is introduced into the cavity:
      a. Equilibrium is reached by osmosis, diffusion, and filtration across the peritoneal membrane.
      b. This occurs between the dialysis solution (dialysate) and the blood.
      c. After equilibrium is established, dialysate is drained from the peritoneal cavity.
      d. The cycle repeats on different schedules, based on patient need and desired results.

   D. Composition of solution: bags come in 1.5% or 4.25% dextrose or sorbitol

   1. Hypertonic 4.25% solution promotes increased fluid removal.
   2. Dialysate composition is similar to that of blood.
   3. Additional substances are added based on client need. These substances include potassium, heparin, other electrolytes, and antibiotics.

TABLE 10-3.
Indications and Contraindications to Peritoneal Dialysis

INDICATIONS	CONTRAINDICATIONS
ARF	Damaged peritoneal membrane
CRF	Abdominal adhesions
Chronic renal insufficiency	Peritonitis (unless reason for use)
Fluid retention	Recent abdominal surgery
Electrolyte imbalance	Perforated bowel
Hemodynamic instability	
Substance intoxications	
Acidosis	
Hypothermia (non-renal causes)	

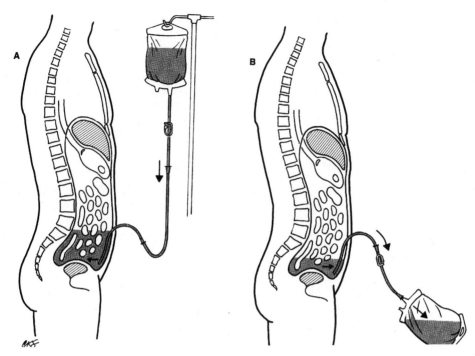

FIGURE 10-3.
Proper positioning of the peritoneal dialysis catheter and dialysate bag during dwelling and draining.

4. These are available in 1- or 2-L bags (actually 1020 mL and 2040 mL).

E. **Procedure: Before starting, the client is asked to void, and a Foley catheter is inserted to prevent accidental bladder perforation (Display 10-4).**
    1. After insertion, the dialysate is quickly infused into the peritoneal cavity at a rate of 10 minutes for 2 L by gravity.

DISPLAY 10-4.
Equipment Needed for Initiating Peritoneal Dialysis

Dialysis solution (dialysate)
Sterile povidone wash
Stylet insertion needle
Peritoneal catheter
Alcohol wipes
Administration tubing
Sterile drape kit

2. The dialysate remains indwelling for a specified time to allow equilibrium to occur, during which time osmosis, diffusion, and filtration occur.
3. Toxins move out of the capillaries.
4. Time varies from "in and out" to an average of 20 minutes.
5. At the end of dwell time, the clamp is opened and the fluid is drained.
6. Total PD time is usually 2–3 days continuously, but may be longer.
7. Periodic blood samples and dialysate samples drawn to monitor progression.

F. Assessment

1. **Observe for signs of bowel/bladder perforation with complaints of abdominal pain that occur immediately after trochar insertion.**
2. **Dialysate output should be straw-colored and clear. Note cloudiness or color change, which may indicate infection.**

G. Nursing diagnoses

1. Risk for Infection
2. Fluid Volume Excess/Deficit
3. Risk for Injury
4. Risk for Decreased Cardiac Output
5. Pain

H. Planning and implementation

1. Maintain accurate I and O via dialysis flow sheet including start time, dwell time, drain time, amounts in and out, and dialysate mixture.
2. Maintain cumulative output positive or negative.
3. Perform daily weights.
4. If abdominal cramping develops during infusion time, temporarily slow down rate until cramps resolve.
5. Keep air out of peritoneal cavity.
6. Keep tubings primed and connections tight.
7. If air is suspected, position patient upright and obtain x-ray.
8. Have patient cough to assist with air removal.
9. Keep dialysate inflow clamp closed and outflow clamp open.
10. For positive fluid balance:
    a. **Correct drainage problems by changing client position and turning side-to-side.**
    b. Decrease fluid intake.
    c. Decrease dwell times.
    d. Suggest use of more hypertonic dialysate.
11. Assess vital signs, respiratory status, and evidence of peripheral edema.
12. Maintain aseptic technique.
13. Clean exit site daily.
14. Clean tubing connections and injection ports with bactericidal solution before adding additive or breaking closed system.
15. Assess for peritonitis as manifested by pain, cloudy outflow, and fever.
16. If infection is suspected, culture fluid and administer antibiotics.

17. Be aware of potential complications:

   a. **Peritonitis is the major complication and usually is due to lack of sterile technique during procedure.**
   b. Protein loss
   c. Hyperglycemia/hyperosmolar coma
   d. Pulmonary edema
   e. Intestinal perforation

I. Evaluation
   1. Patient will maintain fluid balance.
   2. Laboratory studies will remain within acceptable physiologic parameters.
   3. Lung sounds will be clear and will demonstrate sufficient gas exchange.
   4. Catabolism will be decreased.
   5. Infection will be avoided.

J. **Home health considerations: If client needs long-term treatment, he or she may be a candidate for continuous ambulatory peritoneal dialysis (CAPD).**

XIX. Continuous arterial venous hemofiltration (CAVH)

A. Description: process of filtering wastes and removing excess fluid in a patient with renal failure who is hemodynamically unsuitable for hemodialysis or peritoneal dialysis (Fig. 10-4).

B. Description of types
   1. Continuous arteriovenous hemodialysis (CAVHD)
      a. Technically different from other types of dialysis

      b. **Adds a slow (15–30 mL/min) countercurrent dialysate flow on one side of hemofilter, which allows greater clearance of uremic toxins.**
      c. Combines diffusion via dialysate fluid, and convection via production of ultrafiltrate to remove wastes and promote fluid and electrolyte balance.
      d. Requires placement of two large-gauge catheters, arterial and venous.
   2. Continuous venovenous hemodialysis (CVVH)

      a. **Maintained by use of a pump-driven device and a double-lumen central venous catheter**
      b. Between the two catheter ports, a dialysis membrane and dialysate fluid are arranged in a circuit through the catheter
      c. The advantage to this method is the decreased complication rate

   3. **Slow continuous ultrafiltration (SCUF): major goal is excess fluid removal, of 1.5–5 mL/min or 2–7 L/day.**
   4. Continuous arteriovenous hemofiltration (CAVH)
      a. Most effective when used over a period of days early in renal failure
      b. Similar to slow continuous ultrafiltration. It is a continuous process so it is more apt to maintain steady removal of toxins and fluid

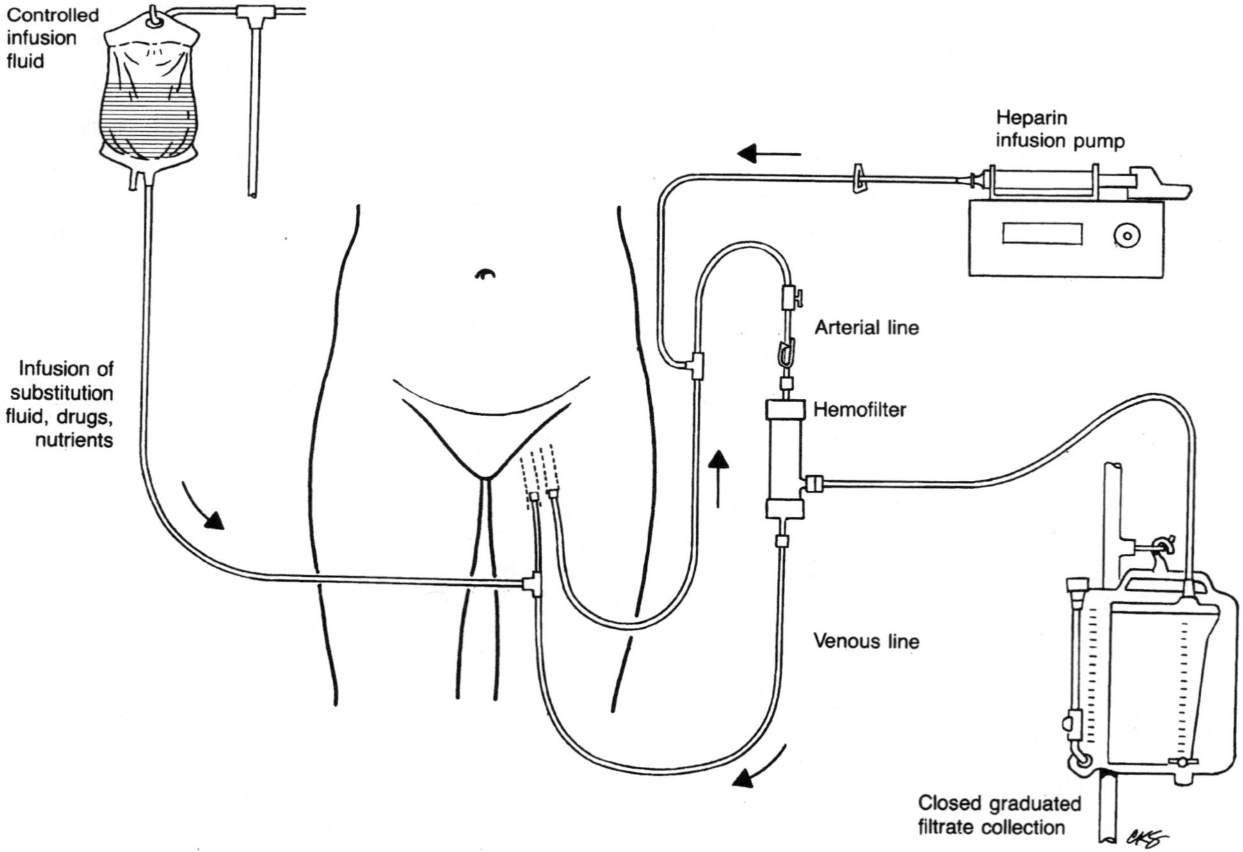

FIGURE 10-4.
Continuous arteriovenous hemofiltration (CAVH) system.

Controlled
infusion
fluid

Heparin
infusion pump

Arterial line

Hemofilter

Venous line

Infusion of
substitution
fluid, drugs,
nutrients

Closed graduated
filtrate collection

420

        c.   Able to remove large amounts of fluid, ranging from 5–20 mL/min or 7–28 L/day)

        d.   **Requires a minimal mean arterial pressure (MAP) of 60 mm Hg**

        e.   Replacement fluid is needed at high ultrafiltration rates, which further dilutes solutes in blood, and contributes to lower overall urea concentration

        f.   **Sufficient clearance of wastes cannot be accomplished in patients who are extremely catabolic**

  C. **Indications**
      1.   Indicated for instances of hypervolemia and/or renal insufficiency
      2.   Refractory CHF with renal insufficiency

  D. **Nursing diagnoses**
      1.   Altered Nutrition: Less than Body Requirements
      2.   Fluid Volume Excess/Deficit
      3.   Risk for Injury
      4.   Decreased Cardiac Output

  E. **Planning and implementation**
      1.   Monitor vital signs and hemodynamic parameters.
      2.   Assess fluid status with hourly I and O and fluid replacement to avoid hypotension.
      3.   Maintain system patency due to clotting:
          a.   Coolness of hemofilter
          b.   Separation of blood in lines
          c.   Decreased ultrafiltration rate
      4.   Maintain intact system to prevent hemorrhage:
          a.   Secure all lines and maintain their visibility
          b.   Restrict patient activity using restraints on affected extremity if absolutely necessary
      5.   Maintain sterile technique when working with system.
      6.   Monitor pulses distal to access site, usually the femoral artery and vein.
      7.   Explain to patient and family reasons for use and expected results.
      8.   Be aware of potential complications:
          a.   Hemorrhage.
          b.   Occlusion of system.
          c.   Infection
          d.   Air in system
          e.   Decreased ultrafiltrate volume

  F. **Evaluation**
      1.   Adequate function of system will allow patient to maintain stable fluid/electrolyte balance.
      2.   Patient will suffer no ill effects of the procedure, such as hemorrhage or infection.

XX. **Organ transplant**
  A. **Description**
      1.   Treatment of choice for many clients with ESRD.
      2.   Provides improved life quality and more cost-effective method of treatment than HD.

B.   Etiology and incidence

1.   Improved surgical techniques and more effective drug immunosuppression have improved survival of both patient and graft.

2.   Nearly 10,000 organ transplants done annually in United States, resulting from complications of:

    a.   Diabetes mellitus

    b.   Hypertension

    c.   Glomerulonephritis

C.   Physiology

1.   Donor may be a cadaver donor or a related living donor.

2.   It is planned so the transplantation and the organ retrieval are performed in adjacent operating rooms.

3.   Cadaver kidney can remain viable for 24–72 hours, depending on storage method.

D.   Assessment

1.   Pretransplant evaluation

    a.   Treatment options: dialysis versus transplantation

    b.   Risk of infection and rejection, life-long immunosuppressant therapy

    c.   Advantages of living-related donor versus cadaver donor (long-term survival is significantly greater with a living-related donor)

    d.   Long-term cost of transplant is much less than lifetime hemodialysis

    e.   Physical examination, diagnostic workup, and laboratory studies

    f.   Rule out any potential infection sources, including dental exam

    g.   Evaluate bladder capacity due to possible prior long-term non-functional bladder

2.   Psychosocial evaluation (also applies to living-related donor):

    a.   Patient ability to adapt, cope successfully, and comply with postoperative regimen

    b.   Also consider social and family history, vocational, educational, and financial constraints

3.   Immunologic assessment

    a.   Blood typing: must be ABO compatible, although not Rh compatible

    b.   Histocompatibility: antigens are responsible for graft rejection

4.   Donor selection

    a.   Identical twins have identical HLA

    b.   Siblings/blood-related family members often are HLA-haploidentical or HLA-identical, which are second best options

    c.   Improved long-term graft survival, fewer postoperative complications, and need for less immunosuppression occur with closer HLA

    d.   Renal angiography to determine which kidney to use

5.   Recipient is dialyzed within 24 hours before surgery.

    a.   May be done by hemodialysis or a continuation of chronic PD.

b. Dialysis is needed to partly reverse uremia, and to assist in hemodynamically stabilizing the recipient.

6. Surgical procedure basics
   a. Extremity with fistula is identified so it will not be used for drawing blood or monitoring BP.
   b. Kidney is placed in cavity constructed in the iliac fossa.
   c. Renal vessels are anastomosed to the iliac vessels.
   d. Donor renal vein is anastomosed to the external iliac vein.
   e. Ureter is anastomosed to recipient bladder.
   f. The non-functional kidney is usually removed only when HTN has been a management problem.

7. Nursing diagnoses
   a. Fear/Anxiety/Powerlessness
   b. Risk for Infection
   c. Risk for Ineffective Management of Therapeutic Regimen
   d. Knowledge Deficit: Organ Transplant
   e. Risk for Injury
   f. Altered Urinary Elimination
   g. Fluid Volume Excess

8. Planning and implementation
   a. Perform preoperative teaching.
   b. Have patient practice deep breathing, turning, and incentive spirometry.
   c. Manage incisional pain and encourage early ambulation.
   d. Implement dietary restrictions.
   e. Explain purposes of postoperative tubes and invasive lines.
   f. Discuss pain management strategies. Be aware that donor pain is very severe.
   g. Monitor vital signs and protect from individuals with infection.

9. Postoperative assessment
   a. Monitor fluid status, I and O, and daily weights.
   b. Immediate diuresis may be up to 1000 mL/hr, with need for hourly fluid replacement. Diuretics may be given to maintain diuresis.
   c. Temporary anuria/oliguria is more common in cadaver transplant, with fluid restriction and diuretics needed as part of the plan of care.
   d. Bladder spasms may occur. Assess for clot obstruction and gently irrigate with sterile water.
   e. Assess for dehydration as manifested by decreased urine output, decreased skin turgor, dry mucous membranes, and swelling over transplant area.
   f. Assess for fluid overload as evidenced by JVD, adventitious breath sounds, S3, and dependent edema.
   g. Monitor for ureteral leak as evidenced by decreased urine output, increased drain output, and serous fluid draining from surgical site.
   h. Assess patency of dialysis access, if the fistula is still in. Listen for bruit and feel for thrill. No use of tourniquets or BP cuffs above vascular access is allowed.

10.   Medications
    a.   Administer antacids and antihistamines to prevent GI irritation.
    b.   Orthoclone OKT3

       ► Assess hydration, weight, and CXR, with volume overload.
       ► Alert MD and prepare for diuretic administration.
       ► Teach that flulike reactions will occur with initial therapy; premedicate with steroids, diphenhydramine, and acetaminophen.

    c.   Cyclosporine: measure dose, place it in glass container, and add a consistent volume and type of diluent just before ingestion.
    d.   Cyclophosphamide: take in the morning; report hematuria STAT, because hemorrhagic cystitis is an adverse reaction; maintain minimum of 2000 mL daily fluid intake.

11.   Acute rejection. Symptoms include:

n   a.   **Decreased urine output, hypertension, low-grade fever**
    b.   Hematuria, increased creatinine, proteinuria

n   c.   **Edema or weight gain >2 lb in 1 day or >5 lb in 2 days**
    d.   Infection: fever, chills, increased WBC, malaise

n   e.   **Often reversible with medication adjustments**

12.   Chronic rejection. Course may sometimes be slowed, but is irreversible.

13.   Hemodynamic assessment
    a.   Monitor vital signs and hemodynamic parameters.
    b.   Assess for intra-abdominal bleeding as evidenced by a firm, distended abdomen, rapidly declining Hgb and Hct, altered mental status, and decreased urine output.
    c.   Prepare for transfusions.
    d.   Monitor renal and hepatic function tests.

14.   Potential complications include:
    a.   Infection/sepsis
    b.   Delayed wound healing/excessive pain
    c.   Immunosuppression
    d.   Vascular problems
    e.   GI disturbances
    f.   Hypertension, hypotension
    g.   Hepatitis
    h.   Electrolyte imbalance

E.   Evaluation
1.   The patient will maintain fluid balance with a functioning new kidney.
2.   The patient will have laboratory studies within acceptable physiologic parameters.
3.   The patient will have clear lungs and will demonstrate sufficient gas exchange.

    4. The patient will develop anabolic response to nutrients.

F. **Home health considerations**
    1. Postoperative care regimen to include fluid and electrolyte monitoring.
    2. Protect from infection and teach client signs and symptoms of infection.
    3. Avoid people with communicable diseases.
    4. Ensure meticulous hygiene and handwashing.
    5. Use sunscreen to prevent sunburn.
    6. Ensure management of medication regimen.
    7. Monitor weight, vital signs, laboratory studies, and urine specimens.
    8. Inform other health care providers about transplant and immunosuppressant use.

Bibliography

Ando, A., Kawata, T., & Hara, Y., (1989). Effects of dietary protein intake on renal function in humans. *Kidney Int* 36(Suppl.), 64.

Bayley, E. W. & Turcke, S. A. (1992). *A comprehensive curriculum for trauma nursing.* Boston: Jones and Bartlett.

Blanford, N. L. (1993). Renal transplantation: A case study of the ideal. *Crit Care Nurse* 13(1), 46–55.

Bove, L. A. (1996). Restoring electrolyte balance: Sodium & chloride. *RN* 58(1), 25–29.

Bove, L. A. (1996). Restoring electrolyte balance: Calcium & phosphorous. *RN* 58(3), 47–52.

Bullock, B. L. & Rosendahl, P. P. (1984). *Pathophysiology: Adaptations and alterations in function.* Boston: Little, Brown.

Carpenito, L. J. (1995). *Nursing care plans & documentation: Nursing diagnoses and collaborative problems* (2nd ed). Philadelphia: J. B. Lippincott.

Ferrin, M. S. (1996). Restoring electrolyte balance: Magnesium. *RN* 58(5), 31–35.

Higley, R. R. (1996). Continuous arteriovenous hemofiltration: A case study. *Crit Care Nurse* 16(5), 37–43.

Horne, M. M., Heitz, U. E., & Swearingen, P. L. (1991). *Fluid, electrolyte, and acid-base balance: A case study approach.* St. Louis: Mosby–Year Book.

Hudak, C. M. & Gallo, B. M. (1994). *Critical care nursing: A holistic approach* (6th ed). Philadelphia: J. B. Lippincott.

Ignatavicius, D. D., Workman, M. L., & Mishler, M. A. (1995). *Medical-surgical nursing: A nursing process approach.* Philadelphia: Saunders.

King, B. A. (1994). Detecting acute renal failure. *RN* 56(3), 34–39.

Marino, P. L. (1991). *The ICU book.* Malvern, PA: Lea & Febiger.

Mitch, W. E. & Wilmore, D. W. (1988). Nutritional considerations in the treatment of acute renal failure. In B.M. Brenner, J. M. Lazarus (Eds.), *Acute renal failure* (2nd ed). New York: Churchill Livingstone.

North American Nursing Diagnosis Association (NANDA). (1996). *Nursing diagnoses: Definitions & classification 1997–1998.* Philadelphia: Author.

Perez, A. (1995). Hyperkalemia. *RN* 58(11), 33–37.

Perez, A. (1995). Hypokalemia. *RN* 58(12), 33–35.

Slomowitz, L. A., Monteon, F. J., & Grosvenor, M. (1986). Energy expenditure in patients with chronic renal failure. *Kidney Int* 30, 741.

Stillwell, S. (Ed.). (1992). *Mosby's critical care nursing reference.* St. Louis: Mosby.

Strohschein, B. L., Caruso, D. M., & Greene, K. A. (1994). Continuous venovenous hemodialysis. *Am J Crit Care* 3(2), 92–99.

Wood, J. M. & Bosley, C. L. Acute postrenal failure: Reversing the problem. *Nursing 95* 25(3), 48–50.

Zaloga, G. P. (1994). *Nutrition in critical care.* St. Louis: Mosby.

STUDY QUESTIONS

1. Which one of the following statements about erythropoietin alpha (Epogen) is true? The drug is:
   a. most effective when given orally three times a week
   b. an alternative to blood transfusions for some clients in renal failure
   c. beneficial when the client in renal failure has low iron levels
   d. contraindicated in hypotensive clients

2. Which one of the following symptoms is normally seen first in a classic post–organ transplant rejection episode?
   a. vomiting
   b. hypertension
   c. increased diuresis
   d. hyperirritability

3. Which one of the following effects is most likely to occur with the use of systemic corticosteroids after a renal transplant?
   a. intensification of the autoimmune response
   b. increased susceptibility to infection
   c. hypertrophy of the adrenal glands
   d. enlargement of the kidneys

4. Which one of the following foods is most likely to be restricted in a diet for a post-renal transplant patient?
   a. applesauce
   b. bananas
   c. bran cereal
   d. spaghetti

5. An insulin-dependent dialysis client is to eat breakfast before her dialysis treatment. She should receive her insulin:
   a. at the regularly prescribed time
   b. immediately before dialysis
   c. during dialysis
   d. immediately after dialysis

6. A client with end-stage renal disease (ESRD) is refusing his aluminum hydroxide gel because he states he has "no indigestion." Your best response is to say:
   a. "I can tell that you know the actions of your medicine."
   b. "The antacid is needed to prevent stomach ulcers from developing."
   c. "The antacid is needed to regulate the calcium level in your blood."
   d. "Your medicines are very irritating to the stomach and may cause nausea if you don't take the antacid."

7. A 40-g protein diet is beneficial for a client in renal failure because it:
   a. limits production of nitrogenous waste products
   b. provides alkaline metabolic end products to combat acidosis
   c. increases gluconeogenesis, thereby supplying the cells with needed glucose
   d. improves appetite by stimulating secretion of gastric juice

8. Which one of the following examples indicates the plasma pH and bicarbonate levels seen in uremia?
   a. increased pH, decreased HCO_3-
   b. decreased pH, increased HCO_3-
   c. decreased pH; decreased HCO_3-
   d. increased pH, increased HCO_3-

9. In comparison with hemodialysis, peritoneal dialysis is:
   a. more sparing of serum protein
   b. less likely to cause serious infection
   c. contraindicated in hemodynamically unstable clients
   d. a relatively simple procedure that is quickly instituted

10. You note that your patient in acute renal failure is experiencing some muscle twitching and lethargy. The ECG currently indicates some dysrhythmias. The client is most likely experiencing
    a. hyperkalemia
    b. hypokalemia
    c. hypercalcemia
    d. hypocalcemia

11. The use of peritoneal dialysis is based on which following scientific principle:
    a. The peritoneum permits transfer of substances only from the interior of a vessel outward.
    b. When the blood pressure is ele-

vated, fluid passes more readily from the blood into the tissues.

c. High molecular weight substances leave the bloodstream and enter the dialysate solution through a semi-permeable membrane.

d. Dissolved particles move across a semi-permeable membrane from a higher to a lower concentration.

12. Before a peritoneal dialysis catheter can be inserted, a Foley catheter must be inserted into the client's bladder to:

a. measure the dialysate that flows from the client's abdomen

b. prevent the bladder from being punctured by the dialysis catheter

c. decompress the abdomen

d. collect lab specimens for culture

13. A peritoneal dialysis cycle may take 10 minutes to infuse, 20 minutes to dwell, and 30 minutes to drain. The purpose of the dwell time is to:

a. give the client a rest time

b. allow time for toxins to move out of the capillaries

c. allow time for glucose to move into the capillaries

d. reduce the work of breathing

ANSWER KEY

1. *Correct response: b*
   Epogen promotes stimulation of bone marrow to produce RBCs with sufficient amounts of iron-containing hemoglobin.
   a. It is given IV or SQ
   c and d. A major contraindication is hypertension, and the client must have normal iron levels in order for the drug to work.
   Application/Physiologic/NA

2. *Correct response: b*
   a. Vomiting may occur, but is not a classic indicator of rejection.
   c. Oliguria or anuria are also apt to occur as the new kidney ceases to function.
   d. Mood swings and irritability are largely related to steroid administration and are not indicative of rejection.
   Knowledge/Physiologic/Assessment

3. *Correct response: b*
   a, b. Steroids decrease the immune response, which is the very reason they are given post–organ transplant. They minimize rejection of the foreign organ.
   c, d. With chronic use, there is atrophy of the adrenal glands but no definite change in kidney size.
   Comprehension/Physiologic/NA

4. *Correct response: b*
   The client must strictly limit high-potassium foods such as bananas, dried fruits, and potatoes.
   a, c, and d. Fruits, bran, and pasta are generally low-potassium sources and are considered "safe" foods for renal clients.
   Comprehension/Physiologic/Planning

5. *Correct response: a*
   Insulin is administered 1/2- to 1 hour before breakfast in all clients to promote maximum absorption and use of nutrients.

Blood sugars are monitored during the hemodialysis procedure, with treatment initiated as needed.
Application/Physiologic/Planning

6. *Correct response: c*
   Although these clients may develop indigestion, the primary reason aluminum hydroxide is administered is to bind phosphorus, which has an inverse relationship to calcium. The ideal result is a normal calcium level.
   Application/Physiologic/Implementation

7. *Correct response: a*
   Protein must be restricted to prevent the build-up of nitrogenous waste products of protein breakdown.
   b, c. Acidosis is a chronic problem, and there is no dietary method to effectively control its development.
   d. Protein does nothing to stimulate gluconeogenesis or stimulate gastric acid secretion.
   Application/Physiologic/Planning

8. *Correct response: c*
   b, c. Because of the renal inability to conserve sodium bicarbonate, the body blood levels are much less than normal, representing an acidotic state.
   a, d. Acidosis is indicated by a low pH.
   Comprehension/Physiologic/NA

9. *Correct response: d*
   Peritoneal dialysis (PD) can be instituted within minutes if necessary, whereas hemodialysis takes from hours to months to institute.
   a, b. PD is more likely to waste protein and to cause peritonitis.
   c. PD is the treatment for clients with hemodynamic instability because it does not cause the rapid fluid shifts that occur during hemodialysis.
   Application/Physiologic/NA

10. *Correct response: a*

Muscle twitching, lethargy, and dys-rhythmias (especially with a tall, tented T wave) are classic findings in hyper-kalemia.

b, c, and d. The opposite is true in hypokalemia (ECG has U waves and nearly flat T waves); hypocalcemia causes Trousseau's and Chvostek's signs.

Analysis/Physiologic/Assessment

11. *Correct response: d*

Diffusion, osmosis, and active transport are all involved in the peritoneal dialysis process, in which particles and water travel from greater to lesser concentrations through a semi-permeable membrane in an attempt to establish equilibrium.

Comprehension/Physiologic/NA

12. *Correct response: b*

Bladder perforation is a likely complication resulting from trochar insertion. The client therefore must void or have a catheter inserted to decrease the chance of this occurring.

a, c. The presence of the catheter is completely separate from the peritoneal dialysis procedure, and only decompresses the bladder, not the entire abdomen.

d. Lab specimens for urinalysis may be obtained through a Foley catheter, but this is not the reason for its insertion prior to the initiation of PD.

Application/Physiologic/Planning

13. *Correct response: b*

a, b. The dwell time is done to promote removal of toxins.

c. Glucose may enter or leave the peritoneal cavity, depending on active transport/diffusion needs.

d. During the dwell time, the person may develop shortness of breath due to increased abdominal pressure owing to presence of dialysate.

Application/Physiologic/Implementation

The Endocrine System

I.   Anatomy and physiology
A.   Structure
1. The endocrine system is composed of highly vascular glands, without ducts, that produce and secrete hormones directly into the bloodstream. This enables a rapid response to hemodynamic and metabolic changes.
2. The major endocrine gland is the pituitary gland or hypophysis, also known as the master gland. It is composed of two lobes, the anterior and the posterior pituitary.
3. These lobes are collectively responsible for maintaining normal serum levels of hormones by sending signals in the form of stimulating hormones to the other endocrine glands.
4. Other endocrine glands include the thyroid, parathyroids, adrenals (cortex and medulla), pancreas, testes, ovaries, mammaries, and the GI tract.

B.   Function
1. The function of the endocrine system is the maintenance of body function regulation in conjunction with the nervous system.
2. The amount of hormones produced and secreted is regulated by feedback control. The body strives to maintain a constant level of each hormone by increasing production/secretion when serum levels fall, and decreasing production/secretion when serum levels are elevated.
3. See Table 11-1, detailing endocrine glands, the hormones they secrete, and their effects.
4. Although it is not an endocrine gland, the hypothalamus is largely responsible for controlling pituitary function via feedback.
   a. The hypothalamus detects a low serum level of a hormone and signals the pituitary.

TABLE 11-1.
Endocrine Glands, Hormones Secreted, and the Effect on Target Glands

PITUITARY HORMONE	TARGET ORGAN	TARGET ORGAN HORMONE	EFFECTS
Thyroid-stimulating hormone (TSH)	Thyroid	Thyroxine	All cells, ↑metabolism
		Thyrocalcitonin	Bones and kidneys, ↓serum calcium
	Parathyroid	Parathyroid hormone (PTH)	Bones, kidneys, and GI tract, ↑serum calcium
Growth hormone (GH)	Bones and muscles	N/A	Carbohydrate, protein, lipid, and calcium metabolism
Adrenocorticotropic hormone (ACTH)	Adrenal medulla	Epinephrine	Cardiac and skeletal muscle, other glands, ↑vasodilation = ↑blood flow to organs, ↑metabolic rate and glucose level
		Norepinephrine	Most organs, ↑peripheral vascular resistance = ↑BP
	Adrenal cortex	Mineral corticoids (aldosterone)	Renal tubules ↑sodium reabsorption and potassium loss, ↑BP
		Glucocorticoids (cortisol)	↑Gluconeogenesis and lipolysis = ↑glucose level, ↓protein synthesis and inflammatory response, ↑sodium retention
		Androgens and estrogens	Development of secondary sex characteristics
Luteinizing hormone (LH)	Ovaries	Progesterone	Responsible for corpus luteum
	Testes	Testosterone	Stimulates development of the male reproductive organs and the growth of bone and muscle; responsible for spermatogenesis
Follicle stimulating hormone (FSH)	Ovaries	Estrogen	Stimulates the development of the female reproductive organs and the proliferation of the endometrium
Prolactin	Mammary glands	N/A	Stimulates milk production
N/A	Pancreas	Glucagon	Liver, ↑blood sugar
		Insulin	All body tissues, ↓blood sugar, regulates fat storage and protein synthesis
		Somatostatin	Pituitary and the pancreas, ↓blood sugar
N/A	Gastrointestinal tract	Gastrin	Gastric glands, ↑GI motility and ↑gastric juice
		Enterogastrin	Gastric glands ↓gastric juice and ↓GI motility
		Secretin	Liver and pancreas, stimulates production of bile and pancreatic juices
		Cholecystokinin	Gallbladder, stimulates the release of bile into the duodenum

433

b. The pituitary gland sends the appropriate stimulating hormone to the corresponding gland.

c. In response, the target gland increases production and secretion of the deficient hormone.

II. The endocrine glands

A. Pituitary gland (hypophysis)

1. The hypophysis is an endocrine gland located at the base of the brain, in the sella turica.

2. It is connected to the hypothalamus by the hypophyseal stalk.

3. The anterior pituitary or adenohypophysis is responsible for stimulating other endocrine glands to secrete hormones (see Table 11-1).

4. The posterior pituitary, or neurohypophysis, is responsible for secreting vasopressin and oxytocin. Oxytocin is the hormone responsible for uterine contractions during childbirth.

B. Thyroid

1. The thyroid is a highly vascular endocrine gland located in the neck anterior to the trachea.

2. It consists of two lobes, one on either side of the trachea, giving it a butterfly-like shape. The lobes are connected in the center by a structure called the isthmus.

3. The function of the thyroid gland is to produce, store, and secrete hormones responsible for regulating cellular metabolism, and to a lesser degree, serum calcium. Thyroid hormone stimulates body growth and increases heart rate and glucose levels along with the metabolic rate.

4. Thyrocalcitonin is secreted by parafollicular cells or "C" cells, and acts on the bones and kidneys to decrease serum calcium levels.

5. Thyroid hormone is produced, stored, and secreted by the follicular epithelial cells and is made up of T_3 (triiodothyronine) and T_4 (thyroxine).

   a. T_3 is converted from T_4 in the peripheral tissues.

   b. T_4 is bound very tightly to plasma proteins and is therefore not as readily available to the cells as is T_3.

   c. A decrease in plasma proteins for any reason will increase the amount of circulating thyroid hormone. This is common in critically ill patients.

C. Parathyroid

1. The parathyroids consist of four small glands located in the posterior thyroid.

2. The major function is to maintain normal serum calcium levels (8.5–10.5 mg/100 mL) by secreting parathyroid hormone (PTH).

3. PTH acts on the following organs to free calcium, raising serum levels of calcium:

   a. Bone: frees calcium from the bones.

   b. Renal: increases calcium (Ca), magnesium (Mg), hydrogen (H), and ammonium resorption from the renal tubules.

   c. Promotes renal excretion of phosphorus, potassium (K), and sodium bicarbonate.

   d. Increases production of active vitamin D, also known as 1,25 dihydroxycholecalciferol.

   e. Gastrointestinal: increases absorption of calcium.

D. Adrenals
  1. Two adrenal glands are located superior to each kidney. Each is made up of an outer layer, the medulla, and an inner layer, the cortex.
  2. Adrenal medulla
      a. The medulla produces catecholamines, composed of dopamine, norepinephrine, and epinephrine.
      b. Epinephrine and norepinephrine increase alertness, metabolic rate, blood and muscle glucose, insulin levels, and free fatty acids.
      c. Epinephrine causes vasodilation and norepinephrine causes vasoconstriction.
      d. Dopamine increases the ionotropic function of the heart, produces renal vasodilation in small amounts, and peripheral vasoconstriction in larger amounts.
  3. Adrenal cortex
      a. The adrenal cortex is composed of three zones:

      ▶ Zona glomerulosa: outermost, secretes mineralcorticoids
      ▶ Zona fasciculata: inner, secretes glucocorticoids
      ▶ Zona reticularis: innermost, secretes androgens and estrogens

      b. Adrenal steroids are degraded by the liver competitively with bilirubin.
      c. Glucocorticoids

      ▶ **Glucocorticoids increase plasma glucose, skeletal muscle endurance, tissue response to glucose, glomerular filtration rate (GFR), and permeability of collecting ducts to free water.**
      ▶ **Glucocorticoids decrease antidiuretic hormone (ADH), number of lymphocytes (which affects humoral and cell-mediated immunity), and size of lymph nodes.**
      ▶ **They contain anti-inflammatory and antihistamine properties**

      d. Mineralcorticoids

      ▶ **Mineralocorticoids increase sodium reabsorption in the collecting ducts and renal tubules. They increase extracellular fluid volume (ECF) and potassium secretion.**
      ▶ **Secretion is stimulated by a decrease in renal perfusion or serum sodium concentration.**

      e. Androgens and estrogens: see Table 11-1

III. Overview of endocrine and metabolic disorders
  A. Assessment
  1. A thorough history should be obtained to include:
      a. Family history of endocrine pathology
      b. Personal history of endocrine pathology
      c. Recent complaints of or changes in activity/sleep, weight gain/loss, appetite, skin/hair amount and consistency, and mental/emotional status
      d. Recent trauma, surgery, radiation, or infection

2. Physical assessment includes:
   a. Overall appearance, weight, body shape, energy level, mental acuity, and mood
   b. Pallor, jaundice, pink skin color
   c. Shape of face, puffy/sunken eyes, dry mucous membranes, goiter
   d. Heart rate/rhythm/sounds, blood pressure (BP), body temperature
   e. Respiratory rate, breath sounds, easy/labored breathing
   f. Soft/distended abdomen, bowel sounds, constipation/diarrhea
   g. Urine output, color, frequency, dysuria

B. Laboratory studies and diagnostic tests
1. Laboratory studies include serum and urine electrolytes, hormones (T_3, T_4, TSH, TRH, ADH, PTH, ACTH), complete blood count (CBC), arterial blood gases (ABG), liver and cardiac enzymes, and gland-specific antibodies
2. CT scan/MRI to identify abscesses, tumors, cysts
3. Nuclear medicine scans such as a thyroid scan using radioactive iodine, which measures overall size, presence of any nodules, and function.
4. Iodine exposure should be limited for a number of days prior to the study as specified by the nuclear medication department. This includes suntan lotions, medications, dietary, IV contrast.
5. Ultrasound is used to measure size and help distinguish tumors from cysts.
6. Hearing and eye exam

C. Nutritional considerations: Syndrome of inappropriate antidiuretic hormone (SIADH)
1. Nutrition support of patients with SIADH directly relates to blood volume.
2. The volume expansion typically associated with SIADH causes dilutional hyponatremia and increased urinary salt loss.
3. Considerations for medical nutrition therapy
   a. The overall goal is to increase the nutrient intake to achieve caloric balance and meet intake needs.
   b. It may be necessary to restrict fluid to as little as 500 mL/day to prevent symptomatic hyponatremia.

D. Nutritional considerations: diabetes mellitus
1. The indications for nutrition support and the daily estimate of caloric, protein, and lipid requirements are similar in diabetic and non-diabetic critically ill patients.
2. Weight loss, stress factors, and the anticipated time that the patient will be unable to meet nutritional needs orally will all influence the need for nutritional support.
3. Consideration must be given to the method of nutrition. If care is not taken, sustained parenteral or enteral nutrition may cause a sustained hyperinsulinemia, which can lead to hepatic dysfunction, affect electrolyte levels, and cause salt and water imbalance.
4. This concern may be addressed by using cyclical nutrition, in which the nutrition is discontinued for a period each day.

5. During parenteral nutrition support, the use of dextrose as the only source of non-protein calories is no longer recommended.

6. Complications can result, such as hepatic lipogenesis, hepatic dysfunction, and hyperglycemia.

7. Administration of a portion of the calories as lipids can minimize these complications.

8. Glycemic control during the transition from parenteral or enteral nutrition to oral intake is often difficult. Conservative use of intermediate-duration insulin and adherence to a regular insulin supplementation algorithm, "sliding scale" insulin, is necessary during the transitional period.

9. Considerations for medical nutrition therapy
   a. The overall goal is to increase the nutrient intake to achieve caloric balance and meet intake needs.
   b. Maintenance of plasma glucose levels between 100 and 200 mg/dL. Once nutritional support is established, plasma glucose levels of 100–150 mg/dL are desirable in stable patients.
   c. Accurate recording of daily weight and fluid balance is essential.
   d. When infusing parenteral nutrition, a portion of the non-protein calories should be from lipids and not solely dextrose.
   e. Before the discontinuation of parenteral nutrition, reduce the infusion rate by 50% and continue for a minimum of 1 hour. Tapering should be slower if large amounts of insulin are present in the parenteral solution.
   f. Unexplained deterioration in glycemic control may be attributed to overfeeding, medication use, or dehydration.

E. Psychosocial implications
1. Patients with endocrine dysfunction may face significant alterations in body image and sexual dysfunction.
2. Fear of the unknown and anxiety related to the diagnosis and treatment modalities are also factors to be considered.
3. Depression may result, particularly if the condition becomes chronic, necessitating long-term management.
4. Impaired work performance may occur because of the disease process, as well as the time off required to ensure optimal treatment.
5. Emotional instability may be a symptom of the disease or a complication of the disease process.

F. Medications used to treat endocrine and metabolic problems (see individual disease processes)

IV. SIADH (Syndrome of inappropriate antidiuretic hormone)

A. Description: a syndrome characterized by the oversecretion of ADH, leading to life-threatening fluid overload and hyponatremia.

B. Etiology and incidence:
1. SIADH may be precipitated by the stress response, interstitial sodium shifts, and edema.
2. Conditions that are associated with SIADH include nephrosis, cirrhosis, Addison's disease, and myxedema.
3. Damage to the posterior pituitary from radiation, infection, contusion, and atrophy can cause SIADH.

4. Because volume receptors responsible for the release of ADH are located in the left atrium or aortic arch, any pulmonary condition (such as pneumonia, tuberculosis, asthma, emphysema, lung cancer, lung abscess, and positive pressure ventilations), and CHF can promote SIADH.

5. Medications that increase renal tubular reabsorption of water, vasopressin, oxytocin, anesthetics, and morphine are associated with SIADH.

C. Pathophysiology

1. Antidiuretic hormone (ADH) is secreted in response to stimuli recognized by the osmoreceptors in the hypothalamus. Some of these stimuli are pain, extracellular fluid, sympathetic nervous system stimulation, and emotional stress.

2. **ADH stimulates water retention and sodium excretion. If ADH is secreted inappropriately (SIADH), severe fluid overload and hyponatremia occur.**

D. Assessment findings

1. Clinical manifestations of SIADH may include:
   a. Confusion, restlessness, feeling of impending doom, and a decreased level of consciousness
   b. Headache, fatigue, weakness, and seizures
   c. Non-edema weight gain, deep tendon reflexes
   d. Anorexia, nausea, vomiting

2. Laboratory studies include:
   a. Decreased serum sodium and osmolarity
   b. Decreased hemoglobin/hematocrit secondary dilution
   c. Increased urine sodium and osmolarity, specific gravity
   d. Increased serum ADH

E. Nursing diagnoses

1. Fluid Volume Excess
2. Altered Protection
3. Risk for Injury

F. Planning and implementation

1. Initiate measures to restore normal fluid balance:
   a. Strictly monitor I and Os.
   b. Measure weight daily.
   c. Adhere to the fluid restriction ordered by the physician, guided by hourly urine output and insensible fluid losses.
   d. Administer Lasix and/or osmotic diuretics as ordered by physician.
   e. Administer frequent mouth care to assist the patient with fluid restriction.

2. Initiate measures to correct electrolyte imbalances:
   a. Monitor electrolytes, especially sodium.
   b. Administer hypertonic sodium as ordered by physician.

3. Maintain measures to protect patient from injury:

   a. **Seizure precautions for severe hyponatremia. Maintain bed in low position with rails up and padded and anticonvulsants available.**
   b. Patient should not be out of bed without nurse in attendance.

        c.   Limit external stimuli.

        d.   Reorient as necessary.

G.   **Evaluation**

      1.   Serum and urine electrolytes and osmolarity are within normal limits.

      2.   The patient remains free from injury.

H.   **Home health considerations: The client will verbally notify the physician of such symptoms as diminished urine output, weight gain, or change in mental status.**

V.   Diabetes insipidus (DI)

A.   **Description: condition associated with extremely high urine output (up to 12 L/day), predisposing the patient to hypovolemia and shock.**

B.   **Etiology and incidence**

      1.   Neurogenic DI results from cerebral inflammation/edema, hypothalamic or pituitary dysfunction, brain tumor, and inadequate amount of ADH.

      2.   Nephrogenic DI results from renal tubule dysfunction. This type does not respond appropriately to ADH.

      3.   DI can also occur secondary to medication administration. Two drugs associated with DI include dilantin, which inhibits secretion of ADH, and lithium, which decreases renal response to ADH.

C.   **Pathophysiology**

      1.   **Failure of the renal tubules to reabsorb water results in very dilute, excessive urine output.**

      2.   ADH secretion is inadequate in neurogenic DI, and the renal tubules do not respond to the ADH that is secreted in nephrogenic DI.

D.   **Assessment findings**

      1.   Clinical assessment is characterized by:

          a.   Polyuria, dry mucous membranes, poor skin turgor, and excessive thirst

          b.   Increased appetite and generalized weakness

      2.   Laboratory results include:

          a.   Increased serum osmolality and sodium, and increased hematocrit/hemoglobin

          b.   Decreased urine osmolality and sodium, and specific gravity

          c.   ADH may be increased or decreased depending on the etiology

E.   **Nursing diagnoses**

      1.   Fluid Volume Deficit

      2.   Risk for Impaired Skin Integrity

F.   **Planning and implementation**

      1.   Monitor I and Os.

      2.   Record daily weights.

      3.   Monitor CBC and electrolytes.

      4.   Administer medications as ordered by physician:

          a.   Desmopressin (DDAVP) 0.1–0.4 mL daily intranasally.

          b.   Aqueous vasopressin 5–10 units SC/2–4 times per day.

          c.   Drug doses are determined by the physician according to daily urine output.

          d.   Monitor for water intoxication.

5.   Monitor vital signs for evidence of hypovolemia/hypovolemic shock, characterized by hypotension, tachycardia, and change in mental status.

6.   Administer fluids as ordered (IV and PO), and replace fluid hourly, if indicated.

7.   **Use caution if administering TPN. Closely monitor glucose. High glucose levels will lead to osmotic diuresis and increased fluid loss.**

8.   **Enteral feedings are hypertonic. Free water should be given; otherwise the feedings will pull fluid into the GI tract, causing increased GI distention and motility, and predisposing the patient to diarrhea and further water loss.**

9.   Monitor patient for skin breakdown.

10.   Administer preventative skin care.

G.   **Evaluation**

1.   The patient will maintain a fluid and electrolyte balance within normal limits.

2.   The patient will not experience any break in skin integrity.

H.   **Home health considerations**

1.   The client will be able to self-administer medications.

2.   The client will verbalize the signs and symptoms of disease exacerbation.

VI.   Thyroid storm (Hyperthyroid crisis)

A.   **Definition: a life-threatening condition secondary to severe hypersecretion of thyroid hormone, resulting in multisystem failure.**

B.   **Etiology and incidence**

1.   Seen following a stressful event in a patient already suffering with hyperthyroidism. Some events include surgery, infection, trauma, serious illness (DKA, hypoglycemia), or an emotional event.

2.   Occurs after thyroid surgery, when there is vigorous manipulation of the gland, which may result in excessive release of hormones.

3.   Can occur in any patient where inadequate control of hyperthyroidism is taking place. This may be in patients who are non-compliant with medication regimen, or who are taking insufficient dosages of antithyroid medication.

4.   **May be associated with contrast studies where iodine is present in the contrast solution. Thyroid utilizes this iodine to increase thyroid hormone production.**

5.   Iatrogenic causes include treatment of hypothyroidism with excessive thyroid hormone.

6.   Primary cause is a TSH-secreting pituitary tumor.

7.   Occurs in women more often than men, usually between the ages of 30–40.

C.   **Pathophysiology**

1.   The pathophysiology is unclear, however two theories are offered:

a.   A stressful event leads to the release of catecholamines, which combine with the already elevated circulating thyroid hormones, causing a synergistic effect.

      b.   A decrease in plasma proteins—which is evident in serious illnesses and trauma—increases free circulating thyroid hormone, which is picked up and used by the cells leading to hypermetabolism.

  2.   An increase in thyroid hormone causes an increase in all metabolic functions affecting every body system.

D. **Assessment findings**

    1.   Clinical manifestations may include:

        a.   Restlessness, agitation, disorientation, tremors, convulsions, coma

        b.   CHF, dyspnea, rales

        c.   Temp >38–41°C.

        d.   Hypertension, heart rate >130 BPM

        e.   Widened pulse pressure

        f.   ECG shows PVCs, PAT, SVT, or A-FIB

        g.   Cardiogenic shock as evidenced by hypotension and circulatory collapse

        h.   S3 heart sound

        i.   Liver failure with symptoms of jaundice and hepatomegaly

        j.   Severe abdominal pain, cachexia, diarrhea, and weight loss

    2.   **The elderly may not experience any symptoms other than CHF and A-Fib.**

    3.   Laboratory findings include:

        a.   Increased T4, RT3U, T3RIA

        b.   Increased alkaline phosphatase, bilirubin, and SGOT, if liver failure is present

        c.   Decreased serum proteins secondary to hypermetabolism

        d.   Increased red cell mass, anemia, lymphocytosis, and neutropenia, secondary to increased O_2 demand

E. **Nursing diagnoses**

    1.   Impaired Gas Exchange

    2.   Decreased Cardiac Output

    3.   Ineffective Thermoregulation

    4.   Altered Nutrition: Less than Body Requirements

    5.   Sleep Pattern Disturbance

    6.   Risk for Injury

F. **Planning and implementation**

    1.   Prepare to administer radioactive iodine:

        a.   **The thyroid pulls the radioactive iodine from the blood stream and is destroyed.**

        b.   It may take more than one dose over a period of months.

        c.   Close monitoring of thyroid levels and physical assessment is essential.

        d.   The patient will eventually need to take synthetic thyroid hormone replacement, and periodic thyroid levels will need to be monitored after stabilization of the thyroid level.

    2.   Prepare patient for thyroidectomy:

        a.   The thyroid may be partially or completely removed, depending on the cause for surgery.

    b.   If the thyroid is completely removed, the patient will be started on thyroid replacement.

    c.   **If the thyroid is only partially removed, hormone replacement may be withheld so that the thyroid gland will be stimulated to produce sufficient thyroid hormone.**

    d.   In both scenarios the patient should be monitored closely for hyper/hypothyroidism.

    e.   **During the postoperative period, the patient also should be monitored for calcium abnormalities due to inadvertent removal of the parathyroid glands and changes in thyrocalcitonin secretion from the thyroid.**

    f.   **Bleeding is a major potential complication of thyroid surgery due to the thyroid's high vascularity. Ensure evaluation of the back of the neck for pooling of blood.**

    g.   **Thyroid storm is a potential life-threatening complication of thyroid surgery due to manipulation of the gland.**

    h.   **A tracheostomy tray also should be at the bedside in the postoperative period, in case of airway obstruction to due swelling.**

3.   Be familiar with the medications commonly used during the treatment of thyroid storm:

    a.   Propylthiouracil (PTU): Prevents conversion of T_4 to T_3 in the peripheral tissues. For hyperthyroidism, a typical dose would initially be 100 mg TID, then decreased to 50–200 mg/day. For thyroid storm: 300 mg q6hr in conjunction with iodide to inhibit the release of thyroid hormone.

    b.   Sodium Iodide: 4–10 mCi PO × 1 (monitor for anaphylaxis)

    c.   Saturated solution of potassium iodide (SSKI): 5 gtts q8hr.

    d.   Methimazole (MMI): Blocks thyroid uptake of iodine, which reduces thyroid hormone production because iodine is necessary for the synthesis of thyroid hormone. For hyperthyroidism: 10 mg TID then decreased to 5–10 mg/daily. (MMI is 10 times stronger than PTU.)

    e.   **Propranolol: Decreases BP and heart rate. 1–3 mg IV or 20–40 mg PO q2hr–q4hr as ordered by physician. (Contraindicated with preexisting asthma or CHF.)**

    f.   Dexamethasone: Facilitates inhibition of T_4 to T_3 conversion. 2 mg PO q6hr, as ordered by physician.

    g.   Digoxin: for control of A-fib and CHF.

    h.   Antipyretics: for control of increased body temperature.

    i.   **Higher doses of all medications may be necessary due to high metabolic rate. Monitor for toxicity as thyroid levels begin to fall.**

4.   Increased O_2 consumption due to hypermetabolism and intercostal muscle weakness, CHF, and pulmonary edema lead to respiratory compromise. Implement measures to improve or maintain adequate gas exchange:

a. Monitor for adventitious breath sounds, labored breathing, and frequent blood gases.

b. Administer diuretics, digoxin, antibiotics, and bronchodilators as ordered.

c. Administer oxygen therapy and pulmonary toilet as ordered.

d. Allow for frequent rest periods.

5. Implement measures to maintain normal hemodynamics.

a. Monitor continuous ECG for rate and rhythm, BP for hypo/hypertension, and hemodynamics for elevated/lowered pressures.

b. Administer IVF, beta blockers, and antipyretics as ordered. Aspirin frees thyroid hormone from proteins, increasing thyroid levels—therefore it is contraindicated in thyroid storm.

c. Apply cooling blankets, ice packs, or tepid baths to reduce body temperature as ordered. Cooling blanket should be tapered off once the body temperature reaches 100.4° F.

6. Implement measures to deliver adequate calories and nutrients:

a. Monitor serum glucose, which may be elevated due to glycogenolysis, impaired insulin secretion, and insulin resistance.

b. Offer frequent feedings, high in calories, protein, and carbohydrates.

c. Limit caffeine due to already increased peristalsis.

d. Monitor daily weights and calorie counts.

7. Implement measures to reduce sleep deprivation:

a. Allow uninterrupted sleep cycles of at least 90–120 minutes.

b. Reduce environmental stimuli as much as possible, limit lights, noise, visitors, activity as necessary.

c. Anticipate and meet comfort needs.

8. Maintain safety measures to prevent injury:

a. Keep call light within easy reach of patient.

b. Instruct patient not to get out of bed without a nurse present, and keep all four bed rails up with bed in low position.

G. Evaluation

1. The patient will maintain adequate gas exchange.

2. The patient will exhibit normal hemodynamics and body temperature.

3. The patient will tolerate adequate nutritional intake to meet metabolic demands.

4. The patient will exhibit no signs of sleep deprivation.

5. The patient will be free of injury during hospital stay.

VII. Myxedema coma

A. Definition: a life-threatening emergency related to severely low levels of thyroid hormone.

B. Etiology and incidence

1. Seen with inadequate thyroid replacement for chronic or autoimmune hypothyroidism, or following thyroid ablation.

2. Also seen secondary to inadequate thyroid hormone related to a dysfunctional pituitary or hypothalamus.

3. Higher incidence in women than men.

4. Occurs in the 4th and 5th decades of life.

5.   Seen in previously controlled hypothyroidism with an added stressor such as infection, trauma, emotional distress, exposure to cold, or sedative use.

C.   Pathophysiology and management

1.   **A lack of thyroid hormone results in a decrease of all metabolic functions, including CNS depression, and heart and respiratory rates leading to hypotension, hypercapnia, and severe hypothermia.**

2.   Edema is caused by a combination of the shock state and deposits of mucopolysaccharides in the subcutaneous tissues over years of hypothyroidism.

D.   Assessment findings

1.   Clinical manifestations of myxedema include:
    a.   Sluggish, lethargic, obtunded coma
    b.   Depressed deep tendon reflexes
    c.   Hypothermia, bradycardia, hypotension
    d.   PCWP and PAP
    e.   Distant heart sounds and a prolonged Q-T interval
    f.   Non-pitting edema and anasarca
    g.   Decreased respiratory rate, respiratory compromise
    h.   Swollen tongue causing airway obstruction
    i.   Diminished bowel sounds, constipation, abdominal distention, ileus
    j.   Decreased urine output, and evidence of renal failure

2.   Laboratory studies include:
    a.   Decreased T_3, T_4, glucose, serum osmolarity, serum sodium
    b.   Increased TSH, urine osmolarity, urine sodium
    c.   Respiratory acidosis

3.   Chest x-ray, which may show evidence of cardiomegaly, pericardial effusion, and CHF

E.   Nursing diagnoses

1.   Impaired Gas Exchange
2.   Fatigue
3.   Fluid Volume Excess
4.   Hypothermia
5.   Altered Nutrition: Less than Body Requirements
6.   Altered Protection

F.   Planning and implementation

1.   Be familiar with the medications commonly used in the treatment of myxedema:
    a.   Thyroxine (T_4, synthroid, levothyroxine): 2 mcg/kg IV over 5–10 minutes, followed by 100 mcg IV daily.

 ▶   **Extreme caution is necessary, especially with cardiac disease.**

 ▶   **The heart muscle oxygen demand and supply is very low during times of hypometabolism. If synthroid therapy is implemented too rapidly, the coronary oxygen demand will be greater than the oxygen supply, and cardiac ischemia will result.**

𝑚 ▸ **Due to decreased GI motility and probable ileus, oral synthroid is not sufficient in myxedema coma.**

    b.   Volume expansion may be necessary to treat hypotension, but due to the risk of dysrythymias vasopressors are usually not given.

    c.   IV glucose for hypoglycemia

    d.   No hypotonic solutions or free water due to hyponatremia

2. Metabolic breakdown of all medications is decreased. Expect to administer lower doses.

3. Institute measures to maintain an adequate gas exchange:
   a. Monitor ABGs, continuous pulse oximetry, breath sounds, and level of respiratory difficulty for impending respiratory failure.
   b. Assess for airway obstruction.
   c. Be prepared to assist with mechanical ventilation.
   d. Assist with pulmonary toilet and position changes as condition warrants.
   e. Administer diuretics as ordered.
   f. CNS depressants are contraindicated in patients with myxedema.
   g. Monitor responsive patients for changes in mental status. Hypoventilation causes hypercapnia, which will induce neurologic changes.

4. Initiate measures to normalize fluid volume excess:
   a. Strictly monitor I and Os, serum sodium, osmolarity, and glucose levels.
   b. Administer IV glucose solutions as ordered to combat hypoglycemia.
   c. Monitor mental status for early signs of water intoxication.
   d. Administer diuretics as ordered, and maintain free water restriction.
   e. IV fluids are usually normotonic, not osmotic, because osmotics would pull the fluid from the intracellular spaces too rapidly, placing a strain on the already weakened heart muscle.
   f. Hypertonic saline is used only for extreme hyponatremia. Mild hyponatremia will normalize with the thyroid levels.
   g. All IV fluids should be administered via an IV pump.
   h. Maintain seizure precautions as hyponatremia precipitates seizures.

5. Initiate measures to maintain a normal body temperature:
   a. Monitor continuous core temperature.
   b. Keep room temperature greater than 75° F if possible.
   c. Provide patient with extra blankets.

𝑚   d.   **Rewarm gradually. Sudden warming will dilate blood vessels, causing a drop in blood pressure, increasing oxygen consumption, and stressing the myocardium.**

6. Implement measures to decrease complications of decreased GI motility:
   a. Assess bowel sounds and abdominal girth
   b. Maintain NPO status if ileus is present.

c. Administer enemas and stool softeners as ordered for constipation.

> ▶ No tap water enemas; the bowel will absorb the water.

G. Evaluation
1. The patient will maintain normal ABGs, with no signs of respiratory distress or changes in mental status.
2. The patient will maintain hemodynamics within normal limits.
3. The patient will maintain a body temperature of 97–99° F.
4. The patient will tolerate an adequate diet to meet metabolic demands.
5. The patient will have regular bowel movements.

VIII.   Hypoparathyroidism
A. Definition: insufficient production/secretion of PTH, resulting in below-normal levels of serum calcium, increased serum phosphate, and neuromuscular excitability. May cause life-threatening cardiac arrythmias or respiratory arrest.
B. Etiology and incidence
1. Related to unintentional removal of the parathyroid glands during thyroid surgery.
2. Also associated with trauma to the parathyroid glands, autoimmune disease or ischemic injury.
3. Hypomagnesemia suppresses PTH function, which may be secondary to malnutrition or alcoholism.
4. Neck cancer is an identified cause.
C. Pathophysiology
1. **Decreased PTH increases calcium excretion and phosphate resorption by the kidneys. There is a reciprocal relationship between calcium and phosphorus.**
2. Calcium resorption from the bones is decreased, as is calcium absorption from the gut.
3. Serum calcium levels then fall below normal levels, leading to neuromuscular excitability.
4. Bicarbonate is reabsorbed by the kidneys, leading to severe metabolic alkalosis.
D. Assessment
1. Clinical manifestations of the patient with hypoparathyroidism may include:
   a. Irritability, mood swings, depression
   b. Neuromuscular excitability, muscle tremors, cramps, numbness, and tingling
   c. Tetany (muscle spasms), tonic-clonic seizures
   d. Chvostek's sign: unilateral lip twitching in response to tapping a finger on the corresponding cheek
   e. Trousseau's sign: corresponding hand trembles/spasms in response to inflation of a blood pressure cuff
   f. Bradycardia, 2nd or 3rd degree heart block
   g. Cardiac arrest secondary to decreased contractility, prolonged S-T and Q-T interval

        h.   Bronchial/laryngeal spasm, wheezing, stridor, labored breathing, respiratory arrest

        i.   Diarrhea, severe abdominal cramps, biliary colic

  2. Lab studies include:

        a.   Decreased PTH, calcium, prothrombin time

        b.   Increased phosphate

        c.   Metabolic alkalosis

        d.   Digoxin level will decrease as serum calcium decreases, and will rise as serum calcium rises. Monitor for digoxin toxicity during calcium replacement.

E. **Nursing diagnoses**

  1. Decreased Cardiac Output

  2. Impaired Gas Exchange

  3. Altered Tissue Perfusion: Cerebral

  4. Altered Nutrition: Less than Body Requirements

F. **Planning and implementation**

  1. Be familiar with medications used in the treatment of hypoparathyroidism:

        a.   Calcium: 1–3 g daily—May be given by slow IV bolus in equally divided doses or by IV drip 10–15 mg/kg over 4–8 hours.

            ► **Rapid IV infusion may cause cardiac arrest due to increased effect of cardiac glycosides.**

            ► **Use large vein and monitor IV site carefully for extravasion; may cause tissue necrosis.**

            ► **Monitor for orthostatic hypotension.**

        b.   Vitamin D: Dose varies with preparation.

        c.   Magnesium, if hypoparathyroidism is secondary to low levels of magnesium.

  2. Initiate measures to stabilize hemodynamics:

        a.   Monitor continuous ECG for bradycardia and 2nd or 3rd degree heart block.

        b.   Keep pacemaker and atropine at bedside and administer as ordered by physician.

        c.   Monitor for hypotension and hemodynamics for decreased cardiac output.

        d.   Administer fluids, calcium, and other medications as ordered by physician.

        e.   Monitor intake and output.

  3. Initiate measures to improve or maintain normal gas exchange:

        a.   **Monitor for stridor, wheezing, or labored breathing.**

        b.   Monitor continuous pulse oximetry and frequent ABGs as ordered.

        c.   Administer bronchodilators as ordered.

  4. Initiate measures to prevent injury and seizures:

        a.   Initiate seizure precautions.

        b.   Monitor frequently for neuromuscular excitability.

        c.   Range of motion relieves the numbness and tingling, and moist heat alleviates some of the pain from spasms.

        d.   Decrease environmental stimuli.

5. Initiate dietary counseling:
   a. High-calcium and high-magnesium, low-phosphate diet as tolerated until serum levels return to normal.
   b. Instruct patient on the symptoms of hypercalcemia, hypocalcemia, and hypomagnesemia.

G. **Evaluation**
   1. The client maintains hemodynamics within normal limits.
   2. The client exhibits adequate gas exchange.
   3. The client is free from seizures and neuromuscular excitability.
   4. The client verbalizes understanding of dietary importance and symptoms of abnormal calcium and magnesium levels.

IX. **Hyperglycemic, hyperosmolar, non-ketotic coma (HHNK)**
   A. Description: a syndrome marked by hyperglycemia, hyperosmolality, and normal or mild ketonemia.
   B. Etiology and incidence
   1. Associated with NIDDM, glucose infusions, and enteral feedings.
   2. The precipitating event is often an illness, physical or emotional stressor, trauma, or surgery.
   3. Medications that increase serum glucose or cause dehydration, such as steroids and diuretics, can contribute to HHNK.
   C. Pathophysiology and management
   1. Serum glucose becomes elevated in a patient with NIDDM, and insulin secretion is not adequate enough to maintain normal serum glucose levels.
   2. Hyperglycemia results and pulls fluid from the intracellular to the extracellular compartments.
   3. Increased fluid load in the extravascular compartment increases renal excretion of fluid, resulting in a loss of fluid and electrolytes, and causing severe dehydration and electrolyte imbalance.
   D. Assessment findings
   1. Clinical manifestations of the patient with HHNK may include:
      a. Polydipsia, polyuria, oliguria, sugar craving, weight loss, dry mucous membrane, poor skin turgor, and pallor
      b. Weakness, fatigue, somnolence, lethargy, and coma
      c. Hypotension, tachycardia, and narrow pulse pressure
      d. Decreased CVP, PCWP, PAP, and CO
      e. ECG changes such as ST and T-wave abnormalities
      f. Decreased temperature with sepsis, and increased temperature with infection or dehydration
      g. Air hunger, labored breathing (no fruity breath)
      h. Nausea/vomiting, abdominal pain
   2. Laboratory findings include:
      a. Increased glucose (800–1200 mg/100 mL); may be as low as 400 mg/100 mL or as high as 4000 mg/100 mL
      b. Initially potassium and magnesium may be normal or elevated, later decreased due to diuresis
      c. Decreased sodium (<130 mEq/L in the late stages)
      d. Decreased phosphorus and calcium
      e. BUN >80 mg/100 mL

      f. **Serum osmolality >400 mOsm/kg**

g. Increased Hct due to hemoconcentration, increased WBCs

h. Mild acidosis on ABGs; pH not usually <7.25

i. Anion gap not usually >15 mmol/L

j. Serum ketones usually normal

E. **Nursing diagnoses**

1. Fluid Volume Deficit

2. Altered Nutrition: Less than Body Requirements

F. **Planning and implementation**

1. Institute measures to maintain a fluid balance within normal limits:

a. Monitor I and Os.

b. Record daily weights.

 c. **The fluid replacement protocol may be as follows; replace half of the deficit over the first 12 hours, and the remaining half over the following 24 hours. NSS may be used until the patient becomes normotensive, then switch to 0.45% saline solution.**

d. **Once the serum glucose level lowers to 250–300 mg/100 mL 0.45% NSS may be changed to D5 and 1/2 NSS.**

e. Monitor closely for hypo/hyperglycemia.

f. Monitor heart rate, B/P, CVP, PAP, PAWP, CO for hypo/hypervolemia.

g. Monitor for ECG changes.

h. Monitor electrolytes and administer supplements as ordered by physician.

2. Initiate measures to maintain a serum glucose level within normal limits:

a. Frequently monitor serum glucose. Hourly finger sticks may be necessary.

b. Cover hyperglycemia with insulin, as ordered by physician.

 c. **Glucose should be lowered gradually to prevent hypoglycemic shock.**

d. These patients may respond strongly to even small doses of insulin, so monitor carefully for signs of hypoglycemia.

G. **Evaluation**

1. The patient's fluid balance will be within normal limits.

2. The patient's serum glucose will be within normal limits.

X. **Diabetic ketoacidosis**

A. Description: an acute complication of insulin-dependent diabetes mellitus (IDDM), or less frequently, non-insulin dependent diabetes mellitus (NIDDM), characterized by hyperglycemia, ketosis, and metabolic acidosis with resultant dehydration and electrolyte imbalance.

B. Etiology and incidence

1. Often DKA is the first presentation of a newly diagnosed, new-onset diabetes mellitus.

2. Occurs as an exacerbation of baseline diabetes in patients with a history of diabetes mellitus.

3. Presents in patients with insufficient insulin replacement.

4. Stressors that may require an increased insulin requirement: infection, trauma, surgery, pregnancy, puberty, and certain medications.

C.   Pathophysiology

1.   DKA is caused by a disproportionate amount of insulin to glucose levels.

2.   Lack of circulating insulin causes the accumulation of glucose in the blood, depriving the cells of glucose needed for energy.

3.   In response to the low cellular glucose, the liver converts its glycogen stores to glucose, further increasing blood glucose levels.

4.   **Glucose levels rise above the renal threshold, spilling into the urine and enabling the glucose to act as an osmotic diuretic.**

5.   Simultaneously, the body begins to draw on its fat stores as a source of energy for the glucose-deprived cells.

6.   Fatty acids are transported to the liver for ketogenesis.

7.   Large amounts of ketones, which are the end-product of fat metabolism, are produced and accumulate in the blood. This process is known as ketosis. Urine spillage is known as ketonuria. This progresses to acidosis.

8.   **In an attempt to correct the acidosis, the lungs blow off the excess hydrogen ions with carbon dioxide (H_2CO_3-carbonic acid) and the kidneys excrete acetoacetate in the urine.**

9.   Respirations deepen and become rapid (Kussmaul's respirations) to rid the body of acetone.

10.   Ketonuria results as the kidneys attempt to clear the body of ketones.

11.   Without insulin, the body's defenses are overwhelmed and increasing acidosis ensues.

12.   Stress hormones, such as cortisol, glucagon, and catecholamines are released, raising the glucose level even further.

13.   Dehydration or osmotic diuresis can occur and severe electrolyte imbalances ensue with sodium, potassium, and chloride primarily affected.

14.   Fluid loss results in hemoconcentration, impeding circulation and causing tissue anoxia and resultant lactic acidosis.

D.   Assessment findings

1.   Physical manifestations of the early stages of DKA may include:

    a.   **Dehydration, causing polyuria, polydipsia, abdominal pain and rigidity, dry mucous membranes, flushed skin, soft eyeballs, and poor skin turgor.**

    b.   Severe electrolyte imbalances may cause nausea and vomiting.

    c.   Weight loss is caused by the body's inability to utilize carbohydrates, thus forcing it to use its fat reserves for energy.

    d.   Kussmaul's respirations

2.   Physical manifestations of the later stages of DKA may include:

    a.   Hypovolemia and ensuing hypotension and oliguria or anuria

    b.   Decreased CVP, PAP, PCWP, CO

    c.   Tachycardia

    d.   Decreased level of consciousness, stupor, and coma

3.   Laboratory findings include:

    a.   Serum glucose >250–300 mg/100 mL

    b.   Arterial pH 6.8–7.3

    c. Serum bicarbonate <15 mEq/L

    d. Serum sodium 130–140 mEq/L

    e. Increased or decreased serum potassium

    f. Decreased serum phosphate

    g. BUN 18–25 mg/mL

    h. Increased serum ketones

    i. Urine ketones >3 mg/24 hours

    j. Serum osmolality (variable)

    k. Serum creatinine possibly elevated

E. Nursing diagnoses

    1. Fluid Volume Deficit

    2. Knowledge Deficit: Diabetic Ketoacidosis

    3. Altered Tissue Perfusion: Cardiopulmonary

    4. Decreased Cardiac Output

    5. Altered Protection

F. Planning and implementation

    1. Be knowledgeable about the medications commonly used to treat DKA, eg, insulin.

        a. **Be aware that a low-dose continuous infusion of regular insulin is the therapy of choice. Mixing 100 U regular insulin in 100 mL/NSS is recommended, producing a 1:1 ratio, thus allowing a more easily prescribed and titrated dose. An IV bolus is usually given, ranging from 0.1–0.3 U/kg body weight, followed by a continuous infusion of 0.1 U/kg/hour.**

        b. **Monitor for a decrease of 50–100 mg/dL/hour in the blood glucose level, indicating proper hydration and insulin therapies. This parameter may be used for titration of the insulin infusion.**

        c. **If the serum glucose level has not changed after the first hour of insulin therapy, it has been recommended to double the insulin infusion rate. It should be noted that large amounts of insulin requirements (>20 U/hr) may indicate inadequate fluid replacement, insulin resistance, or infection.**

        d. **Monitor for rebound hyperglycemia and unresolved acidosis, indicating that insulin therapy was discontinued too early. The decision to stop the insulin infusion should be based on the presence of ketones in the blood or urine.**

        e. Monitor blood glucose levels hourly, and then on an individual basis as ordered.

        f. Be aware that glucose levels should not be lowered more than 50–100 mg/100 mL/hr, due to the risks of cerebral edema and circulatory collapse.

        g. During prolonged hyperglycemia, large quantities of glucose deposits accumulate in the brain. When the blood sugar is lowered too rapidly, water is freed and attracted to the glucose in the brain, creating cerebral edema. DKA causes hypovolemia secondary to osmotic diuresis. Some intravascular volume is retained, however, by the glucose unable to enter the cells, attracting water. If the blood sugar is lowered too rapidly and prior to fluid replacement, the water will follow the glucose into the cells, causing circulatory collapse.

2. Be knowledgeable about the medications commonly used to treat DKA, eg, potassium.

   a. Be aware that the initial potassium level in DKA is a measurement of extracellular potassium, which is an indirect measurement of intracellular levels.

   b. The intracellular level is significantly lower than the serum value. This imbalance occurs because during acidosis the hydrogen ions accumulate in the extracellular fluid, forcing itself into the intravascular fluid.

   c. Conversely, the potassium is forced from the intracellular to the extracellular fluid. Once hydration and insulin therapies are initiated and acidosis begins to resolve, the serum potassium level declines.

   d. This decrease is due to a number of factors: insulin administration causes potassium's reentry into the cells, and increased renal perfusion (from hydration) promotes diuresis and expansion of intravascular volume.

   e. **Potassium replacement may be necessary, but the timing and dosage are very dependent on laboratory values and the patient's renal status. The serum potassium level should be checked every 1–2 hours during the initial phase of treatment.**

3. Be knowledgeable about the medications commonly used to treat DKA, eg, sodium bicarbonate.

   a. Be aware that the routine administration of sodium bicarbonate is currently not recommended. However, in severe acidosis, indicated by an arterial pH of 6.9 or less, sodium bicarbonate is still being used.

   b. It has been recommended that 44 mEq of sodium bicarbonate be administered for a pH of 6.9–7.0 and 88 mEq for a pH <6.9. It is also recommended that an additional 15 mEq/KCL be given for each 44 mEq of bicarbonate as bicarbonate potentiates hypokalemia. Sodium bicarbonate should be infused slowly over several hours.

4. Be knowledgeable about the medications commonly used to treat DKA: Decisions regarding other therapies such as phosphate and magnesium replacement are based on individual preexisting conditions such as nutritional status, pancreatitis, or alcoholism.

5. Implement measures to restore fluid and electrolyte balance:

   a. Administer IV fluids as ordered by physician. Normal saline is usually ordered at the rate of 1–2 L over the first 1–2 hours or until hemodynamically stable, followed with 0.45% NSS at the rate of 150–250 mL/hr.

b. Monitor serum electrolytes; once glucose is <200 mg/dL dextrose should be added to the IV solution to allow for continued insulin administration without inducing hypoglycemia.
   c. Monitor hourly I and Os.
   d. Monitor urine for ketones
6. Implement measures to maintain an adequate cardiac output:
   a. Monitor continuous ECG, vital signs, and hemodynamics.
   b. Administer IV fluids as ordered.
   c. Monitor blood gases.
   d. Monitor for dysrhythmias.
   e. Administer antidysrhythmics as ordered and appropriate.

G. Evaluation
1. The patient will verbalize knowledge about disease process and treatment.
2. The patient will resume a normal fluid/electrolyte balance.
3. The patient will maintain hemodynamics within normal limits.
4. The patient will experience a resolution of any dysrythmias secondary to DKA.

H. Home health considerations
1. The client will verbalize signs and symptoms to report to physician.
2. The patient will exhibit adequate control over diabetes mellitus.

XI. Addisonian crisis
A. Description: a life-threatening exacerbation of Addison's disease, characterized by tachycardia, hypovolemia, hyponatremia, hyperkalemia, and GI distress.
B. Etiology and incidence: Occurs in patients with a history of Addison's disease and recent added stressor such as emotional upheaval, infection, surgery, trauma, hemorrhage, AIDS, or metastatic cancer
C. Pathophysiology
1. The patient with Addison's disease is usually controlled with exogenous steroids which become insufficient during times of added stress.
2. If not treated, a deficiency of mineralocorticoids leads to fatigue, muscle weakness, and sodium depletion, causing hyponatremia, hypovolemia, and potassium retention, resulting in cardiac dysrhythmias.
3. Insufficient amounts of cortisol predisposes the patient to hypoglycemia and decreased mental acuity.

D. Assessment findings
1. Clinical manifestations of addisonian crisis may include:
   a. Lethargy, generalized weakness, fatigue, headache
   b. Tachycardia, hypotension, ECG changes
   c. Decreased CVP, PAP, PCWP, CO
   d. Nausea, vomiting, abdominal pain, diarrhea
   e. Hyperpigmentation of the elbows, hands, knees, and mouth. Seen only with primary Addison's, which is caused by an increase in ACTH

    2. Laboratory findings include:
       a. Decreased sodium, glucose, bicarbonate, serum cortisol
       b. Increased potassium, BUN
       c. Metabolic acidosis
       d. Anemia, lymphocytosis
       e. ACTH may be increased in primary Addison's or decreased in secondary Addison's

E. Nursing diagnoses
    1. Fatigue
    2. Hypovolemia
    3. Altered Protection
    4. Fluid Volume Deficit

F. Planning and implementation
    1. Replace steroids as ordered. Cortisol must be given slowly, as rapid administration may cause anaphylaxis, bronchospasm, and rapid fluid and electrolyte shifts.
    2. Monitor serum glucose levels, especially when fasting. May need IV glucose
    3. Monitor electrolytes and replace sodium and bicarbonate as ordered.
    4. Monitor continuous ECG for cardiac dysrhythmias, and administer medications to reduce potassium if ordered.
    5. Monitor I and Os, and daily weights.
    6. **Monitor heart rate, blood pressure, and hemodynamics for signs of fluid volume depletion and progress with fluid replacement.**
    7. Replace fluids as ordered, usually with D5NSS.
    8. Administer vasoconstrictors as ordered for hypotensive patients. Fluid volume should be replaced before use of vasoconstrictors if possible.
    9. Monitor ABGs to assess progression of metabolic acidosis.

G. Evaluation
    1. The patient will maintain a normal fluid and electrolyte balance.
    2. The patient will not experience hypoglycemia.
    3. The patient will resume normal hemodynamics.

H. Home health considerations
    1. The client will verbalize the signs and symptoms to report to the physician, including any illness or other stressors.
    2. The client will verbalize the importance of compliance with his or her medication and nutritional regimen.

XII. Pheochromocytoma
    A. Description: a chromaffin cell tumor (single or multiple), usually in the adrenal medulla, which secretes inappropriately high amounts of epinephrine and/or norepinephrine.

    Stimulation of this tumor may result in life-threatening high blood pressure and heart rate.

    B. Etiology and incidence
       1. These tumors are rare and usually benign.
       2. There is a familial tendency.
       3. May occur at any age but is more common in the 4th and 5th decades of life.

4. Any physical or emotional stressor may initiate an episode in a patient with a pheochromocytoma. This may include smoking, alcohol use, surgery, illness, trauma, and anesthesia.

C. **Pathophysiology**

1. Most tumors secrete both epinephrine and norepinephrine.
2. Tumors that secrete predominately norepinepherine are characterized by severe hypertension, headache, and hypermetabolism.
3. Epinephrine-secreting tumors present with beta-adrenergic symptoms such as tachycardia, dysrhythmias, palpitations, weakness, anxiety, and tremors.
4. Of patients who present with hypertension, 50% of those have sustained hypertension and 50% are paroxysmal.
5. A sudden secretion of epinephrine occurs and causes peripheral vasodilation. Hypovolemia and hypotension ensue.
6. Sympathetic nervous system is stimulated, causing the release of norepinepherine. Vasoconstriction and hypertension result.

D. **Assessment findings**

1. Clinical manifestations in the patient with a pheochromocytoma may include:
   a. Tremors, anxiety, feeling of impending doom
   b. Raynaud's syndrome; upper extremities become pale, then turn blue, then red
   c. Fever, heat intolerance, flushed skin, diaphoresis, palpitations, syncope, parasthesia
   d. Tachycardia, tachydysrhythmias, hypertension, CHF, rales, angina
   e. Nausea, vomiting, weight loss
   f. Polyuria
2. Laboratory studies include:
   a. Increased glucose
   b. Spot urine for metanephrine (catecholamine derivatives) Must be acquired during or just following an episode.
   c. 24-hour urine for total free catecholamines, total metanephrine, VMA (vanillmandelic acid, a metabolite of epinephrine); see Display 11-1
3. Diagnostic studies: the following diagnostic tests are utilized to locate pheochromocytomas:
   a. Angiogram/IVP
   b. Abdominal/renal CT scan
   c. MRI

E. **Nursing diagnoses**

1. Altered Tissue Perfusion: Renal, Cardiopulmonary, Cerebral
2. Hypovolemia
3. Altered Protection
4. Fear
5. Altered Nutrition: Less than Body Requirements
6. Anxiety

F. **Planning and implementation**

1. The usual treatment for pheochromocytoma is surgical removal of the tumor.
   a. The surgery has a success rate of about 90%.

DISPLAY 11-1.
Considerations for 24-Hour Urine Testing

Urine will not be of use with sporadic episodes; the measurements will level out to near-normal over 24 hours.
Special preparation added to jar before specimen collection.
There will be an altered result with the use of certain foods and medications: caffeine, bananas, nuts, MAO inhibitors, dopamine, quinidine, isoproterenol, alpha-methyldopa, chlorpromazine.

    b.   Preoperative care entails control of the effects of catecholamine secretion with administration of alpha and beta blockers.

    c.   Postoperative care includes assessment of hemodynamics, prevention of complications, and support of body functions until vital signs are returned to normal.

    d.   The major complication of surgery is the secretion of catecholamines and life-threatening hypertension.

2.   Be familiar with the medications commonly used in the treatment of pheochromocytoma:

    a.   Alpha-adrenergic blockers

    ▶ **Phenoxybenzamine: inhibits the release of norepinephrine. The dose is 10 mg q2hr for 2 days, then increase by 10 mg/day until blood pressure is within normal limits.**

    ▶ **Metyrosine: Inhibits synthesis of norepinephrine. 250 mg BID, gradually increasing to maximum dose of 500 mg QID. Side effects include parkinsonian symptoms and sedation. Metyrosine depletes levodopa and dopamine in the CNS.**

    b.   Beta blockers: propanolol and labetolol may be ordered for epinephrine induced tachycardia. Keep heart rate >100.

    c.   Vasodilators and nipride may be ordered to control blood pressure. Continually monitor blood pressure.

3.   Implement measures to insure adequate tissue perfusion to vital organs:

    a.   Adhere to seizure and safety precautions.

    b.   Continuously monitor arterial pressure for paroxysmal or sustained hypertension.

    c.   Administer alpha-adrenergic blockers and vasodilators as ordered.

    d.   Perform neurologic check every hour or more frequently, as necessary.

      e.   Monitor continuous arterial blood pressure for hypotension due to medication regimen, and in the postoperative period due to a decrease in circulating catecholamines.

      f.   Treat with IVF and volume expanders as ordered.

      g.   Monitor heart and lung sounds for CHF and medicate as ordered.

      h.   Continuously monitor heart rate and rhythm for tachycardia and arrhythmias.

      i.   Administer beta blockers and antidysrhythmics as ordered.

      j.   Assess patient for angina related to coronary ischemia.

      k.   Maintain strict I and Os and monitor BUN/creatinine and electrolytes for signs of renal insufficiency.

4.   Implement measures to meet nutritional needs:

      a.   Monitor serum and urine glucose.

      b.   Administer glucose and insulin solutions as ordered.

      c.   Administer small frequent meals with high-calorie, high-nutrition snacks.

      d.   Dietary considerations should include foods that would decrease abdominal distention and constipation.

5.   Provide measures to control anxiety:

      a.   Frequently reassure patient.

      b.   Limit environmental stimuli and visitors as necessary.

6.   Administer alpha and beta blockers as ordered to control nervousness and feelings of impending doom.

G. **Evaluation**

    1.   The patient will maintain adequate perfusion to all vital organs.

    2.   The patient will sustain hemodynamics within normal limits.

    3.   The patient will tolerate a diet adequate to meet nutritional needs.

    4.   The patient will demonstrate control of anxiety levels.

H. **Home health considerations**

    1.   Home health considerations of a client with a pheochromocytoma should include control of blood pressure, heart rate, and anxiety; increased nutritional requirements; knowledge of signs and symptoms that warrant immediate medical attention and immediate notification of physician.

    2.   Teaching should also include measures taken to prevent stimulation of tumor secretion. The patient should:

      a.   Not wear tight clothing.

      b.   Not hold breath or push during a bowel movement.

      c.   Take measures to avoid abdominal distention and constipation.

      d.   Not bend at the waist or pull knees up to the chest.

      e.   Caution a health care worker unfamiliar with his or her history against palpating his or her abdomen.

      f.   Avoid physical stress and learn techniques for handling emotional stress.

Bibliography

Hudak, C. M. & Galo, B. M. (1994). *Critical care nursing: a holistic approach* (6th ed.). Philadelphia: J. B. Lippincott.

Kitabchi, A. E. & Wall, B. M. (1995). Diabetic ketoacidosis. *Med Clin North Am* 79(1), 9–37.

Lebovitz, H. E. (1995). Diabetic ketoacidosis. *Lancet* 345, 767–772.

Lipsky, M. S. (1994). Management of diabetic ketoacidosis. *Am Fam Physician* 49, 1607–1612.

McMahon, M., Manji, N., & Driscoll, D. F. (1989). Parenteral nutrition in patients with diabetes mellitus. Theoretical and practical considerations. *JPEN* 13, 545–553.

North American Nursing Diagnosis Association (NANDA). (1996). *Nursing diagnoses: Definitions & classification 1997–1998.* Philadelphia: Author.

Peragallo-Dittko, V., Godley, K., & Meyer, J. (1993). *A core curriculum for diabetic education* (2nd ed.). Chicago: American Association of Diabetes Educators and the AAOE Education and Research Foundation.

Pomposeli, J. J., Flores, E. A., & Bistrian, B. R. (1988). Role of biochemical mediators in clinical nutrition and surgical metabolism. *JPEN* 12, 212–218.

Wood, R., Bengoa, J., & Sitrin, M. (1985). Calciuretic effect of cyclic versus continuous total parenteral nutrition. *Am J Clin Nutr* 41, 614–619.

Zaloga, G. P. (1994). *Nutrition in critical care.* St. Louis: Mosby.

STUDY QUESTIONS

1. The following lab results would be consistent with SIADH:
   a. Serum sodium (128 mEq/L), serum osmolality (250 mOsm/kg water), urine specific gravity (1.052)
   b. Serum sodium (152 mEq/L), serum osmolality (350 Osm/kg water), urine specific gravity (1.007)
   c. Hematocrit (58%), potassium (4.2 mEq/L), + ketonuria
   d. Hematocrit (40%), urine sodium (20 mEq/L/24 hours), urine osmolality (30 mOsm/kg/water)

2. The following nursing interventions would be inappropriate when caring for the patient with DI:
   a. Administer aqueous vasopressin, 5–10 units SC daily as ordered by physician.
   b. Monitor the patient for a decreased CVP and CO, and tachycardia.
   c. Restrict free water instillation if the patient is receiving enteral feedings.
   d. Replace fluids hourly, cc:cc as ordered by the physician.

3. You receive a patient from the recovery room, status post–partial thyroidectomy with a temperature of 104.9° F, BP 180/90, HR 148. One hour ago his temperature was 99.5° F, BP 120/70, HR 105. Which of the following orders would not be appropriate?
   a. Give two aspirin PO now and q4hr PRN for temperature >101.5° F or pain.
   b. Propranolol 3 mg IV x 1 now, followed by 30 mg PO q3hr.
   c. Dexamathasone 2 mg PO q6hr.
   d. Oxygen 4 L by nasal cannula; notify physician of pulse oximetery <94%.

4. Assessment findings for the patient in thyroid storm may include the following:
   a. Somnolence, swollen tongue, abdominal distention, non-pitting edema
   b. 2nd degree heart block, wheezing, Chovstek's sign, mood swings
   c. Temperature 102.0° F, hypotension, polydipsia, tachycardia
   d. Disorientation, increased T_4, rales, abdominal pain

5. Which of the following nursing diagnoses would not be appropriate for the patient with myxedema?
   a. Alteration in mental status
   b. Alteration in nutrition: less than body requirements
   c. Impaired gas exchange
   d. Fluid volume deficit

6. PTH is responsible for maintaining a normal serum calcium level by:
   a. Increasing calcium resorption from the bones
   b. Decreasing calcium absorption from the gut
   c. Increasing calcium excretion from the kidneys
   d. Increasing phosphorus resorption from the kidneys

7. Which of the following patient histories correlates with HHNK?
   a. IDDM, recent bronchitis, able to tolerate three 3 meals a day during illness.
   b. Young athlete, training for the Olympics, eating 7 high-calorie, high-nutrition meals a day for the last 6 months.
   c. NIDDM, recent strep infection, able to tolerate liquids such as water ice, milkshakes, and juices.
   d. 50-year-old female with no history of DM, admitted to the hospital for a cholecystectomy, IVF of D5 and .045% sodium chloride at 125 mL/hr.

8. You would expect to see the following hemodynamics in the patient with addisonian crisis:
   a. CVP (10), PCWP (23), CO (8)
   b. CVP (0), PCWP (5), CO (3)
   c. CVP (4), PCWP (12), CO (5)
   d. CVP (3), PCWP (23), CO (3)

9. The following lab results might be seen in the patient with addisonian crisis:

a. Serum glucose (54 mg/100 mL), serum potassium (6.0 mEq/L), bicarbonate (15 mEq/L)
b. Serum glucose (110 mg/100 mL), serum potassium (5.0 mEq/L), bicarbonate (24 mEq/L)
c. Serum sodium (128 Meq/L), serum osmolality (250 mOsm/kg water), urine sodium (250 mEq/L/24 hours)
d. Serum calcium (7.2 mg/100 mL), serum phosphorous (7.0 mEq/L), PTH (1 pg/mL)

10. Which of the following nursing diagnoses does not apply to the patient with DKA?
    a. Alteration in tissue perfusion
    b. Alteration in hemodynamics
    c. Potential for cardiac dysrhythmias
    d. Alteration in fluid balance: fluid overload

11. Polyuria, polydipsia, abdominal pain, and fruity odor to breath are classic symptoms of
    a. HHNK
    b. Myxedema
    c. DKA
    d. Hypoparathyroidism

12. When treating the patient in DKA with an insulin drip, a drop in the glucose level averaging 200 mg/100 mL/hr indicates:
    a. The rate of the insulin drip is too high.
    b. The rate of the insulin drip is too low.
    c. The insulin drip is at the correct rate.
    d. The patient may be experiencing insulin resistance.

ANSWER KEY

1. *Correct response: a*

   SIADH causes water retention and sodium excretion, resulting in hyponatremia, hypo-osmolality, and an increased urine specific gravity due to concentrated urine.

   b. These lab results are consistent with DI.

   c. Hct would be decreased in SIADH due to hemodilution, potassium is within normal range, and ketonuria is consistent with DKA.

   d. Decreased Hct is consistent with SIADH but urine sodium and osmolality would be increased, not decreased, in SIADH due to concentrated urine.

   Comprehension/Physiologic/NA

2. *Correct response: c*

   Enteral feedings are hypertonic and pull water into the bowel, exacerbating dehydration and causing abdominal distention and diarrhea.

   a. This is an appropriate order.

   b. The patient with DI should be assessed a low CO and CVP with tachycardia; these findings would indicate hypovolemia.

   d. This is an appropriate intervention for the patient with DI.

   Application/Physiologic/Intervention

3. *Correct response: a*

   According to the history and symptoms, this patient is in thyroid storm; ASA is contraindicated because it frees T_4 from proteins, increasing thyroid levels.

   b, c, d. These are appropriate orders for the patient in thyroid storm.

   Analysis/Physiologic/Implementation

4. *Correct response: d*

   Signs and symptoms are consistent with thyroid storm.

   a. These symptoms are consistent with myxedema.

   b. These symptoms are indicative of hypoparathyroidism.

   c. These symptoms are consistent with HHNK (hypotension due to hypovolemia), thyroid storm causes hypertension until the patient develops cardiogenic shock.

   Knowledge/Physiologic/Assessment

5. *Correct response: d*

   Patients with myxedema experience fluid overload due to decreased contractility of the heart.

   a. This is an appropriate diagnoses; these patients may be somnolent to comatose.

   b. These patients may appear overweight, but they are unable to metabolize nutrients properly and are therefore malnourished.

   c. Respiratory rate, respiratory center, and respiratory effort are all diminished in myxedema.

   Analysis/Physiologic/Planning

6. *Correct response: a*

   The function of PTH is to increase serum calcium levels when they are low. One of the ways this is accomplished is by the resorption of calcium from the bones to the bloodstream.

   b. PTH increases calcium reabsorption from the gut.

   c. PTH decreases calcium excretion from the kidneys.

   d. PTH increases renal excretion of phosphorus; calcium and phosphorus have a reciprocal relationship.

   Knowledge/Physiologic/NA

7. *Correct response: c*

   Precipitating factors for HHNK include anything that would raise the glucose level higher than the body's insulin levels can tolerate, but low enough to prevent ketonemia.

   a. This patient would be at a higher risk for developing DKA.

b. This person may actually need seven meals a day to meet his nutritional requirements.

d. This patient has no history of DM; D5 and 0.45% sodium chloride at 125 mL/hr should not cause her to develop HHNK.

Analysis/Physiologic/Assessment

8. **Correct response: b**

Sodium depletion due to loss of mineralocorticoids in addisonian crisis contributes to hypovolemia demonstrated by the low hemodynamics.

a. These pressures would indicate hypervolemia.

c. These are normal hemodynamics.

d. CVP demonstrates a normal blood return to the heart, the elevated PCWP and decreased CO indicate left ventricular failure.

Comprehension/Physiologic/Assessment

9. **Correct response: a**

Decreased cortisol predisposes to hypoglycemia, decreased mineral corticoids leads to potassium retention, and decreased bicarbonate causes metabolic acidosis.

b. These are normal lab values.

c. These values may indicate SIADH.

d. These lab values are consistent with hypoparathyroidism.

Comprehension/Physiologic/Assessment

10. **Correct response: d**

Increased glucose levels produce osmotic diuresis, causing hypovolemia.

a, b. Severe fluid loss leads to hemoconcentration and a decreased CO, causing a state of poor tissue perfusion.

c. Osmotic diuresis promotes severe electrolyte imbalances, predisposing patient to cardiac dysrrhythmias.

Analysis/Physiologic/Planning

11. **Correct response: c**

Osmotic diuresis in DKA causes polyuria, which causes dehydration and electrolyte imbalances, leading to polydipsia and abdominal pain. The fruity odor to breath is secondary to the lungs trying to rid the body of acetone.

a. There is no fruity odor to the breath in HHNK, because the body produces enough insulin to prevent ketonemia.

b. The classic signs of myxedema include severe hypothermia, bradycardia, hypotension, and somnolence.

d. Hypoparathyroidism would produce neuromuscular excitability with Chovstek's and Trousseau's signs, bradycardia, and bronchial spasms.

Knowledge/Physiologic/NA

12. **Correct response: a**

b, c. The goal is to reduce the glucose level by 50–100 mg/100 mL/hr to prevent hypoglycemia.

d. Insulin resistance would be evident in a patient requiring an insulin drip exceeding 20 units/hr.

Application/Physiologic/Implementation

The Female Reproductive System

I.   Anatomy and physiology
A.   Structures: External female genitalia
1.   Vulva: also known as the pudenda, the vulva is the term used to designate all external visible structures from the pubis to the perineum.
2.   Mons pubis: also known as the mons veneris, the mons pubis is the fatty cushion that lies over the anterior symphysis pubis.
3.   Clitoris: a small cylindrical, erectile body lying within the anterior portion of the vulva.
4.   Labia majora and labia minora: rounded folds of tissue covered with skin that converge at the mons pubis and extend downward. The labia minora lie within the labia majora.
5.   Vestibule: This is the area bordered by the labia minora, extending from the clitoris downward. The vestibule contains the openings of the urethra, two Skene's ducts of the paraurethral glands, the vaginal orifice, and two ducts of Bartholin's glands.
6.   Urethra: a vertical slit that lies just above the vaginal opening, about 4 cm long, leading to the bladder neck.
7.   Vaginal opening: located at the inferior portion of the vestibule, it varies greatly in size and shape.
8.   Perineum: the region of the genital area that lies between the vulva and the anus.

B.   Structures: Internal female reproductive organs
1.   Vagina: serves as the excretory duct of the uterus, female copulation organ, and birth canal for the infant. The vagina is a tube lined with rugae that is able to distend markedly during childbirth.
2.   Uterus: the uterus is located in the lower pelvis, and lies between the urinary bladder and the rectum.
   a.   The upper portion is the body or corpus. The lower portion is the cervix.
   b.   The dome-shaped upper segment is located between the insertion of the fallopian tubes and is called the fundus.
   c.   The uterus contains three layers:

   ► Perimetrium or outer layer
   ► Myometrium or thick muscle layer
   ► Endometrium or inner layer

3.   Fallopian tubes: two tubes extending from the uterus to the ovaries.
4.   Ovaries: paired organs that develop and produce ova and secrete steroid sex hormones; they lie on either side of the uterus.

C.   Functions
1.   Uterus:
   a.   The endometrium is replaced once a month in anticipation of conception.
   b.   The uterus helps to provide the endometrium for the implantation of a fertilized ovum.
   c.   Within the uterus, a placenta is formed, which will nourish the developing fetus during pregnancy.
   d.   The uterus also develops musculature that protects the fetus and contracts during labor to expel the infant.
2.   Ovaries: produce the eggs necessary for fertilization and secrete steroid sex hormones.

3. Fallopian tubes: transport sperm to the ova and the ova to the uterus; these serve as a passageway for the fertilized ovum to the uterus.

II. Overview of female reproductive pathology

A. Assessment

1. Obstetric/gynecologic history should include information about:
   a. Previous pregnancies—GTPAL
   b. Gravida (G): how many pregnancies in total, including miscarriages, abortions, ectopic pregnancies, multiple gestations, normal vaginal deliveries, cesarean sections, and premature deliveries
   c. Para: subdivided into term (T) deliveries and preterm (P) deliveries
   d. Abortion (A): either elective or spontaneous abortion
   e. Living (L): the number of children living presently.

2. Menstrual history should include age of first menstruation, length of average cycle, and number of days of normal menstrual flow. Information regarding the first day of last period and whether the last period was within normal limits should be obtained. This is to ascertain expected date of delivery (EDD) or due date.

3. Expected date of delivery: from the first day of her last menstrual period (LMP) to her expected due date is 280 days: 40 weeks, 10 lunar months, or 9 calendar months.

4. Obstetric history should include:
   a. Types of previous deliveries, spontaneous vaginal deliveries (SVD) or cesarean section (C/S). Should also obtain dates of previous deliveries and weights of babies at birth.
   b. Medical problems associated with previous pregnancies, such as pregnancy induced hypertension (PIH), and gestational diabetes mellitus.
   c. Medical problems associated with previous deliveries, such as cephalopelvic disproportion, premature delivery, and placental abruption.
   d. Previous contraception use.
   e. History of or present sexually transmitted diseases.

5. General health history should include information on:
   a. Age
   b. Race
   c. Occupation
   d. Allergies
   e. Medication taken at present or as needed
   f. History of, or present use of tobacco, alcohol or "street" drugs
   g. Previous surgery
   h. Medical problems, especially hypertension, diabetes, seizures, heart problems, or asthma
   i. Family history, especially any history of congenital anomalies in both the pregnant patient's and father of the baby's families.

6. Psychosocial assessment should include information regarding:
   a. Family structure and support network
   b. Pregnant woman's personal feelings about the pregnancy

        c. Relationship with father of the baby
        d. Anticipation and preparation for the infant
        e. Financial impact on the family
        f. Nutritional assessment

    7. Physical exam should be complete and systemic, with particular attention paid to pulmonary and cardiac systems.

B. Laboratory studies

    1. Human chorionic gonadotrophin (HCG) is a hormone detected in maternal blood or urine. HCG concentration is about 100 mIU/mL at first missed menstrual period and doubles every 2 days until 10 weeks' gestation, then it drops sharply.

    2. Factors affecting interpretation of test results:
        a. Multiple gestation
        b. Hydatidiform mole
        c. Missed abortion
        d. Unknown or irregular menstrual cycle

    3. Hemoglobin (Hgb) and hematocrit (Hct) should be obtained for detection of anemia.

    4. Blood type including type, Rh, and antibody titer tests.

    5. Rubella screening.

    6. Serology is used to screen and diagnose for syphilis.

    7. Hemoglobin electrophoresis is used to detect genetic hemoglobin disorders such as sickle cell anemia and thalassemias.

    8. Hepatitis screening.

    9. HIV testing.

    10. Routine urinalysis.

    11. Diabetes screening (done at 24–28 weeks).

C. Diagnostic testing

    1. Ultrasonography: lst trimester testing
        a. Non-invasive
        b. Identifies ectopic pregnancy or blighted ovum
        c. Provides image of fetus, placenta, and uterus
        d. Assesses gestational age
        e. Evaluates congenital anomalies
        f. Confirms suspected multiple gestation
        g. Evaluates fetal growth
        h. Diagnostic evaluation of vaginal bleeding
        i. Diagnostic evaluation of pelvic mass
        j. Used in combination with amniocentesis and chorionic villus sampling
        k. Four weeks after LMP gestational sac can be seen
        l. Seven weeks after LMP fetal cardiac activity seen
        m. Accurately dates pregnancy between 7–13 weeks after LMP by measuring crown–rump length (CRL) of fetus

    2. Ultrasonography: 2nd trimester testing
        a. Assesses gestational age
        b. Diagnoses multiple gestation
        c. Assesses fetal growth
        d. Placental location
        e. Identifies structural abnormalities of the fetus
        f. Guides amniocentesis and fetoscopy

g. Interpretation:

  ▸ Between 16–20 weeks gestation, biparietal diameter (BPD) is used to assess gestational age

  ▸ Serial sonograms can be used to assess fetal growth when there is a concern over whether fetus is too large or too small

3. Ultrasonography: 3rd trimester testing
   a. Fetal position
   b. Estimates fetal size
   c. Placental location
   d. Evidence of placental abruption
   e. Guide for amniocentesis

4. Amniocentesis: aspiration of amniotic fluid from the amniotic sac within the uterus through the maternal abdomen for the purpose of analysis.
   a. In an Rh-negative mother this can test for elevated bilirubin levels.
   b. Culture and sensitivity studies can be done if amnionitis is suspected.
   c. Fetal lung maturity tests can be done if complications indicate a premature delivery.
   d. L/S ratio: a 2:1 ratio of lecithin to sphingomyelin indicates fetal lung maturity, usually after 35 weeks.
   e. Phosphatidylglycerol: the presence of this indicates positive fetal lung maturity. It is reported as PG+.

5. Biophysical profile (BPP): Ultrasound and electronic fetal monitoring used to evaluate 5 parameters. Uses a scoring system with a 2 being normal and a 0 being absent or abnormal.
   a. Fetal breathing movements
   b. Gross body movements
   c. Fetal tone
   d. Reactive fetal heart rate (electronic fetal monitoring)
   e. Qualitative amniotic fluid volume

6. Electronic fetal monitoring
   a. Assesses fetal heart rate and pattern.
   b. Assesses frequency, duration, and intensity of contractions.
   c. Internal fetal scalp electrode and/or intrauterine pressure catheter can be used if membranes have ruptured and the need is indicated.

D. Nutritional considerations
   1. Pregnancy-induced hypertension, eclampsia, and pre-eclampsia in the critically ill patient have essentially the same nutrition care needs.
   2. Intake requirements should be established to meet the recommended daily allowances (RDAs).
   3. Sodium restrictions are no longer indicated, as the disease mechanisms are not thought to be related to sodium intake. A bland or low-sodium diet that is not accepted by the patient may reduce oral intake, placing the patient at risk for nutrient deficiency.
   4. It is important to meet the patient's RDAs for all nutrients—especially calcium, as it has been isolated in recent studies as having potential clinical benefits.

5. Considerations for medical nutrition therapy
   a. The overall goal is to increase the nutrient intake to achieve caloric balance and meet intake needs.
   b. Calories and nutrients should not be restricted.
   c. When oral intake is established, a regular diet with additional dairy (calcium) intake is the therapy of choice.

E. Psychosocial implications—assessment should include the following:
   1. Woman's response to pregnancy.
   2. Her beliefs of normal healthy behavior in pregnancy and labor.
   3. How childbearing will affect her life.
   4. Presence or lack of family, and/or father of the baby support.
   5. Cultural norms.
   6. Risks associated with early and delayed childbearing.

F. Commonly used medications.
   1. Prenatal vitamin/mineral supplements are recommended.
   2. Iron supplementation: 30–60 mg every day throughout the pregnancy to early postpartum period is often prescribed to reduce the risk of iron deficiency anemia.

III. Ruptured ectopic pregnancy

A. Description: fertilized ovum implants outside the uterine cavity, with the fallopian tube being the most common site. Other sites include the abdomen, cervix, ovary, and wall of the uterus. When the structure surrounding the growing embryo can no longer expand, a ruptured ectopic pregnancy occurs. This is a surgical emergency.

B. Etiology and incidence: Highest incidence in patients with the following:
   1. History of pelvic inflammatory disease (PID)
   2. Tubal surgery
   3. Use of an intrauterine device (IUD)
   4. Infertility
   5. Endometriosis
   6. 1 in 59 pregnancies reported to the Centers for Disease Control and Prevention in 1987 were ectopic.

C. Assessment
   1. Physical assessment should be directed toward evaluation of:
      a. Abdominal or pelvic pain ranging from soreness to cramping.
      b. Pain is generally present before rupture.
      c. **With acute rupture, pain is sharp and diffuse.**
      d. Shoulder pain may result from diaphragmatic irritation by a hemoperitoneum.
      e. Vaginal bleeding: may or may not be present. It is usually light and results from uterine decidual slough.
      f. Unilateral adnexal mass may be present.
      g. Nausea and vomiting, which occurs occasionally before and frequently after rupture.
      h. Dizziness, fainting, pallor.
      i. Rapid pulse after rupture, which occurs secondary to pain and blood loss.

     j.   Blood pressure is increased before rupture and drops after rupture.

     k.   Respirations may be rapid due to pain.

  2.   Diagnostic testing should include:

     a.   Culdocentesis: a needle is placed transvaginally into the cul-de-sac, and the area is aspirated. A positive result is when non-clotting blood is obtained during aspiration.

     b.   Ultrasonography: transabdominal or endovaginal is done to evaluate:

        ► Presence of adnexal mass
        ► Fluid in the cul-de-sac
        ► Absence of intrauterine gestation
        ► May be completely normal in up to 20% of women with ectopic pregnancy

     c.   Laparoscopy allows for direct visualization of pelvic structures; used to diagnose and treat ectopic pregnancy.

  3.   Laboratory findings:

     a.   White cell count >15,000/mL
     b.   Red cell count low if blood loss is large
     c.   Sedimentation rate slightly elevated
     d.   HCG: positive

D. **Nursing diagnoses**

  1.   Altered Tissue Perfusion: Renal, Cardiopulmonary
  2.   Pain
  3.   Grief
  4.   Fear
  5.   Knowledge Deficit: Ruptured Ectopic Pregnancy

E. **Planning and implementation**

  1.   **Surgery: a ruptured ectopic pregnancy requires immediate surgical exploration:**

     a.   Salpingostomy is indicated for a ruptured ectopic gestation without extensive tubal damage.
     b.   Salpingectomy is indicated for a ruptured ectopic gestation with extensive tubal damage, or when future fertility is of no concern.

  2.   Administer analgesics as ordered.
  3.   Ensure administration of parenteral fluids only and NPO before surgery. Clear liquids or diet as tolerated may be administered after surgery.
  4.   If patient is Rh-negative, RhoGAM is given.
  5.   Wound care—observe for:

     a.   Redness
     b.   Pain
     c.   Swelling
     d.   Drainage

  6.   Be aware of potential complications:

     a.   Hemorrhage
     b.   Shock
     c.   Infection

        d.   Decreased fertility

        e.   Increased risk for future ectopic pregnancies

F.   **Evaluation**

    1.   Patient is pain-free.

    2.   Patient demonstrates progress in grieving process.

    3.   Patient performs self-care activities.

    4.   Patient verbalizes understanding of home care instructions.

G.   **Home health considerations**

    1.   The client and family should have a thorough understanding of required wound care and recognition of infection.

    2.   Activity as tolerated.

    3.   Emphasize importance of prevention of pregnancy for 2–4 months, or as indicated by physician.

IV.   Ruptured uterus

A.   **Description: a ruptured uterus often occurs in the thinned-out lower uterine segment, and may also occur along previous uterine scars.**

    1.   Complete: rupture extends through the entire uterine wall, with contents extruded into the abdominal cavity.

    2.   Incomplete: rupture extends through the endometrium and myometrium, with peritoneum surrounding the uterus remaining intact.

B.   **Etiology and incidence**

    1.   **Traumatic uterine rupture: associated with a previous uterine scar and application of excessive force during labor**

    2.   Trauma from instruments:

        a.   Forceps delivery

        b.   High vacuum extraction

    3.   Excessive fundal pressure or tumultuous labor

    4.   Violent bearing-down efforts

    5.   Shoulder dystocia

    6.   Internal version

    7.   Forceps rotation

    8.   Induced uterine hypertonicity from oxytocin infusion

    9.   Manual removal of placenta

   10.   Spontaneous uterine rupture

   11.   Previous uterine surgery

   12.   Cesarean section

   13.   Myomectomy

   14.   Salpingectomy

   15.   Curettage

   16.   Grand multiparity combined with the use of oxytocin

   17.   Cephalopelvic disproportion, malpresentation, or hydrocephalus

   18.   Incidence: 1 in 1500 deliveries

   19.   Responsible for 5% of maternal deaths; 50% of deliveries status post–uterine rupture result in fetal demise

C.   **Assessment**

    1.   Assess for signs and symptoms of impending uterine rupture as evidenced by:

        a.   Restlessness, anxiety, severe lower abdominal pain

        b.   Lack of progress in dilatation or fetal descent

        c.   Palpable ridge of uterus above the symphysis pubis

        d.   Retraction ring, an indentation across the lower abdominal wall, between the upper and lower uterine segments with tenderness above the symphysis

        e.   Tetanic contractions

  2.   Incomplete uterine rupture is characterized by:

        a.   Tenderness or pain in the abdomen associated with increasing uterine irritability before the onset of labor

        b.   Small amounts of vaginal bleeding

        c.   Increasing abdominal pain and tenderness as labor progresses, not associated with uterine contractions

        d.   Rebound tenderness of the abdomen

        e.   Excessive abdominal distention

        f.   Retraction ring across lower abdomen

        g.   Thinning and ballooning of lower uterine segment, similar to a full bladder

        h.   Lack of cervical dilatation

  3.   Complete uterine rupture is characterized by:

        a.   Intense, sharp, stabbing, or tearing pain in the lower abdomen

        b.   Palpation of fetal parts outside the uterine wall

        c.   Abrupt termination of uterine contractions

        d.   Ascent of presenting part when compared to previous vaginal examination

        e.   Gross hematuria from bladder damage

        f.   Rapid signs of fetal distress or cessation of fetal heart tones

        g.   Signs and symptoms of maternal hypovolemic shock

D. **Nursing diagnoses**

  1.   Fluid Volume Deficit

  2.   Altered Tissue Perfusion: Cardiopulmonary

  3.   Pain

  4.   Anxiety

  5.   Knowledge Deficit: Uterine Rupture

  6.   Altered Family Process

E. **Planning and implementation**

  1.   Attempt to deliver the fetus before demise:

        a.   Vaginal delivery is not attempted if signs of possible uterine rupture are present.

        b.   If symptoms of uterine rupture are not severe, emergency cesarean delivery with repair of uterine tear may be attempted.

        c.   If symptoms of uterine rupture are severe, emergency laparotomy is performed to immediately deliver the fetus, establish homeostasis, and repair the uterine tear.

  2.   Stop maternal hemorrhage:

        a.   Repair of uterine tear may be attempted

        b.   Hysterectomy may be required

  3.   Prepare for surgery:

        a.   Continuous monitoring of maternal blood pressure, pulse and respirations

        b.   Continuous monitoring of fetal heart rate, if present

        c.   Insertion of a central venous pressure catheter to assess blood loss and monitor effects of fluid and blood replacement

        d.   Indwelling urinary catheter inserted

        e.   Blood gases to assess maternal acidosis

  4.   Oxygen administration and maintenance of an open airway.

  5.   Type and screen/cross in preparation for blood administration.

  6.   Administer medications and anticipate general anesthesia for emergency surgery.

  7.   Administer postoperative pain medications as ordered.

  8.   Ensure administration of parenteral fluids and blood products as indicated.

  9.   Perform wound care and observe for:

        a.   Redness

        b.   Pain

        c.   Swelling

        d.   Drainage

  10.   Assess for potential complications

        a.   Maternal: hemorrhage, hypovolemic shock, possible need for hysterectomy

        b.   Fetal: shock, anemia, hypoxia, death

F.   **Evaluation**

  1.   The patient experiences no postoperative surgical complications.

  2.   Pre-surgical dietary and elimination patterns are resumed.

  3.   Patient performs self-care activities.

  4.   Pain is controlled with comfort measures and medication as needed.

  5.   Patient verbalizes understanding of need for emergency surgery.

  6.   Patient verbalizes understanding that childbearing is no longer possible, if hysterectomy has been performed.

  7.   The patient demonstrates adaptive response related to self concept.

  8.   The patient demonstrates understanding of home care instructions and follow-up care.

G.   **Home health considerations**

  1.   Wound care and assessment of infection are understood and performed.

  2.   Activity as tolerated.

  3.   Reinforce the need to abstain from intercourse, tampons, and douching for 6 weeks, or as indicated by physician.

  4.   Avoid constipation.

  5.   Avoid lifting and driving for 6 weeks, or as indicated by physician.

  6.   Ensure planned rest periods.

  7.   Ensure proper nutrition and increased fluids.

  8.   Keep postpartum appointment, which is usually 1 to 2 weeks after delivery.

  9.   Home health nurse may remove staples at first visit.

V. **Placenta abruption**

  A.   **Description: the complete or partial separation of a normally implanted placenta from its uterine implantation site before the delivery of the fetus. Variations include:**

    1.   External hemorrhage: bleeding between the membranes and uterus that escapes through the cervix and appears externally.

    2.   Concealed hemorrhage: Bleeding behind the placenta, but its margins remain intact.

3. Placenta completely separated, but the membranes retain their attachment to the uterine wall.
4. Blood enters the amniotic cavity after breaking through the membranes.
5. Fetal head is tightly engaged in the lower uterine segment, and the blood cannot make its way past.

B. Etiology and incidence
1. The primary etiology is unknown. Potential causes include:
   a. Trauma
   b. Short umbilical cord
   c. Sudden decompression of the uterus
   d. Uterine anomaly or tumor
   e. Pregnancy-induced or chronic hypertension
   f. Pressure by the enlarged uterus on the inferior vena cava
2. Other known or suspected risk factors include:
   a. Poor weight gain
   b. Cigarette smoking
   c. Cocaine use
   d. Diabetes
   e. Amnionitis
   f. Fetal anomalies
   g. High parity
3. Incidence: Occurs in 0.5%–4% of pregnancies. Women with a history of abruption have a 10%–20% increased risk with subsequent pregnancies.

C. Assessment
1. Signs and symptoms are extremely variable and depend on the extent and location of the abruption. In 25% of cases diagnosis is made after a normal delivery, when examining the placenta.
2. Vaginal bleeding may be from scant to frank hemorrhage.
3. Uterine contractions may be mild to extremely painful and tumultuous. You may see coupled contractions with no return to resting tone.
4. The uterus is tender to palpation, especially over the area of the placenta.
5. Persistent lower back pain, particularly with a posterior placenta, may occur.
6. Fetal monitoring may reveal loss of variability or late decelerations.
7. Rarely, maternal hypotension or shock may present.
8. Disseminated intravascular coagulation (DIC) is associated with severe hemorrhage.
9. Fetal distress is characterized by:
   a. Tachycardia
   b. Prolonged bradycardia
   c. Loss of baseline variability
   d. Repetitive late decelerations
   e. Severe variable decelerations
10. The diagnosis is made by:
   a. Clinical findings listed above

b.   Ultrasound may clarify diagnosis in 25%–50% of cases

c.   Pathologic examination of the placenta after delivery

D.   Nursing diagnoses

1.   Pain

2.   Knowledge Deficit: Placenta Abruption

3.   Fluid Volume Deficit

4.   Altered Tissue Perfusion: Placenta, Neonate

5.   Fear

6.   Anxiety

E.   Planning and implementation

1.   Prevent shock and maintain adequate blood volume and oxygenation.

2.   Prevent perinatal asphyxia.

3.   Immediate delivery is indicated with the following conditions:

a.   Term pregnancy

b.   Continuous intense bleeding

c.   Maternal DIC

d.   Persistent fetal distress

4.   Vaginal delivery may be attempted if:

a.   Mother not in shock

b.   Fetal heart rate pattern normal

c.   Continuous fetal heart rate monitoring is available

d.   Unit is able to perform immediate cesarean delivery

5.   Cesarean delivery is indicated if there is:

a.   Brisk bleeding

b.   Fetal distress

c.   Maternal shock

6.   Preterm gestation: physician must weigh the risks of preterm delivery versus the risk that the abruption may compromise the fetus.

7.   Delay delivery until fetal maturity is attained.

a.   Use amniocentesis to test for fetal lung maturity

b.   Betamethasone, a corticosteroid, is given to reduce the risk of respiratory distress syndrome in the fetus. The dose is 12 mg IM q12hr–q24hr times 2 doses.

c.   Maternal bed rest in hospital setting.

8.   Fetal monitoring may include:

a.   Nonstress test

b.   Biophysical profile

c.   Serial ultrasounds to assess fetal growth rate

9.   Delivery usually occurs within 2 weeks due to repeated bleeding and contractions, spontaneous rupture of membranes, and persistent fetal distress.

10.   Ensure adequate pain relief.

11.   Ensure optimal wound care and observe for evidence of infection.

12.   Be aware of potential maternal complications:

a.   Hemorrhagic shock

b.   Hypovolemia

c.   Renal failure

d.   Couvelaire uterus: extravasation of blood into the uterine musculature and beneath the serosa of the uterus

        e.   DIC: release of placental thromboplastin into the maternal circulation can initiate DIC. See Chapter 13 for diagnosis and management of DIC.

    13.   Be aware of the fetal complications:

        a.   Hypoxia

        b.   Hypovolemia

        c.   Complications from a premature delivery

F.   **Evaluation**

    1.   Maternal homeostasis is maintained and a viable newborn is delivered.

    2.   There are no postoperative surgical complications if cesarean delivery is performed.

    3.   Patient performs self-care activities.

    4.   Presurgical dietary and elimination patterns resumed if cesarean delivery.

    5.   Pain is controlled with comfort measures and medication as needed.

    6.   Patient verbalizes understanding of need for emergency surgery.

    7.   Patient demonstrates adaptive response related to self-concept.

    8.   Patient demonstrates understanding of home care instructions and follow-up care.

G.   **Home health considerations**

    1.   Wound care and assessment are performed if cesarean delivery was done.

    2.   Activity as tolerated.

    3.   Reinforce no intercourse, tampons, douching for 6 weeks, or as indicated by physician.

    4.   Avoid constipation.

    5.   Avoid lifting and driving for 6 weeks or as indicated by physician.

    6.   Planned rest periods.

    7.   Stress importance of proper nutrition and increased fluids.

    8.   Ensure medications are taken as ordered, especially iron supplements.

    9.   Keep postpartum appointment, usually 1 to 2 weeks after delivery.

    10.   Home health nurse may remove staples at first visit.

VI.   **Eclampsia**

    A.   **Description: the addition of grand mal seizures to either mild or severe preeclamptic syndrome.**

        1.   Preeclampsia: referred to as pregnancy-induced hypertension (PIH), primarily affects very young women or women over 35 in their first pregnancy, usually during the last trimester.

        2.   In multiparas, preeclampsia may be associated with multiple gestation, fetal hydrops, chronic hypertension, diabetes, and coexisting renal disease.

        3.   It is subdivided into mild or severe, and is diagnosed by the classic triad of hypertension, proteinuria, and edema

        4.   Eclampsia: includes the symptoms of preeclampsia along with seizure.

    B.   **Etiology: No definite causes have been identified. Listed below are some common theories.**

        1.   Immunologic factor or deficiency: either excessive compatibility or incompatibility between mother and fetus.

        2.   Prostaglandin: imbalance between vasodilators PGE_2 and prostacyclin, and the vasoconstrictor PGR series and thromboxanes.

3. Uteroplacental ischemia: preeclampsia seen more frequently in the following conditions, in which there is also increased distention of the uterine wall:
    a. Women in their first pregnancy with a large baby
    b. Multiple pregnancy
    c. Polyhydramnios
    d. Hydatidiform mole
4. Incidence: approximately 7% of all pregnancies experience some form of hypertension, and 1%–4% of preeclamptic cases develop eclampsia.

C. **Assessment**
1. Preeclampsia
    a. Mild

        ► BP 140/90–160/110, or systolic increase >30 mm Hg and diastolic increase >15 mm Hg.
        ► Proteinuria 1+ to 2+ (<5 g/24 hr)
        ► Pathologic edema of the hands and face

    b. Severe

        ► BP >160/110
        ► Proteinuria 3+ to 4+ (>5 g/24 hr)
        ► Pathologic edema of the hands and face

    c. Oliguria (less than 400 mL/24 hr)
    d. Altered consciousness, headache, scotomata, or blurred vision due to cerebral edema
    e. Pulmonary edema or cyanosis
    f. Epigastric or right upper quadrant pain secondary to hepatic edema and stretching of Glisson's capsule (this is a classic warning sign of imminent seizure)
    g. Significantly altered liver function
    h. Significant thrombocytopenia
    i. Hyperflexion, clonus
    j. Nausea, vomiting
2. Eclampsia: along with the symptoms listed above for preeclampsia, eclampsia includes the development of seizure or coma in a patient without an underlying neurologic or febrile origin. Seizures may occur before, during, or after labor.

D. **Nursing diagnoses**
1. Altered Protection
2. Fluid Volume Excess
3. Altered Tissue Perfusion: Cerebral, Cardiopulmonary, Fetal, Renal
4. Fluid Volume Deficit
5. Impaired Gas Exchange
6. Knowledge Deficit: Eclampsia
7. Fear
8. Anxiety
9. Altered Family Processes

E. **Planning and implementation**
1. **The only "cure" for preeclampsia/eclampsia is delivery, with lab values usually returning to normal within 48 hours.**

2. Indications for delivery include:
   a. Worsening hypertension
   b. Increased proteinuria
   c. Compromised fetus
   d. Nonreactive non-stress test
   e. Positive contraction-stress test
   f. Poor results of biophysical profile
   g. L/S ratio may be used to determine fetal lung maturity if time allows
   h. Induction of labor with IV oxytocin when no fetal distress
   i. Cesarean section in cases of severe preeclampsia/eclampsia, especially with a cervix that cannot be induced
3. Administer antihypertensives as ordered:
   a. Reduces maternal morbidity and mortality associated with cerebral vascular accidents.

    b. Reduces perinatal morbidity and mortality associated with intrauterine growth retardation, placental infarcts, and placental abruption.
   c. Maternal BP >160/110 treated with intravenous hydralazine.
   d. Nitroprusside is used for very critical situations.
   e. For long-term control, an oral antihypertensive can be used, eg, Aldomet.

 4. Administer anticonvulsant therapy as ordered: seizure prophylaxis is instituted in all preeclamptics during labor and delivery and continued for 12–24 hours following delivery.
5. Be aware that magnesium sulfate is the agent of choice for seizures. It is a neuromuscular sedative that decreases the amount of acetylcholine produced by motor nerves and blocks neuromuscular transmission.
   a. Prophylactic loading: 5 g each buttock, IM or 4 g over 10–20 minutes IV
   b. Maintenance: 5 g/4 hr IM or 1–2 g/hr IV
   c. Therapeutic (for treatment of seizures): 1 g/min IV until seizure controlled; 4–6 g maximum (Display 12-1)

 6. Calcium gluconate 1 g IV is the antidote and should be kept at the bedside. Signs of magnesium toxicity include:
   a. Diminished reflexes, especially patellar

DISPLAY 12-1.
Serum Magnesium Levels (mg/dL)

1.2–1.8	Normal
3–8	Therapeutic
8–10	CNS depression
12–17	Respiratory depression
13–17	Coma
19–20	Cardiac arrest

b.   Hypotension
c.   Muscle flaccidity
d.   Respiratory paralysis
e.   Decreased renal function
f.   Circulatory collapse

7. **Administer furosemide 40 mg IV (slow push) to treat pulmonary edema resulting from eclamptic seizures, as ordered by physician. It may conceal the degree of hypovolemia and oliguria. It is usually given after delivery.**

8.   Valium 10 mg IV push for treatment of seizures.

9.   During the intrapartum phase ensure:
   a.   Careful assessment of maternal and fetal well-being
   b.   Physical assessment of the mother should include:

   ▶ Blood pressure readings in supine and left lateral position
   ▶ Weight and level of edema noted
   ▶ Deep tendon reflexes evaluated
   ▶ Urinary output and proteinuria checked
   ▶ Respiratory assessment
   ▶ Check for signs of coagulopathy such as petechiae, ecchymosis, oozing of venipunctures and hematuria
   ▶ Ensure quiet non-stimulating environment

   c.   Fetal assessment should involve continuous fetal monitoring

10.   During the seizure, implement the following:
   a.   Maintain patent airway.
   b.   Protect patient from injury.
   c.   Turn patient on her side to reduce risk of aspiration.
   d.   Nasopharyngeal airway or nasal trumpet kept at bedside. Once it is inserted, tubing can be used for suctioning or oxygen administration.
   e.   Administer oxygen at 8–12 L/minute by mask to maximize fetal oxygenation.
   f.   Administer medications as ordered.
   g.   Ensure delivery as soon as stable.

11.   Be aware that 25% of eclamptic seizures occur after delivery. All of the above measures are instituted except for interventions related to the fetus.

12.   Additional antihypertensives may be substituted for hydralazine as fetal safety is no longer an issue.

13.   Seizure prohylaxis or treatment is usually continued for 12–24 hours postpartum.

14.   Be aware of potential complications:
   a.   Fetal—placental insufficiency and ischemia related to vasoconstriction and abruption. The fetus may also be stressed by medications given to the mother. A preterm or growth-retarded fetus is at serious risk.
   b.   Maternal—DIC, cerebral edema, cerebral petechial hemorrhages, major cerebral hemorrhage, liver dysfunction, hemorrhage, acute renal failure, and adult respiratory distress syndrome.

F. Evaluation
   1. Homeostasis is maintained.
   2. Adequate cardiac output and tissue perfusion are maintained.
   3. Fetal distress is prevented.
   4. A viable newborn is delivered.
   5. Permanent renal, liver, pulmonary, and CNS dysfunction are prevented.
   6. Emotional support for patient and her family are provided.

G. Home health considerations
   1. Blood pressure monitoring and assessment of vaginal bleeding should be continued in the home setting.
   2. Evaluation of CNS, renal, and respiratory functions should also be continued.
   3. Assess family coping mechanisms.

VII. HELLP syndrome

 A. Description: HELLP syndrome is a variant of severe preeclampsia. Maternal and perinatal outcome may be poor when this syndrome is present, and it may occur in the absence of significant hypertension, proteinuria, or edema. It is characterized by:

   1. **Hemolysis**
   2. **Elevated liver enzymes**
   3. **Low platelets**

 B. Laboratory evaluation should include evaluation of:
   1. Hemolysis on blood smear
   2. Elevated bilirubin
   3. Elevated LDH
   4. Abnormal liver enzymes
   5. Low platelet count

 C. Treatment: Treat as with DIC. Ensure safe delivery, offer supportive measures, and administer blood products as needed.

Bibliography

Burrows R., Hunter D., & Andrew M. (1987). A prospective study investigating the mechanism of thrombocytopenia in preeclampsia. *Obstet Gynecol* 70, 334–338.

Cunningham F., MacDonald P., & Gant N. (1989). *Williams' obstetrics.* Norwalk, CT: Appleton & Lange.

Daddario, J. B. (1989). Trauma in pregnancy. *J Perinat Neonat Nurs* 3(2), 14–22.

Katz V. I., Dotters D. J., & Droegemueller, W. (1986). Perimortem cesarean delivery. *Obstet Gynecol* 68, 571–576.

Mahlmeister, L. R. & May, K. A. (1990). *Comprehensive maternity nursing.* Philadelphia: J.B. Lippincott.

NAACOG, The Organization for Obstetric, Gynecologic, and Neonatal Nurses (1991). *Standards for the nursing care of women and newborns* (4th ed.). Washington: NAACOG.

North American Nursing Diagnosis Association (NANDA). (1996). *Nursing diagnoses: Definitions & classification 1997–1998.* Philadelphia: Author.

Shannon D. M. (1987). HELLP syndrome: A severe consequence of pregnancy-induced hypertension. *J Obstet Gynecol Neonat Nurs* 16, 395–402.

STUDY QUESTIONS

1. A laboring patient is being given magnesium sulfate for treatment of her severe PIH because it:
   a. induces efficient uterine contractions
   b. decreases blood pressure by direct action on the kidneys
   c. reduces the activity at the neuromuscular junction and helps prevent convulsions
   d. prevents preterm labor, a serious complication of PIH

2. When is a patient diagnosed as eclamptic?
   a. when her BP is 180/110
   b. when she experiences pulmonary edema
   c. when she has generalized edema, especially of the hands and face
   d. when she experiences convulsions

3. All of the following are signs of a ruptured ectopic pregnancy except:
   a. sharp and diffuse pain
   b. profuse vaginal bleeding
   c. unilateral adnexal mass
   d. nausea and vomiting

4. A laboring patient is experiencing anxiety, and pain in the lower abdomen, although her contractions are no longer showing on the monitor, and the fetal head is now higher in the pelvis than the previous exam. The most likely cause of this is:
   a. incomplete uterine rupture
   b. complete uterine rupture
   c. partial placental abruption
   d. complete placental abruption

5. The primary etiology of placental abruption is:
   a. sudden decompression of the uterus
   b. trauma
   c. pregnancy-induced hypertension
   d. unknown

6. A patient was admitted to the hospital for bed rest with the diagnosis of suspected partial placental abruption at 32 weeks' gestation. The decision to deliver her will be made if any of the following conditions occur, except:
   a. spontaneous rupture of membranes, bloody fluid
   b. amniocentesis showing immature fetal lungs
   c. repeated bleeding and contractions
   d. persistent fetal distress

7. A patient with severe preeclampsia has a serum magnesium level of 13.6 and is experiencing difficulty breathing. She would be given:
   a. Valium 10 mg IV push
   b. magnesium sulfate 5 g IM each buttock, or 4 g over 10–20 minutes
   c. calcium gluconate 1 g IV
   d. IV hydralazine

8. Fetal distress would probably be present in all of the following situations except:
   a. abruption
   b. ectopic pregnancy
   c. eclampsia
   d. ruptured uterus

9. Preeclampsia in the multiparous pregnant patient is associated with all of the following conditions except:
   a. multiple gestation
   b. diabetes
   c. hyperthyroidism
   d. glomerulonephritis

10. A potential complication of eclampsia, DIC is characterized by:
    a. hyperfibrinogenemia
    b. bradycardia
    c. hypertension
    d. thrombocytopenia

ANSWER KEY

1. Correct response: c
Magnesium sulfate reduces seizure activity by acting at the neuromuscular junction.
a. MgSO$_4$ does not enhance uterine contractions.
b. A decrease in blood pressure is an added benefit.
d. Does not prevent preterm labor.
Comprehension/Physiologic/Implementation

2. Correct response: d
Eclampsia occurs when the patient has convulsions in addition to the symptoms of preeclampsia.
a. This would indicate severe preeclampsia.
b. This would indicate severe preeclampsia.
c. This would indicate mild preeclampsia.
Knowledge/Physiologic/Assessment

3. Correct response: b
Vaginal bleeding may or may not be present. If it is present it will be scant and due to uterine sloughing.
a, c, d. All are symptoms of a ruptured ectopic pregnancy.
Knowledge/Physiologic/Assessment

4. Correct Response: b
These are signs of a complete uterine rupture.
a, c, d. Uterine contractions are present with an incomplete uterine rupture, partial and complete placenta abruption.
Analysis/Physiologic/Evaluation

5. Correct response: d
The primary etiology of placenta abruption is unknown.
a, b, c. All may cause placenta abruption.
Knowledge/Physiologic/NA

6. Correct response: b
Normal finding at 32 weeks' gestation. Supplemental O$_2$ not necessary.

a. Indicates hemorrhage, resulting in increased O$_2$ consumption.
c, d. Increased stress to fetus, lowering chances of survival.
Application/Physiologic/Evaluation

7. Correct response: c
Calcium gluconate is the antidote to magnesium sulfate.
a. Valium would further depress her respiratory center.
b. This patient is already experiencing magnesium toxicity.
d. Hydralazine would have no effect on the magnesium level.
Analysis/Physiologic/Implementation

8. Correct response: b
Ectopic pregnancy occurs within the first three weeks of pregnancy, before the fetus develops.
a, c, d. These disorders occur in the last trimester of pregnancy and impair circulation to the fetus.
Application/Physiologic/Planning

9. Correct response: c
Preeclampsia has not been associated with hyperthyroidism.
a, b, d. Definitive causes of preeclampsia are unknown, but there is an increased risk in multipara women with renal pathology, multiple gestation, and diabetes.
Knowledge/Physiologic/NA

10. Correct response: d
Thrombocytopenia is evident in DIC.
a. Fibrinogen levels are low in DIC.
b. The patient with DIC would be tachycardic.
c. The patient with DIC would be hypotensive.
Knowledge/Physiologic/NA

Multisystem Pathology

I. **Abdominal anatomy review**
   A. Peritoneum: the internal lining of the abdominal cavity
   B. Peritoneal cavity
      1. The peritoneal cavity has a potential space that contains peritoneal
         fluid.
      2. Purposes of the peritoneal fluid
         a. Lubrication for organ movement
         b. Barrier to infection
      3. Layers
         a. Parietal: lines anterolateral and posterior abdominal walls
         b. Visceral: covers surface of the abdominal viscera

C. **Surfaces and organs contained in/bordered by peritoneum (Fig. 13-1)**
    1.   Intraperitoneal surface is completely covered by the peritoneum.
        a.   The organs within the peritoneum include the spleen, liver, gall bladder, stomach, pancreas, and large and small intestines.
        b.   The mesenteric surface is a double-layered fold of peritoneum that contains the vascular supply to each organ.
    2.   The retroperitoneal surface lies behind the parietal peritoneum.
        a.   The organs in this area include the kidneys and pancreas.
        b.   Only one surface is joined to the peritoneum.
    3.   Extraperitoneal area comprises organs outside the peritoneum, including the bladder, rectum, and uterus.

II. **Review of skin**
  A. **Structure**
    1.   Epidermis: outermost layer
        a.   Consists of primarily epithelial cells
        b.   Contains keratin to limit fluid loss and melanin for skin color
    2.   Dermis: middle layer. It contains blood vessels, sensory receptors, portions of hair follicles, sebaceous glands, and sweat gland ducts
    3.   Hypodermis: contains subcutaneous fat. It also contains sweat gland roots and hair follicle roots. It lies over fascia, muscles and organs.
  B. **Function**
    1.   Serves as a first-line barrier against infection.
    2.   Serves to conserve body fluids to prevent dehydration and maintain fluid balance.
    3.   Controls temperature regulation by allowing for evaporation of water from the sweat glands.

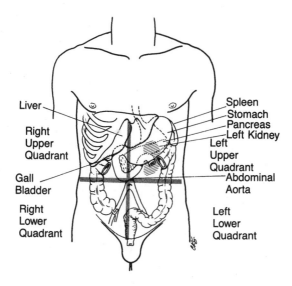

FIGURE 13-1.
Location of organs in abdominal quadrants.

4. Excretes wastes in the form of urea.
5. Secretes substances from the sebaceous glands to soften and lubricate the skin.
6. Produces vitamin D by interaction between sunlight and cholesterol compounds.

C.   Nutritional considerations

1. There is an emerging consensus that early nutritional support benefits moderately and severely injured patients. It is now believed that unless nutrition support is provided within the first 24 to 48 hours, hypermetabolism induced by the injury stress response can seriously deplete endogenous substrate stores.

2. Nutritional requirements vary according to the degree of injury and resulting hypermetabolism. There is some debate as to the optimal route of substrate delivery (ie, enteral vs. parenteral).

3. Recent basic clinical research seems to advocate using the gut if at all possible. Enteral nutrition prevents gastrointestinal mucosal atrophy, attenuates the injury stress response, maintains immunocompetence, and preserves normal gut flora.

4. Because of the increased rates of amino acid catabolism and protein synthesis during the acute stage, protein needs are elevated.

5. The elevation in protein synthetic rate accounts for some of the increase in energy expenditure experienced by patients recovering from surgery or trauma.

6. As the patient recovers, protein and energy requirements tend to level off.

7. Considerations for medical nutrition therapy
   a. The overall goal is to increase the nutrient intake to achieve caloric balance and meet intake needs.
   b. Maintain accurate documentation of intake and output and daily weights. Note that fluid retention may cause a false low value in serum protein concentrations, because of dilution and extravasation from intravascular to interstitial spaces.
   c. Monitor electrolytes and replace as required.
   d. Do not rule out enteral feedings in the obtunded patient who is at risk for aspiration. The presence of nausea, secretions, and changes in intracranial pressure do not preclude enteral feedings, if appropriate precautions are taken. Nutrient-dense formulas with 1.5–2.0 kcal per mL are helpful when low-volume feeding is necessary.
   e. Following GI surgery, dumping syndrome, which is characterized by rapid gastric emptying, is experienced in some patients. It can be addressed with small frequent meals, no concentrated sweets, and caffeine omitted from the diet.

III.   Motor vehicle accident (MVA)

A.   Mechanism of injury: blunt

1. Acceleration/deceleration occurs when there is an increased velocity of a moving body followed by a decreased velocity.

2. MVA factors
   a. Vehicle hits object
   b. Occupant impacts inside of vehicle

    c.   Internal organs and tissues impact against rigid body structures

   3.   Crushing/compression occurs when there is squeezing together of organs

   4.   Shearing occurs when two oppositely directed parallel forces come into play

B.   **Mechanism of injury: penetrating**

   1.   Stab wounds: low-velocity damage caused by sharp cutting edge, with little secondary trauma

   2.   Injury pathway is determined by:

     a.   Victim's position

     b.   Attacker's position

     c.   Attacker's gender (men usually stab upward, women downward)

     d.   Weapon used

   3.   Impalements

     a.   Low-velocity injuries

     b.   Impaled objects should not be removed until emergency equipment ready

IV. Gunshot wounds

A.   **Basic principles**

   1.   Impact velocity depends on distance between firearm and victim.

   2.   At medium and high velocities, the missile has an explosive effect and creates a temporary passage in the tissue along its course.

   3.   Sudden formation of this track displaces adjacent organs and vascular structures.

   4.   High-velocity missiles drag external contaminants into the wound, thereby causing contamination.

B.   **Three wounding mechanisms**

   1.   Laceration is the result of penetration and severance of tissue by a sharp, moving object.

   2.   Tissue disruption is due to the missile's kinetic energy. The greater the energy lost by the bullet in the tissue, the greater the amount of tissue damage.

   3.   Muzzle blast

     a.   Cloud of hot gas and burning powder are present at the muzzle immediately after firing and extend outward 1–3 feet.

     b.   It is a factor in tissue injury only when the gun is in physical contact.

C.   **Extent of damage is based on:**

   1.   Density and compressibility of the tissue damaged. The denser the tissue the more damage occurs.

   2.   The velocity of the missile. A greater velocity causes more damage.

   3.   Amount of ammunition in contact with tissue. This refers to whether it is a straight-through hit or internal shattering takes place.

D.   **Types of guns**

   1.   Low-velocity

     a.   handguns and some rifles

     b.   cavity 2–3× missile diameter

        2. High-velocity
            a.   military assault rifles
            b.   cavity 3–4× missile diameter
        3. Shotguns
            a.   low-velocity pellets
            b.   injury is related to distance from which it was fired

V. Head injury (see Chapter 2)
VI. Chest injury (see Chapter 4)
VII. Abdominal injury (see Table 13-1)
    A.   Structure: Divided into 4 or 9 quadrants to identify internal organs (Display 13-1)
    B.   Pathophysiology
        1. Injury to the abdominal organs and structures, plus hemorrhage and organ necrosis, result in the release of digestive enzymes into the peritoneal cavity.
        2. There is also the risk of a possible spill of virulent bacterial contents of the bowel into the peritoneum.
        3. Release of organ excretions can result in fluid collection, which provides an optimal culture media for abscess development.
        4. This often causes impaired digestive function with a resulting catabolic state. The end result is severe nutritional deficiencies.
    C.   Blunt injuries
        1. The spleen and lower colon are injured most often.
        2. Can occur by direct and indirect mechanisms of injury.

        3. Results in sudden increased intra-abdominal pressure from trauma, which can rupture hollow organs.
        4. Crushing effect is exerted on the space between the abdominal wall and vertebrae.

        5. Deceleration can create a shearing force, which may damage both hollow and solid viscera.
    D.   Penetrating injuries
        1. Suspect an abdominal injury when penetration occurs as high as the fourth intercostal space (ICS) anteriorly and the seventh laterally.
        2. Abdominal contents may be damaged through penetration of the anterior and lower chest, flank, and lower back.
        3. Search for exit wound(s) and check every possible wound. Locate entrance and exit wounds. If there is no exit wound, then diagnostics/surgery are required to find the bullet.
        4. With stab wound injuries, determine the size, shape, length, and type of object used.
        5. Pain and blood loss are the major nursing concerns:
            a.   Volume loss results in hemodynamic changes, such as decreased BP and increased heart rate.
            b.   Solid visceral injury and infections, or enzymatic irritation may cause pain.
            c.   May be present at onset or delayed hours to days.
            d.   Determine whether pain is localized or referred.
            e.   Pain from the hemoperitoneum may be referred to shoulder tips.
            f.   Testicular pain is compatible with retroperitoneal injury.

TABLE 13-1.
Damage Caused by Trauma to Abdominal Organs

ORGAN/TYPE	ETIOLOGY	ASSOCIATED FINDINGS	DIAGNOSTIC FINDINGS	COMPLICATIONS	COLLABORATIVE/NURSING MANAGEMENT
Liver (solid)	Blunt/penetrating usually vehicular cause mortality usually due to hemorrhage	Left lower rib fractures	Guarding; + DPL; RUQ pain; abnormal liver, coagulation studies	DIC, clotting abnormalities; sepsis; hepatic failure	Hemostatic agents; drainage; suturing/ligation; resection
Pancreas (solid)	Blunt/penetrating delayed diagnosis most frequent cause of mortality	Abdominal, liver, spleen, vascular injuries	Signs and symptoms may occur hours post-injury; epigastric pain, tenderness, guarding; + DPL (with retroperitoneal bleed); + Grey-Turner's sign	Fistula; pseudocyst; abscess; diabetes mellitus, pancreatitis	Drainage for 8–14 days; possible resection; note impaired fat/fat-soluble and glucose metabolism; hypocalcemia; meperidine used—causes less sphincter spasm than MSO₄
Spleen (solid)	Blunt/penetrating seen with left lower chest wounds, usually vehicular cause due to deceleration effects	Left lower rib fractures, vascular and thoracic injuries	Kehr's sign, + DPL	Sepsis: pneumococcemia; subdiaphragmatic abscess	Blood replacement; partial/total splenectomy; bedrest
Stomach (hollow)	Penetrating most common	Thoracic, renal, other abdominal injuries	Heme + gastric drainage; pain LUQ		Closure of wound
Small intestine (hollow)	Penetrating most common; blunt increasing with seatbelt use, handlebars, shearing forces	Thoracic, renal, other abdominal injuries	Fever, jaundice, RLQ or epigastric pain	Ileus; peritonitis; ischemic bowel syndrome	Closure of wound; possible resection, vagotomy, antrectomy, gastrojejunostomy; ileostomy
Large intestine (hollow)	Penetrating most common; blunt increasing with seat belt use	Thoracic, renal, other abdominal injuries	+DPL; minimal symptoms until peritonitis develops; pain/tenderness on rectal exam	Ileus; peritonitis; ischemic bowel syndrome	Colostomy; debridement; peritoneal irrigations to remove fecal material
Kidney (solid)	Blunt/penetrating; may cause dissection of renal blood vessels from renal motion after injury-associated findings	Lower rib fractures, other abdominal injuries	Hematuria; flank pain; bruise at ribs 11–12	Renal failure, undetected retroperitoneal bleed	Bedrest; nephrectomy if other kidney functioning

489

DISPLAY 13-1.
Abdominal Quadrants and Relevant Organs

> RUQ: Liver, gallbladder, duodenum, pancreas, right kidney, right adrenal gland, hepatic flexure of colon
>
> LUQ: Stomach, spleen, left kidney, left adrenal gland, pancreas, splenic flexure of colon
>
> RLQ: Cecum, appendix, right ovary and tube, bladder (if distended), uterus (if enlarged), right spermatic cord, right ureter
>
> LLQ: Sigmoid colon, left ovary and tube, bladder (if distended), uterus (if enlarged), left permatic cord, left ureter

E. Assessment (Display 13-2)

  1. Physical assessment parameters consistent with intra-abdominal injury include:

  a. Rigid abdomen: boardlike hardness from intramuscular bleeding or peritoneal inflammation/hollow organ contents

  b. Guarding: automatic movement by the client to protect abdomen

  c. Back pain may be indicative of retroperitoneal bleeding

  d. Presence of generalized/specific pain or tenderness

  e. Abdominal distention from free air or blood collection, with loss of bowel sounds

  f. Rebound tenderness: pain on release of pressure during palpation

  g. Splinting and thoracic breathing

  h. Hematuria

  i. Vital sign changes, dyspnea, and nausea/vomiting. Thirst is the first signal of hypovolemia and may indicate hemorrhage.

    j. All of these are signs and symptoms of irritation by spilling of bowel contents, digestive enzymes, urine, bile, and/or blood into abdominal cavity

DISPLAY 13-2.
Assessment of Trauma

> Time and mode of injury
>
> Amount of vehicle damage
>
> Did client impact steering wheel?
>
> Whether and what type of restraints used
>
> Position of client in vehicle
>
> Type of instrument
>
> Range from which gun fired
>
> Type of instrument used in stabbing
>
> Blood loss

2. Symptoms of peritonitis include:
   a. Diffuse abdominal pain
   b. Guarding and rigidity
   c. Elevated temperature
   d. Elevated WBC count

   m e. **Onset of peritonitis may be insidious, because small lacerations may be painless if leakage is minimal**

3. Laboratory tests that should be evaluated are:
   a. Serum amylase: increased when there are leaks into the peritoneal cavity. If elevation occurs immediately after trauma, this may indicate secondary injury.
   b. Hemoglobin and hematocrit: these provide information on acute blood loss.
   c. Leukocytes
   d. Type and screen/crossmatch
   e. BUN/creatinine, urinalysis
   f. Electrolytes, blood glucose

4. Radiologic tests
   a. Flat, erect, and lateral abdomen x-rays
   b. Intravenous pyelogram (IVP)
   c. CT scan/MRI
   d. Paracentesis: invasive method for assessing intra-abdominal bleeding

   ▸ Contraindicated in pregnancy, abdominal wall hematoma, prior abdominal surgical scar.
   ▸ The procedure involves inserting a trocar into the abdomen and aspirating fluid.

   ▸ **20 mL bright red blood is considered a positive result. The test is stopped and the client is taken immediately to operating room if a positive tap occurs.**

   ▸ Negative results DO NOT prove absence of intra-abdominal injury.
   ▸ Four quadrant "tap" may be necessary. This involves tapping into different abdominal areas.

5. Peritoneal lavage (a more accurate test):

   m a. **Ensure that bladder is empty**
   b. Nasogastric tube (NGT) PRN to decompress the stomach
   c. Abdominal prep
   d. Used to assess penetrating as well as blunt trauma
   e. Unreliable for retroperitoneal injuries
   f. The procedure involves the use of one site, 1–3 cm below umbilicus at midline. If there is no free blood, one liter lactated Ringers/NSS is instilled and released by gravity drainage.
   g. Clear outflow is considered a negative test
   h. Pink/straw outflow is a weakly positive test
   i. Bloody outflow is a strongly positive test

m   j.   Associated problems include intra-abdominal blood vessel rupture, accidental GI tract puncture, accidental puncture of rectus abdominus muscle, and a false-negative result.

F.   **Nursing diagnoses for the trauma patient**
1.   Fluid Volume Deficit
2.   Impaired Gas Exchange
3.   Impaired Tissue Integrity
4.   Risk for Infection
5.   Anxiety/Fear/Powerlessness
6.   Ineffective Airway Clearance
7.   Pain
8.   Ineffective Individual/Family Coping

G.   **Planning and implementation**

m   1.   **Assess respiratory status including rate, rhythm, depth, breath sounds, work of breathing, use of accessory muscles, ABGs, and pulse oximetry.**
2.   **Assess for hypoxemia, which is manifested by tachycardia, tachypnea, restlessness, diaphoresis, headache, lethargy, confusion, and pallor.**
3.   Replace volume as ordered with crystalloids and/or colloids.
4.   Monitor vital signs and hemodynamic parameters.
5.   Maintain body alignment with repositioning q2hr.
6.   Maintain humidification and oxygen therapies.
7.   Anticipate and prepare for possible intubation.
8.   Maintain patent IV line.
9.   Change dressings per order and assess drainage for color, odor, consistency, and amount.
10.   Monitor laboratory tests.
11.   Maintain and assist with chest tube insertion.
12.   Monitor gastric suction for blood.
13.   Monitor for dysrhythmias.

m   14.   **Assess anxiety level and intervene appropriately.**
15.   Encourage attendance at support groups if chemical abuse/dependency involved.

H.   **Evaluation**
1.   The patient will maintain optimal fluid balance.
2.   The patient will maintain adequate oxygenation and normal acid–base balance.
3.   Existing wounds will heal and no additional breakdown will occur.
4.   No signs or symptoms of infection will be present.
5.   Effective airway clearance will be attained.
6.   The patient will effectively communicate needs and concerns.
7.   The patient and family will progress through grieving stages toward acceptance of altered body image.
8.   The patient and family will demonstrate tracheostomy care, using clean technique.

9. The patient will verbalize basic understanding of pathophysiology of disease, necessary life-style adjustments, and medications.

10. The patient will experience reduced anxiety/fear as evidenced by calm and trusting appearance, and verbalization of fears and concerns.

VIII. **Chest trauma**

    A. Description

        1. Chest trauma is any traumatic injury to the chest.

        2. It is considered life threatening because it results in the loss of a patent airway, change in intrathoracic pressure, destruction of bones, muscle, and nerves of the thorax, blood loss, and alteration in cardiac function.

        3. It can lead to cardiopulmonary failure, hypovolemic shock, and death.

    B. **Etiology: chest trauma can be caused by a motor vehicle accident (MVA), gunshot wound, stab wound, etc.**

    C. Assessment

        1. Loss of negative pressure in the chest leads to collapse of the lung and buildup of air in the intrathoracic cavity

        2. A mediastinal shift, which is movement of the heart, great vessels, trachea, and esophagus toward the unaffected side, may occur.

            a. Due to increasing pressures from air and blood in the intrathoracic cavity.

            b. Shift to the unaffected side results in compression of inferior and superior vena cavae, leading to reduced venous return to the heart.

            c. Ultimately leads to a decrease in cardiac function and output.

            d. Shift also compresses the unaffected lung and distorts the shape of the trachea and bronchus, leading to decreased air movement into the unaffected lung.

        3. Blood loss directly into the chest cavity further impairs pulmonary and cardiac function. It also leads to hypovolemia and shock.

    D. **Classification of thoracic injuries**

        1. Blunt

            a. A closed chest injury results from direct impact. It may deform the chest and may press the sternum against the spinal column.

            b. This results from falls, being hit by something, or contact sports.

            c. Mechanisms include:

                ▶ Acceleration/deceleration

                ▶ Shearing

                ▶ Compression/decompression.

            d. Compression increases the intravascular pressure of all structures in the thorax, and may result in vascular damage and bleeding.

e. Acceleration/deceleration injuries cause the greatest damage to the vascular system (eg, when the car stops rapidly, and the victim's torso continues forward until stopped by an immovable object).

   2. Penetrating

      a. Define the area of injury by determining the entrance and exit sites

      b. Causes include bullets and other ballistics, knives, etc.

 c. **Wound is not always in a straight line. It may not exit, it may not be sterile, and it may injure underlying abdominal organs. When a knife is the weapon, do not remove the blade from the wound. It may be providing a mechanical tamponade.**

E. Rib fractures

   1. Incidence: most common in athletes and in the elderly

   2. Assessment

      a. History of chest trauma

      b. Increased pain on inspiration leading to shallow breathing

      c. Local pain and crepitus over the fracture site

      d. Diagnosis is confirmed with chest x-ray (CXR)

   3. Complications

 a. **A high injury (ribs 1–3) is associated with a high mortality, due to laceration of the subclavian artery or vein. 25% of patients will have a punctured lung or pneumothorax; 20% will have a hemothorax; and 30% will have both.**

      b. A low injury (ribs 9–12) may result in injuries to the kidneys, spleen, and liver.

   4. Interventions

      a. Ensure rest, heat, and analgesia.

      b. Have patient cough and deep breathe, and change position frequently.

      c. For severe pain or compromised ventilation, may employ a nerve block.

      d. Chest strapping is not done any more because it decreases ventilation, which may lead to atelectasis and pneumonia.

      e. Healing occurs within 3–6 weeks.

F. Flail chest

   1. Definition: two or more adjacent rib fractures or detached sternum that floats freely in the thorax

   2. Pathophysiology

 a. **The flail segment moves paradoxically. On inspiration the flail segment sinks inward, because atmospheric pressure is greater than intrathoracic pressure. Air movement into the lungs is therefore decreased on that side. This can contribute to hypoxemia and hypercapnia, leading to acidosis.**

        b.   On expiration, the segment will bulge outward, due to intrathoracic pressure now being greater than atmospheric pressure.

  3.   Associated injuries

        a.   **The cough mechanism is inhibited, allowing the buildup of secretions.**

        b.   **There may be a mediastinal shift leading to reduced cardiac output, hypotension, and shock.**

        c.   **There may also be evidence of a myocardial or pulmonary contusion, alveolar atelectasis, and hemothorax.**

  4.   Diagnosis

        a.   Observation of flailing chest

        b.   Shortness of breath

        c.   Chest x-ray

  5.   Interventions

        a.   Clear airway.

        b.   Relieve pain.

        c.   Stabilize flail with sandbags.

        d.   **May need to intubate and stabilize with PEEP.**

        e.   May need to treat contusions with steroids and diuretics.

        f.   Replace lost blood volume with albumin or blood products.

G.   **Pneumothorax**

  1.   Description: air in the thorax.

        a.   Tension pneumothorax: air trapped in the thorax due to ruptured alveoli or penetrating wound that sealed shut. Buildup of pressure may result in shifting of mediastinum and severe respiratory distress.

        b.   Open pneumothorax: opening in the chest wall that allows air to pass freely in and out of the thoracic cavity.

        c.   Sucking wound: open pneumothorax is sometimes referred to as a sucking wound, due to the noise of air moving back and forth.

        d.   **Mediastinal flutter: the back and forth movement of the mediastinum with each inspiration and expiration. It interferes seriously with cardiac function.**

  2.   Etiology

        a.   Can occur secondary to ruptured alveoli from emphysema or high ventilation pressures

        b.   Penetrating wound

  3.   Pathophysiology

        a.   Buildup of air in the thorax collapses the lung

        b.   This causes a mediastinal shift leading to respiratory distress, hypoxemia, and hypoxia

  4.   Assessment

        a.   History of sudden onset of chest pain

        b.   Absence of breath sounds on the affected side

        c.   Asymmetric chest movement of the affected side

        d.   Shortness of breath, air hunger, tachycardia, tachypnea, syncope, and diaphoresis

e.   Displacement of the trachea toward the unaffected side

f.   Enlarged neck veins due to compression of superior vena çava

g.   Patient complains of "crunching with each heartbeat" due to mediastinal air accumulation

h.   Crepitus (subcutaneous emphysema)

i.   Change in level of consciousness (LOC)

5.   Diagnosis

a.   Physical examination

b.   CXR

6.   Interventions

a.   Chest tube placement

b.   High-flow O_2

c.   If the wound is an open wound, cover completely with a cloth, heel of the hand, or petrolatum gauze (at end expiration) until a chest tube can be inserted.

d.   Tell the patient to inhale and strain against a closed glottis to reexpand the lung and eject air from the thorax.

H.   Hemothorax

1.   Definition: blood in the pleural space

2.   Pathophysiology

a.   The blood presses on the lungs and heart and interferes with normal function.

b.   It takes up space usually needed for lung expansion and cardiac filling.

c.   Signs and symptoms are the same as for pneumothorax, with the addition of signs and symptoms of hypovolemia and shock. These include hypotension, tremors, and cold and clammy skin.

3.   Interventions

a.   Shock is treated with IVs and colloids.

b.   Manage hemothorax with a chest tube insertion and oxygen administration.

I.   Pulmonary contusion

1.   Description: blunt trauma to lung parenchyma, resulting in local hemorrhage and edema.

2.   Pathophysiology

a.   Abnormal accumulation of fluid and protein in the interstitial and intra-alveolar spaces.

b.   Interferes with gas exchange, leading to hypoxemia and hypercapnia.

c.   Bruising on the side opposite to the point of impact is called a contrecoup contusion.

3.   Assessment

a.   Tachycardia and chest pain

b.   Tachypnea, hypoxia, and blood-tinged secretions

c.   Respiratory acidosis

    4. Interventions
        a. Maintain airway and breathing
        b. Administer oxygen and analgesics as indicated.
        c. May need fluid restriction, antibiotics, intubation, and steroids

J. **Cardiac contusion**
    1. Description: bruising of the heart muscle due to blunt trauma or CPR
    2. Assessment
        a. Shortness of breath
        b. Hypotension, tachycardia

        c. **Cardiogenic shock in severe contusion**
        d. **Dysrhythmias and ST and T-wave changes on ECG**
        e. Increased cardiac enzymes
    3. Interventions: same as for an acute myoardial infarction

K. **Cardiac tamponade**
    1. Description: blood in the pericardial sac.
    2. Etiology
        a. Penetrating wound or blunt trauma to the chest wall
        b. Cancer
        c. Renal failure
    3. Pathophysiology

        a. **Exerts pressure on the heart and takes up space the heart needs for diastolic filling.**
        b. **Leads to decreased stroke volume and cardiac output.**
    4. Assessment
        a. Decreasing blood pressure and pulse pressure

        b. **Distant heart sounds, distended neck veins**
        c. Pulsus paradoxus (systolic pressure drops and fluctuates with respiration)
    5. Intervention
        a. Pericardiocentesis
        b. Repair injuries if present

L. **Nursing diagnoses for chest trauma**
    1. Ineffective Breathing Pattern
    2. Impaired Gas Exchange
    3. Ineffective Airway Clearance
    4. Decreased Cardiac Output

M. **Planning and implementation**
    1. Assessment:

        a. **ABCs are a priority.**
        b. **Assess color, rate, depth, symmetry, and chest movement.**
        c. **Check carotid pulse rate and quality.**
        d. **Assess skin temperature and presence of diaphoresis.**
        e. **Interventions to maintain ABCs may be needed at this time.**
        f. **MAST trousers are contraindicated for the treatment of shock in chest injuries.**

2. Inspect:
    a. Wound for size, location, ecchymosis, abrasions, and lacerations
    b. For signs of internal trauma such as distended neck veins, narrow pulse pressure, tracheal deviation, and retractions
3. Auscultate: heart and lung sounds for diminished sounds or unequal lung sounds
4. Palpate for subcutaneous emphysema, broken ribs, and tenderness.
5. Interventions:
    a. Assist physician and respiratory therapist to place and maintain airway and breathing.
    b. Assist with maintaining circulation.
    c. Assist with placement of chest tubes and repair of chest wounds.
    d. Document actions.

IX. Burns

A. **Description: tissue injury caused by a transfer of energy from a heat source to the body. Results from direct thermal injury, exposure to irritating chemicals, radiation, or contact with an electrical current (Table 13-2).**

B. **Etiology and incidence**
1. Causes over 10,000 fatalities each year in the United States.
2. Usually occurs in the home and may be due to careless smoking.
3. Children and those over age 70 are at greatest risk for death from burns.

 4. **Most burns are preventable.**

C. **Chemical burns**
1. Specific chemical action will cause progressive tissue damage until chemical is removed or inactivated.

 2. **Treat ideally within the first hour. Continuously irrigate for 30 minutes and remove contaminated clothing.**

D. **Electrical burns**
1. Factors that determine extent of tissue damage and complications are listed in Table 13-3.
2. Types of electrical injury (Display 13-3)
3. Treatment: turn off current, remove client, and call for help.

E. **Toxic epidermal necrolysis syndrome (TENS, Stevens-Johnson syndrome): exfoliative drug reaction, often due to allergic reaction to penicillin and sulfa drugs.**

F. **Pathophysiology of burns: immediately post-injury (first 24 hours)**
1. Hypovolemia from plasma leaking out of vascular compartment into interstitial tissue is the primary event in the immediate post-injury phase.
2. Damage to the skin allows fluid (water, electrolytes, and protein) to shift interstitially to develop edema and intravascular dehydration.
3. Initial sympathetic nervous system signs and symptoms of compensatory shock, quickly leading to decreased CO.

TABLE 13-2.
Burn Types and Characteristics

BURN TYPE	SUPERFICIAL PARTIAL THICKNESS (First Degree)	DEEP PARTIAL THICKNESS (Second Degree)	FULL THICKNESS (Third Degree)
Area damaged	Epidermis only	Epidermis and part of dermis	Epidermis, dermis, and possibly hypodermis
Characteristics	Epidermal erythema; little or no edema; dry, intact skin without blisters; soothed by cooling	Erythema; blanching on pressure; hair remains; blisters increasing in size; minimal to moderate edema with oozing; underlying tissue mottled pink/white; sensitive to cold	Dry; no blisters or blisters that do not increase in size; red, black, white charred eschar; leathery texture; no blanching on pressure; blood vessels may be visible
Causes	Scald, flash flame, contact, chemical, ultraviolet light (sunlight)	Scald, flash flame, contact, chemical, ultraviolet light (sunlight); prolonged contact with hot surface (tar, heating pad)	Scald, flash flame, contact, chemical, electrical, tar
Pain/Temperature	Very painful with rapid heat loss	Severe pain with rapid heat loss	minimal to no pain
Healing time	2–5 days without scarring; possible discoloration will have peeling	Spontaneously in about one month; sometimes needs grafting; possible scarring and pigment changes	Large areas need grafting, which may take several months to complete; small areas eventually heal from the edges; scarring, with loss of shape and function

TABLE 13-3.
Factors Affecting Injury

CHEMICAL BURNS	ELECTRICAL BURNS
Strength/concentration	Type of current
	Voltage and amperage
Quantity	Resistance
	Current pathway
Method and length of contact	Duration of contact
Extent of skin/tissue penetration	
Mechanism of action	

DISPLAY 13-3.
Types of Electrical Injury

True: current passes directly through body; entrance and exit wounds
Arc: Burn current courses outside body (flash) from contact point to ground
Flame: Burn (secondary item ignites clothing)

4.   Release of smooth muscle vasoconstricting agents, such as catecholamines, thromboxane, and serotonin decrease alveolocapillary perfusion and increase PVR.
5.   Activation of the stress response promotes release of glucagon, cortisol, and catecholamines, which further increase metabolic rate, resulting in negative nitrogen and potassium balances, hyperinsulinemia, insulin resistance, and sodium retention.
6.   Increased anaerobic metabolism leads to accumulation of lactic and pyruvic acids, which results in metabolic acidosis.
7.   Intravascular hemolysis results in cell damage that may cause hyperkalemia due to release of potassium from ICF to ECF compartments.
8.   Increased blood viscosity occurs secondary to the increased proportion of RBCs compared with plasma. This leads to increased afterload and decreased peripheral blood flow.

9.   **This can account for a loss of up to 50% of circulating blood volume. This decreases tissue perfusion and produces an imbalance of O_2 supply and demand.**

G.   **Pathophysiology of burns: 24–36 hours post-injury**
1.   Fluid and electrolytes start returning to the intravascular space, enhancing tissue perfusion.
2.   Capillaries become intact, thus reestablishing osmotic pressure to pull fluids back into blood vessels.
3.   Diuresis occurs because of the increased GFR secondary to increased intravascular volume.
4.   Hypernatremia and hyperosmolality may occur because of sodium returning to the intravascular beds.
5.   Hypokalemia may result from increased aldosterone, diuresis, and return of potassium into the intracellular spaces.
6.   During the recovery phase, the cardiac output may increase to 2–3 times normal, with signs of hypermetabolism and increased oxygenation needs.

7.   **This hyperdynamic and hypermetabolic state peaks within 1–2 1/2 weeks after injury.**

H.   **Assessment**
1.   Burn severity is categorized as either major, moderate, or minor (Display 13-4).
2.   Determination of categories (Display 13-5):
     a.   Rule of nines: assigns percentages to various body areas. It is a fast and convenient method for determining extent of in-

DISPLAY 13-4.
American Burn Association Burn Classification

Major Burn Injuries

Partial-thickness (second-degree) burns over 25% TBSA adult or over 20% TBSA child

Full thickness (third-degree) burns involving 10% or more TBSA

All burns of hands, face, eyes, ears, feet, or perineum

All inhalation injuries

Electrical burns

All burns with associated complications of fractures or other trauma

All high-risk patients (those with pre-existing pulmonary, renal, or cardiovascular disease)

Moderate Burn Injuries

Partial-thickness burns over 15%–25% TBSA adult or 10%–20% TBSA child

Full-thickness burns of 2%–5% TBSA

Burns not involving eyes, ears, face, hands, feet, or perineum

Minor Burn Injuries

Partial-thickness burns over less than 15% TBSA adult or less than 10% child

Full-thickness burns of 2% TBSA or less

---

       jury, but does not account for differences in body proportions among age groups (Fig. 13-2).

    b.   Lund and Browder chart: correlates TBSA percentage with age

3. Renal function tests

4. Muscle damage assessment

5. Neurovascular compromise as characterized by respiratory changes, PaO_2 decrease, and restlessness

6. Gastrointestinal system effects may involve development of a paralytic ileus and abdominal distention. These put the client at risk for aspiration. Patients may also develop Curling's ulcer, a hemorrhagic gastritis that needs emergency treatment.

DISPLAY 13-5.
Determination of Burn Categories for Admission
to Burn Unit

Burn depth

Length of contact and heat generated

Partial-thickness and full-thickness percentage

Burn location: "special" areas (face, hands, feet)

Cosmetic or functional deformity (joint range-of-motion)

Burn size: % TBSA of both partial- and full-thickness burns

Risk factors: electrical burns, fractures, age

Inhalation injury

Pre-existing disorders

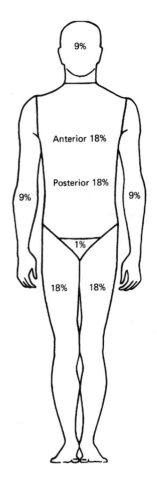

FIGURE 13-2.
The *rule of nines* method for determining percentage of body area with burn injury.

I.   Fluid resuscitation
    1.   Parkland formula estimates fluid needs during first 24 hours post-burn (Display 13-6).
    2.   Urine output is the best measure of fluid resuscitation effectiveness.

J.   Wound care
    1.   Control environmental infection by administration of tetanus prophylaxis, use of sterile technique, and cultures as needed.
    2.   Application of topical antimicrobials.

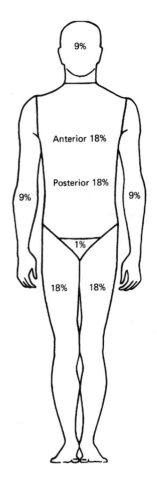
    3.   **Systemic antimicrobials are only given for evidence of systemic, not local, infection.**
    4.   Hydrotherapy to soften eschar, remove topical agents, and assist with debridement.
    5.   Escharotomy to relieve respiratory distress and prevent circulatory occlusion.
    6.   Fasciotomy is used for deep burns. It is used to assess what muscle remains functional.
    7.   Debridement is the removal of eschar.

DISPLAY 13-6.
Parkland Formula for Fluid Needs 24 Hours Post-Burn

> 4 mL × weight (kg) × % TBSA burned
> Give 1/2 in first 8 hours
> Give 1/4 in second 8 hours
> Give 1/4 in third 8 hours

8. Dressings (see Table 13-4)
9. Aggressive wound care involves the staged removal of eschar to a bleeding base, with dressings and frequent grafting needed.
10. Debridement
    a. Removal of necrotic tissue/eschar to expose healthy tissue.
    b. The goal is to remove contaminated tissue, protect the client from sepsis, and remove eschar in preparation for grafting and wound healing.
    c. Natural debridement: bacteria at the juncture of burned and viable tissue causes dead tissue to separate spontaneously.
    d. Mechanical: use of scissors and forceps to separate and remove eschar.
    e. Surgical: excision of skin down to fascia or "shaving" of skin layers down to viable tissue.
11. Temporary wound closure
    a. Allograft: grafting of skin from one individual to another of the same species. Most commonly uses human cadaver skin. It usually takes 3–5 weeks before host rejection occurs.
    b. Xenograft/heterograft: use of skin from another species (eg, pig skin).
    c. Amnion: uses materials from human placentas.
    d. Synthetic dressings: man-made skin substitutes.

TABLE 13-4.
Types of Burn Dressings, Benefits, and Problems

EXPOSURE (OPEN METHOD): WOUNDS OPEN TO AIR	DRY OCCLUSIVE	PARTIAL EXPOSURE (MOST COMMON)
Needs reverse isolation	Limits observation (thick bandages) and mobility	Thin layer (not used for hands or feet)
Needs warm room	Assists with graft stabilization	Covered with thin gauze layer and antimicrobial cream (heat loss)
Easy visibility of wound		
No painful dressing change		No painful dressing change
Increased mobility		Increased mobility
Easy assessment		Easy assessment

e.   Biosynthetic skin substitutes: These are permeable to antimicrobials and can be left in place for 2 weeks until the area is ready for grafting.

 f.   Other substances are cultured human epithelial cells, and artificial skin.

12.   Permanent wound closure

    a.   Autografting: graft transferred from one site to another from the same individual to provide permanent coverage for full-thickness injuries.

    b.   Donor sites include the buttocks and thighs.

    c.   Full-thickness burns need partial-thickness grafting to minimize scarring.

    d.   Cannot graft onto bone, must graft only onto tissue.

    e.   Order of grafting is to provide for survival, function, then appearance.

    f.   Types of grafts are either split-thickness or full-thickness.

    g.   Application can be of sheets or "postage stamp" pieces that can be expanded to form a meshwork over burned area, or left as is to form unions with each other.

    h.   **Donor site skin is treated as a partial-thickness burn. The site may be reused after healing occurs.**

    i.   Wound healing disorders include the formation of scars, keloids, failure to heal, contractures, and non-function.

K.   Nursing diagnoses

  1.   Impaired Gas Exchange

  2.   Impaired Tissue Integrity

  3.   Pain

  4.   Altered Nutrition: Less than Body Requirements

  5.   Risk for Injury

  6.   Risk for Infection

  7.   Ineffective Individual/Family Coping

  8.   Anxiety/Fear/Powerlessness

  9.   Ineffective Thermoregulation

 10.   Knowledge Deficit: Burns

L.   Planning and implementation

  1.   **Assess TBSA burned.**

    a.   **Identify and document location and assess wound depth.**

    b.   **Note intact areas, presence of pain, and adherent items.**

    c.   **Take photos for later comparison (if permitted by hospital/client).**

  2.   Assess anxiety level and intervene appropriately.

  3.   Evaluate I and O trends, reporting decreases in urine output. Massive increases during the acute phase should also be noted.

  4.   Monitor carboxyhemoglobin levels.

  5.   Assess for inhalation injury as characterized by coughing up of soot, singed nasal hairs, and burns around the mouth or neck.

  6.   Maintain patient NPO and insert NGT to decrease risk of aspiration.

7. Elevate affected extremities above level of the heart.
8. Promote active/passive ROM to affected extremities hourly.
9. Maintain therapies to prevent contractures and minimize disfigurement.
10. Assess gastric pH and report if under 5. Administer antacids and histamine antagonists as ordered.
11. Monitor vital signs and hemodynamic parameters.
12. Prevent nosocomial infection by leaving blisters intact for natural barrier protection.
13. Change dressings per order and assess drainage for color, odor, consistency, and amount.
14. Use as few invasive lines as possible to minimize infection risk.
15. Immobilize graft sites to prevent trauma.
16. Maintain protective isolation.
17. Perform wound cultures and biopsies as ordered.
18. Monitor antimicrobial topical agent.
19. Use radiant heat to maintain body temperature.
20. Administer medications for pain, and antibiotics specific to cultured organism.
21. **Narcotic analgesics are often rotated in clients with burns to decrease the development of tolerance.**
22. Teach alternate pain control methods: guided imagery, music therapy, relaxation techniques.
23. **Medicate for pain before daily dressing changes.**
24. **Be prepared to assist with emergency fasciotomy/escharotomy to relieve compression of nerves or blood vessels, especially with burns of chest or circumferential burns, to prevent compartment syndrome effectiveness.**
25. **Monitor for compartment syndrome.**
26. Pad pressure areas and apply splints as needed.
27. Assess respiratory status and administer oxygen therapies as indicated.
28. Anticipate and prepare for possible intubation.
29. Explain all care activities and keep explanations simple.
30. Refer to other support systems such as social services and chaplaincy as needed.
31. Involve significant others in care as early as possible.
32. Prepare family for initial visit and go with them to greet patient.
33. Stress to family the need for patient to perform ADLs as possible, even if it causes pain.

M. Evaluation

1. The patient's hemodynamic parameters, vital signs, LOC, and urine output return to normal.
2. Burns are accurately assessed and unburned skin remains intact.
3. The patient remains infection-free, as evidenced by normal temperature, WBC, and wound healing.
4. The patient maintains normal fluid volume, as evidenced by normal BP, urine output over 30 mL/hr, and normal vital signs.

5. The patient maintains effective breathing pattern, airway clearance, and tissue perfusion.
6. The patient verbalizes relief/ability to tolerate pain.
7. The patient and family progress through grieving stages toward acceptance of altered body image.
8. The patient is able to verbalize basic understanding of pathophysiology of burns, necessary life-style adjustments, and correct use of medications.
9. The patient demonstrates progressive healing of existing wounds without additional breakdown.
10. No complications will develop.
11. The patient will develop an anabolic state with progressive tolerance of nutritional intake with supplements.
12. The patient will perform progressively more self-care activities.
13. The patient will be able to integrate altered body image and begin to develop a realistic self-image.

N. Home health considerations
1. Rehabilitation begins with admission. The goal is to assist the client to return to pre-burn activity levels and societal function.
2. Wound care
   a. Cover open wounds with gauze.
   b. Keep moisturized with lanolin-based cream to prevent drying and cracking.
   c. Avoid sun exposure of newly grafted skin.
3. Positioning
   a. In opposite direction of expected contracture.
   b. Splinting may be used to maintain length of soft tissue joint structure.
   c. Exercise is indicated until optimal joint motion and scar maturation occur.
4. Pressure dressings
   a. Aid in circulation, cover and protect scars, and minimize hypertrophic scarring.
   b. Scar-prevention garments to be worn 23 hours a day for up to 18 months.
5. Discuss fire safety/burn prevention, but do not be judgmental or place blame on client.
6. Encourage diet that is high in protein, vitamin C, and zinc to promote wound healing.
7. Refer to support groups and community agencies.

X. Frostbite

A. Description and etiology: trauma from exposure to freezing temperatures that causes localized freezing of tissue fluids in cells and intracellular spaces, resulting in vascular damage.

B. Predisposing factors
1. Age extremes, pre-existing disorders
2. Poor nutrition/inadequate heat production
3. Increased risk of damage with exposure to ears, nose, hands, and feet.
4. Substance abuse, fatigue.

C. Assessment findings
    1. Early warning signs/symptoms are a dull, aching of exposed areas, leading to loss of flexibility. Ultimately this results in loss of sensation of the affected area.
    2. Skin at the site appears white or whitish-blue and mottled, and is cool to the touch.
    3. Injury extent is not always initially apparent.

D. Nursing diagnoses
    1. Impaired Tissue Integrity
    2. Pain
    3. Risk for Injury
    4. Risk for Infection
    5. Knowledge Deficit: Frost Bite

E. Planning and implementation
    1. Give analgesics before starting treatment.
    2. Remove constrictive clothing, and handle extremity gently.
    3. Rewarming should be done to decrease amount of tissue loss.
    4. Rewarming is best done by use of a whirlpool, with immersion until the tips of the injured area start to flush.
    5. Wrap sterile gauze between the affected digits PRN.
    6. Elevate extremity to control edema.
    7. Do not rub or massage area, as this may cause further tissue damage.
    8. Cover with blankets, warming blanket, or use radiant warmer.
    9. Monitor vital signs and hemodynamic parameters.
    10. Administer warmed IVs, peritoneal fluid, and Foley installations PRN.
    11. Supply heated, humidified oxygen PRN.
    12. Administer tetanus prophylaxis.
    13. Evaluate for transfer to burn unit.
    14. Be aware of possible surgical interventions:
        a. Debridement: decreases infection
        b. Escharotomy: allows for normal circulation and joint movement
        c. Fasciotomy: releases pressure on muscles, nerves, and blood vessels

F. Evaluation: The patient will be restored to maximum function by the completion of rehabilitation.

XI. Hypothermia
  A. Description: less than normal body temperature
  B. Etiology and incidence
    1. Should be considered whenever history, client behavior, and/or weather conditions indicate possible abnormal heat loss.
    2. Risk factors (Display 13-7)
  C. Pathophysiology
    1. Body compartments involved in heat transfer include:
        a. Shell = skin, subcutaneous tissue
        b. Core = body

DISPLAY 13-7.
Common Risk Factors in Hypothermia Development

Alcohol ingestion	Age extremes
Medications	Outdoor exposure
Trauma	Cold exposure
Flawed thermoregulation	Homelessness

2. Factors that affect heat transfer from the body to the environment include:
   a. Body surface area (BSA)
   b. Peripheral vasomotor tone
   c. Quantity of subcutaneous tissue

3. **The hypothalamus is the normal thermostat ("set point"), but excessive heat loss causes failure to adjust quickly enough.**

4. Compensatory mechanisms unsuccessfully try to maintain internal temperature. These include shivering, blood shunting to core organs, decreased temperature, and decreased metabolism.

5. **Shivering: most effective heat production method, but results in**
   a. **2–5-fold increase in oxygen consumption and cardiac workload**
   b. **400%–500% increase in metabolic demands**
   c. **Increased CO_2 production**
   d. **Cutaneous vasoconstriction**
   e. **Eventual lactic acidosis**

6. Types of heat transfer
   a. Conduction: direct heat transfer from body to cooler objects without motion
   b. Convection: transfer of heat by circulation
   c. Radiation: transfer of heat between skin and environment
   d. Evaporation: wet skin results in heat loss by losing moisture into the environment

D. Types, stages, and assessment findings
   1. Types
      a. Intentional: needed for surgery to protect the heart, decrease metabolic needs, and provide blood-free operative field
      b. Inadvertent: side effect of cold operating room/PACU
      c. Accidental: unintentional; from trauma, weather, substances, or exposure
   2. Formula for calculating temperature in either Fahrenheit or Celsius (Display 13-8)
   3. Stages of hypothermia (see Table 13-5)
      a. Thermal blankets are ineffective unless the periphery is vasodilated.

DISPLAY 13-8.
Formula for Calculating Temperature in Either
Fahrenheit or Celsius

$$[°C = (°F - 32) (5/9); °F = (°C) (9/5) + 32]$$

𝄞 b.   **May not respond to drugs until warmer, therefore do
not stop resuscitation efforts until temperature is 95° F
without return of pulse.**

E.   Nursing interventions

𝄞 1.   **Monitor temperature closely.**

2.   Monitor vital signs, hemodynamics, and ECG

3.   Institute general warming measures:

a.   Increase room temperature.

b.   Provide blankets around body, especially head and feet.

c.   Warm beverages/foods as tolerated. Institute specific warming measures (Display 13-9).

F.   Evaluation

1.   Patient returns to acceptable body temperature without development of complications.

2.   Patient understands that avoidance of temperature extremes is ideal and largely preventable.

𝄞 3.   **"No one is dead until warm and dead."**

XII.   Disseminated intravascular coagulopathy (DIC)

A.   Description: disorder in which bleeding and clotting occur simultaneously due to a cascade of events resulting from the abnormal, sequential, systemic activation of both the coagulation and fibrinolytic systems.

TABLE 13-5.
Stages and Manifestations of Hypothermia

MILD-(90–95°F)	MODERATE (85–89°F)	SEVERE (UNDER 85°F)
Increased pulse, respirations blood pressure, cardiac output.	Shivering stops.	Respirations decrease.
Decreased level of consciousness.	Stuporous; decreased pain sensation.	Unresponsive.
Decreased manual dexterity.	Decreased heart rate, respirations, blood pressure, and cardiac output.	Pupils fixed and dilated.
Shivering occurs as initial respons against heat loss: shunts warm blood from extremities to core.		May have undetectable/absent pulse (PEA), BP, and respirations. Increased urine output. Absent bowel sounds.
		Leads to coagulation changes and acid–base imbalances.

DISPLAY 13-9.
Warming Fluids for Hypothermia

> Peritoneal dialysis
> Bladder irrigations
> Intravenous fluids, radiant warmer
> Hemodialysis extracorporeal ("ECMO" is bypass-type machine)
>
> **REMEMBER* to do all of these slowly to prevent rewarming shock or hyperthermia!

1. Results in the inappropriate, accelerated consumption of coagulation factors, thus leading to hemorrhage.
2. Occurs secondary to some other abnormality and is associated with infection, neoplasms, obstetric complications, tissue trauma, and burns.

B. Normal coagulation

1. The balance maintained between clot formation and clot dissolution
2. The initial response after injury:
   a. Attainment of hemostasis by vasoconstriction, which reduces blood flow
   b. Platelets adhere to the damaged endothelial lining of the vessel and secrete catecholamines and platelet adhesive factors
   c. Binding of additional free platelets, forms a platelet plug
   d. Catecholamines induce the further release of adhering substances
3. Clot formation
   a. After this initial response, the coagulation system takes over.
   b. Fibrin, the final product of coagulation, joins with the platelet aggregate to strengthen the hemostatic plug at the bleeding site.
   c. The sequence is activated by either the intrinsic or extrinsic pathways.
   d. The intrinsic pathway begins with factor XII activation after blood contacts exposed foreign surfaces.
   e. The extrinsic pathway begins when thromboplastin (lipoprotein released by injured tissues) joins with factor X in blood.
   f. Factor X is the first step on the common pathway.
   g. After this, prothrombin is converted to thrombin, and fibrinogen is converted to fibrin. Factor XIII is the final factor needed to produce a solid clot.
4. Clot dissolution: involves conversion of plasminogen to plasmin, which acts on both fibrinogen and fibrin degradation products (FDPs or FSPs).

C. Etiology and incidence

1. Associated with at least a 25% mortality rate.

2.   **Sepsis is the major trigger for DIC development. It is also a complication of other disorders such as shock, surgical procedures, respiratory distress syndrome, trauma, obstetrical disorders, neoplasms, transfusion reactions, etc.**

D.   Pathophysiology
1.   Vascular endothelium disruption activates the intrinsic pathway, and tissue damage causes activation of the extrinsic system, with the release of large amounts of thromboplastin.
2.   Continued endothelial and tissue injury promote intravascular clotting and fibrinolysis as a result of decreased perfusion.
3.   DIC occurs with coagulation system activation and overproduction of normal defense mechanisms.
4.   Overproduction of coagulation factors causes release of excess fibrin, causing small thrombi to develop in the microcirculation.
5.   Thrombi obstruct blood flow, resulting in peripheral ischemia and organ injury.
6.   Rapid clot formation also exhausts the supply of platelets, fibrinogen, and other clotting factors, leading to uncontrolled bleeding
7.   RBC hemolysis and resulting ischemic tissue damage may also occur.
8.   Widespread clotting causes thrombocytopenia due to continuous platelet aggregation.
9.   Clotting factors I, II, V, and VIII become depleted because they are used up faster than they can be replenished.
10.   The body begins lysing thrombi in a useless attempt to restore flow to the microcirculation. This leads to release of FDPs, which have anticoagulant properties and contribute to bleeding.
11.   Rapid secondary activation of the fibrinolytic system produces FDPs, which decreases serum fibrinogen
12.   The anticoagulant action of FDPs further interferes with actions of thrombin, fibrin, and platelets.

    13.   **The combination of the above responses leads to diffuse bleeding.**

E.   Assessment
1.   Bleeding from three unrelated sites strongly suggests developing DIC.
2.   Bleeding from venipuncture/injection sites, mucous membranes, drain sites, stoma sites, and incisions is also common.
3.   Assess for the development of ecchymosis, petechiae, or acrocyanosis.
4.   May also note abdominal tenderness, diarrhea, heme+ stools, and emesis.
5.   Renal symptoms include oliguria, anuria, and hematuria.
6.   Pulmonary involvement is manifested by crackles, dyspnea, cyanosis, and hemoptysis.
7.   A change in LOC, disorientation, and restlessness may also occur.
8.   Laboratory studies (Display 13-10)
    a.   Presence of FDPs indicates the body's attempt to stop intravascular clot formation.

DISPLAY 13-10.
Laboratory Findings in DIC

PT prolonged
PTT prolonged
TT prolonged
Fibrinogen decreased
FDPs greater than 10
D-dimer assay elevated
Hgb/Hct decreased
Platelets decreased

      b.   FDPs prevent normal platelet function and add to the lack of coagulation.

m   c.   **Elevated D-dimer assay indicates that the body has attempted to break down internal clots.**

F.   **Nursing diagnoses**
    1.   Fluid Volume Deficit
    2.   Risk for Injury
    3.   Impaired Gas Exchange
    4.   Altered Tissue Perfusion: Cardiopulmonary, Renal, Cerebral
    5.   Decreased Cardiac Output
    6.   Impaired Tissue Integrity
    7.   Risk for Infection
    8.   Anxiety/Fear/Powerlessness

G.   **Planning and implementation**
    1.   Diagnose and treat the primary disease process.
    2.   Maintain life support and prevent the development of shock and acidosis.

m   3.   **Identify those at risk. This may include patients with shock, trauma, pregnancy, renal/liver dysfunction, sepsis, and blood disorders.**
    4.   Monitor hemodynamic parameters including vital signs, and cardiopulmonary measurements.
    5.   Assess for the presence of petechia, ecchymoses, epistaxis, bleeding gums, bleeding at venipuncture, incision, stoma, or drainage sites.
    6.   Note trends in laboratory values, especially those related to clotting.
    7.   Monitor trends in respiratory parameters.
    8.   Implement methods to prevent tissue trauma and unnecessary bleeding.
    9.   Apply pressure to bleeding sites.
   10.   Do not disturb clots.

11. Avoid IM injections and use smallest gauge needle. Draw blood from central lines as possible.

12. Alert others to bleeding precautions.

13. Prevent pressure areas by turning and positioning patient frequently and gently.

 14. **Do not use a BP cuff, as this could result in subdermal bleeding.**

15. Secure all drainage tubes to prevent unnecessary pulling and irritation.

16. Alleviate anxiety by explaining all procedures and activities.

 17. **Assess hands and feet for coldness and acral cyanosis. These are clearly defined areas of gray-purple mottling due to clot formation in small vessels of the extremities.**

18. Elevate legs 15–30 degrees to prevent venous stasis and watch for unilateral swelling (DVT).

19. Monitor heparin and blood component therapy.

20. Prevent and/or treat acidosis.

21. Administer medications as ordered and appropriate:

     a. **Heparin: may be used to interrupt cycle of thrombin release, fibrin deposition, clotting factor activation, and additional thrombin release. You must weigh the risk of hemorrhage with the supposed benefits.**

     b. **Replacement of clotting factors: platelets, fresh frozen plasma (FFP), cryoprecipitate (Factor VIII).**

22. Assess respiratory status and intervene appropriately.

23. Monitor vital signs and hemodynamic parameters.

H. Evaluation

 1. **Side effects of heparin treatment are reduced through monitoring and early intervention.**

2. There is a reduced incidence of bleeding and hematoma development.

3. The patient is able to maintain optimal fluid balance, normal BP, and UOP greater than 30 mL/hr.

4. The patient is able to maintain optimal gas exchange.

5. The patient is able to maintain adequate oxygenation and normal acid–base balance.

6. Existing wounds show no evidence of bleeding.

7. The patient experiences reduced anxiety/fear, as evidenced by calm and trusting appearance, and verbalization of fears and concerns.

XIII. Adult respiratory distress syndrome (ARDS)

A. Description

 1. **A progressive, acute pulmonary injury causing damage to the alveolocapillary membrane, resulting in acute respiratory failure.**

2. Mortality is over 50% without prompt treatment.

3. Survival is dependent on:

a.   Extent of original injury
b.   Effectiveness of supportive measures
c.   Prevention of further pulmonary injury

B.   Etiology and incidence

1.   **Approximately 95% of cases develop within 24–72 hours after the onset of the predisposing condition.**
2.   Indirect lung injury occurs with sepsis, which is the primary precipitating factor, major trauma, shock, multiple blood transfusions, DIC, extensive burns, drug overdose, and pancreatitis.
3.   Direct lung injury occurs with aspiration of gastric contents, pneumonia, oxygen toxicity, fat/air embolism, pulmonary contusion, and inhalation injury.
4.   Any disorder causing a low-flow perfusion state places a patient at risk for ARDS.

C.   Pathophysiology

1.   Damage to the capillary endothelium and alveolar Type I gas exchange cells occurs secondary to direct or indirect lung injury.
2.   This results in cell membrane disruption.
3.   This also results in the release of lysosomal enzymes, and precipitates platelet aggregation.
4.   Swelling and retraction of the basement membrane cells occurs.
5.   This causes a pulmonary capillary leak.
6.   Plasma moves interstitially, resulting in interstitial and alveolar edema
7.   The process of diffusion between the alveoli and capillaries is disrupted. This leads to:
     a.   Decreased compliance

     b.   **Decreased O_2 diffusion**
     c.   **Bronchiolar edema and congestive atelectasis**
8.   Surfactant is inactivated. This causes increased fluid and plasma protein leakage, resulting in atelectasis, decreased compliance, and increased work of breathing.
9.   Hyaline membrane formation contributes to development of interstitial fibrosis, which increases diffusion barrier, thus increasing shunting and decreasing compliance.

D.   Assessment

1.   **Assess respiratory rate, rhythm, depth, breath sounds, sputum characteristics, frequency of suctioning ABG results, I and O, PA pressures, PCWP, and CO.**
2.   In the early phase of ARDS, dyspnea, tachypnea, and hyperventilation are noted.
3.   In the late phase, respiratory distress, tachycardia, and hypertension may occur.
4.   Cyanosis is a rare and late finding.
5.   Assess LOC for restlessness, apprehension, and agitation.
6.   **Signs and symptoms of decreased cerebral O_2 perfusion include tachypnea leading to dyspnea, crackles, decreased breath sounds, thin, frothy sputum, chest wall movements, and use of accessory muscles.**

7. Assess skin color for:

    a. **Central cyanosis: due to decreased arterial saturation. Cyanosis is seen around the lips, mouth and mucus membranes.**

    b. **Peripheral cyanosis: due to decreased venous saturation. Seen at nailbeds and tip of the nose.**

8. Laboratory results (Display 13-11)

    a. ABGs: early respiratory alkalosis leading to respiratory acidosis.

    b. The hallmark of ARDS is a hypoxemia refractory to increasing levels of oxygen. An FiO_2 >0.5 with a PaO_2 of <50 indicates shunting.

    c. Pulse oximetry (SpO_2) <90–92%, SvO_2 <60%, and $EtCO_2$ progressively lower due to CO_2 retention, all signs of ARDS.

9. Respiratory parameters (see Display 13-11)

    a. Amount of hypoxia (PaO_2)

    b. Amount of PEEP needed

    c. Lung compliance

    d. Degree of infiltrates

10. **CXR will show diffuse bilateral pulmonary infiltrates. This is considered a classic "white-out" without localized area of involvement.**

E. Nursing diagnoses

1. Ineffective Airway Clearance
2. Impaired Gas Exchange
3. Ineffective Breathing Patterns
4. Fear/Anxiety/Powerlessness
5. Ineffective Individual/Family Coping

F. Planning and implementation

1. **Provide respiratory support to decrease hypoxemia, increase compliance, decrease pulmonary HTN, promote return of acceptable V/Q matching, and decrease alveolar inflammation.**
2. Treat the underlying cause.
3. Prevent complications.
4. Decrease respiratory effort by placing patient in Fowler's position, spacing of care, and suctioning.
5. Monitor respiratory parameters and ventilator settings.
6. Perform frequent respiratory assessments.
7. Promote active exercise of respiratory muscles.

DISPLAY 13-11.
Respiratory Parameters in ARDS

FRC:	decreased
Compliance:	decreased
V/Q ratio:	decreased

ℳ 8. Decrease risk of aspiration and promote chest expansion with nasogastric tube PRN.

9. Implement mechanical ventilation. Ideally keep FiO_2 under 0.5 to prevent oxygen toxicity:
   a. Conventional methods
   b. Other methods: pressure control ventilation (PCV), inverse ratio ventilation (IRV), high-frequency ventilation (HFV), permissive hypercapnia, PEEP (PEEP maintains alveolar hyperinflation at low oxygen tensions to minimize atelectasis)

10. Promote comfort.
    a. Sedation PRN. You may also need concurrent paralytic agents in some patients.
    b. Decrease pain, especially postoperatively.
    c. Teach client to breath *with* machine.

ℳ 11. Promote normal sleep patterns as possible by spacing care to allow for 90-minute biologic sleep periods, especially at night.

12. Decrease anxiety and fear.
    a. Explain care activities.
    b. Explain ICU environment sounds.
    c. Encourage liberal visiting hours, based on unique client needs.
    d. Develop alternate communication methods with clients receiving mechanical ventilation.

13. Establish and maintain adequate hydration:
    a. Monitor I and O.
    b. Maintain PCWP 10–15mm Hg.
    c. Account for insensible fluid losses from NGT, ETT, diaphoresis.
    d. Administer free water with enteral feedings.
    e. Promote anabolism.
    f. Supply nutritional supplements.
    g. Establish enteral feedings, if possible, with elevated head of bed.
    h. Recognize and account for hypermetabolic needs.

14. Prevent additional infection.
    ℳ a. Administer antibiotics per order and around-the-clock.
    b. Be aware of nosocomial transfer to susceptible clients.
    c. Provide skin care to prevent breakdown.
    d. Change peripheral IV sites per CDC guidelines/institutional protocol.

15. Administer medications as ordered and appropriate:
    a. Aerosolized surfactant: decreases alveolar surface tension, increases compliance, therefore believed to decrease shunting.
    b. Anti-inflammatory agents: corticosteroids, ibuprofen.
    c. Nitric oxide (NO): inhalation causes pulmonary vasodilation with minimal systemic effects. This may decrease mortality by decreasing pulmonary hypertension.

G. **Evaluation**
   1. The patient will be able to breathe spontaneously with satisfactory respiratory parameters.
   2. The patient will be able to maintain effective airway clearance by being able to expectorate secretions when coughing.
   3. The patient will exhibit a decrease in adventitious breath sounds and use of accessory muscles.
   4. The patient will have a return to normal hemodynamic parameters, vital signs, LOC, urine output, normoactive bowel sounds, airway patency.
   5. The patient will experience reduced anxiety/fear as evidenced by calm and trusting appearance, and verbalization of fears and concerns.
   6. The patient will verbalize basic understanding of pathophysiology of disease, necessary life-style adjustments, and correct use of medications.
   7. There will be a return to normal hemodynamic parameters, vital signs, LOC, urine output, active bowel sounds, and airway patency.

XIV. **Multiple organ dysfunction syndrome (MODS)**

   A. **Description:** a syndrome that occurs when more than one system/organ cannot support its activities. MODS is not a disease that affects a single organ or system.
   B. **Etiology and incidence**
      1. Mortality is up to 90%, despite early diagnosis and treatment.
      2. Preexisting factors: see Display 13-12.
      3. Increasing in frequency due to increased survival rates from massive insults to the body (eg, trauma, myocardial infarction, shock, etc.).
   C. **Pathophysiology**
      1. Infection (sepsis), persistent inflammation, and ischemia are present. These are the 3 "I's" of MODS.
      2. Normally, mediators help the body withstand and recover from injury, but with severe injuries, responses cannot stop.
      3. There is stimulation of the inflammatory–immune response (IIR).
         a. This is an injury-induced pathway with abrupt or gradual onset.

DISPLAY 13-12.
Factors Influencing the Development of MODS

Gram-negative sepsis (#1 risk)
Immunosuppressants
Traumatic injury
Sleep deprivation
Immunosuppression
Malnutrition
Over 65 years of age
Blood transfusions

       b.   Results in sympathetic nervous system stimulation and release of catecholamines.

       c.   Causes endothelial damage.

       d.   The endothelial lining promotes coagulation, thus there is an increased tendency for embolus development.

       e.   Complement activation occurs. Complement's major function is to induce inflammation.

       f.   **The goal of inflammation is to protect the body, limit injury extent, and promote healing at the damaged site.**

4.   Other mediators involved in the IIR are WBCs, platelets, T cells, B cells, and histamine.

5.   Cumulative effects

       a.   **Maldistribution of circulating volume**

       b.   **Oxygen supply/demand imbalance**

       c.   **Alterations in metabolism**

6.   **Respiratory failure is the number one early postoperative problem, due in part to alveoli–capillary membrane changes. The lung often is the first organ to fail in MODS.**

7.   Altered perfusion, related to small microvasculature emboli and respiratory insufficiency; causes initial shunting of blood to major organs until compensatory mechanisms fail.

8.   Altered hepatic protein synthesis and glucose production occur.

9.   A hyperdynamic state leads to initial increased CO, which increases renal blood flow with resulting polyuria.

10.   Continuation causes dehydration and the development of shock with decreased renal blood flow and renal failure.

11.   Initial thermoregulation shows hyperthermia, leading to hypothermia as IIR is unable to supply enough components to combat infection/inflammation.

12.   Metabolic effects include:

       a.   Glucose: initially increased until the development of insulin resistance, necessitating increased gluconeogenesis, which leads to increased lactate production and lactic acidosis.

       b.   Protein: catabolism causes negative nitrogen balance and proteinuria.

       c.   Coagulation system: DIC or primary bleeding problem.

       d.   Accelerated coagulation causes development of emboli, which the body tries to break down.

       e.   Production of anticoagulants degrades the clot, resulting in formation of FDPs.

       f.   Body cannot get rid of FDPs fast enough, with resultant generalized bleeding.

13.   **"Snowball" effect as systems overwork to get rid of internal clots, while simultaneously prohibiting external coagulation.**

D. **Assessment**

    1.   Early MODS is characterized by:

       a.   Vasodilation and decreased PVR with normal BP

       b.   CO increases to maintain blood pressure

c. Hypovolemia begins due to increased capillary permeability and interstitial fluid losses

d. Skin is warm, pink, and dry, which is related to vasodilation

e. Increasing temperature with shaking chills, although the reverse may occur in the elderly or in those who are immunosuppressed

f. Hyperventilation results in respiratory alkalosis

g. Signs of tissue hypoxia manifest due to oxyhemoglobin dissociation curve principles. Hemoglobin is reluctant to release oxygen to cells.

2. Late stage manifestations of MODS:

a. Hypotension occurs because cardiac output cannot keep up with the expanding intravascular space and continued capillary leakage.

b. In response to hypotension, PVR is increased via catecholamine release due to sympathetic nervous system stimulation.

c. Pulse becomes weak and thready.

d. ST and T-wave changes on ECG indicate decreased myocardial perfusion.

e. Cold, moist, pale skin and development of mottling and cyanosis.

f. Hematologic alterations begin to show.

g. Hypoxia and decreased perfusion are evident.

h. Metabolic acidosis develops due to lactic acidosis resulting from anaerobic metabolism, with further decreased perfusion.

 i. **Cell death and organ failure increases due to decreased available cellular energy and generalized acidotic state.**

E. Nursing diagnoses

1. Risk for Infection
2. Impaired Gas Exchange
3. Impaired Tissue Integrity
4. Ineffective Airway Clearance
5. Altered Nutrition: Less than Body Requirements
6. Fluid Volume Deficit
7. Ineffective Individual/Family Coping
8. Anxiety/Fear/Powerlessness
9. Ineffective Thermoregulation

F. Planning and implementation

 1. **Maintain ventilatory support to optimize oxygen saturation and decrease work of breathing.**

 2. **Assess respiratory status including rate, rhythm, depth, breath sounds, work of breathing, use of accessory muscles, ABGs, and pulse oximetry.**

3. Maintain humidification and oxygen therapies.

 4. **Assess for hypoxemia, which is characterized by tachycardia, tachypnea, restlessness, diaphoresis, headache, lethargy, confusion, and pallor.**

𝕟 5. **Optimize CO with fluids, increased inotropes, and vasoactive agents.**
6. Optimize hemoglobin.
7. Prevention/early detection of primary infection or stimulus of IIR.
8. Ensure good handwashing to prevent nosocomial pneumonia.
9. Maintain aspiration assessment/prevention.
10. Monitor for dysrhythmias.
11. Monitor vital signs and hemodynamic parameters.

𝕟 12. **Assess for evidence of impaired tissue oxygenation, such as changes in mental status and restlessness.**
13. Monitor for signs/symptoms of hypovolemia including oliguria, thirst, dry tongue, and tachycardia.
14. Monitor I and O, including insensible fluid losses.
15. Assess the GI system for abdominal distention, decreased/absent bowel sounds, and abdominal girth.
16. Check nasogastric drainage and stools for occult blood.
17. Provide nutrition/metabolic support.
    a. Support organ structure and function.
    b. Support metabolic pathways.
    c. Maintain positive nitrogen balance.
    d. Provide enteral feeding if possible.

𝕟   e. **Note that if patients are NPO long-term, translocation of bacteria from the gut into circulation can occur.**
18. Administer medications as ordered:
    a. Antibiotics: broad-spectrum until organism identified
    b. Antacids, histamine antagonists, sucralfate
    c. Assess gastric pH and report if under 5
    d. Analgesics/anti-anxiety agents; sedate as needed and ordered to decrease metabolic needs
    e. Anti-inflammatories
    f. Vasoactive medication combinations
    g. Oxygen-free radical scavengers (mannitol, allopurinol)
    h. Steroids: not proven to be beneficial

𝕟 19. **Be aware of future trends in therapy to inhibit the acute in-flammatory response and decrease the systemic inflammation that contributes to progression in MODS.**
    a. Cyclosporine versus FK-586
    b. Monoclonal/polyclonal antibodies

G. **Evaluation**
1. The patient will have a return to normal hemodynamic parameters, vital signs, LOC, urine output, active bowel sounds, and airway patency, and wounds will be kept clean.
2. The patient will remain infection free, as evidenced by normal temperature, WBC, and wound healing.
3. The patient will maintain normal fluid volume, as evidenced by normal BP, urine output over 30 mL/hr, and normal VS.
4. The patient will maintain an effective breathing pattern, airway clearance, and tissue perfusion.
5. The patient will verbalize relief/ability to tolerate pain.

6. The patient will verbalize a basic understanding of pathophysiology of MODS, necessary life-style adjustments, and correct use of medications.
7. The patient will maintain optimal fluid balance, oxygenation, and acid–base balance.
8. The patient will develop an anabolic state with progressive tolerance of nutritional intake with supplements.

XV. Physiology of shock

A. **Description: a syndrome that results in inadequate tissue perfusion, decreased cellular oxygenation, and cellular death. It is usually recognized by the classic symptoms of restlessness, disorientation, hypotension, rapid, thready pulse, tachypnea with increasing dyspnea, cold, clammy skin, and oliguria.**

B. **Etiology and incidence: see specific types of shock (neurogenic/spinal, cardiogenic, septic, hypovolemic, anaphylactic)**
    1. The usual infection sites are the genitourinary, GI, and pulmonary systems.
    2. Specific causes include invasive procedures, immunosuppression, and trauma.
    3. Nosocomial causes include humidifiers, mechanical ventilators, sinks, irrigating fluids, and cut flowers.

C. **Pathophysiology**
    1. The body attempts to maintain hemodynamic stability, so baroreceptors stimulate catecholamine release from SNS, resulting in:
        a. Increased total PVR, HR, and cardiac contractility
        b. Increased CO and BP, with improved tissue perfusion
    2. Increased BP by vasoconstriction stimulates aldosterone release:
        a. Decreased RBF due to renal arteriolar vasoconstriction stimulates RAA
        b. Increased ADH secretion is stimulated by decreased CO, and causes water retention and arteriolar constriction, increasing volume and BP
    3. Constricted arterioles cause fluid to go from interstitial space into intravascular space, further increasing circulating blood volume.
    4. Blood vessels eventually are unable to maintain vasoconstriction. Vasodilation leads to decreased PVR and blood pressure
    5. Decreased tissue perfusion results in anaerobic metabolism and lactic acidosis.
        a. Acids act as vasodilators, further decreasing venous return and blood flow to tissues.
        b. Hypoxia and acidosis cause histamine and lysosomal enzyme release into extracellular space, resulting in weakened capillary membrane and increased capillary permeability.
    6. Fluid shifts from intravascular to interstitial space, further decreasing blood volume and venous return.
    7. This results in sluggish blood flow and pooling of blood in vessels, leading to clumping and embolus formation.
    8. **Myocardial depressant factor (MDF) is released from the ischemic pancreas, which leads to decreased pumping ability of heart.**

9. Overall ischemic changes include:
   a. **Acute renal failure**
   b. **Adult respiratory distress syndrome**
   c. **Altered metabolic function and coagulopathies because of effect on the liver**
   d. **Release of vasodilating endotoxins, which contribute to shock progression because of effect on the GI tract**
   e. **Confusion, lethargy, and coma secondary to CNS effects**

XVI. Septic shock

A. Description: a life-threatening condition caused by bloodstream invasion by a variety of organisms. It is characterized by decreased systemic vascular resistance (SVR) and altered distribution in vascular volume OR an inadequate state of tissue perfusion. Circulation of endotoxin results in increased capillary permeability and decreased SVR.

B. Etiology and incidence
   1. Sepsis occurs in about 1% of hospitalized patients, with septic shock accounting for a mortality rate approaching 50%, despite aggressive treatment.
   2. Sepsis refers to the presence of pathogenic microorganisms or their toxins in the bloodstream.
   3. Sepsis syndrome is the systemic response to sepsis. This is characterized by tachycardia, fever/hypothermia, tachypnea, and inadequate organ perfusion, decreased mental status, hypoxemia, decreased urine output, or increased serum lactate
   4. Septic shock refers to the sepsis syndrome accompanied by hypotension.

C. Pathophysiology
   1. The body's defense mechanisms stimulate a generalized inflammatory response, which then generates various chemical mediators that may play a role in the multiple alterations occurring with septic shock.
   2. These result from hemodynamic and metabolic events triggered in part by the invading microorganism and by the host's defense system.
   3. Gram-negative bacteria is the most common cause. Staphylococci, streptococci, pneumococci, and clostridia are also frequent contributors to septic shock.
   4. Gram-negative bacteria have endotoxins that produce negative biochemical changes and cause mediator activation that contributes to the development of the shock state.
   5. Gram-negative organisms contain toxins within their cell walls and release them only after cell death.
   6. Gram-positive organisms may also be involved. These produce exotoxins that trigger immune mediators.

D. Assessment (see Table 13-6)
   1. Early stage
      a. Vasodilation leads to decreased PVR and decreased SVR, while BP remains within normal limits due to compensatory increase in CO.

TABLE 13-6.
Comparison of Symptoms: Hyperdynamic (Early)
vs. Hypodynamic (Late) Septic Shock

EARLY	LATE
Higher blood pressure	Hypotension
Tachypnea	Tachypnea
Tachycardia	Tachycardia
Restlessness/feeling of impending doom	Additional decreased level of consciousness
Warm, dry skin	Cool, clammy skin
Respiratory alkalosis	Respiratory acidosis
Shaking	Chills
Rapid hyperthermia	Oliguria
	Coagulation abnormalities

    b.   Hypovolemia begins due to the inflammatory response causing increased capillary permeability, resulting in loss of intravascular volume.

    c.   Inflammatory response mediators are activated and infiltrate the lung tissue and vasculature, resulting in increased capillary permeability.

    d.   Skin is warm, pink, and dry related to vasodilation; increasing temperature with shaking chills.

    e.   The initial pulmonary response is bronchoconstriction, resulting in pulmonary hypertension and increased work of breathing.

    f.   Hyperventilation results in respiratory alkalosis.

2.   Late stage

    a.   **Hypotension develops as cardiac output declines due to increasing vascular space expansion and capillary leakage.**

    b.   Increased PVR and SVR due to catecholamine release secondary to sympathetic nervous system stimulation, in response to hypotension.

    c.   Pulse becomes weak and thready.

    d.   Skin becomes cold, moist, pale, with the developing of mottling and cyanosis.

    e.   Signs of tissue hypoxia and hypooxygenation occur due to hemoglobin, which is reluctant to release oxygen to cells.

    f.   Platelet abnormalities, due to indirect platelet aggregation from endotoxins and subsequent release of vasoactive substances, may occur.

    g.   Circulating platelet aggregates cause obstruction of blood flow and compromised cellular metabolism.

h. Endotoxin or bacterial infectious process itself activates the coagulation system and eventually leads to depletion of clotting factors, which may progress to disseminated intravascular coagulation.

i. Progressive inability to use glucose, protein, and fat as energy sources.

j. Hyperglycemia occurs due to increased gluconeogenesis and insulin resistance, which prevents the uptake of glucose into the cell.

k. Eventually hypoglycemia results, as glycogen stores are depleted and there are insufficient supplies of proteins and fats to meet body's increasing metabolic demands.

l. Protein and fat breakdown eventually results in ketoacidosis and lactic acidosis.

E. **Nursing diagnoses**
1. Decreased Cardiac Output
2. Impaired Gas Exchange
3. Risk for Infection
4. Altered Tissue Perfusion: Cardiopulmonary, Renal, Cerebral
5. Altered Nutrition: Less than Body Requirements
6. Fluid Volume Deficit
7. Impaired Gas Exchange
8. Anxiety/Fear/Powerlessness
9. Ineffective Airway Clearance

F. **Planning and implementation**
1. Assess skin turgor, color, temperature, chills, and peripheral pulses.
2. Culture/sensitivity of any possible sources of infection.
3. Obtain peak and trough blood levels with ordered dose of antibiotic.
4. Monitor antibiotic toxicity, especially with use of aminoglycosides.
5. Must identify and treat the infection sources—therefore administer broad-spectrum antibiotic therapy intravenously until causative organism is identified.
6. Provide measures to decrease hyperthermia: hypothermia blanket, environmental cooling, tepid baths, decreasing metabolic needs.

7. **Observe for signs/symptoms of hypovolemia such as oliguria, thirst, dry tongue, and tachycardia. Must monitor I and O, including insensible fluid losses.**

8. Restore intravascular volume to reverse hypotension:

   a. **Guided by hemodynamic parameters**
   b. **Administer fluids and monitor patient hemodynamic responses**

9. Maintain adequate cardiac output:
   a. Administer and monitor vasoactive IV drugs
   b. Titrate vasoactive drugs based on response and development of potentially dangerous side effects (Display 13-13)

10. **Assess respiratory status and monitor for the development of hypoxia.**
11. Ensure adequate ventilation and oxygenation.

DISPLAY 13-13.
Vasoactive Drugs Used in Treating Shock

	Desired Action in Shock	**Disadvantages**
Sympathomimetics		
Dopamine (Intropin)	Improve contractility, increase stroke volume, increase cardiac output	Increase oxygen demand of the heart
Dobutamine (Dobutrex)		
Epinephrine (Adrenaline)		
Vasodilators		
Nitroprusside (Nipride)	Reduce preload and afterload, reduce oxygen demand of heart	Cause hypotension
Nitroglycerine (Tridil)		
Vasoconstrictors		
Phenylephrine (Neo-Synephrine)	Increase blood pressure by vasoconstriction	Increase afterload, thereby increasing cardiac workload; compromise perfusion to skin, kidneys, lungs, GI tract
Methoxamine (Vasoxyl)		

       a.   Ensure airway patency, augment ventilation, and ensure adequate oxygenation.

       b.   Maintain PaO_2 of at least 80 mm Hg

       c.   Mechanical ventilation with PEEP

12.   Ensure adequate nutrition.

13.   Be aware that steroid use remains controversial.

 14.   **Be aware that shivering may cause increased tissue hypoxia by increasing metabolic demand. Chlorpromazine/thorazine may be necessary to decrease shivering.**

15.   Be aware of potential complications:

       a.   Adult respiratory distress syndrome (ARDS)

       b.   50% risk of developing DIC

       c.   MODS

       d.   Oxygen toxicity

G.   **Evaluation**

   1.   The patient will be able to maintain effective airway clearance.

   2.   Cause of infection is identified and appropriate treatment initiated.

   3.   The patient will be able to maintain optimal fluid balance.

   4.   The patient will be able to maintain adequate oxygenation and normal acid–base balance.

   5.   Effective airway clearance will be maintained.

   6.   The patient will be able to effectively communicate needs and concerns, demonstrating reduced anxiety/fear as evidenced by verbalization of fears and concerns.

H.   **Home health considerations**

   1.   Protect client from nosocomial infection (environmental and normal flora).

   2.   Keep environment dry.

3. Indwelling urinary catheters
   a. Keep above floor level, but do not raise bag above bladder level.
   b. Maintain continuity of drainage system.
   c. Irrigate catheter only if absolutely necessary, using equipment once, then discarding.
   d. Prevent obstructions (kinks) in the tubing.
   e. Maintain perineal hygiene.
4. IV catheters
   a. Change site according to hospital policy/CDC guidelines.
   b. Dressing changes according to hospital policy/CDC guidelines
   c. Handwashing and use of sterile technique as required.

XVII. Hypovolemic shock

A. **Description: a decrease or loss of circulating fluid volume (blood, plasma, water) that results in inadequate systemic tissue perfusion.**

B. **Etiology and incidence**
   1. Hypovolemic shock is the most common type of shock. It is often associated with other causes of decreased tissue perfusion.
   2. Occurs from actual loss of fluid volume, such as occurs with hemorrhage, vomiting, and diarrhea.
   3. Hemorrhagic shock often occurs after trauma, GI bleeding, or rupture of organs/aneurysms.
   4. Often associated with trauma, but other risks include hemorrhage at a fracture site (hip, femur), postoperative blood loss, bleeding postpartum, renal/retroperitoneal bleeding, and GI bleeding.
   5. Stages of hypovolemic shock and major symptomatology are listed in Table 13-7.

C. **Pathophysiology**

   1. **Begins with loss of circulating fluid secondary to decreased body water. Causes include:**
      a. Vomiting and/or diarrhea, diabetic acidosis, diabetes insipidus

TABLE 13-7.
Stages of Hypovolemic Shock
and Major Symptomatology

CLASS	PERCENTAGE OF BLOOD LOSS	TOTAL MAJOR SYMPTOMS
Class I	Up to 15%	Few clinical signs
Class II	15–30%	BP stable, tachycardia
Class IIIq	30–40%	Worsening tachycardia, BP
Class IV	>40%	Immediate threat to life

          b.   Excessive use of diuretics, adrenal insufficiency, heat exhaustion, obstruction, hemorrhage, plasma shifts

   2.   Compensatory mechanisms allow the body to lose up to 10% of circulating blood volume with minimal signs/symptoms of fluid loss.

          a.   The body senses decreased intravascular volume, so the sympathetic nervous system stimulates catecholamine release to maintain cardiac output via vasoconstriction.

          b.   The body also channels fluid from extravascular areas into the vasculature, and stimulates the release of antidiuretic hormone and aldosterone to help retain water and sodium.

          c.   Urine output is a measure of renal blood flow, which depends on CO.

   3.   In patients with hemorrhagic hypovolemia, blood vessels at the hemorrhage site go into spasm in an attempt to stop the bleeding, while platelets adhere to the endothelial walls of damaged vessels and initiate clotting.

          a.   This is reflected in the hematocrit. Early in the hemorrhagic state, the Hct is normal due to loss of equal percentages of RBCs and plasma.

          b.   The Hct drops as the vascular space is reexpanded with fluid and BP may approach normal, but there still are inadequate RBCs available to carry oxygen and nutrients.

          c.   Vasoconstriction consequently shunts blood from the periphery to vital organs.

          d.   If continued, this results in multiple organ dysfunction.

   4.   Early respiratory alkalosis occurs until enough lactic acid accumulates to produce a metabolic acidosis.

D.   Assessment

   1.   **Assess for degree of tachycardia. The faster the heart rate, the more bleeding is occurring.**

   2.   **Patients receiving certain medications, especially beta blockers or calcium channel blockers, may not develop the tachycardia that normally develops with shock.**

   3.   Decreasing CO, CVP, and increasing SVR occur as blood is shunted from the periphery into the core.

   4.   There is initial piloerection as blood is shunted away from the extremities to the center of body, progressing to cold, clammy skin as sympathetic tone decreases vasoconstriction.

   5.   Narrowing of the pulse pressure occurs as bleeding continues.

   6.   **Decreased arterial blood pressure appears only after 30% or more blood volume has been lost.**

E.   Nursing diagnoses

   1.   Fluid Volume Deficit

   2.   Impaired Gas Exchange

   3.   Decreased Cardiac Output

   4.   Impaired Tissue Integrity

   5.   Anxiety/Fear/Powerlessness

   6.   Ineffective Airway Clearance

7.   Pain
8.   Ineffective Individual/Family Coping

F.   Planning and implementation

1.   Monitor I and O, including insensible fluid losses.
2.   Assess for signs and symptoms of hypovolemia.
3.   Restore intravascular volume to reverse hypotension:
   a.   Guided by hemodynamic parameters.
   b.   Administer fluids and monitor patient hemodynamic responses.
   c.   Maintain adequate cardiac output.
   d.   Administer and monitor effects of vasoactive intravenous drugs.
   e.   **Titrate vasoactive drugs based on response and development of potentially dangerous side effects.**
4.   Types of crystalloids/colloids to be administered:
   a.   Lactated Ringer's has electrolytes, but normal saline solution is also used.
   b.   Replace blood, platelets, plasma: type and crossmatch, usually with PRBCs, unless massive hemorrhage necessitates whole blood replacement.
   c.   One unit of packed cells raises the hematocrit about three percentage points.
   d.   FFP is used as a volume expander.
   e.   Albumin.
   f.   Dextran/Hespan: hypertonic colloidal solution that produces an immediate expansion of plasma volume by drawing fluid from interstitial to intravascular spaces.
5.   Use fluid warmer/rapid infusion therapy to maintain core temperature near normal.
6.   **Vasopressors should be used only after fluid volume is adequately replaced, because they may increase blood pressure but do not treat the cause of hemorrhagic shock.**
7.   Note changes in Hgb and Hct. Hct decreases as fluids are given due to dilution. It decreases 1% per liter of LR/NSS used.
8.   **Prevent blood loss by controlling bleeding source; apply pressure as needed.**
9.   Place in modified Trendelenburg: head flat with body flat, legs elevated to 30 degrees, with knees straight to promote venous return.
10.   **Assess respiratory status and monitor for evidence of hypoxia.**
11.   Ensure adequate ventilation and oxygenation.
   a.   Maintain airway patency and administer supplemental oxygen.
   b.   Maintain PaO_2 of at least 80 mm Hg.
   c.   Mechanical ventilation with PEEP.
12.   Administer nutritional supplements as needed.
13.   Assess skin turgor, color, temperature, and peripheral pulses.
14.   Warm fluids before infusion.
15.   Monitor cardiac output and Swan-Ganz measurements.

𝄞 16. Monitor arterial blood gases: initial respiratory alkalosis progressing to metabolic acidosis.

17. Monitor laboratory and diagnostic data:

𝄞 a. **Increased serum sodium indicates hypovolemia due to dehydration**

b. Hyperkalemia secondary to administration of large amounts of blood, or development of acute renal failure

𝄞 c. **Increased BUN reflects dehydration, while creatinine remains WNL in absence of concomitant renal dysfunction**

d. Serum lactate (normal 5–15 mg/100 mL) levels increase with additional anaerobic metabolism; levels correlate with the degree of shock

e. ECG: tachycardia, nonspecific S-T segment or T-wave changes from decreased coronary blood flow

18. Hourly urine output assessment:

𝄞 a. **Under 30 mL/hr is sign of decreased renal perfusion**

b. Urine specific gravity: greater than 1.010 indicates fluid depletion and renal function is normal, as the system tries to conserve fluids

c. Urine osmolality

19. Be aware of potential complications:

a. Adult respiratory distress syndrome (ARDS)

b. 50% risk of developing DIC

c. MODS

d. Oxygen toxicity

G. Evaluation

1. The patient will maintain optimal fluid balance via use of crystalloids and/or colloids.

2. The patient will maintain adequate oxygenation and normal acid–base balance for client.

3. Source of blood loss will be identified and bleeding stopped.

4. The patient will experience reduced anxiety/fear as evidenced by calm and trusting appearance.

5. The patient will maintain effective airway clearance.

6. The patient will maintain optimal fluid balance.

XVIII. **Spinal/neurogenic shock (see Chapter 3)**
XIX. **Cardiogenic shock (see Chapter 4)**
XX. **Anaphylactic shock (see Chapter 9)**
XXI. **Toxic shock syndrome**

A. Description: an acute, severe febrile illness, usually caused by *Staphylococcus aureus* and manifested by a macular palmar rash and hypotension, which may result in shock if undiagnosed and untreated.

B. Etiology and incidence: occurs most often in young, healthy menstruating women using tampons at the time of the event, although there are instances of occurrence in men and in nonmenstruating women who have staphylococcal colonization of mucous membranes.

C. Pathophysiology

1. Most often caused by *Staphylococcus aureus* (coagulase-positive), which is part of the normal flora of skin and mucous membranes.

2. Increasing incidence of methicillin-resistant *S. aureus* infections as cause.

3. Progression of untreated symptoms the same as that of general shock.

D. **Assessment**

 1. Characterized by fever, syncope, hypotension, vomiting, and watery diarrhea.

2. Characterized by inflammation of mucous membranes, and a macular or petechial skin rash, with sloughing of the skin of hands and feet.

E. **Nursing diagnoses**

1. Fluid Volume Deficit
2. Impaired Gas Exchange
3. Impaired Tissue Integrity
4. Risk for Infection
5. Anxiety/Fear/Powerlessness
6. Ineffective Airway Clearance
7. Pain
8. Ineffective Individual/Family Coping

F. **Planning and implementation**

 1. Assess respiratory status and evaluate for development of hypoxemia.

2. Replace volume as ordered with crystalloids and/or colloids.

3. Use fluid warmer/rapid infuser therapy to maintain core temperature near normal.

4. Titrate vasopressors per blood pressure measurements.

5. Identify source of infection and remove if possible.

6. Record daily weights, intake and output.

7. Monitor vital signs and hemodynamic parameters.

8. Place in modified Trendelenburg: head flat with body flat, legs elevated to 30 degrees, with knees straight to promote venous return.

9. Be aware of potential complications:
   a. Septic shock
   b. MODS

G. **Evaluation**

1. The patient will maintain adequate oxygenation and normal acid–base balance.

2. The patient will show no signs or symptoms of infection.

3. The patient will maintain optimal fluid balance.

4. The patient will experience reduced anxiety/fear as evidenced by calm and trusting appearance, and verbalization of fears.

H. **Home health considerations: Teach proper tampon use such as absorbency, maximum time to remain inserted, signs and symptoms of another attack, and use of sanitary pads.**

Bibliography

Bayley, E. W. & Turcke, S. A. (1992). *A comprehensive curriculum for trauma nursing.* Boston: Jones and Bartlett.

Bove, L. A. (1996). Restoring electrolyte balance: Sodium & chloride. *RN* 59(1), 25–29.

Bove, L. A. (1996). Restoring electrolyte balance: Calcium & phosphorous. *RN* 59(3), 47–52.

Bullock, B. L. & Rosendahl, P. P. (1984). *Pathophysiology: Adaptations and alterations in function.* Boston: Little, Brown.

Byers, J. F. & Flynn, M. B. (1996). Acute burn injury: A trauma case report. *Crit Care Nurse* 16(4), 55–65.

Carpenito, L. J. (1995). *Nursing care plans & documentation: Nursing diagnoses and collaborative problems* (2nd ed.). Philadelphia: J. B. Lippincott.

Cerra, F. B. (1987). Hypermetabolism, organ failure, and metabolic support. *World J Surg* 11(2), 173–181.

Conforti Cordisco, M. E. (1994). Fighting DIC. *RN* 57(8), 37–41.

Ferrin, M. S. (1996). Restoring electrolyte balance: Magnesium. *RN* 59(5), 31–35.

Flavell, C. M. Combating hemorrhagic shock. *RN* 54(12), 26–31.

Hosada, N., Nishi, M., & Nakaguwa, M. (1989). Structural and functional alterations in the gut of parenterally or enterally fed rats. *J Surg Res* 47, 129.

Hudak, C. M. & Gallo, B. M. (1994). *Critical care nursing: A holistic approach* (6th ed.). Philadelphia: J. B. Lippincott.

Lickley, H. L. A., Track, N. S., & Vranic, M. (1978). Metabolic responses to enteral and parenteral nutrition. *Am J Surg* 135, 172.

Marino, P. L. (1991). *The ICU book.* Malvern, PA: Lea & Febiger.

North American Nursing Diagnosis Association (NANDA). (1996). *Nursing diagnoses: Definitions & classification 1997–1998.* Philadelphia: Author.

Perez, A. (1995). Hyperkalemia. *RN* 58(11), 33–37.

Shaw, J. H. F. & Wolfe, R. R. (1989). An integrated analysis of glucose, fat, and protein metabolism in severely traumatized patients. *Ann Surg* 209, 63.

Zaloga, G. P. (1994). *Nutrition in critical care.* St. Louis: Mosby.

STUDY QUESTIONS

SCENARIO: Ms. Dolma Sproat, a 57-year-old female, was admitted to your unit yesterday after sustaining a gunshot wound to the abdomen. She underwent surgical repairs of her small bowel and left kidney. Vital signs have been stable postoperatively, ranging from T: 36.8°C–37.6°C PO; pulse 92–100 beats per minute without ectopy; respirations 16–20/minute on oxygen via 4 L/min nasal cannula; BP = 130–152/86–92; O_2 saturation is between 95%–98%

Your latest assessment findings are as follows: T = 39°C PO, pulse 116 (ST without ectopy); respirations 28/min with some use of accessory muscles; BP 150/90.

Ms. Sproat is awake and oriented ×3, but is becoming increasingly restless and agitated. Bibasilar crackles have also developed, and her oxygen saturation has dropped to 92%. In addition, she has no bowel sounds (NGT intact), and her Foley catheter is draining 30–35 mL/hour of cloudy yellow urine

Because of her history and your assessment findings, you suspect that Ms. Sproat is developing ARDS.

1. Which one of the following ABG results is most likely to be found in a client developing early ARDS?
   a. pH = 7.49; $PaCO_2$ = 32 ; PaO_2 = 80 ; HCO_3- = 24
   b. pH = 7.40; $PaCO_2$ = 46 ; PaO_2 = 80 ; HCO_3- = 25
   c. pH = 7.26; $PaCO_2$ = 52 ; PaO_2 = 74 ; HCO_3- = 30
   d. pH = 7.50; $PaCO_2$ = 28 ; PaO_2 = 74 ; HCO_3- = 19

2. The reason for the answer to question #1 is:
   a. Metabolic acidosis is an early indicator for ARDS.
   b. Metabolic alkalosis is an early indicator for ARDS.
   c. Respiratory acidosis is an early indicator for ARDS.
   d. Respiratory alkalosis is an early indicator for ARDS.

3. Which one of the following statements about the development of ARDS is CORRECT?
   a. The lung injury always starts in the pulmonary vasculature.
   b. Increased surfactant production results in alveolar blockage and atelectasis.
   c. Decreased surfactant production results in decreased pulmonary capillary permeability.
   d. Acute lung injury (pulmonary or non-pulmonary) precipitates the disorder.

4. Which of the following assessment findings puts Ms. Sproat at increased risk for developing ARDS?
   a. status post–gunshot wound with spillage of bowel contents
   b. cloudy yellow urine via Foley catheter
   c. age 57 years
   d. elevations in TPR and BP

5. Which one of the following is a positive result of using PEEP in the treatment of ARDS?
   a. cardiac output increases
   b. large airways open
   c. shunting increases
   d. alveoli open

6. Following multiple trauma, you would suspect internal bleeding in a client who exhibits:
   a. blood coming from the wounds
   b. complaints of thirst and tachycardia
   c. complaints of back pain and headache
   d. a drop in pulse and an increase in blood pressure

7. Peritoneal lavage can identify intra-abdominal bleeding from all of the following organs except the:
   a. small intestine
   b. stomach
   c. spleen
   d. kidney

8. Which one of the following statements best describes the pathophysiology occurring during the development of a tension pneumothorax?
   a. Air enters the pleural space with each inspiration through a defect in the chest wall. The air becomes trapped, causing a pressure buildup as the air accumulates.
   b. Air enters the pleural space with each inspiration through a defect in the chest wall. During expiration, air leaves through the same defect causing constant shifting of thoracic structures.
   c. Air enters the pleural space without apparent cause, increasing the negative intrapleural pressure and causing collapse of lung tissue.
   d. Air enters the pleural space due to a rupture of the pleural membrane. Blood quickly accumulates and compresses lung tissues resulting in decreased oxygenation.

9. Burn wounds tend to heal in positions of non-function and:
   a. extension
   b. opposition
   c. contraction
   d. abduction

10. Rank, in order, the priorities for burn wound grafting:
    a. survival, function, appearance
    b. appearance, survival, function
    c. function, survival, appearance
    d. survival, appearance, function

11. Mr. Collins has sustained second and third degree burns over 65% TBSA. His blood pressure drops rapidly after admission to the hospital primarily because of:
    a. severe pain
    b. psychogenic shock
    c. internal hemorrhage
    d. hypovolemic shock

12. Which one of the following patients is most likely to develop multiple organ dysfunction syndrome (MODS)? The patient with:
    a. ARDS caused by pneumothorax
    b. acute renal failure caused by nephrotoxic drug administration
    c. gram-negative sepsis caused by a urinary tract infection
    d. hypovolemia caused by massive hemorrhage

ANSWER KEY

1. **Correct response: a**
   Early ARDS is often indicated by respiratory alkalosis as the person attempts to combat metabolic acidosis by "blowing off" CO_2.
   b, c, and d. Because this is an early finding, the renal system has not had time to begin compensating for the decreased CO_2, so the bicarbonate level will be normal.
   Comprehension/Physiologic/Assessment

2. **Correct Response: d**
   Respiratory alkalosis is present in the early stage of ARDS due to hyperventilation as the person attempts to "blow off" CO_2.
   a and b. The renal system does not have any effect on the bicarb in the early stage.
   c. Because the patient will be hyperventilating, alkalosis (not acidosis) ensues.
   Knowledge/Physiologic/NA

3. **Correct Response: d**
   a. Primary lung injury or pulmonary injury that arises from a secondary disorder (hypovolemic shock) precipitates ARDS development.
   b and c. The disorder may start anywhere in the pulmonary system, and causes decreased surfactant production and increased pulmonary capillary permeability.
   Comprehension/Physiologic/NA

4. **Correct Response: a**
   Sepsis is the major risk factor for the development of ARDS.
   b. Cloudy yellow urine may indicate sepsis as well, but this is not the most likely precipitating factor in the case of Mrs. Sproat.
   c and d. Age itself is not a primary reason, nor are elevations in vital signs.
   Comprehension/Physiologic/Assessment

5. **Correct Response: d**
   PEEP maintains alveolar hyperinflation at low oxygen tensions to minimize atelectasis.
   a. Because of the positive pressure exhibited by PEEP, cardiac output decreases.
   b. PEEP affects the alveoli, not the large airways.
   c. More effective alveolar function decreases shunting.
   Comprehension/Physiologic/Evaluation

6. **Correct Response: b and c**
   a. Any client with obvious bleeding may also have internal bleeding, but there must be more information to make this determination.
   b. Occult bleeding is usually indicated by complaints of thirst and compensatory sympathetic changes in vital signs (increased pulse, increased respiratory rate, and initial increased blood pressure).
   c. Back pain and headache may also signal retroperitoneal or intracranial bleeding.
   d. A decreased BP and increased pulse may signify hemorrhage.
   Analysis/Physiologic/Assessment

7. **Correct Response: d**
   Peritoneal lavage can detect bleeding coming from within the abdomen or abdominal wall, but it cannot reliably detect retroperitoneal bleeding that may come from the kidneys or pancreas.
   Knowledge/Physiologic/Assessment

8. **Correct Response: a**
   The accumulation of air within the pleural space eventually causes excessive positive pressure and a tension pneumothorax.

b, c, and d. There need be no intrinsic chest wall defect, and pleural membrane rupture causes a hemothorax.
Knowledge/Physiologic/Assessment

9. Correct Response: c
Without aggressive physical therapy, burn wounds will eventually form contractures, which are flexion problems.
Comprehension/Physiologic/NA

10. Correct Response: a
The client must survive the burn, then must be able to use the affected area as effectively as possible in the environment. Cosmetic repair is also important, but is necessarily the lowest priority.
Comprehension/Safe care/Planning

11. Correct Response: d
Burns result in massive fluid shift from the intravascular to the interstitial spaces, resulting in hypovolemic shock.

a. Pain is more likely to increase blood pressure.
b. Psychogenic shock does occur with massive burns, but does not contribute to the initial physiologic responses in the acute shock state.
c. Burn wounds do not cause hemorrhage; if massive bleeding occurs, it is due to a secondary complication or other injury.
Comprehension/Physiologic/Assessment

12. Correct Response: c
Although all of these clients are at risk of developing MODS, the most common precipitating factor is gram-negative sepsis, which most often arises from a urinary tract infection.
Application/Physiologic/Assessment

COMPREHENSIVE TEST—QUESTIONS

1. Where is the correct placement for lead V4 when doing an ECG?
   a. 4th ICS, right sternal border
   b. 5th ICS, mid axillary line
   c. 4th ICS, left sternal border
   d. 5th ICS, mid-clavicular line

2. Your patient's ECG shows elevated S-T in leads V1–V4 and ST depression in leads II, III, and AVF. You realize that this indicates:
   a. hyperkalemia
   b. anterior injury
   c. lateral infarction
   d. posterior injury

3. An anterior MI is an occlusion of the:
   a. LAD
   b. RCA
   c. circumflex
   d. all of the above

4. A pacemaker set on the demand mode at the rate of 70 BPM will fire:
   a. continuously at 70 BPM
   b. sporadically as long as the natural heart rate stays above 70 BPM
   c. only if the natural heart rate falls below 70 BPM
   d. every time the patient's atria contract

5. S-T elevation in leads V1, V2, V3, and V4 would indicate:
   a. anterior infarct
   b. lateral ischemia
   c. posterior infarct
   d. anterior injury

6. Identify the rhythm in Figure 1:
   a. bigeminy
   b. A-flutter
   c. normal sinus rhythm
   d. sinus tachycardia

7. S-T elevation in leads II, III, and AVF would indicate:
   a. inferior infarct
   b. lateral ischemia
   c. posterior infarct
   d. anterior injury

8. Identify the rhythm in Figure 2:
   a. bigeminy
   b. A-flutter
   c. normal sinus rhythm
   d. PAT

Answer sheet provided on page 548

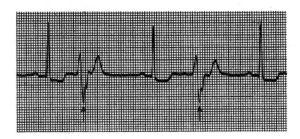

FIGURE 1.

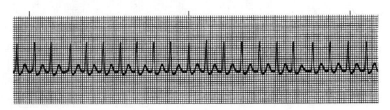

FIGURE 2.

9. While awaiting the implantation of a permanent pacemaker for second-degree heart block, your patient has a transcutaneous temporary pacemaker applied. He is somewhat disoriented, but you note that every time you turn him on his left side he cries out and asks why you are hurting him. The most likely explanation for this may be:
   a. He is suffering from ICU psychosis, a temporary disorder that will resolve spontaneously after being transferred out of ICU.
   b. He was abused as a child and you remind him of his abusive parent.
   c. He is suffering from digoxin toxicity.
   d. When he turns, the pacemaker fails to sense and he receives a shock.

10. You should prepare the patient with Guillain Barré to:
   a. go home in a few days
   b. be a paraplegic for the rest of his life
   c. possibly be intubated in the next few days until his illness resolves
   d. be sent to a nursing home after the acute stage of his illness

11. Plasma pheresis is beneficial:
   a. when used daily for up to 2 months
   b. at separating and discarding antibodies
   c. in the treatment of autonomic dysreflexia (AD)
   d. when used in conjunction with hemodialysis

12. Tensilon 2 mg every 2 minutes until and adequate response is seen is given for:
   a. myasthenia crisis
   b. Guillain-Barré
   c. cholinergic crisis
   d. autonomic dysreflexia

13. Which of the following lab values does not correlate with HELLP syndrome?
   a. increased platelets
   b. increased liver enzymes
   c. decreased Hgb
   d. hemolysis

14. PTH is responsible for each of the following actions except:
   a. increased GI absorption of calcium
   b. promoted excretion of potassium
   c. increased renal resorption of calcium
   d. decreased serum levels of calcium

15. Which of the following catecholamines does not match the listed properties?
   a. Dopamine: vasoconstriction (in large amounts), vasodilation (in small amounts), and increased ionotropic function of the heart
   b. Epinephrine: vasoconstriction, increased heart rate, increased blood glucose
   c. Norepinephrine: vasoconstriction, thereby raising blood pressure
   d. All of the above.

16. Identify the rhythm in Figure 3:
   a. bigeminy
   b. A-flutter
   c. normal sinus rhythm
   d. sinus tachycardia

17. Which of the following statements about pancuronium (Pavulon) is true?

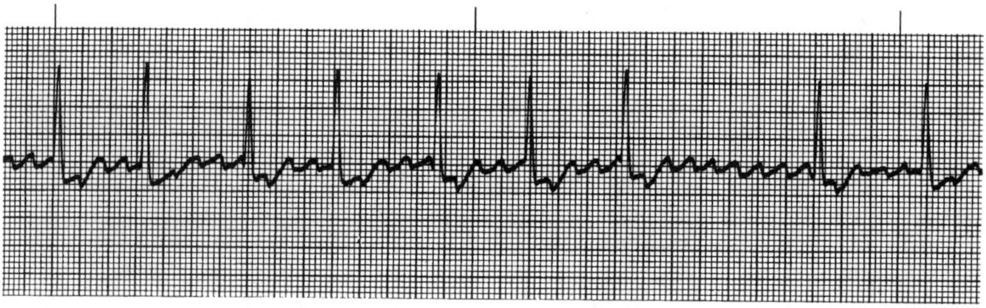

FIGURE 3.

a. Sedation is a necessary adjunct to treatment with Pavulon.

b. Pavulon has no contraindications.

c. The patient being treated with Pavulon should also be on tube feeds due to inability to swallow.

d. You will know that the patient is awake when the patient opens his eyes.

18. If peritoneal dialysate does not readily drain from the abdominal cavity into the drainage bag, the initial nursing intervention is to:

a. Run more fluid into the peritoneal cavity to increase intra-abdominal pressure.

b. Change the client's body position by moving her from side-to-side.

c. Disconnect the drainage tubing and irrigate the catheter with 50 mL of NSS.

d. Assist the client to a standing position and direct her to cough forcefully.

19. Mr. Rivera's K+ level is 5.8 mEq/L before his morning hemodialysis, which he receives three times a week. He asks you why his daily digoxin dose was increased from 0.125 mg to 0.25 mg. Your best response is to say:

a. "Increasing the digoxin will help to push the K+ back into your body cells and decrease your K+ blood levels."

b. "Because of your kidney failure and high K+ level, you need more digoxin to get the same cardiac effects."

c. "Your morning digoxin level was 1.8 mEq/L, which is too low for someone receiving hemodialysis, so the dose was increased."

d. "The digoxin dose is often increased on the day of dialysis so that some of the medication will remain in your system after your treatment."

20. The primary objective of hemodialysis is to:

a. remove excess extracellular fluid

b. prevent cardiotoxic effects from low serum potassium levels

c. decrease serum concentrations of toxic wastes

d. increase circulating blood volume

21. A bloody return from a paracentesis may indicate:

a. peritonitis

b. lacerate liver

c. urosepsis

d. placenta previa

22. Which of the following symptoms would correlate with a tension pneumothorax?

a. hypotension, decreased CO, mediastinal shift to the left

b. hypertension, increased CO, mediastinal shift to the right

c. no change in vital signs, midline trachea

d. tachycardia, hypotension, no tracheal deviation

23. Each of the following would be appropriate nursing interventions for the patient with hypothermia except:

a. Allow shivering to increase the core temperature.

b. Apply warming blankets.

c. Administer warmed IVF.

d. Be aware that no one is "dead" until "warm and dead."

24. An appropriate nursing intervention for a patient with eclampsia would be to:

a. Administer magnesium sulfate 1–2 g/hr/IV.

b. Monitor for respiratory depression.

c. Prepare to administer Valium 10 mg/IV for seizure activity.

d. All of the above.

25. A patient is admitted with DKA. Pre-insulin drip lab values are as follows: serum glucose 739 mg/100 mL, serum potassium 3.8 mEq/L, serum ketones 4.5 mg/dL, and magnesium 1.8 mEq/L. The nurse should monitor the patient for development of the following:

a. hypermagnesemia

b. hypokalemia

c. ketonemia

d. hyperglycemia

26. Glucose should be added to the IVF of a patient with DKA when serum glucose reaches:
    a. 300–350 mg/100 mL
    b. 100–150 mg/100 mL
    c. 200–250 mg/100 mL
    d. The patient in DKA should not have glucose in the infusion.

27. Potential risks for lowering serum glucose levels too rapidly in the patient with DKA include:
    a. cerebral edema
    b. circulatory collapse
    c. hypoglycemia
    d. all of the above

28. Abnormal metabolism in MODS causes:
    a. production of low carbon dioxide levels
    b. consumption of large amounts of oxygen
    c. breakdown of carbohydrates into glucose
    d. positive nitrogen balance (anabolism)

29. In a patient experiencing angina pectoris, the ECG should reveal:
    a. prolonged Q-T interval
    b. prolonged P-R interval
    c. S-T depression
    d. S-T elevation

30. Renal failure secondary to hypovolemia would be considered:
    a. prerenal
    b. intrarenal
    c. postrenal
    d. hyponephrosis

31. The purpose of erythropoietin is to:
    a. increase vitamin B12 levels
    b. increase Hct
    c. decrease renal hypertension
    d. increase folic acid availability

32. Any of the following pathologies may cause rhabdomyolysis except:
    a. alcoholic coma
    b. status epilepticus
    c. heroin overdose
    d. first day postoperative patient with a history of smoking

33. The body's response to MODS is always the result of:

a. pathologic events stimulated by the release of endotoxin
b. controlled mediator release
c. feedback mechanisms that slow mediator release
d. events that normally help the body recover from an insult

34. Catecholamines (epinephrine and norepinephrine) act to:
    a. decrease blood pressure
    b. promote coagulation
    c. trigger vasodilation
    d. increase heart rate

35. Your patient's ABGs reveal an acidic pH, an acidic CO_2, and a normal bicarbonate level. Which one of the following indicates this acid–base disturbance?
    a. respiratory acidosis
    b. respiratory alkalosis
    c. metabolic acidosis
    d. metabolic alkalosis

36. Ms. Marge Collins is admitted to your unit after suffering from severe diarrhea (over 1000 mL per day) for 2 days. Which of the following respiratory findings do you expect to find?
    a. increased rate and depth
    b. decreased rate and depth
    c. increased rate and decreased depth
    d. decreased rate and increased depth

37. What assessment finding of a patient with acute pancreatitis would indicate a bluish discoloration around the umbilicus?
    a. Grey-Turner's sign
    b. Homans's sign
    c. Rovsing's sign
    d. Cullen's sign

38. You are assessing a patient with a diagnosis of hepatitis B. Which of the following signs and symptoms would best help identify this diagnosis?
    a. light-colored urine
    b. asterixis
    c. hepatosplenomegaly
    d. elevated alpha-fetoprotein

39. Which of the following responses by a patient with an acute myocardial infarction would indicate that additional teaching is needed? "I will . . .

a. ... gradually increase my activities."

b. ... put nitroglycerin under my tongue when I get chest pain."

c. ... call my doctor if I have any changes in my pulse."

d. ... stop taking my medication for a day if I have any problems."

40. A patient has massive left ventricular failure. A nursing priority would be to assess for signs and symptoms of (a):

a. cardiogenic shock

b. Dressler's syndrome

c. ventricular aneurysm

d. interventricular septal rupture

41. Which one of the following is most likely to cause respiratory alkalosis?

a. airway obstruction (biting on endotracheal tube)

b. pulmonary edema from receiving too much intravenous fluid in a short time period

c. excessive tidal volume in a mechanically ventilated patient

d. overuse of antacids, especially those containing aluminum hydroxide

42. Mrs. Edna Haas has been receiving mechanical ventilation because of an exacerbation of COPD. Which one of the following statements about ventilator weaning is correct, based on her latest ABG results of pH = 7.40; $PaCO_2$ = 42; PaO_2 = 80; and HCO3− = 24? Weaning from the ventilation is:

a. Indicated; her normal ABGs indicate readiness.

b. Not indicated; her respiratory acidosis must be corrected for stimulation of her respiratory drive.

c. Not indicated; her normal PaO_2 and $PaCO_2$ will decrease her respiratory drive.

d. Indicated; her respiratory acidosis will stimulate her respiratory drive.

43. Which one of the following problems is most likely when a client has a 30-minute period of hyperventilation?

a. respiratory acidosis

b. respiratory alkalosis

c. compensated respiratory acidosis

d. compensated respiratory alkalosis

44. Which one of the following meals is best for a client with chronic respiratory insufficiency?

a. roast pork, baked beans, applesauce, skim milk

b. grilled hamburger, French fries, cole slaw, whole milk

c. baked chicken, buttered lima beans, pineapple chunks, skim milk

d. baked fish, lettuce and tomato salad, orange slices, whole milk

45. When preparing cyclosporine, an immunosuppressant agent, for a liver transplant patient, you must be aware that this drug is:

a. administered in a glass container

b. administered IV bolus over 20 to 30 minutes

c. directly infused via the hepatic artery

d. used as rescue therapy in acute rejection

46. A patient with severe cirrhosis of the liver develops hepatorenal syndrome. Which of the following nursing assessment data would support this?

a. oliguria and azotemia

b. metabolic alkalosis

c. decreased urinary concentration

d. weight gain of <1 lb/week

47. A clinical manifestation of acute pancreatitis is epigastric pain. Your nursing intervention to facilitate relief of pain would place the patient in a:

a. knee-chest position

b. semi-Fowler's position

c. recumbent position

d. low-Fowler's position

48. Which phase of hepatitis would the nurse incur strict precautionary measures at?

a. icteric

b. non-icteric

c. post-icteric

d. pre-icteric

49. Which one of the following statements is true when assessing the oxygen needs of the anemic client?

a. Pulse oximetry is just as accurate as arterial blood gases.

b. Arterial blood gas tests are more accurate than pulse oximetry.

c. Both arterial blood gas tests and pulse oximetry are equally accurate.

d. Pulse oximetry should never be used.

50. Your client's ventilator alarm begins sounding continuously. Which one of the following is the correct initial response?

a. Call respiratory therapy STAT.

b. Suction the client.

c. Assess the client.

d. Check the ventilatory tubing for kinks or water.

51. Synchronized intermittent mandatory ventilation (SIMV):

a. helps to maintain diaphragmatic strength

b. ensures that the client receives the same tidal volume with every breath

c. allows the client to speak during spontaneous breathing

d. may cause discomfort if the client tries to exhale during the mandatory inhalation time

52. The assist-control (A/C) mode of mechanical ventilation:

a. allows for spontaneous breathing at lower tidal volumes

b. prevents the client from initiating a breath

c. ensures that the client receives the same tidal volume with each breath

d. promotes maximum alveolar inflation throughout both inspiratory and expiratory cycles

53. Percutaneous transluminal coronary angioplasty would NOT be recommended for a patient with:

a. cardiogenic shock

b. unstable angina responsive to treatment

c. coronary artery bypass graft closure

d. reocclusion after thrombolytic therapy

54. A patient is admitted with a cardiac contusion as a result of a motor vehicle accident. Your assessment reveals muffled heart sounds, pulsus paradoxus, and hypotension. Based on these findings the nurse would prepare the patient for a:

a. pericardectomy

b. pericardial window

c. chest tube insertion

d. pericardiocentesis

55. Which of the following admission data would support placement on a heart transplantation list? A patient with a history of:

a. Printzmetal's angina

b. coronary artery occlusion

c. cardiomyopathy

d. Dressler's syndrome

56. A patient is being treated for hepatic encephalopathy. Based on your knowledge of this disease, the laboratory tests you would closely monitor would be:

a. partial thromboplastin time

b. fibrinogen split products

c. direct and indirect bilirubin

d. ammonia levels

57. Which one of the following is most important when teaching the family of the client receiving mechanical ventilation?

a. Discourage them from placing the client's personal items at the bedside because these are potential sources of infection.

b. Reinforce the danger of accidentally disconnecting ventilatory tubes when standing at the bedside.

c. Encourage them to touch the client and speak to her about daily events, even if she does not appear to be responsive.

d. Reinforce the need to promote a positive outlook, even if the prognosis is poor.

58. Your client is placed on mechanical ventilation after having a right-sided partial pneumonectomy. Which one of the following positions promotes optimal oxygenation for this client?

a. left side–lying

b. semi-Fowler's

c. supine

d. right side–lying

59. Your client has been diagnosed with left lower lobe pneumonia. You expect breath sounds in this lobe to be:
 a. hyperresonant
 b. bronchial
 c. clear
 d. absent

60. Your client is on an aminophylline drip. His morning theophylline level is 15 mcg/mL. Your first action is to:
 a. Notify the physician; the client probably needs a higher dosage.
 b. Notify the physician; the client probably needs a lower dosage.
 c. Request that the physician switch the client to oral theophylline.
 d. Leave the results on the chart so the physician can see them on her next visit.

61. Which nursing intervention would NOT be included for a post–transesophageal echocardiography patient?
 a. Immediately feed the patient; she is hungry.
 b. Remind the patient that her throat will be sore.
 c. Inform the patient that the physician will tell her the results of the test.
 d. Inform the patient to tell the nurse if she has any chest pain.

62. A priority nursing intervention for a patient with a dissecting thoracic aneurysm would be:
 a. Prepare the patient for chest tube insertion.
 b. Monitor urinary output.
 c. Administer nitroprusside sodium (Nipride).
 d. Administer dopamine hydrochloride.

63. A nursing diagnosis for a patient with cardiomyopathy (CMP) is Ineffective Breathing Pattern. Your nursing care would include:
 a. Report urinary output <50 mL/hr.
 b. Monitor vital signs q4hr after activity.
 c. Report a weight gain over 2 lb.

 d. Assess for jugular vein distention and dependent edema.

64. Which of the following should be at the bedside of a postoperative coronary artery bypass graft (CABG) patient?
 a. temporary pacer box
 b. hemostats to clamp the chest tubes
 c. warming blanket
 d. intraaortic balloon pump (IABP)

65. Which one of the following is the most common initial finding in a client with a pulmonary embolus (PE)?
 a. sudden severe dyspnea and chest pain
 b. chest pain with unequal chest expansion
 c. petechiae over the upper chest and shoulders
 d. gradually ascending leg pain

66. Your client asks you why he needs to have a ventilation-perfusion (V/Q) scan. Your most accurate response is to say, "The test will help to determine. . .
 a. . . . if there is a blood clot in your lung tissue."
 b. . . . if there is a blood clot in one of the large vessels of your lungs."
 c. . . . whether you may need mechanical ventilation to help more oxygen get into your circulation."
 d. . . . if your lungs can get enough oxygen when you breathe."

67. Mr. Burns, a client with emphysema, was recently extubated. His latest arterial blood gase tests (ABGs) are pH = 7.36; $PaCO_2$ = 49; PaO_2 = 72; and HCO3– = 29. Until you can report these results to the physician, you should:
 a. Call anesthesia STAT for possible reintubation.
 b. Place Mr. Burns on oxygen at 5 L/min to correct his hypoxia.
 c. Continue with routing care; these results are probably normal for Mr. Burns.
 d. Place Mr. Burns in high-Fowler's position; improved gas exchange will decrease his $PaCO_2$.

68. Nineteen-year-old Juan Lopez has been receiving mechanical ventilation for 24 hours because of emergency surgery that resulted in a thoracotomy. Which one of the following statements is correct, based on Juan's latest ABG results of pH = 7.43; $PaCO_2$ = 36; PaO_2 = 86; and HCO3– = 24? Weaning from the ventilator is

a. Indicated; his normal ABGs indicate readiness.

b. Not indicated; his respiratory alkalosis must be corrected to stimulate his respiratory drive.

c. Not indicated; his normal PaO_2 and $PaCO_2$ will decrease his respiratory drive, predisposing him to the development of ARDS.

d. Indicated; his respiratory alkalosis will stimulate his respiratory drive.

69. An AIDS-related condition that causes purplish macular or papular lesions on the extremities and can invade internal organs is called:

a. Burkitt's lymphoma

b. herpes simplex virus

c. Kaposi's sarcoma

d. candidiasis

70. What is the most common cause of an acute myocardial infarction?

a. coronary artery spasm

b. atherosclerotic plaques

c. stress thallium 20l test

d. platelet aggregation

71. The physician orders pain medication for an AMI patient. Which of the following medications would you anticipate administering to the patient?

a. diltiazem

b. Inderal

c. nitroglycerin

d. morphine sulfate

72. A patient is receiving a thrombolytic agent. Which of the following laboratory tests would you evaluate first?

a. increased prothrombin time and partial thromboplastin time

b. increased hemoglobin and hematocrit

c. decreased erythrocyte sedimentation rate

d. decreased white blood cell count

73. Which one of the following must be part of the teaching plan for a client receiving isoniazid (INH)?

a. The urine will turn reddish-brown.

b. The development of a rash is not of concern.

c. Periodic chest x-rays are needed.

d. Periodic liver function tests are needed.

74. Which one of the following treatment measures has the highest priority for a client with tuberculosis?

a. taking medications as prescribed

b. having sufficient rest

c. eating nourishing diet

d. living where there is clean, fresh air

75. Your HIV-negative client is started on a multiple drug regimen for treatment of TB. He needs to know that the average length of time for effective chemotherapy is:

a. 1–6 months

b. 9–12 months

c. 12–18 months

d. 16–24 months

76. Which one of the following statements about *Mycobacterium tuberculosis* is true?

a. It can be transmitted by droplet nuclei, blood, or urine.

b. It is able to lie dormant within the body for up to 2 weeks.

c. It is preventable with anti-tuberculin vaccination.

d. It requires oxygen to survive.

77. Your client diagnosed with AIDS is taking the drug zidovudine (Retrovir). He must be monitored for which one of the following side effects?

a. anemia

b. hypokalemia

c. hypoglycemia

d. lymphocytopenia

78. Which one of the following statements is it appropriate to use when teaching your asymptomatic, HIV-positive, pregnant client?

   a. "You should seriously consider terminating the pregnancy because your baby will carry the HIV virus."

   b. "There is a chance that your baby will test negative for HIV."

   c. "You will have to take AZT during your pregnancy in order to have an HIV-negative baby."

   d. "What kinds of support services will help you to care for the baby once you develop AIDS?"

79. Cervical node biopsy results that confirm the diagnosis of Hodgkin's disease reveal the presence of:

   a. Epstein-Barr cells

   b. Reed-Sternberg cells

   c. Bence Jones proteins

   d. small oat cell proteins

80. Which one of the following is an appropriate nursing intervention for a client with severe bone marrow depression from treatment of multiple myeloma?

   a. Test urine and stool for the presence of occult blood.

   b. Take rectal temperatures to assess for the development of infection.

   c. Encourage a diet high in calcium to increase bone marrow activity.

   d. Encourage activity to promote the return of calcium from the blood vessels into the bones.

81. A Mantoux (PPD) tuberculin test reveals an induration of 15 mm, which indicates that:

   a. Active disease is present.

   b. There was contact with the tubercle bacillus.

   c. Preventive treatment must be initiated.

   d. The reaction is doubtful and should be repeated

82. Which one of the following is the primary reason for the recent outbreaks of multi-drug resistant tuberculosis (MDR-TB)?

   a. increased incidence of AIDS, which makes effective treatment of TB impossible

   b. lack of compliance with prior antitubercular medication treatment, resulting in the development of new TB strains

   c. increased incidence of homelessness, which makes direct observational therapy (DOT) difficult to maintain

   d. lack of TB research funding, due to the greater need to find a cure for HIV/AIDS

83. The diagnosis of *M. tuberculosis* is confirmed by:

   a. the presence of mycobacterium tuberculosis in a sputum culture

   b. the presence of acid-fast bacilli in a sputum smear

   c. three consecutive monthly chest x-rays

   d. three PPD tests that yield indurations of 10 mm or greater

84. Which one of the following vitamins is needed during treatment with the drug isoniazid (INH)?

   a. vitamin B1

   b. vitamin B2

   c. vitamin B6

   d. vitamin B12

85. Fever, cough, and chest pain are symptoms related to which opportunistic infection?

   a. Kaposi's sarcoma (KS)

   b. *Pneumocystis carinii* pneumonia (PCP)

   c. cytomegalovirus (CMV)

   d. cryptosporidiosis

86. Mr. Cruz is admitted to your floor with malnutrition, anorexia, and AIDS. When the physician tells you that he is considering the use of TPN for Mr. Cruz, your best response is to say:

   a. "TPN is an appropriate nutritional option for most clients with AIDS and persistent diarrhea."

   b. "Parenteral nutrition is not as effective a nutritional therapy as is enteral feeding."

c. "TPN should only be used for those clients who cannot tolerate enteral feedings because of malabsorption problems."

d. "The use of TPN may have some drawbacks, but it seems to be the best option for Mr. Cruz."

87. Which one of the following statements is most appropriate when teaching the client with cryptosporidium enteritis?

a. "You may need intravenous nutrition (TPN) because there is no cure for your severe diarrhea."

b. "You need to give us a stool specimen so that the physician can order appropriate, curative antibiotics."

c. "You will probably be started on Amphotericin B intravenously to kill the cryptosporidium protozoa."

d. "As long as you continue to eat a variety of foods and take vitamin-mineral supplements, you need not worry about the diarrhea."

88. Planning care for the client with AIDS is based on the understanding that:

a. AIDS indicates an infection with human immunodeficiency virus (HIV) only.

b. Human immunodeficiency virus and at least two opportunistic infections are present.

c. Clients with AIDS always have multiple concurrent infections.

d. Human immunodeficiency virus and a CD4 lymphocyte count under $200/mm^3$ are present.

89. A client with tuberculosis is no longer considered infectious after:

a. 1 week of treatment with at least four antitubercular medications

b. 2 weeks of treatment with two antitubercular medications

c. three consecutive negative sputum specimens

d. repeat PPD tests show no additional induration

90. Which one of the following measures helps to decrease hypercalcemia?

a. use of IV NSS or LR

b. use of thiazide diuretics

c. promotion of bedrest

d. all of the above

91. Signs and symptoms of superior vena cava (SVC) syndrome include all of the following except:

a. edema of head and neck

b. dyspnea

c. hypertension

d. chest pain

92. An HLA-matched allogeneic bone marrow transplant means that:

a. The donor and recipient are siblings.

b. The donor and recipient are not necessarily related.

c. The donor and recipient are identical twins.

d. More information is needed to answer the question.

93. Which one of the following persons is most likely to become infected with HIV?

a. A 19-year-old woman with multiple sexual partners who use condoms.

b. A 44-year-old impotent IV drug abuser who does not share needles.

c. A 56-year-old post-menopausal woman who has one HIV-infected long-term male sexual partner.

d. A 25-year-old male who has one HIV-infected long-term female sexual partner.

94. Your anemic patient verbalized concern about receiving blood from "someone who has the HIV virus." Which one of the following is the most appropriate initial response?

a. "You can have family members donate blood if it will make you feel better about receiving a transfusion."

b. "You can refuse to receive a blood transfusion if you are afraid of contracting AIDS."

c. "Don't worry, you cannot get AIDS from a blood transfusion."

d. "Although all blood is tested for the HIV antigen, there is no guarantee that a unit of blood is free of these antibodies."

95. Mr. Carter, who is gay, admits to you that he has been unfaithful to his lover during their 5-year relationship. Which one of the following questions should be asked first?
    a. "Have you used condoms with nonoxynol-9 during these affairs?"
    b. "Have you been tested for HIV?"
    c. "Is your lover aware of your unfaithfulness?"
    d. "What makes you bring up this topic?"

96. The most chronic sign associated with HIV infection is:
    a. persistent generalized lymphadenopathy.
    b. *Pneumocystis carinii* pneumonia
    c. cryptosporidiosis
    d. Kaposi's sarcoma

97. Whch of the following describes the sequence of progression in anaphylactic shock?
    a. bronchospasm, increased capillary permeability, smooth muscle constriction
    b. increased capillary permeability, bronchospasm, hypotension
    c. increased capillary permeability, smooth muscle constriction, hypotension
    d. Any of the above may occur, depending on the initial stimulus.

98. Which one of the following is the final step in the attack of HIV on the immune system?
    a. encounters and invades a T4 cell
    b. is engulfed by the phagocyte
    c. fuses its RNA with the host cell's DNA
    d. is replicated by the host cell

99. Which one of the following is the most precise indicator for the diagnosis of AIDS?
    a. CD4 cell count below $200/mm^3$
    b. positive HIV test (ELISA)
    c. positive western blot test
    d. positive p24 antigen test

100. Mr. Eldorado has been HIV-positive for the past 2 years and currently is admitted for persistent diarrhea. His CD4 count is $600/mm^3$, which is a decrease from his $800/mm^3$ level of a year ago. You anticipate that Mr. Eldorado:
    a. is at high risk for AIDS because his CD4 count is under $800/mm^3$
    b. may develop more frequent opportunistic infections as his CD4 count decreases
    c. will be started on PCP prophylactic therapy based on his current CD4 count
    d. will be diagnosed with AIDS based on his present CD4 count and the CDC definition of the disease

Answer Sheet for Comprehensive Exam

With a pencil, blacken the circle under the option you have chosen for your correct answer.

	A	B	C	D		A	B	C	D		A	B	C	D
1.	○	○	○	○	22.	○	○	○	○	43.	○	○	○	○
2.	○	○	○	○	23.	○	○	○	○	44.	○	○	○	○
3.	○	○	○	○	24.	○	○	○	○	45.	○	○	○	○
4.	○	○	○	○	25.	○	○	○	○	46.	○	○	○	○
5.	○	○	○	○	26.	○	○	○	○	47.	○	○	○	○
6.	○	○	○	○	27.	○	○	○	○	48.	○	○	○	○
7.	○	○	○	○	28.	○	○	○	○	49.	○	○	○	○
8.	○	○	○	○	29.	○	○	○	○	50.	○	○	○	○
9.	○	○	○	○	30.	○	○	○	○	51.	○	○	○	○
10.	○	○	○	○	31.	○	○	○	○	52.	○	○	○	○
11.	○	○	○	○	32.	○	○	○	○	53.	○	○	○	○
12.	○	○	○	○	33.	○	○	○	○	54.	○	○	○	○
13.	○	○	○	○	34.	○	○	○	○	55.	○	○	○	○
14.	○	○	○	○	35.	○	○	○	○	56.	○	○	○	○
15.	○	○	○	○	36.	○	○	○	○	57.	○	○	○	○
16.	○	○	○	○	37.	○	○	○	○	58.	○	○	○	○
17.	○	○	○	○	38.	○	○	○	○	59.	○	○	○	○
18.	○	○	○	○	39.	○	○	○	○	60.	○	○	○	○
19.	○	○	○	○	40.	○	○	○	○	61.	○	○	○	○
20.	○	○	○	○	41.	○	○	○	○	62.	○	○	○	○
21.	○	○	○	○	42.	○	○	○	○	63.	○	○	○	○

	A	B	C	D
64.	○	○	○	○
65.	○	○	○	○
66.	○	○	○	○
67.	○	○	○	○
68.	○	○	○	○
69.	○	○	○	○
70.	○	○	○	○
71.	○	○	○	○
72.	○	○	○	○
73.	○	○	○	○
74.	○	○	○	○
75.	○	○	○	○
76.	○	○	○	○

	A	B	C	D
77.	○	○	○	○
78.	○	○	○	○
79.	○	○	○	○
80.	○	○	○	○
81.	○	○	○	○
82.	○	○	○	○
83.	○	○	○	○
84.	○	○	○	○
85.	○	○	○	○
86.	○	○	○	○
87.	○	○	○	○
88.	○	○	○	○

	A	B	C	D
89.	○	○	○	○
90.	○	○	○	○
91.	○	○	○	○
92.	○	○	○	○
93.	○	○	○	○
94.	○	○	○	○
95.	○	○	○	○
96.	○	○	○	○
97.	○	○	○	○
98.	○	○	○	○
99.	○	○	○	○
100.	○	○	○	D

COMPREHENSIVE TEST—ANSWER KEY

1. *Correct response: d*
Lead V4 placement is at the 5th ICS, midclavicular line.
- **a.** This is the correct placement for lead V1.
- **b.** This is the correct placement for lead V6.
- **c.** This is the correct placement for lead V2.

Knowledge/Safe care/Assessment

2. *Correct response: b*
An anterior injury will be evident with elevated S-T in the anterior leads (V1–V4) and S-T depression in the reciprocal leads (II, III, AVF).
- **a.** Hyperkalemia is evident in peaked P and T waves.
- **c.** Lateral injury is evident in S-T elevation in leads I, AVL, V5 and V6, with reciprocal changes in leads II, III, and AVF.
- **d.** Posterior injury would be evident in predominant R waves in leads VI–V2.

Application/Physiologic/Assessment

3. *Correct response: a*
An anterior MI is an occlusion of the LAD.
- **b.** An occlusion of the RCA would cause a posterior or inferior MI.
- **c.** An occlusion of the circumflex would cause a posterior or lateral MI.

Knowledge/Physiologic/NA

4. *Correct response: c*
A pacemaker set on demand mode will only fire if the patient's heart rate falls below the set rate.
- **a.** This indicates a fixed rate; it will fire at 70 BPM no matter what the patient's heart rate is.
- **b.** No functioning pacemaker fires sporadically.

- **d.** This indicates a ventricular pacemaker set to fire after the P wave. This would be used in a patient with a functioning SA node with a lower block.

Knowledge/Safe care/NA

5. *Correct response: a*
S-T elevation is indicative of myocardial infarction. Leads V1–V4 are the anterior leads.
- **b.** The lateral leads are leads I, AVL, V5, and V6. Ischemia is signified by T-wave inversion.
- **c.** The posterior changes are exactly opposite the anterior ones because the posterior of the heart is directly behind the anterior. Therefore, a posterior infarct would be indicated by V1–V2 depression.
- **d.** Anterior injury is signified by S-T and T wave inversion in leads V1–V4.

Knowledge/Physiologic/Assessment

6. *Correct response: a*
Bigeminy is indicated by a PVC every other beat.
- **b.** A flutter has more than one visible P wave to every QRS. These QRSs are wider than normal.
- **c.** NSR would have a P wave followed by a QRS and then a T wave.
- **d.** Sinus tachycardia has normal P waves followed by normal QRSs at a rate greater than 100 beats per minute.

Knowledge/Physiologic/Assessment

7. *Correct response: a*
S-T elevation is indicative of myocardial infarction. Leads II, III, and AVF are the inferior leads.
- **b.** The lateral leads are leads I, AVL, V5, and V6. Ischemia is signified by T-wave inversion.

c. The posterior changes are exactly opposite the anterior ones because the posterior of the heart is directly behind the anterior. Therefore, a posterior infarct would be indicated by V1–V2 depression.

d. Anterior injury is signified by S-T and T-wave inversion in leads V1–V4.

Application/Physiologic/Assessment

8. *Correct response: d*
   PAT (paroxysmal atrial tachycardia) is defined as a rate greater than 150–250 BPM, originating in the atria. P:P and R:R are regular.
   a. Bigeminy is indicated by a PVC every other beat.
   b. A flutter has more than one visible P wave to every QRS (these QRSs are wider than normal).
   c. NSR would have a P wave followed by a QRS and then a T wave.

Knowledge/Physiologic/Assessment

9. *Correct response: d*
   When he turns, the pacemaker may move away from the heart and fail to sense his natural rhythm.
   a, b. If every time you turn him the same thing happens, that would indicate a stimulus for his response.
   c. Digoxin is contraindicated in heart block; the classic signs of digoxin toxicity include nausea, vomiting, bradycardia, and visual disturbances.

Analysis/Physiologic/Evaluation

10. *Correct response: c*
    The ascending paralysis in Guillain-Barré may ascend past the respiratory and cranial nerves.
    a, b. Guillain-Barré may effect the patient for as long as 6 months to 1 year.
    d. This patient will need rehabilitation after recovery but can expect to eventually regain all body functions.

Comprehension/Physiologic/Planning

11. *Correct response: b*
    Plasma pheresis separates, discards antibodies in such disorders as Guillain-Barré and myasthenia gravis.

a. Plasma pheresis is used only 3–4 times, 1–2 days apart, during the onset of symptoms.

c, d. Plasma pheresis is not indicated for AD and hemodialysis is not indicated for Guillain-Barré or myasthenia gravis.

Knowledge/Physiologic/NA

12. *Correct response: a*
    Tensilon is the treatment for myasthenia crisis.
    b. Tensilon has no effect on Guillain-Barré.
    c. Cholinergic crisis is caused by an overdose of anticholinesterase (tensilon), treatment is to hold medications.
    d. The treatment for AD is to remove the "trigger."

Knowledge/Physiologic/Intervention

13. *Correct response: a*
    HELLP syndrome is characterized by hemolysis, elevated liver enzymes, and low platelets. Post-delivery care includes supportive measures and administration of blood products.

Knowledge/Physiologic/Assessment

14. *Correct response: d*
    PTH acts to increase serum calcium levels.
    a. This is correct.
    b, c. PTH promotes renal excretion of phosphorous, potassium, and sodium bicarbonate and increases renal resorption of calcium, magnesium, and hydrogen, raising the serum levels of each.

Knowledge/Physiologic/NA

15. *Correct response: b*
    Epinephrine causes vasodilation, not vasoconstriction.
    a, c. Functions and catecholamines are accurate.

Knowledge/Physiologic/NA

16. *Correct response: b*
    A flutter has more than one visible P wave to every QRS (these QRSs are wider than normal).

a. Bigeminy is indicated by a PVC every other beat.

c. NSR would have a P wave followed by a QRS and then a T wave.

d. Sinus tachycardia has normal P waves followed by normal QRSs at a rate greater than 100 BPM.

Knowledge/Physiologic/Assessment

17. Correct response: a
Pavulon is a neuromuscular blocking agent. When used appropriately the patient will be completely, temporarily paralyzed but will feel pain and will need continuous sedation to decrease the anxiety associated with being unable to move.

b. Pavulon is contraindicated in an unventilated patient. It is also contraindicated in patients with myasthenia gravis.

c. Tube feeds are contraindicated with pavulon due to the potential for a paralytic ileous. Nutrition should be via IVF.

d. The patient's eyelids will be paralyzed. If he is able to open his eyes, he is undermedicated.

Knowledge/Physiologic/Intervention

18. Correct response: b
a. Running more fluid into the peritoneum will result in additional positive cumulative balance and respiratory distress.

c. The drainage tubing should never be disconnected without the physician's order and should not forcefully be flushed.

d. Changing positions is helpful, but encouraging the client to stand lowers the level of the dialysate due to gravity and the cough could dislodge the catheter.

Application/Safe care/Intervention

19. Correct response: b
Renal failure leads to chronic hyperkalemia, which increases resistance to cardiac glycosides. Additional medica-

tion is needed to maintain a therapeutic level of 1.8–2.4mEq/L

Application/Physiologic/Intervention

20. Correct response: c
The major reason for hemodialysis is to enhance release of toxins that cannot be removed by the kidneys.

a, c. Removal of fluid is a secondary benefit.

d. The client in renal failure will be hyperkalemic.

Knowledge/Physiologic/NA

21. Correct response: b
Paracentesis is useful in determining intra-abdominal bleeding.

a, c. Does not indicate peritonitis or urosepsis.

d. Contraindicated in pregnancy.

Comprehension/Physiologic/Evaluation

22. Correct response: a
A tension pneumothorax causes pressure in the chest, resulting in a decreased CO and hypotension with a trachea deviated away from the pressure.

b. BP and CO would be decreased, and a mediastinal shift could be to the right or left, depending on the location of the pneumothorax.

c. These are normal parameters.

d. A variety of disorders may cause tachycardia and hypotension.

Application/Physiologic/Assessment

23. Correct response: a
Shivering increases cardiac workload, O_2 consumption, metabolic demands, and CO_2 production

b, c, d. These are appropriate nursing interventions.

Application/Physiologic/Intervention

24. Correct response: d
a. $MgSO_4$ is the drug of choice to prevent seizure activity in eclamptic patients.

b. Respiratory depression is a side effect of $MgSO_4$.

c. During seizure activity administration of Valium is an appropriate intervention.

*Comprehension/Physiologic/
Implementation*

25. *Correct response: b*
The insulin will carry the potassium into the cells with the glucose; potassium replacement may be necessary.

  a. Some magnesium will be lost during diuresis; magnesium replacement may be necessary.

  c, d. This patient already has elevated levels of ketones and glucose; the insulin drip should reduce both levels.

Application/Physiologic/Assessment

26. *Correct response: c*
Dextrose is necessary at this point to prevent a hypoglycemic episode.

  a. This glucose level is still to high for a glucose infusion to be appropriate.

  b. This patient is at risk for a sudden hypoglycemic event.

  d. Dextrose should be added to IV infusions when the serum glucose level reaches 200–250 mg/100 mL.

Application/Physiologic/Implementation

27. *Correct response: d*

  a. During prolonged hypoglycemia, large quantities of glucose deposits accumulate in the brain. When the blood sugar is lowered too rapidly, water is freed and attracted to the glucose in the brain, creating cerebral edema.

  b. DKA causes hypovolemia secondary to osmotic diuresis. If the blood sugar is lowered too rapidly and prior to fluid replacement, the water will follow the glucose into the cells causing circulatory collapse.

  c. Rapid reduction in glucose levels predispose the patient to hypoglycemia.

Application/Physiologic/Evaluation

28. *Correct response: b*
The use of large amounts of oxygen during hypermetabolism and the resulting anaerobic metabolism lead to high carbon dioxide production, ineffective glucose utilization, and negative nitrogen balance (catabolism).

Knowledge/Physiologic/NA

29. *Correct response: c*
Anginal pain results from cardiac ischemia and is manifested as S-T depression on an electrocardiogram.

  a. A prolonged Q-T interval is associated with an acute myocardial infarction, hypocalcemia, antidysrhythmic drugs (quinidine, procainamide, amiodarone), ventricular tachycardia, and sudden death.

  b. A prolonged P-R interval (greater than 0.20 second in duration) is associated with first-degree heart block.

  d. S-T elevations occur during pain episodes associated with Prinzmetal's angina.

Analysis/Physiologic/Assessment

30. *Correct response: a*
Prerenal failure results from a decrease in renal perfusion.

  b. Intrarenal failure results secondary to an inflammatory process effecting the glomeruli.

  c. Postrenal failure is caused by an obstruction of the urinary system from the calyces to the urethra.

  d. This is not a type of renal failure.

Knowledge/Physiologic/NA

31. *Correct response: b*

  b. Erythropoietin is used to increase Hct.

  a, d. Vitamin B12 and folic acid are necessary for erythropoietin to be effective.

  c. Erythropoietin is contraindicated in hypertension; it may further elevate BP.

Knowledge/Physiologic/NA

32. *Correct response: d*

  a, b, c. Rhabdomyolysis is caused by any activity resulting in muscle breakdown.

d. This patient has no risk factors for rhabdomyolysis.

Knowledge/Physiologic/NA

33. **Correct response: d**
The major problem in the successful treatment of multiple organ dysfunction syndrome is the need to treat the cause but not destroy the body's normal inflammatory responses.
a, b, c. Endotoxin may be a factor in some cases, but all are characterized by uncontrolled, rapid mediator release.

Comprehension/Physiologic/NA

34. **Correct response: d**
a, c, d. These sympathetic nervous system agents promote the "fight-or-flight" response, which leads to increases in vital sign measurements.
b. Catecholamines are not greatly involved in the clotting process.

Knowledge/Physiologic/NA

35. **Correct response: a**
An acidic pH (under 7.35) indicates acidosis, as does an acidic CO_2 (over 45) and bicarbonate (under 22).
b, d. Alkalosis is indicated by a pH above 7.45, CO_2 under 35, and bicarbonate of over 26.

Comprehension/Physiologic/Assessment

36. **Correct response: a**
Severe diarrhea often results in metabolic acidosis, so the respiratory system compensates by increasing rate and depth to "blow off" excess acid.
b, c, d. Decreasing rate and/or depth would perpetuate the acidotic state.

Analysis/Physiologic/Assessment

37. **Correct response: d**
Cullen's sign is associated with pancreatitis when a hemorrhage is suspected.
a. Grey-Turner's sign is ecchymosis in the flank area suggesting a retroperitoneal bleed.
b. Homans' sign elicits calf pain with dorsiflexion of the foot and suggests a deep vein thrombosis.
c. Rovsing's sign is associated with ap-

pendicitis, when pain is felt with pressure at McBurney's point.

Application/Physiologic/Assessment

38. **Correct response: c**
Hepatosplenomegaly results from inflammation of the liver, portal hypertension, and interrupted bile flow.
a. Dark-colored urine is seen in hepatitis.
b. Asterixis or liver flaps are jerking muscular movements or muscle tremors seen in hepatic encephalopathy. These movements are elicited by extension of the fingers and dorsiflexion of the wrist.
d. Elevated alpha-fetoproteins are seen in cancer of the liver.

Knowledge/Physiologic/Assessment

39. **Correct response: d**
This response indicates that the patient needs additional reinforcement regarding medications.
a, b, c. The patient accurately verbalizes information.

Comprehension/Health promotion/ Evaluation

40. **Correct response: a**
Massive left ventricular damage causes inadequate coronary and systemic perfusion resulting in cardiogenic shock.
b. Dressler's syndrome is treated symptomatically and usually subsides within a few days to weeks.
c. Ventricular aneurysm may lead to left ventricular failure if the aneurysm is not surgically treated.
d. Interventricular septal rupture may lead to left ventricular failure if surgical repair is not performed after the patient is stabilized.

Knowledge/Physiologic/Assessment

41. **Correct response: c**
a, b. Mechanical or fluid obstruction to the airway, such as that caused by biting on an endotracheal tube, and fluid overload result in respiratory acidosis due to buildup of carbon dioxide.

d. Overuse of antacids leads to metabolic, not respiratory, acidosis.
Knowledge/Physiologic/NA

42. Correct response: c
These ABG results are considered to be within normal limits for a client without respiratory disease; Mrs. Haas cannot be weaned successfully because she most likely will stop breathing because of lack of hypoxic stimulus.
a, b, d. A client with COPD has adjusted to a normally high level of carbon dioxide and a lower than normal oxygen level.
Analysis/Physiologic/Evaluation

43. Correct response: b
Rapid respirations "blow off" carbon dioxide, creating respiratory alkalosis.
c, d. Thirty minutes of hyperventilation is an insufficient amount of time for the kidneys to begin to make adjustments in bicarbonate levels, so the result is an uncompensated respiratory alkalosis.
Comprehension/Physiologic/Evaluation

44. Correct response: b
Clients with respiratory insufficiency need diets that require less energy to digest, such as those higher in fats and lower in carbohydrates.
Application/Health promotion/Planning

45. Correct response: a
Intermittent infusion cyclosporine is stable for 12 hours at room temperature in a glass container and 6 hours in a polyvinylchloride container when mixed with 0.9% NaCl.
b. Fluorouracil (5-fluorouracil, 5-FU) may be used as a direct infusion through the hepatic artery via an implantable pump to prolong survival and improve the quality of life. It is also used as adjuvant therapy after therapy.
c. Methylprednisolone (Solu-Medrol) is a steroid given parenterally that decreases the production of activated T-helper cells and cytotoxic cells, decreasing the antigenic activity of the graft. Intravenous boluses (40 to 100 mg) must be given over 20 to 30 minutes.
d. OKY3 (orthoclone-OKT3) is prophylactically used for rejection via intravenous bolus and is used as rescue therapy in acute rejection episodes when other rejection efforts have failed.
Knowledge/Safe care/Implementation

46. Correct response: a
Hepatorenal syndrome is a functional disorder resulting from a redistribution of renal blood flow. Oliguria and azotemia occur abruptly as a result of this complication.
b. Excess organic acids are not being excreted by the damaged kidneys, resulting in an elevated concentration of hydrogen ions; decreased pH occurs, causing metabolic acidosis.
c. Concentration of the urine is increased with decreased renal function.
d. With renal insufficiency, significant weight gain is expected due to fluid retention.
Comprehension/Physiologic/Assessment

47. Correct response: a
Flexion of the trunk lessens the pain and decreases restlessness.
b, c, d. These positions do not decrease pain.
Comprehension/Physiologic/Intervention

48. Correct response: d
Pre-icteric is the infective phase and precautionary measures should be strictly enforced. However, patients are not always diagnosed during this phase. Consequently the disease may be transmitted during this phase.
a, c. Precautionary measures should already be instituted in these phases.
b. There is no such phase.
Application/Safe care/Planning

49. Correct response: b
The process of pulse oximetry relies on infrared assessment of capillary saturation. The machine cannot detect what

substance the capillaries are saturated with. For example, CO poisoning could result in a normal SpO_2.

   a, c. Pulse oximetry is a guideline that correlates well when a person has no concurrent hematologic or respiratory problems, but is relatively ineffective otherwise. In the case of an anemic client, the pulse oximetry reading is usually normal because oxygen is fully saturated on the inadequate number of Hgb molecules, although the arterial O_2 measurement would indicate hypoxemia.

Application/Physiologic/Implementation

50. *Correct response: c*
The initial response to any client problem is to assess the person and the situation, then determine the rest of the priority needs.

Application/Safe care/Assessment

51. *Correct response: a*
   b. describes assist-control ventilation
   c. depends on type of endotracheal tube cuff
   d. occurs with IMV without synchronization

Knowledge/Safe care/NA

52. *Correct response: c*
   a. describes SIMV or IMV
   b. describes CMV
   d. describes the rationale for use of PEEP

Knowledge/Physiological/NA

53. *Correct response: b*
This procedure is not performed if the patient is responsive to medical treatment.
   a, c, d. These are indications for a percutaneous transluminal coronary angioplasty.

Comprehension/Physiologic/Evaluation

54. *Correct response: d*
A pericardiocenteses is an immediate evacuation of accumulated fluid in the pericardial sac. This is an emergency procedure that is necessary for symptomatic patients.

   a, b. These procedures may be performed for recurrent pericardial effusion. They is usually performed to relieve compression of the heart in recurrent pericarditis.
   c. Chest tubes are inserted for patients with a hemothorax or pneumothorax, a flail chest, and with open heart surgery.

Application/Physiologic/Planning

55. *Correct response: c*
Terminal end-stage cardiomyopathy may require cardiac transplantation. Many patients with dilated (congestive) cardiomyopathy die awaiting heart transplantation.
   a. Prinzmetal's angina results from a coronary artery spasm and is relieved with sublingual nitroglycerin.
   b. A coronary artery bypass graft would be the treatment of a coronary artery occlusion.
   d. Dressler's syndrome is a complication of an acute myocardial infarction and is usually self-limiting.

Comprehension/Health promotion/ Evaluation

56. *Correct response: d*
Elevated ammonia levels are in the blood of patients with hepatic encephalopathy. Changes in this level would indicate appropriate treatment. Neomycin enemas, oral lactulose, and a restricted or low-protein diet are treatments for hepatic encephalopathy.
   a, b. These coagulation studies are increased with liver disease and do not directly affect the treatment of hepatic encephalopathy.
   c. Bilirubin, both direct and indirect, are increased with liver disease and do not directly affect the treatment of hepatic encephalopathy.

Analysis/Physiologic/Assessment

57. *Correct response: c*
Communication with all clients is essential, especially in the critical care area, where the overwhelming sensory stimuli are completely alienating and

the sound of the family may be the only familiar thing in the environment.

a, b. Personal items in moderation are encouraged to allow the client to have some sense of "personal space." Teaching about possible hazards of equipment should be kept general and presented calmly. The family should focus on the person in the bed and not on the machinery.

d. A positive outlook promotion may or may not be appropriate, depending on the particular situation. Keep in mind, however, that many clients are aware of the severity of their conditions and may resent false reassurance.

Application/Psychosocial/Intervention

58. *Correct response: a*
"Good lung down" is the general guiding principle when positioning the client with a partial pneumonectomy.

b, c. The opposite is true if the person has had a total pneumonectomy. Semi-Fowler's and supine positions may be utilized, but should be limited because oxygenation will not be as effective in these positions.

Application/Physiologic/Implementation

59. *Correct response: b*
Bronchial breath sounds are normally heard only over the anterior chest in the area of the large airways. An area of posterior consolidation, such as occurs with pneumonia, will cause the anterior bronchial sounds to be transmitted posteriorly.

a. Hyperresonant sounds occur over areas with air distention; sounds are absent if there is no air exchange.

Comprehension/Physiologic/Assessment

60. *Correct response: d*
Normal theophylline level is 10–20 mcg/mL

Analysis/Physiologic/Assessment

61. *Correct response: a*
Before the test is performed, a local anesthetic is sprayed in the patient's throat to inhibit the gag reflex. Therefore, you must check for a gag reflex before feeding the patient.

b, c, d. These are appropriate nursing interventions.

Application/Safe care/Implementation

62. *Correct response: c*
The blood pressure mube be rapidly decreased to limit the dissection. Nitroprusside reduces preload and afterload and causes vasodilation.

a. Chest tube insertion would not limit the dissection.

b. Monitoring urinary output is always an appropriate nursing intervention but it is not a priority at this time.

d. Dopamine hydrochloride would cause peripheral vasoconstriction or increase renal perfusion depending on dose.

Application/Physiologic/Implementation

63. *Correct response: c*
Weight gain greater than 2 lb indicates excess fluid and could lead to pulmonary edema.

a. Urinary output less than 30 mL/hr should be reported; it indicates renal insufficiency.

b. Vital signs should be monitored after all activity to assess for pulmonary edema and decreased cardiac output.

d. Jugular vein distention and dependent edema are symptoms of right-sided heart failure. Left-sided heart failure symptoms include dyspnea on exertion, orthopnea, crackles, S3 heart sounds.

Analysis/Physiologic/Planning

64. *Correct response: a*
A temporary pacer may be used to increase heart rate or synchronize the atria and ventricles if heart block or sinus bradycardia are present.

b. Chest tube clamping is contraindicated.

c. This intervention requires a physician's order or may be contraindicated.

d. An intra-aortic balloon pump is instituted by a physician and maintained by nursing staff.

Application/Physiologic/Implementation

65. *Correct response: a*
   b. indicates flail chest
   c. indicates fat embolus
   d. indicates DVT

Knowledge/Physiologic/Assessment

66. *Correct response: b*
This statement is the simplest to understand and the most accurate explanation of the test.

a, c are false.

d is indirectly correct, but is not the best choice.

Knowledge/Physiologic/Planning

67. *Correct response: c*
These blood gases are typical of a client with COPD. The pH is normal, and the PaCO$_2$ and HCO3– are both elevated (HCO3– is a long-term compensatory mechanism). The PaO$_2$ is probably quite tolerable to this client, who depends on hypoxia to stimulate the respiratory drive.

Analysis/Physiologic/Evaluation

68. *Correct response: a*
This is a young, previously healthy man who needed a brief period of mechanical ventilation postoperatively. His normal ABGs indicate readiness for successful weaning.

Analysis/Safe care/Evaluation

69. *Correct response: c*
   a. Burkitt's lymphoma affects the lymphatic system.
   b. HSV causes painful vesicles internally and externally.
   d. Candidiasis results in a cream-to-yellowish thick coating on mucous membranes.

Knowledge/Physiologic/NA

70. *Correct response: b*
Atherosclerotic plaques deposit in the coronary arteries, blocking blood flow to the myocardial tissue.
   a. Coronary artery spasms are triggered by atherosclerotic plaques.
   c. This is a diagnostic test that detects ischemic or infarcted areas of the heart.
   d. Platelet aggregation is a physiologic mechanism that is triggered as a result of tissue necrosis.

Knowledge/Physiologic/NA

71. *Correct response: d*
Morphine sulfate is the drug of choice for rapid pain relief and is also used to reduce anxiety. Morphine controls pain by binding to the opiate receptors in the CNS. It produces vasodilation, thereby decreasing venous return to the heart. Consequently it decreases the workload of the heart.
   a. Calcium channel blockers are not used for pain relief. Diltiazem hydrochloride decreases the work of the heart by decreasing myocardial contractility, relaxing smooth muscle, and dilating coronary arteries.
   b. Inderal, a beta blocker, blocks stimulation of beta-1 and beta-2 receptor sites, decreasing the heart rate, blood pressure, AV conduction, and myocardial oxygen consumption.
   c. Nitroglycerin may be administered several ways. Given intravenously it dilates the coronary arteries, and produces a more rapid effect of preload and afterload reduction, with resultant decreased myocardial oxygen consumption.

Knowledge/Physiologic/Implementation

72. *Correct response: a*
Prothrombin time and partial thromboplastin time indicate a decrease in the clotting mechanism and can lead to bleeding.

b. An increase in hemoglobin and hematocrit indicates polycythemia, dehydration, and COPD.

c. A decrease in erythrocytes and sedimentation rate can indicate sickle cell anemia and liver disease.

d. A decreased white blood cell count can indicate aplastic anemia and viral infections.

Analysis/Physiologic/Evaluation

73. *Correct response: d*

Hepatotoxicity may develop from INH use.

a, b. Rifampin changes urine color. The development of a rash may signal early hypersensitivity and perhaps discontinuation of the drug.

c. Chest x-rays are part of the follow-up for clients with tuberculosis, but are not related to pharmacotherapy.

Knowledge/Health promotion/Planning

74. *Correct response: a*

Clients with tuberculosis must adhere to their medication regimens to avoid MDR-TB development.

b, c, d. Rest, nourishment, and fresh air are helpful adjuncts, but are not always possible in urban environments. All of these answers are appropriate for all persons.

Knowledge/Health promotion/Planning

75. *Correct response: b*

Length of treatment varies from about 6 months for prophylaxis post-exposure to up to 2 or more years for someone who is immunosuppressed. However, 9–12 months is the average pharmacotherapy time.

Knowledge/Health promotion/Planning

76. *Correct response: d*

M. tuberculosis is an aerobic organism. It can only be transmitted by droplet nuclei, not by blood or urine.

b. It is able to lie dormant in the body for many years.

c. There is no definite anti-tuberculin vaccination. BCG vaccine has not proven to provide immunity against the bacillus.

Knowledge/Physiologic/NA

77. *Correct response: a*

Anemia is the most serious adverse effect of zidovudine use.

b, c, d. Potassium generally is not affected, and lymphocytopenia is not a normal result of zidovudine use.

Knowledge/Physiologic/Planning

78. *Correct response: b*

b, c. Nearly one-half of infants born to HIV-infected mothers will remain HIV-negative, although zidovudine treatment drastically reduces risk.

a. Moral issues such as abortion are not part of the nurse's role in this situation, and false advice is tantamount to lying to the client.

d. Although support services for many new mothers may be an appropriate consideration, the presence of HIV does not mean that the mother is in danger of imminent death; she may remain AIDS-free for many years.

Knowledge/Physiologic/Planning

79. *Correct response: b*

Reed-Sternberg cells are found with Hodgkin's disease.

a. Epstein-Barr bodies are found with mononucleosis and other disorders.

c. Bence Jones proteins are found with multiple myeloma.

d. Small oat cell proteins are associated with oat cell carcinoma.

Knowledge/Physiologic/Assessment

80. *Correct response: d*

Increasing activity will help calcium return to the bones, which is particularly important for the client with multiple myeloma, owing to chronic hypercalcemia.

a. Testing urine and stools for occult blood is also appropriate, although it is focused more on platelet functioning than it is on bone marrow depression per se.

b. Rectal temperatures and procedures that could irritate mucosa should be avoided.

c. These patients are already hypercalcemic.

Application/Physiologic/Intervention

81. *Correct response: b*

An induration of greater than 10 mm indicates contact with the tubercle bacillus. Any induration is suspect if the person is immunocompromised.

a, c. This positive finding does not indicate the presence of active disease. Confirmation of *M. tuberculosis* in sputum is needed. Therefore no immediate pharmacotherapy is necessarily indicated.

d. False-positive reactions rarely (if ever) occur.

Application/Health promotion/NA

82. *Correct response: b*

Lack of compliance with pharmacotherapy is the major factor influencing the increase in development of MDR-TB.

a. Incidence of AIDS or other immunodeficiency state makes treatment more difficult at times, but not impossible.

c. Homelessness and lack of adequate DOT therapy are factors that affect compliance and indirectly the development of MDR-TB.

d. Decreased research funding has thwarted efforts to develop more resistant medications but is not the major factor.

Knowledge/Health promotion/NA

83. *Correct response: a*

The only practical definitive test is the presence of *M. tuberculosis* in a sputum culture.

b. The presence of AFB signifies acid-fast bacillus only, which may be other varieties of mycobacterium.

c, d. Chest x-rays and PPD tests are guideline tests; they do not provide definite confirmation of tuberculosis.

Knowledge/Health promotion/NA

84. *Correct response: c*

Vitamin B6 (pyridoxine) is essential to prevent the peripheral neuritis that develops with INH therapy, although all B vitamins are important in general nutrition.

Comprehension/Physiologic/Planning

85. *Correct response: b*

a. KS is a cancer.

c. CMV usually affects the retina/GI tract.

d. Cryptosporidiosis produces profuse diarrhea.

Knowledge/Physiologic/Assessment

86. *Correct response: c*

Malabsorption is the only reason that TPN must be used for this client.

a. The presence of diarrhea may lead to TPN if nutritional needs are not being met, but is not the initial nutritional source.

b. Enteral nutrition is just as effective as TPN and has less potential for lethal effects.

Comprehension/Physiologic/Planning

87. *Correct response: a*

If diarrhea adversely affects nutritional intake, TPN may be the only option.

b, c. There is no cure for cryptosporidium enteritis.

Application/Physiologic/Intervention

88. *Correct response: d*

a. The presence of HIV in isolation does not mean the person has AIDS.

c. Many clients do not develop multiple concurrent opportunistic infections.

Knowledge/Physiologic/NA

89. *Correct response: c*

Three consecutive negative sputum specimens for *M. tuberculosis* indicate a noninfectious state.

a, b. Current CDC recommendations are for two weeks of treatment with at least four antitubercular medications before a person is considered "noninfectious" with *M. tuberculosis*.

d. Once a person has a positive PPD test, the test results will always be positive as long as normal immunity is present.

Knowledge/Health promotion/ Evaluation

90. *Correct response: a*
The use of IV NSS or LR helps to decrease hypercalcemia.
b. Thiazide diuretics conserve calcium.
c. Bedrest promotes calcium release from bones and encourages its entry into the bloodstream.
Comprehension/Physiologic/Implementation

91. *Correct response: c*
Occlusion or compression of the SVC affects blood flow to the upper extremities, head, and neck, but does not generally affect systemic BP.
Physiologic/Comprehension/Assessment

92. *Correct response: b*
a. HLA matching can occur between compatible siblings or other compatible persons.
c. This is a syngeneic match.
Knowledge/Physiologic/NA

93. *Correct response: c*
Statistics show that females who are sexually active with males and do not use safer sex practices are at higher risk for HIV than are males in general or those who practice safer sex.
Knowledge/Health promotion/NA

94. *Correct response: d*
There is never a guarantee that a particular unit of blood is free of all possible diseases, but the risk of contracting HIV from such exposure is minimal.
a. Family members can donate blood, although this may provide the client with false comfort that these persons are HIV–.
b. The client also can refuse a blood transfusion or any other procedure, but should be fully aware of the pros and cons of doing so before making such a decision.
Knowledge/Safe care/Intervention

95. *Correct response: d*
Choice d is the only response that is open. All of the others, although pertinent to the client's overall history, are making the assumption that the client is discussing HIV/AIDS, which cannot be inferred from his question.
Comprehension/Psychosocial/Intervention

96. *Correct response: a*
PCP, cryptosporidiosis, and Kaposi's sarcoma are all opportunistic infections that occur as the CD4 count declines.
Knowledge/Physiologic/Assessment

97. *Correct response: d*
a. Smooth muscle constriction results in bronchospasm but is not limited to the pulmonary system.
b. As a result of secondary exposure to a toxin, the inflammatory response begins by increasing systemic capillary permeability.
c. Hypotension eventually occurs as a result of the body's response to the toxin.
Comprehension/Physiologic/Assessment

98. *Correct response: d*
HIV initially encounters and invades a T4 cell, at which time the HIV is engulfed by the phagocyte. The HIV is then able to fuse its RNA with the host cell's DNA, ending with replication of the newly created HIV strain by the host cell.
Knowledge/Physiologic/NA

99. *Correct response: a*
The ELISA, western blot, and p24 antigen test are indicators of HIV status, but do not qualify development into AIDS. Only the CD4 cell count of under 200/mm3 is diagnostic for AIDS.
Knowledge/Physiologic/Assessment

100. *Correct response: b*

Lowered immunity presents increased opportunities for opportunistic infections.

a. The client with HIV is always at some risk for the development of AIDS, but the amount of risk cannot be determined.

c. PCP prophylaxis is currently started when the CD4 count drops below $500/mm^3$

d. He does not have AIDS, based on the CDC definition of the disease.

Knowledge/Physiologic/Evaluation

Index

References with *t* denote tables; *f* denote figures; *d* denote displays